FIRST AID

FOR THE®
PEDIATRIC
BOARDS

TAO LE, MD, MHS

Assistant Clinical Professor of Pediatrics and Medicine
Division of Allergy and Clinical Immunology
University of Louisville

WILBUR LAM, MD

Clinical Fellow
Division of Pediatric Hematology/Oncology
Department of Pediatrics
University of California, San Francisco

SHERVIN RABIZADEH, MD, MBA

Chief Resident, Pediatrics
Fellow, Pediatric Gastroenterology
Johns Hopkins University Hospital

ALAN SCHROEDER, MD

Division of Pediatric Critical Care
Department of Pediatrics
Stanford University

KIMBERLY VERA, MD

Chief Resident, Pediatrics
Johns Hopkins University Hospital

McGraw-Hill
MEDICAL PUBLISHING DIVISION

New York / Chicago / San Francisco / Lisbon / London / Madrid / Mexico City
Milan / New Delhi / San Juan / Seoul / Singapore / Sydney / Toronto

This book was set in Electra LH by Rainbow Graphics.
The editor was Catherine A. Johnson.
The production supervisor was Phil Galea.
Project management was provided by Rainbow Graphics.
Quebecor Dubuque was printer and binder.

This book is printed on acid-free paper.

To the contributors to this and future editions, who took time to share their knowledge, insight, and humor for the benefit of residents and clinicians.

and

To our families, friends, and loved ones, who endured and assisted in the task of assembling this guide.

CONTENTS

AUTHORS

REBECCA BLANKENBURG, MD, MPH

Clinical Instructor, General Pediatrics
Lucile Packard Children's Hospital
Stanford University Medical Center
Neurology

JULIE BOKSER, MD

Department of Pediatrics
University of California, San Francisco
Dermatology

DANIEL R. BROWN, MD, PhD

Pediatric Rheumatology Fellow
Boston Children's Hospital
Allergy, Immunology, and Rheumatology

MARIA KARAPELOU BROWN, MD

Attending Physician, Pediatric Emergency Department
St. Agnes Hospital, Baltimore, MD
The Musculoskeletal System and Sports Medicine

ALBERT CHAN, MD

Clinical Instructor
Lucile Packard Children's Hospital
Stanford University Medical Center
Neonatology

CURTIS CHAN, MD, MPH

Medical Epidemiologist
San Francisco Department of Public Health
Clinical Instructor, Department of Pediatrics
University of California, San Francisco
Preventive Pediatrics, Ethics, and Epidemiology

RONALD D. COHN, MD

Assistant Professor of Pediatrics and Neurology
McKusick-Nathans Institute of Genetic Medicine
Director, Johns Hopkins Center for Hypotonia
Human Genetics and Development

ALLISON GEORGE AGWU, MD

Clinical Fellow
Divisions of Adult/Pediatric Infectious Diseases
Johns Hopkins University
Infectious Disease

GREGORY H. GORMAN, MD, MHS

Fellow, Pediatric Nephrology
Johns Hopkins University
The Renal System

DAVID HARRILD, MD, PhD

Fellow in Pediatric Cardiology
Boston Children's Hospital
Harvard Medical School
Cardiology

SANJAY JAIN, MD

Instructor, Pediatric Infectious Diseases
Johns Hopkins University School of Medicine
Infectious Disease

NANCY KIM, MD

Pediatric Cardiology Fellow
Stanford University
Cardiology

RYAN MILLER, MD

Fellow Instructor, Pediatric Endocrinology
Johns Hopkins University School of Medicine
Endocrinology

NEAL ROJAS, MD

Fellow, Developmental Behavioral Pediatrics
Boston Children's Hospital
Department of Pediatrics
Harvard Medical School
Growth, Development, and Behavior

ELIZABETH TAN ROSOLOWSKY, MD

Division of Endocrinology
Boston Children's Hospital
Endocrinology

DEBBIE SAKAGUCHI, MD

Clinical Fellow
Division of Pediatric Hematology/Oncology
Department of Pediatrics
University of California, San Francisco
Hematology; Oncology

AMY SAROFF, MD

Department of Pediatrics
Franklin Square Hospital Center
Adolescent Health

KARIN SALIM, MD

Fellow, Division of Pediatric Critical Care
Department of Pediatrics
Lucile Packard Children's Hospital
Stanford University Medical Center
Emergency and Critical Care Medicine

SHANNON S. SULLIVAN, MD

Clinical Fellow, Pediatric Pulmonary
University of California San Francisco
The Pulmonary System

SENIOR REVIEWERS

LAURIE ARMSBY, MD

Assistant Professor
Division of Pediatric Cardiology
Doernbecher Children's Hospital
Oregon Health Sciences University

ANNA L. BRUCKNER, MD

Assistant Professor of Dermatology and Pediatrics
Stanford University School of Medicine

CLIFFORD CHIN, MD

Associate Professor of Pediatrics
Division of Pediatric Cardiology
Stanford University

PATRICIA DeRUSSO, MD

Assistant Professor
Department of Pediatrics—Gastroenterology
Johns Hopkins University

JONATHAN ELLEN, MD

Associate Professor of Pediatrics and Adolescent Medicine
Johns Hopkins School of Medicine

SUSAN FURTH, MD, PhD

Associate Professor of Pediatrics
Johns Hopkins University School of Medicine

ROBERT E. GOLDSBY, MD

Assistant Professor of Pediatrics
Division of Pediatric Hematology/Oncology
University of California, San Francisco

LOUISE GREENSPAN, MD

Pediatric Endocrinologist
Kaiser Permanente, San Francisco

ADA HAMOSH, MD, MPH

Clinical Director, Institute of Genetic Medicine
Scientific Director, OMIM
Associate Professor, Pediatrics
Johns Hopkins University School of Medicine

SHANNON E. G. HAMRICK, MD

Assistant Professor, Neonatal-Perinatal Medicine
University of California, San Francisco

TERI M. McCAMBRIDGE, MD

Assistant Professor of Pediatrics
Primary Care Sports Medicine
Johns Hopkins School of Medicine

DENNIS NIELSON, MD

Pulmonology Division, Department of Pediatrics
University of California, San Francisco

LESLIE PLOTNICK, MD

Professor of Pediatrics, Endocrinology
Johns Hopkins School of Medicine

ANIL SAPRU, MD

Critical Care Division, Department of Pediatrics
University of California, San Francisco

ALISON SCHONWALD, MD

Assistant in Medicine Instructor
Harvard Medical School

JONATHAN B. STROBER, MD

Assistant Clinical Professor, Neurology & Pediatrics
University of California, San Francisco

ALAN UBA, MD

Associate Clinical Professor
University of California, San Francisco

With *First Aid for the*® *Pediatric Boards*, we hope to provide residents and clinicians with the most useful and up-to-date preparation guide for the American Board of Pediatrics (ABP) certification and recertification exams. This new addition to the *First Aid* series represents an outstanding effort by a talented group of authors and includes the following:

- A practical exam preparation guide with resident-tested test-taking and study strategies
- Concise summaries of thousands of pediatric board–testable topics
- Hundreds of high-yield tables, diagrams, and illustrations
- Key facts in the margins highlighting "must know" information for the boards
- Mnemonics throughout, making learning memorable and fun
- Mini-cases that illustrate how pediatric concepts may be tested on the exam

We invite you to share your thoughts and ideas to help us improve *First Aid for the*® *Pediatric Boards.* See How to Contribute, p. xv.

Louisville	Tao Le
San Francisco	Wilbur Lam
Baltimore	Shervin Rabizadeh
Palo Alto	Alan Schroeder
Baltimore	Kimberly Vera

ACKNOWLEDGMENTS

This has been a collaborative project from the start. We gratefully acknowledge the thoughtful comments and advice of the residents, international medical graduates, and faculty who have supported the authors in the development of *First Aid for the*® *Pediatric Boards*.

For support and encouragement throughout the process, we are grateful to Thao Pham and Selina Bush. Thanks to our publisher, McGraw-Hill, for the valuable assistance of their staff. For enthusiasm, support, and commitment to this challenging project, thanks to our editor, Catherine Johnson. For outstanding editorial work, we thank Andrea Fellows. A special thanks to Rainbow Graphics for remarkable production work.

Louisville	Tao Le
San Francisco	Wilbur Lam
Baltimore	Shervin Rabizadeh
Palo Alto	Alan Schroeder
Baltimore	Kimberly Vera

HOW TO CONTRIBUTE

To continue to produce a high-yield review source for the pediatric board exam, you are invited to submit any suggestions or corrections. We also offer **paid internships** in medical education and publishing ranging from three months to one year (see next page for details). Please send us your suggestions for

- Study and test-taking strategies for the pediatric boards
- New facts, mnemonics, diagrams, and illustrations
- Low-yield topics to remove

For each entry incorporated into the next edition, you will receive a $10 gift certificate, as well as personal acknowledgment in the next edition. Diagrams, tables, partial entries, updates, corrections, and study hints are also appreciated, and significant contributions will be compensated at the discretion of the authors. Also let us know about material in this edition that you feel is low yield and should be deleted.

The preferred way to submit entries, suggestions, or corrections is via electronic mail. Please include name, address, institutional affiliation, phone number, and e-mail address (if different from the address of origin). If there are multiple entries, please consolidate into a single e-mail or file attachment. Please send submissions to:

firstaidteam@yahoo.com

NOTE TO CONTRIBUTORS

All entries become property of the authors and are subject to editing and reviewing. Please verify all data and spellings carefully. In the event that similar or duplicate entries are received, only the first entry received will be used. Include a reference to a standard textbook to facilitate verification of the fact. Please follow the style, punctuation, and format of this edition if possible.

The author team is pleased to offer part-time and full-time paid internships in medical education and publishing to motivated physicians. Internships may range from three months (e.g., a summer) up to a full year. Participants will have an opportunity to author, edit, and earn academic credit on a wide variety of projects, including the popular *First Aid* series. Writing/editing experience, familiarity with Microsoft Word, and Internet access are desired. For more information, e-mail a résumé or a short description of your experience along with a cover letter to **firstaidteam@yahoo.com**.

Guide to the ABP Examination

INTRODUCTION

For residents, the American Board of Pediatrics (ABP) certification exam is the culmination of three years of hard work. For practicing physicians, it becomes part of the maintenance of certificate. However, the process of certification and recertification does not simply represent another in a series of expensive tests. To patients and their parents, it means that you have attained the level of clinical knowledge and competency required to provide good clinical care. In fact, parents are typically aware of a pediatrician's board-certification status.

In this chapter we talk more about the ABP exam and provide you with proven approaches to conquering the exam. For a detailed description of the exam, visit **www.abp.org** or refer to the *Booklet of Information (ABP Policies and Procedures)*, which can also be found on the ABP Web site.

ABP—THE BASICS

How Do I Register to Take the Exam?

You can register for the exam online at www.abp.org. The registration fee in 2006 was $1350. The regular registration deadline is typically in February of that year. If you miss the application deadline, a $245 nonrefundable late fee is also tacked on. Check the ABP Web site for the latest registration deadlines, fees, and policies.

What If I Need to Cancel the Exam or Change Test Centers?

The ABP currently provides partial refunds if a written cancellation is received before certain deadlines (typically in August). You can also change your test center with a written request before a specific deadline. Check the ABP Web site for the latest on the ABP's refund and cancellation policy and procedures.

How Is the ABP Test Structured?

The ABP certification exam is currently a **two-day** paper-based test administered at about 30 test centers around the country. The exam is divided into four 3-hour blocks during those two days. During the time allotted for each block, you can answer test questions in any order as well as review responses and change answers. Examinees cannot go back and change answers from previous blocks.

What Types of Questions Are Asked?

All questions are **single-best-answer** type only. You will be presented with a scenario and a question followed by multiple options. Most questions on the exam are vignette based. A substantial amount of extraneous information may be given, or a clinical scenario may be followed by a question that could be answered without actually requiring that you read the case. As with other board exams, there is no penalty for guessing. Between 5% and 10% of the questions require interpretation of photomicrographs, radiology studies, photographs of physical findings, and the like. It is your job to determine which information is superfluous and which is pertinent to the case at hand.

The majority of patients will be aware of your certification status.

Register before February to avoid the late fee.

Most questions are case based.

Most questions are relevant to the practice of general pediatrics and the clinical science behind it. Only a small portion will focus on basic science principles. Question content is based on a content "blueprint" developed by the ABP that contains **34 topic areas** (see Table 1-1). This blueprint may change from year to year, so check the ABP Web site for the latest.

How Are the Scores Reported?

Passing scores are set before exam administration, so your passing is not influenced by the relative performance of others taking the test with you. Scoring and reporting of test results may take up to three months.

TABLE 1-1. ABP Content Breakdown

TOPIC AREA	%
Infectious diseases	5.0
Allergy and related disorders	4.5
Fetus and newborn infant	4.5
Growth and development	4.5
Disorders of the blood and neoplastic disorders	4.0
Ear, nose, and throat disorders	4.0
Gastrointestinal disorders	4.0
Neurologic disorders	4.0
Nutrition and nutritional disorders	4.0
Preventive pediatrics	4.0
Respiratory disorders	4.0
Skin disorders	4.0
Fluid and electrolyte metabolism	3.5
Endocrine disorders	3.5
Cardiovascular disorders	3.5
Musculoskeletal disorders	3.5
Genetics and dysmorphology	3.0
Renal disorders	3.0
Adolescent medicine and gynecology	3.0
Psychosocial issues and problems	3.0
Collagen vascular and other multisystem disorders	2.0
Sports medicine and physical fitness	2.0
Disorders of cognition, language, learning, and attention	2.5
Critical care	2.0
Emergency care	3.0
Pharmacology	2.0
Genital system disorders	1.5
Metabolic disorders	1.5
Poisoning and environmental exposure to hazardous substances	1.5
Substance abuse	1.5
Basic science	1.0
Ethics	1.0
Disorders of the eye	1.0
Statistics	1.0

Your score report will give you a "pass/fail" decision, the overall number of questions answered correctly with a corresponding percentile, and the number of questions answered correctly with a corresponding percentile for the primary and cross-content subject areas note in the blueprint. Between 2002 and 2004, **81%** of first-time examinees passed on the first attempt. The ABP Web site also lists pass rates that are specific to training programs in the United States and Canada.

THE RECERTIFICATION EXAM

The recertification exam is one part of the Program for Maintenance of Certification in Pediatrics (PMCP). The test is a computerized exam with 200 questions administered over a half day at a Prometric testing center. It is administered year round, except July and August. Many of the testing centers are open Saturdays. The exam fee in 2006 was $1250. Historically, pass rates have ranged from 92% to 100%. A score of 75% or better on the ABP Knowledge Self-Assessment is a good predictor of passing.

TEST PREPARATION ADVICE

The good news about the ABP exam is that it tends to focus on the diagnosis and management of diseases and conditions that you have likely seen as a resident and that you should expect to see as an internal medicine specialist. Assuming that you have performed well as a resident, *First Aid* and a good source of practice questions may be all you need to pass. However, consider using *First Aid* as a **guide** and using multiple resources, including a standard textbook, Pediatrics Review and Education Program (PREP) questions and explanations, *Pediatrics in Review*, journal review articles, and a concise electronic text such as *UpToDate* as part of your studies. Original research articles are low yield and very new research (i.e., research conducted less than 1–2 years before the exam) will not be tested. In addition, there are a number of high-quality board review courses offered around the country. Board review courses are very expensive but can help those who need some focus and discipline.

Ideally, you should start your preparation early in your **last year of residency,** especially if you are starting a demanding job or fellowship right after residency. Cramming in the period between the end of residency and the exam is **not advisable.**

As you study, concentrate on the **nuances of management,** especially for difficult or complicated cases. For **common diseases,** learn both common and **uncommon presentations;** for **uncommon diseases,** focus on **classic presentations** and manifestations. Draw on the experiences of your residency training to anchor some of your learning. When you take the exam, you will realize that you've seen most of the clinical scenarios in your three years of wards, clinics, morning reports, case conferences, or grand rounds.

Other High-Yield Areas

Focus on topic areas that are typically not emphasized during residency training but are board favorites. These include:

- Topics in outpatient specialties (e.g., allergy, dermatology, ENT, ophthalmology)

- Formulas that are needed for quick recall (e.g., alveolar gas, anion gap, creatinine clearance)
- Basic biostatistics (e.g., sensitivity, specificity, positive predictive value, negative predictive value)
- Adverse effects of drugs

TEST-TAKING ADVICE

By this point in your life, you have probably gained more test-taking expertise than you care to admit. Nevertheless, here are a few tips to keep in mind when taking the exam.

- For long vignette questions, read the question stem and scan the options, and **then** go back and read the case. You may get your answer without having to read through the whole case.
- There's no penalty for guessing, so you should **never** leave a question blank.
- Good pacing is key. You need to leave adequate time to get to all the questions. Even though you have two minutes per question on average, you should aim for a pace of 90–100 seconds per question. If you don't know the answer within a short period, make an educated guess and move on.
- It's OK to **second-guess** yourself. Research shows that our "second hunches" tend to be better than our first guesses.
- Don't panic with "impossible" questions. They may be **experimental questions** that won't count. Again, take your best guess and move on.
- Note the age and race of the patient in each clinical scenario. When ethnicity is given, it is often relevant. Know these well, especially for more common diagnoses.
- Questions often describe clinical findings rather than naming eponyms (e.g., they cite "tender, erythematous bumps in the pads of the finger" instead of "Osler's nodes" in a febrile adolescent).

Never, ever leave a question blank! There's no penalty for guessing.

TESTING AND LICENSING AGENCIES

American Board of Pediatrics
111 Silver Cedar Court
Chapel Hill, NC 27514
919-929-0461
Fax: 919-929-9255
www.abp.org

Educational Commission for Foreign Medical Graduates (ECFMG)
3624 Market Street, Fourth Floor
Philadelphia, PA 19104-2685
215-386-5900
Fax: 215-386-9196
www.ecfmg.org

Federation of State Medical Boards (FSMB)
P. O. Box 619850
Dallas, TX 75261-9850
817-868-4000
Fax: 817-868-4099
www.fsmb.org

NOTES

CHAPTER 2

Adolescent Health

Amy Saroff, MD
reviewed by Jonathan Ellen, MD

The first sign of puberty in girls is the growth spurt, which usually begins at 9 years of age and peaks between the ages of 11½ and 12.

The average age of menarche in the United States is 12 years.

The first sign of puberty in boys is scrotal and testicular growth, which usually begins at 10–12 years of age.

The male growth spurt usually begins at 11 and peaks at approximately 13½ years of age.

ADOLESCENT PHYSICAL DEVELOPMENT

Tables 2-1 and 2-2 outline the characteristics of female and male sexual maturation and growth.

ADOLESCENT PSYCHOSOCIAL DEVELOPMENT

Adolescence can be divided into three major stages: early, middle, and late.

Early Adolescence

- Refers to those 11–14 years of age.
- Physically characterized by growth spurt and by the development of 2° sexual characteristics.
- Fatigue and easy embarrassability are often seen.
- Major issues include **body image,** self-concept, and self-esteem.
- Characterized by **concrete thinking**—inability to consider the consequences of one's actions.

Middle Adolescence

- Refers to those 15–17 years of age.
- 2° sexual development is complete for girls but is ongoing for boys.

TABLE 2-1. Adolescent Female Sexual Maturation

STAGE	BREAST DEVELOPMENT	PUBIC HAIR
I	Preadolescent	Preadolescent
II	Breast bud (11 years)	Sparse, long, slightly pigmented downy hair (12)
III	Continued enlargement, no contour separation (12 years)	Darker, coarser, and more curled (12.5)
IV	Secondary mound, projection of areola and papilla (13 years)	Hair resembles adult, distributed less than adult and not to medial thighs (13)
V	Mature stage (15 years)	Mature stage (14.5)

Adapted, with permission, from Stead LG, Stead SM, Kaufman MS. *First Aid for the Pediatrics Clerkship.* New York: McGraw-Hill, 2004:278.

TABLE 2-2. Adolescent Male Sexual Maturation

STAGE	BREAST DEVELOPMENT	PUBIC HAIR
I	Preadolescent	Preadolescent
II	Enlargement of scrotum and testes, darkening of scrotum and texture change (12 years)	Sparse, long, slightly pigmented downy hair (13.5)
III	Enlargement of penis (13 years)	Darker, coarser, and more curled (14)
IV	Increase in penis breadth and development of glans (14 years)	Hair resembles adult, distributed less than adult and not to medial thighs (14.5)
V	Mature stage (15 years)	Mature stage (15)

Adapted, with permission, from Stead LG, Stead SM, Kaufman MS. *First Aid for the Pediatrics Clerkship.* New York: McGraw-Hill, 2004:278.

- Major issues include **autonomy and independence**, which often → parental conflict.
- Dating and sexual experimentation often begin.
- Thinking moves to formal operation with the capacity for **abstract thought.**

Late Adolescence

- Describes those ≥ 18 years of age.
- Operative thinking is firmly established.
- Major issues include **education** and **intimate dating relationships.**

HEALTH SUPERVISION

Clinical services for adolescents should include screening for high-risk social and medical problems. Routine annual health visits are recommended for this purpose.

Psychosocial Screening

Psychosocial screening can elicit information about high-risk behaviors such as sexual activity, drug abuse, suicidal thoughts, and poor school performance. The **HEADSS** screen is a quick tool with which to assess patients for high-risk social behaviors:

- Home: Who lives with the patient?
- Education: How is the patient doing in school?

> *Assessment for high-risk social behaviors—HEADSS*
>
> **H**ome?
> **E**ducation?
> **A**ctivities?
> **D**rug use?
> **S**exual activity?
> **S**uicidal ideation?

> *Assessment for alcohol abuse— CAGE*
>
> **C**ut back?
> **A**dverse effects?
> **G**uilty?
> "**E**ye opener"?

- Activities: What are the patient's interests outside of school?
- Drug use: Is the patient using controlled substances?
- Sexual activity: Is the patient sexually active?
- Suicidal ideation: Is the patient considering suicide?

The **CAGE** questionnaire can be used to screen for significant alcohol abuse:

- Have you ever felt the need to **C**ut down on alcohol or drug use?
- Have you ever experienced any **A**dverse effects from drinking, such as blacking out or fights with friends?
- Do you ever feel **G**uilty about your drug or alcohol use?
- Do you ever need an "**E**ye opener" or a drink before noon?

Teens with a nonfasting cholesterol > 170 mg/dL should have a fasting lipid panel.

Medical Screening

A complete physical exam with height, weight, body mass index (BMI), and BP should be obtained.

LABORATORY EVALUATION

- **STD screening:**
  - A Pap smear should be obtained annually in all sexually active teens.
  - Nucleic acid amplification tests for chlamydia and gonorrhea infection should be performed via urine or cervical swab for all symptomatic patients as well as every 6–12 months for sexually active teens.
  - Teens with a history of STDs or high-risk sexual behavior should be screened for HBV, syphilis, and HIV.
- **Cholesterol screening:**
  - The American Heart Association recommends that the following groups be screened for hypercholesterolemia:
    1. Those with a ⊕ **family history of conditions associated with atherosclerosis,** including having a parent, grandparent, or first-degree aunt or uncle with a history of MI, angina pectoris, peripheral vascular disease, cerebrovascular disease, sudden cardiac death, or documented coronary atherosclerosis before age 55.
    2. Those with a ⊕ **family history of high parental cholesterol (> 240 mg/dL).**
    3. Those with a **condition associated with an ↑ risk of CAD,** such as diabetes, obesity, or hypertension.
  - Screening should begin with a nonfasting cholesterol for all teens except those in group 1, who should have a fasting lipid panel.
  - Table 2-3 outlines the appropriate management of hypercholesterolemia in teens.

TABLE 2-3. Management of Hypercholesterolemia in Adolescents

LDL (mg/dL)	INTERVENTION
> 130	Diet and exercise.
> 190	Diet, exercise, and medication.
> 160 and screened under group 1	Diet, exercise, and medication.

IMMUNIZATIONS

The following immunizations are recommended for adolescents:

■ A complete series of three HBV vaccines.
■ A tetanus-diphtheria booster > 5 years after the fourth DTaP.
■ Varicella vaccine.
■ Rubella vaccine for previously unimmunized females.
■ Meningococcal vaccine for those living in dormitories.
■ HAV vaccine for those living in high-risk areas.
■ Influenza vaccine may be considered.
■ Pneumococcal vaccine for the immunocompromised.

CONSENT AND CONFIDENTIALITY

■ Minors may give consent for their own medical care if they are living apart from their parents, are themselves the parent of a child, or are in the armed services.
■ If they are ≥ 15 years of age, "mature minors" may give consent for care and can also give informed consent for low-risk procedures.
■ In many states, minors of any age may give consent for HIV testing; for the testing and treatment of STDs and other issues surrounding sexual health; and for the treatment of substance abuse and other mental health issues.

ADOLESCENT GYNECOLOGY

A 14-year-old girl complains of painless but unpredictable menses. She denies sexual activity and has a normal physical exam, normal hemoglobin, and a ⊖ β-hCG. She underwent menarche one year ago. How should she be treated? These are most likely anovulatory cycles; no treatment is needed.

1° Amenorrhea

Defined as the absence of menses by 16 years of age. Important historical facts to elicit include recent weight change, headaches, visual changes, abdominal pain, difficulty urinating, stressors, and excessive exercise. Pertinent aspects of family history include maternal age at menarche or a history of constitutional delay of puberty. Etiologies of 1° amenorrhea are as follows:

■ **Chromosomal:** Table 2-4 outlines chromosomal abnormalities associated with amenorrhea.
■ **Congenital anatomic lesions:**
  ■ Include outflow tract obstructions such as **transverse vaginal septum** and **imperforate hymen.**
  ■ Symptoms include **cyclic abdominal or pelvic pain** that may be associated with back pain, together with nausea, bloating, and difficulty urinating 2° to vaginal distention.
  ■ Physical exam may reveal a **bluish, bulging hymen** and a perirectal mass from hematocolpos.
■ **Hypothalamic dysfunction:**
  ■ Abnormal GnRH secretion → absent LH surge and subsequent anovulation.
  ■ Can be caused by stress, eating disorders, and extreme exercise.
  ■ Examination is often significant for low BMI and bradycardia.

TABLE 2-4. **Chromosomal Abnormalities Involving Amenorrhea**

SYNDROME	KARYOTYPE	DEFECT	ANATOMY	LABS/TREATMENT
Complete androgen insensitivity syndrome	46,XY	Testosterone resistance 2° to an androgen receptor defect.	Phenotypic female; testes are present; no upper tract female structures; **thelarche but no adrenarche** at puberty.	**High serum testosterone.** Pelvic ultrasound shows absence of upper vagina, uterus, and fallopian tubes. Excise testes in light of ↑ risk of testicular cancer.
Vanishing testes syndrome	46,XY	Early gonadal failure (< 8 weeks' gestation); late gonadal failure (> 8 weeks' gestation).	**Early:** Phenotypic female because of gonadal streaks. **Late:** Male genitalia are seen at birth, but 2° sexual characteristics fail to develop.	High LH/FSH. Excise testicular remnants in light of ↑ risk of gonadal cancer (e.g., gonadoblastoma, dysgerminoma).
Ullrich-Turner syndrome	46,XY	A deletion/mutation in the testis-determining factor on Y chromosome.	Phenotypic female with both upper and lower tract structures intact.	Diagnose with DNA hybridization.
5α-reductase (5AR) deficiency	46,XY	An enzyme defect in converting testosterone to dihydrotestosterone (DHT).	Phenotypic female until puberty, when virilization occurs.	High testosterone-to-DHT ratio. Mutation analysis of 5AR gene.
Turner syndrome	45,XO	**Early ovarian failure.**	Female internal and external genitalia are seen.	Estrogen and cyclic progesterone therapy to stimulate pubertal development.
Kallmann syndrome	46,XX	A defect in the synthesis and/or release of LHRH.	Phenotypic female and will not develop 2° sexual characteristics; will also have **anosmia.**	Administer synthetic LHRH.
Mayer-Rokitansky-Küster-Hauser syndrome	46,XX	Uterine agenesis and absence of the upper two-thirds of the vagina. Ovaries, fallopian tubes, breasts, pubic hair, and hormone patterns are normal.	Phenotypic female.	Diagnose via pelvic ultrasound and MRI +/− laparoscopy.

- CNS tumors:
  - Include prolactinoma, craniopharyngioma, dysgerminoma, and Langerhans cell histiocytosis.
  - Symptoms include **headaches** and **visual field defects.**
  - Evaluation includes prolactin level and brain MRI.
- **Ovarian:** Includes 1° ovarian failure and polycystic ovarian syndrome (PCOS).

- **Endocrine:** Includes virilization disorders such as adrenal hyperplasia as well as Cushing syndrome.
- **Physiologic delay of puberty:**
  - A diagnosis of exclusion.
  - Must assess for a family history of delayed puberty.
- **Pregnancy.**

EXAM

Examination should include height, weight, Tanner stage, and an external genital exam to evaluate hymen, clitoral size, pubertal hair development, and vaginal depth.

DIAGNOSIS

Guidelines for the diagnosis of 1° amenorrhea are as follows (see also Figure 2-1):

- If the physical exam is abnormal, obtain a pelvic ultrasound to evaluate for the presence of ovaries, uterus, and cervix.
- In patients without müllerian structures, a karyotype and testosterone level should be obtained.
- In patients with müllerian structures and no evidence of congenital anatomic lesions, β-hCG, LH, FSH, and karyotype should be considered.

Having a withdrawal bleed in response to a medroxyprogesterone challenge points to normal anatomy and estrogen levels.

Pregnancy should always be considered as an etiology for both 1° and 2° amenorrhea.

2° Amenorrhea

Absence of menses for > 3 cycles or > 6 months in women who were previously menstruating. Potential etiologies are outlined in Table 2-5.

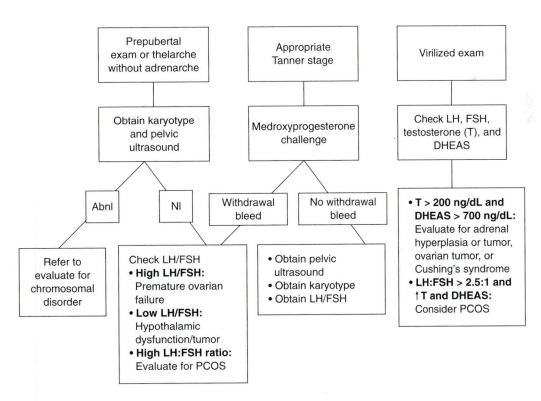

FIGURE 2-1. Evaluation of 1° amenorrhea.

13

ADOLESCENT HEALTH

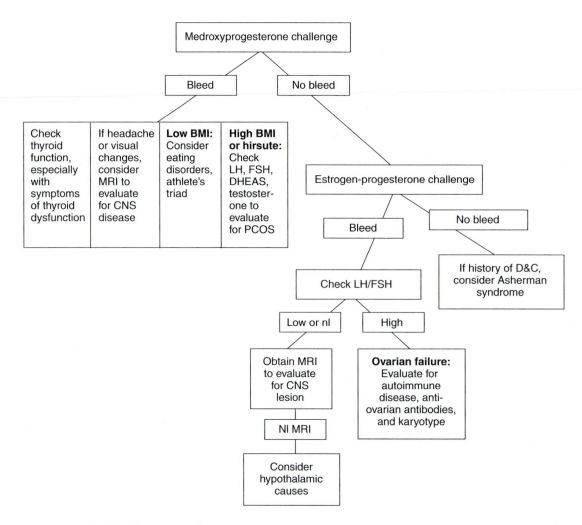

FIGURE 2-2. Evaluation of 2° amenorrhea.

Pregnancy must be ruled out first in all cases of 2° amenorrhea even if sexual activity is denied.

DIAGNOSIS

Evaluation includes LH, FSH, testosterone, DHEAS, prolactin, and TFTs in conjunction with a medroxyprogesterone challenge (see Figure 2-2). A brain MRI and pelvic ultrasound may be indicated.

Dysfunctional Uterine Bleeding (DUB)

Abnormal vaginal bleeding during menstrual cycles in the absence of ovulation. There are several subtypes.

- **Menorrhagia:** Excessive or prolonged blood loss occurring at regular intervals.
- **Metrorrhagia:** Irregular bleeding from the uterus between cycles.
- **Menometrorrhagia:** Irregular or excessive bleeding during menstruation and between menstrual cycles.
- **Anovulatory bleeding:** Unpredictable endometrial bleeding of variable flow and duration.

EXAM

- Consider weight and BMI.
- Evaluate for abnormal bruising, acanthosis nigricans, and hirsutism.

TABLE 2-5. Etiologies of 2° Amenorrhea

DISORDER	HISTORY/PHYSICAL EXAM	LABS/IMAGING	TREATMENT
Functional hypothalamic amenorrhea	Assess for recent weight change, including **low body weight/BMI,** low body fat, and brittle hair.	FSH is often higher than LH (similar to prepubescence). Low serum estradiol.	Evaluate for eating disorders such as anorexia nervosa and for high stress; consider referral for counseling.
Female athlete triad	Assess amount of exercise/ weight loss.	DEXA scan for osteoporosis.	Nutritional counseling, calcium supplementation, OCPs; consider counseling.
Pituitary disease (e.g., prolactinoma)	Headaches, visual changes, galactorrhea.	↑ prolactin on two separate measurements. Obtain an MRI.	Refer to neurosurgery.
Infiltrative diseases (e.g., Langerhans cell histiocytosis, lymphoma)	Headaches, visual changes.	Obtain an MRI. Bone marrow aspirate/ biopsy.	Refer to neurosurgery and oncology.
Thyroid disorders	**Hyperthyroidism:** Weight loss, tachycardia, palpitations, exophthalmos. **Hypothyroidism:** Weight gain, fatigue, myxedema.	Obtain TFTs.	**Hyperthyroidism:** Antithyroid therapy such as propylthiouracil (PTU)/methimazole or radioactive iodine/surgery. **Hypothyroidism:** Levothyroxine.
PCOS	Weight gain, hirsutism, acne, male-pattern alopecia, voice deepening, acanthosis nigricans.	LH:FSH ratio is usually > 2.5:1; prolactin mildly ↑; androgens (including testosterone, DHEAS) ↑. Consider pelvic ultrasound to image ovaries. Screen for dyslipidemia and DM with fasting blood sugar and lipid panel.	**OCPs** reduce levels of circulating androgen and reestablish cycles. **Weight loss** can often help improve insulin resistance; medications such as metformin can treat hyperinsulinism. Antiandrogen medications include spironolactone and flutamide.
Asherman syndrome	History of uterine instrumentation (e.g., D&C).	Hysterosalpingography and hysteroscopy.	Hysteroscopic lysis of intrauterine adhesions.
Drug effect (e.g., antipsychotics)		Hyperprolactinemia.	

ADOLESCENT HEALTH

15

Menstrual cycles that are accompanied by an ↑ in mucous cervical secretions, menstrual cramps, breast tenderness, and appetite and mood changes are likely ovulatory.

Anovulatory cycles are common in the first 2–3 years after menarche.

Dysmenorrhea is the most common single cause of school and job absence among females.

- Perform a pelvic exam to evaluate for estrogenization of vaginal mucosa as well as for foreign bodies, condylomata acuminata, cervicitis, and uterine/adnexal tenderness.

DIFFERENTIAL

- **Prepubertal:** Trauma, foreign body, vulvovaginitis, precocious puberty, ovarian cyst, tumor or neoplasm of the vagina or cervix.
- **Pubertal:** Anovulatory cycles, STDs, OCP use, hematologic disorders (e.g., von Willebrand disease, leukemia), endocrine disorders (e.g., thyroid disease, diabetes, adrenal insufficiency, Cushing syndrome), pregnancy, eating disorders, PCOS, cervical or uterine polyps/fibroids/ovarian cyst, tumors or neoplasms of the cervix or vagina.

DIAGNOSIS

- CBC, thyroid studies, LH, FSH, DHEAS.
- Culture/PCR for gonorrhea and chlamydia infection.
- Vaginal wet prep to evaluate for trichomonads and "clue cells."
- β-hCG.
- Pelvic ultrasound or MRI if there is a concern for uterine or ovarian abnormalities.

TREATMENT

- Anovulatory cycles require no treatment unless they are persistent or associated with significant anemia.
- **Mild DUB:** Iron supplementation, NSAIDs, and OCPs can be considered.
- **Moderate DUB:** Associated with a ↓ in hemoglobin (Hb < 12); should be treated with iron supplementation and OCPs.
- **Acute severe DUB:** A monophasic OCP should be given q 6 h until the bleeding stops, which usually occurs within 24–48 hours. OCPs can then be tapered down to daily dosage. The patient should remain on OCPs for 3–6 months. If anemia is severe (Hb < 9) or there is hemodynamic instability, inpatient admission for IV estrogen is indicated. DDAVP may be necessary.

Dysmenorrhea

Pelvic pain associated with menstruation; can be 1° or 2°. Distinguished as follows:

- **1° dysmenorrhea:** Pelvic pain during menstruation without pelvic pathology. Usually develops 6–12 months after menarche. Pain may precede menstrual flow by two days and lasts for 24–72 hours after start of flow.
- **2° dysmenorrhea:** Pelvic pain during menstruation 2° to a specific pathology.

SYMPTOMS/EXAM

Bilateral lower abdominal pain that may radiate to the lower thighs or back.

DIFFERENTIAL

UTI, PID, uterine or ovarian tumor.

TREATMENT

- NSAIDs are first-line therapy; OCPs can also be considered.
- Supportive care includes reducing caffeine and sugar and ensuring regular sleep and exercise.

Vulvovaginal Candidiasis

Most frequently caused by *Candida albicans*. Risk factors include antibiotic use, diabetes, pregnancy, and HIV.

SYMPTOMS/EXAM

Presents with vaginal pruritus or burning, vulvar erythema, dyspareunia, and a cottage cheese–like, odorless vaginal discharge.

DIAGNOSIS

Yeast or pseudohyphae can be visualized with application of 10% KOH to vaginal secretions (see Figure 2-3).

TREATMENT

- Topical application of clotrimazole.
- Oral fluconazole × 1 dose.

Sexually Transmitted Diseases (STDs)

Risk factors include multiple partners (≥ 2 partners within the last six months) and inconsistent barrier contraception use. The presentation, diagnosis, and treatment of STDs commonly found in adolescents are outlined in Table 2-6.

PELVIC INFLAMMATORY DISEASE (PID)

Encompasses many inflammatory disorders of the reproductive tract, including endometritis, salpingitis, tubo-ovarian abscess, and pelvic peritonitis. Pathogens include *Neisseria gonorrhoeae* (50% of cases), *Chlamydia trachomatis* (20–35% of cases), and endogenous flora of the lower genital tract, including anaerobes, *Haemophilus influenzae*, enteric gram-⊖ rods, and *Streptococcus agalactiae*.

SYMPTOMS

- Usually occurs during or immediately after menses.
- Presents with intense cramping, pelvic pain, and abnormal bleeding and vaginal discharge.

Bacterial vaginosis is caused by the replacement of normal vaginal flora with a high concentration of Gardnerella vaginalis *and* Mycoplasma hominis.

Adolescents infected with N. gonorrhoeae *are often coinfected with* C. trachomatis. Treatment should therefore be given for both.

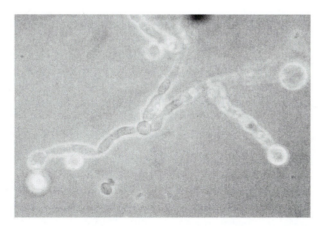

FIGURE 2-3. Pseudohyphae of candidiasis seen on vaginal secretions under KOH.

(Reproduced, with permission, from Wolff K, Johnson RA, Suurmond D. *Fitzpatrick's Color Atlas & Synopsis of Clinical Dermatology*, 5th ed. New York: McGraw-Hill, 2005:717.) (Also see Color Insert.)

TABLE 2-6. Common STDs in Adolescents

STD	MALE PRESENTATION	FEMALE PRESENTATION	DIAGNOSIS	TREATMENT	COMPLICATIONS
Gonorrhea	Urethritis, prostatitis, dysuria, purulent penile discharge.	Cervicitis, intermenstrual bleeding, purulent cervical discharge, dysuria, frequent urination.	Intracellular gram-$\ominus$ diplococci in urethral and endocervical secretions; DNA or enzyme immunoassay (EIA) probe; culture in Thayer-Martin medium.	Ceftriaxone × 1 dose, cefixime × 1 dose, or ciprofloxacin × 1 dose.	Disseminated gonorrhea with migratory polyarthritis, PID, Fitz-Hugh–Curtis syndrome.
Chlamydia	Urethritis, prostatitis, epididymitis, watery penile discharge; asymptomatic in 25–50% of cases.	Cervicitis +/− endocervical discharge and cervical bleeding; asymptomatic in 50% of cases.	DNA probe, tissue culture, EIA, monoclonal antibody, PCR or ligase chain reaction.	Doxycycline × 7 days, azithromycin × 1 dose, ofloxacin × 7 days, or erythromycin × 7 days.	PID, salpingitis, perihepatitis, acute Reiter's syndrome.
HSV	**"Punched-out"** ulcers with a flat edge and a yellow-gray base on the penis, perineum, perianal region, mouth, lips, or pharynx.	**"Punched-out"** ulcers with a flat edge and a yellow-gray base on the vulva, introitus, vagina, cervix, perineum, perianal region, mouth, lips, or pharynx.	Tzanck prep shows multinucleated giant cells; tissue culture, DNA probe testing.	1° : Acyclovir × 7–10 days. **Recurrent:** Treatment must be started during the prodromal phase or during the first two days after lesions appear; acyclovir × 5 days.	Complications are rare in immunocompetent individuals but may include recurrent neuralgias, encephalitis, and meningitis in the immunocompromised.
Trichomoniasis	Typically asymptomatic, or may present with urethritis, dysuria, and mild pruritus.	Vaginitis associated with a **frothy, watery gray-green discharge;** cervicitis with red, punctate strawberry cervix; urethritis.	Motile trichomonads on wet mount of vaginal secretions or spun sediment of urine.	Metronidazole × 1 dose.	
Bacterial vaginosis		Foul-smelling gray-white discharge that adheres to the vaginal walls.	Presence of **"clue cells"** on wet prep (see Figure 2-4); vaginal pH > 4.5 plus whiff test revealing fishy odor of vaginal discharge after addition of 10% KOH.	Metronidazole × 7 days or metronidazole gel BID × 5 days.	↑ risk of postabortion PID.

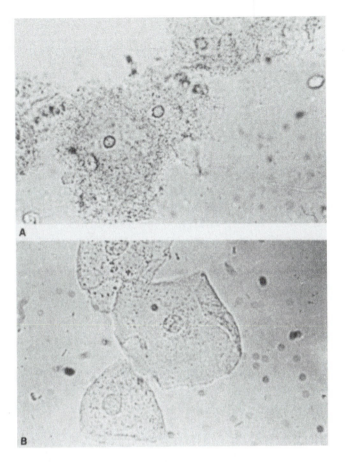

FIGURE 2-4. Vaginal epithelial "clue cells."

Clue cells (A) with a granular appearance are contrasted with normal cells (B). (Reproduced, with permission, from Kasper DL et al. *Harrison's Principles of Internal Medicine*, 16th ed. New York: McGraw-Hill, 2005:767.)

EXAM/DIAGNOSIS

- **Minimal criteria:** Lower abdominal tenderness, cervical motion tenderness, adnexal tenderness.
- **Additional criteria:** Temperature > 38.2°C, abnormal cervical or vaginal discharge, ↑ ESR, laboratory evidence of endocervical gonorrhea or chlamydia.
- **Elaborate criteria:** Histopathologic evidence of endometritis on biopsy, tubo-ovarian abscess on imaging, laparoscopic abnormality consistent with PID.

TREATMENT

- Hospitalization should be considered under the following conditions:
  - When a surgical condition such as appendicitis cannot be excluded.
  - In the presence of tubo-ovarian abscess, pregnancy, immunodeficiency, or nausea and vomiting that would prevent tolerance of oral antibiotics.
  - When the patient cannot follow up with a health care provider within 72 hours of treatment onset.
- Inpatient treatment includes cefoxitin or cefotetan plus IV doxycycline.
- Outpatient treatment includes doxycycline × 14 days plus ceftriaxone IM × 1 dose.

COMPLICATIONS

Peritonitis, tubo-ovarian abscess, perihepatitis with adhesion, ↑ risk of ectopic pregnancy, sterility.

SYPHILIS

SYMPTOMS/EXAM

- **1° syphilis:** Presents with chancre, a painless, flat ulcer with a raised, rolled border that is seen at the site of infection (see Figure 2-5). Common sites include the penis, vulva, introitus, vagina, cervix, perineum, perianal region, lip, and tongue. The lesion commonly presents 10–90 days after infection. It lasts 2–6 weeks and then spontaneously resolves.
- **2° syphilis:** Constitutional symptoms include fever, sore throat, headache, and arthralgias. Skin manifestations include condylomata lata, alopecia, and a rash on the palms and soles. Symptoms occur six weeks to six months after the chancre has cleared and persist for two weeks.
- **3° syphilis:** Gummas of bone, skin, and viscera; aortitis. Manifestations occur 15 years after onset of infection.

DIAGNOSIS

- Nontreponemal tests such as RPR and VDRL are used as a screen.
- Treponemal tests such as FTA-ABS are used to confirm a ⊕ screen.
- Darkfield microscopy shows spirochetes on scrapings from the chancre.

TREATMENT

1° and 2° syphilis are treated with benzathine penicillin G IM × 1 dose.

Genital ulcers are a cofactor in HIV transmission. All patients with syphilis should be screened periodically for HIV.

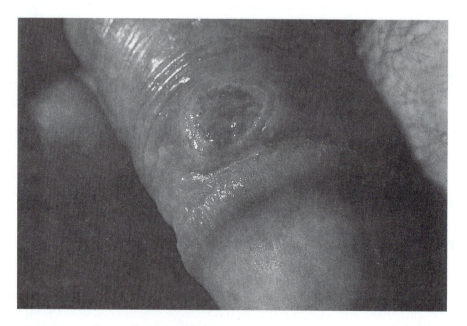

FIGURE 2-5. Chancre in primary syphilis.

(Reproduced, with permission, from Wolff K, Johnson RA, Suurmond D. *Fitzpatrick's Color Atlas & Synopsis of Clinical Dermatology*, 5th ed. New York: McGraw-Hill, 2005:915.) (Also see Color Insert.)

HUMAN PAPILLOMAVIRUS (HPV)

HPV causes genital warts, also called condylomata acuminata, as well as cervical dysplasia. Types 6 and 11 are most frequently found in genital warts; types 16 and 18 are most frequently detected in cervical dysplasia.

SYMPTOMS/EXAM

- Verrucous lesions can be found on the penis, urethra, or rectum in males and on any genital mucosal surface in females.
- Lesions are painless.
- Cervical infection can be visualized by applying 5% acetic acid solution, which → a whitening of the affected tissue.

DIAGNOSIS

Cervical dysplasia is diagnosed by Pap smear. Dysplasia is graded on a continuum from atypical squamous cells of undetermined significance (ASCUS) to low-grade squamous intraepithelial lesions (LSILs) to high-grade squamous intraepithelial lesions (HSILs).

TREATMENT

- Genital warts can be treated topically with 25% podophyllin or trichloroacetic acid.
- Lesions can recur.
- ASCUS found on a Pap smear requires a repeat Pap smear in 3–6 months.
- Persistent ASCUS, LSILs, or HSILs require referral for colposcopy.

COMPLICATIONS

- Genital warts often proliferate during pregnancy.
- HPV can be passed on to infants during delivery → laryngeal papillomatosis.
- **Cervical cancer.**

HPV is the most frequent etiology of abnormal Pap smears.

Some 25% of ASCUS cases will progress to dysplasia.

Breast Masses

Some common etiologies of breast masses are delineated in Table 2-7.

SYMPTOMS/EXAM

Assess for tenderness, skin and nipple changes, ↑ mass size, failure of the mass to ↓ in size over 2–3 menstrual cycles, and the presence of nipple discharge.

DIAGNOSIS

Breast ultrasound is useful in distinguishing cystic from solid masses.

TREATMENT

Observation, FNA, or excisional biopsy, depending on the pathology.

Contraception

Table 2-8 outlines common contraceptive methods used among adolescents.

Fibroadenoma is the most common breast mass in adolescents and is seen in 70–95% of biopsies.

*Mammography is **not** indicated in the diagnosis of breast masses owing to the high density of fibrous breast tissue in adolescents.*

TABLE 2-7. Differential Diagnosis of Breast Masses in Adolescents

CONDITION	PHYSICAL EXAM	LABS/IMAGING	TREATMENT
Fibroadenoma	A round, well-demarcated, mobile, nontender mass, often found in the upper outer quadrant.	Breast ultrasound reveals a smooth-margined mass that is homogeneous and hypoechoic.	May observe for 4–6 months, but if there is no involution or if enlargement occurs, excisional biopsy is indicated.
Giant juvenile fibroadenoma	The mass is > 5 cm in diameter and doubles in size within 3–6 months.	Breast ultrasound.	Excisional biopsy.
Cystosarcoma phyllodes	A rapidly growing, painless, multilobular, nonfixed lesion +/– bloody nipple discharge and skin discoloration.	Breast ultrasound. If malignant, it metastasizes to the lung, so chest CT may be indicated.	Wide-margin excisional biopsy. If malignant, radiation, chemotherapy, and hormone treatment are required.
Adenocarcinoma	A painless, hard, immobile mass adherent to the chest wall or skin +/– peau d'orange skin change, nipple retraction or discharge, or lymphadenopathy.	Breast ultrasound to distinguish cystic from solid tumors. Labs include alkaline phosphatase, hydroxyproline, and CEA to look for metastases.	Surgery, radiation, and chemotherapy, depending on the pathology.
Simple cyst	Masses are tender and spongy, with worsening of symptoms premenstrually. Typically, lesions spontaneously resolve within 2–3 menstrual cycles.	Breast ultrasound.	Observe for 3–6 months; if no resolution, FNA.
Fibrocystic change	Firm, mobile, cordlike abnormalities found diffusely throughout the breast. Often there is cyclic tenderness.		Biopsy may be required if there is a dominant mass present. OCPs may be tried to inhibit ovulation.
Breast abscess	A tender, cystic, warm, fluctuant mass with overlying erythema.	FNA; consider a blood culture if the patient is febrile.	Incision and drainage; antibiotics to cover *S. aureus;* warm compresses and analgesics.

TABLE 2-8. Common Methods of Contraception in Adolescents

METHOD	ADVANTAGES	DISADVANTAGES	SIDE EFFECTS
Abstinence	100% effective.	None.	None.
Condoms	The only method that protects against STDs.	Deteriorate with age and heat exposure; consistent use is poor among teens.	None.
Diaphragm	Convenient, as it is easily transported.	Higher failure rate than condoms or hormones; may be difficult for teens to insert properly; no STD protection.	↑ risk of UTIs; some studies show an ↑ risk of toxic shock syndrome.
OCPs	Inhibit ovulation and thicken cervical mucus; highly effective in preventing pregnancy when properly used. ↓ anemia, ovarian and endometrial cancer risk, and ectopic pregnancy risk.	No STD protection; teens may easily forget to take. Other medications (e.g., antibiotics) may ↓ efficacy.	Headaches, hypertension, and hypercoagulability, especially in smokers.
Contraceptive patch	Same mechanism as OCPs; highly effective in preventing pregnancy. Patch must be changed only once per week, so it is easier for teens to remember than daily OCPs.	No STD protection.	Same as for OCPs. May be less effective in obese teens.
Depo-Provera	Highly effective in inhibiting ovulation; requires only one IM shot every three months. Associated with ↓ menstrual flow, ↓ anemia, ↓ menstrual pain, ↓ risk of endometrial and ovarian cancer, and ↓ risk of ectopic pregnancy.	No STD protection.	Irregular bleeding, weight gain, ↓ bone density, possible dyslipidemias.
Emergency contraception	Effective in preventing ovulation and attachment of fertilized egg if taken within 72 hours of unprotected intercourse.	No STD protection; may delay ovulation up to 10 days.	Nausea and vomiting.

ADOLESCENT HEALTH

Spontaneous separation of the labia usually occurs in labial adhesions.

> A four-month-old girl presents for a well-child visit. During diaper changes, the mother has discovered that she cannot separate the child's labia to clean, and she is very concerned. What do you advise the mother? Reassure her that the condition usually resolves; no treatment is needed.

Labial Adhesions

Defined as a fusion of the labia minora that typically occurs in girls from two months to six years of age. Most cases are 2° to poor hygiene and vulvar irritation. Other etiologies include severe diaper dermatitis and estrogen deficiency.

SYMPTOMS/EXAM

Inability to separate the labia minora.

TREATMENT

No treatment is necessary if the patient has normal urinary and vaginal drainage. Children who do not have adequate urinary and vaginal drainage may require the application of an estrogen-containing cream for several weeks. Forceful separation of the adhesions is contraindicated because trauma to the tissue may occur, causing the adhesions to re-form.

Vulvovaginitis

Inflammation of the vagina and/or vulva. Etiologies are as follows:

- **Nonspecific:** Responsible for most cases. Exam shows lack of labial development and unestrogenized mucosa, often due to poor hygiene, bubble baths, shampoos, or tight clothing such as tights or leotards.
- **Infectious:** Etiologic agents include pinworms, respiratory pathogens (especially *Streptococcus pyogenes* and *Candida*), and STDs such as *N. gonorrhoeae*, *C. trachomatis*, and *Trichomonas vaginalis*.
- **Foreign bodies:** Chronic vaginal discharge associated with a foul odor and intermittent bleeding; the most common irritant is toilet paper.
- **Polyps or tumors:** Sarcoma botryoides arises near the introitus and may involve the hymen, urethra, and anterior vaginal wall. Peak incidence in girls occurs at 2–5 years of age.
- **Congenital anomalies:** Ectopic ureter → chronic wetness and 2° vulvar irritation.
- **Dermatologic: Lichen sclerosus** manifests as itching, discharge, and possible bleeding. On physical exam, vulvar tissue displays a **white onion-skin lesion with whitened skin circumscribing the vulvar and perianal areas.** Punctate hemorrhage may be seen on the affected skin. Treat with high-potency topical corticosteroids for two weeks. If left untreated, the condition may → long-term sexual dysfunction 2° to scarring.

SYMPTOMS/EXAM

Patients present with an erythematous, painful vulva or vagina.

TREATMENT

Dependent on the etiology.

Physiologic Leukorrhea

Defined as an intermittent discharge that results from estrogen stimulation. The discharge typically begins several months prior to menarche.

SYMPTOMS/EXAM

Discharge is usually clear or white, with a watery to mucoid consistency. Wet mount shows mucus and epithelial cells only.

TREATMENT

No treatment is necessary.

Newborns who appear to have bilateral cryptorchidism should be evaluated for congenital adrenal hyperplasia.

GENITOURINARY DISORDERS IN MALES

Cryptorchidism

Refers to undescended testicles; may be unilateral or bilateral. Occurs in 2–5% of term infants and is more common among preterm infants. Subtypes are as follows:

- **True cryptorchidism:** The testicle has stopped along its normal path of descent. Many of these testes will descend into the scrotum within the first year of life.
- **Ectopic cryptorchidism:** The testes have descended into an abnormal position. The most common site is the superficial inguinal pouch. Surgery is required.
- **Retractile testes:** These testes can be milked down into the scrotum after fatiguing the cremasteric muscle. No surgical intervention is required.

SYMPTOMS/EXAM

Inability to palpate testes in the scrotum.

TREATMENT

Orchiopexy, or the surgical pinning of the testicle in the scrotum, is indicated for true cryptorchidism at one year of age. Ectopic cryptorchidism can be repaired as soon as the diagnosis is made.

COMPLICATIONS

Neoplasms, infertility or subfertility, torsion, trauma.

Scrotal/Testicular Masses

Scrotal and testicular masses have numerous etiologies, including inguinal hernia, hydrocele, varicocele, spermatocele, testicular tumor, testicular torsion, torsion of the appendix testis, epididymitis, and orchitis.

INGUINAL HERNIA

Occurs when the processus vaginalis fails to atrophy → a communication between the peritoneal cavity and the scrotum. This allows for the passage of bowel into the scrotum.

SYMPTOMS

Inguinal fullness or bulging with ↑ intra-abdominal pressure such as that associated with crying, coughing, or prolonged standing.

EXAM

- Palpation of bowel in the external inguinal ring or scrotum.
- Auscultation of bowel sounds in the scrotum.

TREATMENT

Surgical repair.

COMPLICATIONS

- Herniated bowel loop may → partial bowel obstruction.
- Incarceration, or inability to reduce the hernia, causes complete bowel obstruction and necrosis.

HYDROCELE

Scrotal masses due to hydroceles can be transilluminated.

Defined as a fluid collection within the tunica vaginalis or processus vaginalis. In a communicating hydrocele, there is free flow of fluid between the tunica and the peritoneal cavity. In a noncommunicating hydrocele, the fluid is confined to the scrotum. Hydroceles can form acutely in response to trauma, epididymitis, orchitis, tumor, or torsion.

SYMPTOMS/EXAM

- Nontender scrotal swelling.
- Fluid may disappear overnight and then recollect during the day in a communicating hydrocele.

DIAGNOSIS

Doppler ultrasound may be necessary to confirm the diagnosis.

TREATMENT

Surgical repair is required for communicating hydroceles. Expectant management is all that is necessary for most noncommunicating hydroceles. Sclerotherapy can be used in children > 2 years of age. Surgical treatment for noncommunicating hydroceles may be needed if the scrotum is tense and impairing blood supply to the testes.

VARICOCELE

Defined as a scrotal mass caused by tortuous dilatation of the pampiniform venous plexus. Most 1° varicoceles are left sided because the left spermatic vein enters the left renal vein at a 90° angle, which → ↑ pressure. 2° varicoceles result from mechanical venous obstruction such as IVC thrombus, right renal vein thrombosis, or retroperitoneal tumor.

SYMPTOMS/EXAM

- Palpation of a scrotal mass that feels like a bag of worms.
- ↑ size with standing or Valsalva.
- 1° varicoceles disappear when the patient is supine, but 2° varicoceles do not.

TREATMENT

1° varicoceles are managed expectantly unless examination reveals testicular pain, ↓ testicular volume, or an excessively large size, in which case surgical ligation is indicated. For 2° varicoceles, it is necessary to diagnose and treat the underlying cause.

SPERMATOCELE

Defined as a sperm-filled cyst that develops from the epididymal tubules.

SYMPTOMS/EXAM

A painless nodule is palpated posterior and superior to the testis. The mass is distinct from the testis and may be transilluminated.

TREATMENT

Most cases are followed expectantly. Surgical excision can be used for painful spermatoceles.

 A 12-year-old boy presents to the ER with acute onset of severe left testicular pain. The testicle is swollen and tender. What is the next step in evaluation? Emergent testicular ultrasound with Doppler.

TESTICULAR TORSION

Defined as twisting of the testes or, more precisely, of the spermatic cord.

SYMPTOMS

- Sudden onset of scrotal pain; can be spontaneous or associated with exercise or trauma.
- Nausea and vomiting may be seen.

EXAM

- Tender, swollen testicle.
- Elevation of the testicle does not relieve pain.
- Absent ipsilateral cremasteric reflex.

DIFFERENTIAL

Epididymitis, orchitis.

DIAGNOSIS

- The first line is scrotal Doppler ultrasound documenting ↓ perfusion.
- Technetium 99m demonstrates ↓ perfusion.

TREATMENT

- Emergent surgical correction is necessary, as irreversible infarction occurs within 5–6 hours.
- Bilateral fixation is done during the surgery because the opposite side is at risk for future torsion.

EPIDIDYMITIS

Inflammation of the epididymis due to urethritis, UTI, prostatitis, tumor, urologic instrumentation, mumps or other viral infection, or bacterial infection. Most cases are due to chlamydia or gonorrhea infection or are idiopathic.

SYMPTOMS

Gradual or sudden onset of epididymal pain; swelling of the scrotum and/or epididymis.

EXAM

- Tenderness and swelling of the epididymis and/or scrotum is noted on exam.
- Elevation of the testicle ↓ pain.
- The cremasteric reflex is intact.

DIAGNOSIS

- Obtain a UA and culture.
- Obtain a urethral culture for chlamydia and gonorrhea infection.
- Scrotal Doppler ultrasound is normal.

TREATMENT

Bed rest with cold compresses, scrotal elevation, analgesics; antibiotics for chlamydia/gonorrhea.

TESTICULAR CANCER

Most commonly a seminoma or embryonal carcinoma.

SYMPTOMS

Approximately 10% of cases present with pain.

EXAM

- Presents as a painless, firm testicular mass that does not transilluminate.
- Reactive hydrocele may develop.

DIAGNOSIS

- Biopsy the mass.
- Imaging for staging.
- Obtain serum markers such as β-hCG and α-fetoprotein.

TREATMENT

- Treatment options include orchiectomy of the affected testicle, retroperitoneal lymph node dissection, and chemotherapy/radiation.

Persistence of inflammation for > 14 days suggests a coexisting testicular tumor. This is seen in 10% of cases of epididymitis.

- Prognosis depends on tumor type. The best prognosis is seen with seminoma, which is associated with a 90% five-year survival rate.

Priapism

Persistent painful erection that may be due to sickle cell crisis, leukemia, urethritis, bladder stones, spinal cord injury, mumps, pelvic tumor, medication, or idiopathic causes.

TREATMENT

- Give supportive care such as ice packs.
- Erections lasting > 1–2 hours require hospitalization and urologic consultation.
- Surgical reestablishment of the drainage pathway may be required.

COMPLICATIONS

Erections lasting > 24 hours result in infarction → fibrosis and ultimately impotence.

MENTAL HEALTH

Depression

Has a 2:1 female predominance in postpuberty. There is a peak in late adolescence. Some 4–6% of adolescents suffer from depression. Subtypes are as follows:

- **Major depressive disorder:** Characterized by depressed or irritable mood or ↓ interest or pleasure that lasts for at least two weeks.
- **Dysthymic disorder:** Less severe depression involving chronic symptoms and lasting at least one year.

Some 25–75% of youth with depression suffer from comorbid anxiety disorders.

SYMPTOMS

- **Neurovegetative symptoms:** Disordered eating, disordered sleeping, difficulty concentrating, ↓ energy, anhedonia, hopelessness, suicidal ideation.
- **Psychosomatic complaints:** Abdominal pain, headaches, chest pain.
- **Other:** Change in school performance; withdrawal from family and friends; may self-medicate with drugs or alcohol.

DIFFERENTIAL

Eating disorders, thyroid disorders, substance abuse, anemia.

TREATMENT

- SSRIs for 6–12 months are the treatment of choice.
- Psychotherapy may be of benefit.
- Assessment of suicide risk is imperative.

Suicide

- The third leading cause of death among adolescents.
- Attempts are more prevalent among females, but completion is more prevalent among males 15–19 years of age.

- **Exam/Dx:**
  - Must evaluate for suicidal thoughts and plan as well as for previous attempts, including intent and lethality.
  - Some 80% of suicide attempts and 90% of suicides are associated with a history of psychiatric disorders, most commonly depressive disorders, substance abuse, conduct disorder, or anxiety disorder.
  - Gay, lesbian, and bisexual teens are at ↑ risk, as are those with firearms in the home.
- **Tx:** Includes psychiatric inpatient or day-hospital treatment, "no-suicide" contracts, pharmacologic therapy for underlying depression or anxiety, and identification and treatment of substance disorders.

Substance Abuse

Risk factors include a family history of abuse, familial discord, inconsistent parental supervision, easy availability of substances, use of substances at an early age, drug use in peer group, ADHD, learning disorders, and behavioral disorders such as conduct disorder.

SYMPTOMS

Changes in dress and personal hygiene, ↑ moodiness or irritability, ↓ communication with friends and family, deterioration in school performance, frequent detention for disruptive behavior, sexually promiscuous behavior.

EXAM

May present with weight loss, track marks on skin, or nasal mucosal injection with or without rhinorrhea.

DIAGNOSIS

Drug screening should not be carried out without the patient's consent; forced screening with parental consent undermines the therapeutic alliance. Consent should be waived only if the patient is not competent or seems to be at high risk of incurring serious harm that could be avoided if the substance were identified.

TREATMENT

- Substance abuse counselors.
- Self-help groups such as Narcotics Anonymous and Alcoholics Anonymous.
- Contract for avoidance and monthly follow-up for adolescents who have begun to experiment.

COMPLICATIONS

A high rate of relapse exists and is an expected part of recovery.

Anorexia Nervosa

- An eating disorder characterized by a distorted body image and an intense fear of becoming fat. More common among adolescent white females from middle-to-upper socioeconomic groups.

- **Sx:** May present with obsessive dieting with voluntary food limitation; intense fear of weight gain and distorted body image; amenorrhea; and refusal to maintain a BMI ≥ 17.5.
- **Exam:** Chronic findings include brittle hair and nails, lanugo, bradycardia, and hypothermia.
- **Tx:** Multidisciplinary treatment approach includes supportive care, behavioral therapy, and antidepressants.

Bulimia Nervosa

An eating disorder characterized by uncontrolled bingeing and purging. As with anorexia nervosa, it is more common among white, middle/upper-class females.

SYMPTOMS

- Recurrent episodes of binge eating characterized by the following:
    - Eating a quantity of food that is larger than most people would eat in a similar period of time and circumstance.
    - Lack of control of the eating behavior.
- Other pathologic measures of weight control, including self-induced vomiting, laxative and diuretic abuse, and excessive exercise.
- Binge eating occurs at least twice a week for three months.
- Self-image is overly influenced by weight.

EXAM

May present with salivary gland enlargement, dental enamel erosion, **Russell's sign** (calluses over the dorsa of the fingers), posterior pharyngeal abrasions, facial petechiae and scleral hemorrhage, stress fractures, and weight fluctuations.

TREATMENT

- Supportive care.
- **Psychotherapy:** Individual, group, family.
- Antidepressants, including SSRIs.

Amenorrhea precedes weight loss in 25% of patients, is concurrent with weight loss in 50%, and occurs after weight loss in 25%.

Most patients with bulimia are overweight or weigh within the normal range.

ADOLESCENT HEALTH

CHAPTER 3

Allergy, Immunology, and Rheumatology

Daniel R. Brown, MD, PhD
reviewed by Laurie Armsby, MD

Many allergies are immune or hypersensitivity reactions that are classified according to time of onset and mechanism, as delineated in the Gell and Coombs classification system (see Table 3-1).

Urticaria and Angioedema

Urticaria is an edematous lesion of the superficial epidermis that is caused by IgE-, complement-, or direct stimulation–mediated degranulation of mast cells → pruritic wheals. **Angioedema** is a similar type of edema that occurs in deeper layers of the skin → more diffuse swelling. Both are type I immune reactions. Chronic urticaria and angioedema are defined by persistence for > 6 weeks.

SYMPTOMS/EXAM

- Pruritus is the most common presenting symptom.
- Individual lesions last < 24 hours.
- In 50% of patients with acute urticaria, a trigger can be identified (e.g., foods, insects, medications, viruses, physical stimuli).
- Fewer than 10% of patients with chronic urticaria have a known trigger.
- Physical urticaria has distinct syndromes whose presentations vary:
    - **Cold:** Reactions can be immediate or delayed and can be associated with systemic symptoms such as wheezing or hypotension.
    - **Cholinergic:** Heat, exercise, or stress can trigger urticaria and systemic symptoms.
    - **Solar:** Occurs within minutes of exposure to particular wavelengths of light.

DIFFERENTIAL

- **Pigmented urticaria:** Mastocytoma similar to a nevus → hives when stroked.
- **Hereditary angioedema:** The absence of C1q inhibitor → painful, nonpruritic episodes of edema involving the extremities, bowel, or larynx.
- **Urticarial vasculitis:** Vasculitic lesions that can resemble urticaria, but lesions last > 24 hours and heal with pigment change.
- **Serum sickness:** A drug reaction consisting of fever, urticaria, and arthritis.

> **Gell and Coombs classification system—ACID**
>
> **A**naphylactic—type I
> **C**ytotoxic—type II
> **I**mmune complex—type III
> **D**elayed hypersensitivity—type IV

Patients with severe cold-induced urticaria can develop anaphylaxis while swimming in cold water.

TABLE 3-1. Gell and Coombs Classification of Immune Reactions

TYPE	TIMING	MECHANISM	EXAMPLES
Type I	Minutes	Cross-linking of IgE on mast cells.	Anaphylaxis, urticaria.
Type II	Hours	Cytotoxic antibody.	Hemolytic anemia.
Type III	Hours	Immune complex deposition with activation of complement.	Serum sickness.
Type IV	Days (24–72 hours)	T-cell mediated.	Contact dermatitis.

DIAGNOSIS

- Skin-prick testing or blood radioallergosorbent testing (RAST) for antigen-specific IgE can help confirm allergic triggers when suggested by history. Random "across-the-board" testing is not useful owing to a high false-$\oplus$ rate.
- Antithyroid antibodies are $\uparrow$ in some patients and suggest autoimmune urticaria.
- Obtain AST and ALT to screen for urticaria associated with viral hepatitis.
- Complement levels are low in urticarial vasculitis and serum sickness.

TREATMENT

- Antihistamines, including H_2 blockade, are the mainstays of therapy.
- Low-dose steroids and low-dose cyclosporine are second-line agents because of their side effects.

Anaphylaxis

Widespread mast cell degranulation $\rightarrow$ a severe, life-threatening allergic reaction that usually occurs within minutes of exposure to an offending agent.

SYMPTOMS

- Presents with pruritus, a feeling of impending doom, dysphagia (a "lump in the throat"), nausea or vomiting, and dyspnea.
- A history of exposure to a specific trigger (drugs, foods, insects, latex) is usually recognized, but cross-contamination occasionally $\rightarrow$ unrecognized exposures.

EXAM

Examination reveals urticaria, swelling of the tongue and lip, wheezing and stridor, and hypotension (anaphylactic shock).

DIFFERENTIAL

Other causes of shock (septic, cardiogenic, hypovolemic), asthma exacerbations, hereditary angioedema, anxiety attacks.

DIAGNOSIS

- Diagnosed by history and exam.
- Tryptase, a mast cell enzyme, is $\uparrow$ for hours after an attack.

TREATMENT

- ABCs, **IM epinephrine early,** H_1 and H_2 blockers.
- Corticosteroids may prevent late-phase or biphasic reactions.
- Epinephrine injectors (e.g., EpiPen) for self-administration in the event of future attacks.
- Avoid repeat exposure; for drugs, desensitization can provide temporary tolerance.
- Immunotherapy for anaphylaxis 2° to insect allergy.

COMPLICATIONS

- Organ damage due to hypoperfusion.
- Patients with atopy or asthma have more severe outcomes.

Penicillin is the only drug for which there is a sufficient number of metabolites to provide adequate sensitivity for skin testing.

Desensitization does not work for serum sickness, Stevens-Johnson syndrome, hemolytic anemia, and other non-IgE-mediated forms of drug reaction.

Drug Reaction

Some 90% of drug reactions—including overdose, side effects, idiosyncratic reactions, and drug-drug interactions—are due to the pharmacologic properties of drugs; only 10% are due to an immune-mediated response and are considered drug allergy. Risk factors for drug allergy include a first-degree relative with such an allergy, allergy to another drug, parenteral administration, and short or frequent courses of medication. Many drug reactions are classified by the Gell and Coombs system (see Table 3-1); others include the following:

- **Stevens-Johnson syndrome** (also see the Dermatology chapter): Presents with sloughing of the skin, oral mucosa, and conjunctiva.
- **Morbilliform reactions:** Common with ampicillin or amoxicillin and do not require discontinuation of medication.

DIAGNOSIS

- Skin-prick testing is effective only for type I reactions, and sensitivity is limited, as testing for drug metabolites is often impossible (with the exception of **penicillin**).
- Eosinophilia is occasionally seen in type I reactions.

TREATMENT

- Eliminate the offending drug.
- If medication must be used, desensitization can be performed for type I–mediated reactions before each course of therapy.

A six-year-old boy is treated for a URI and bilateral otitis media with cefaclor. Seven days later he develops a temperature of 38.4°C, mild abdominal pain, arthralgias, puffy hands and feet, and a diffuse rash that is more prominent in the lower extremities. The rash consists of pruritic, erythematous wheals that blanch with pressure. The boy also has a macular area of erythema in the web spaces of his hands and feet. Labs are as follows: WBC count 7.5 (60% neutrophils, 32% lymphocytes, 5% monocytes, 2% eosinophils), Na 137, K 4.2, Cl 103, HCO_3 24, BUN 12, and creatinine 0.5. UA is 1.018 with 2+ protein and is otherwise normal. C3 is 65 (80–170), C4 10 (15–45), and IgA 75 (50–150). What is the diagnosis, and what is the appropriate treatment? This is serum sickness that is most likely 2° to viral infection or cefaclor. The presentation is similar to Henoch-Schönlein purpura except that the rash described above is urticaria and not palpable purpura. Another diagnostic aid is the low complement level, which occurs because of consumption from immune complex deposition. Treatment is supportive; if symptoms are severe, NSAIDs or glucocorticoids can be used.

Serum Sickness

A vasculitic syndrome caused by deposition of immune complexes (a type III immune response) commonly in response to a drug (typically penicillin, cefaclor, or infused immunoglobulin) or a viral infection.

- Symptoms appear after antibodies are created, typically 7–12 days or up to three weeks after exposure to the offending agent.
- Presents with a triad of **fever, urticaria,** and **arthritis.**
- Abdominal pain is also common.
- Patients generally appear quite ill.

DIFFERENTIAL

SLE, polyarteritis nodosa.

DIAGNOSIS

Diagnosed by history, low C3 and C4, and proteinuria.

TREATMENT

- Withdraw the offending agent.
- The condition is self-limited, resolving in 7–10 days.
- Symptomatic treatment with antihistamines, NSAIDs, or prednisone.

Food Reaction

The most common offending foods are milk, soy, peanuts, tree nuts, shellfish, fish, and wheat.

SYMPTOMS/EXAM

- IgE-mediated reactions occur within two hours and take the form of urticaria, wheezing, vomiting, and hypotension.
- Food-induced enterocolitis syndrome is usually due to soy or milk protein and is not IgE mediated; it presents with bloody diarrhea and profuse vomiting.
- Food may → a flare of atopic dermatitis.

The food responsible for most adverse reactions is milk protein.

DIAGNOSIS

- The gold standard is a double-blind, placebo-controlled food challenge.
- Skin testing is sufficiently sensitive to rule out IgE-mediated immune reactions, but false-⊕ reactions are common.

TREATMENT

- Eliminate the offending food from the diet.
- Hydrolyzed formula is less allergenic.
- Patients with food allergy should carry epinephrine in the event of accidental exposure.

Skin and RAST tests cannot be used to detect food-induced enterocolitis syndrome because this syndrome is not IgE mediated.

COMPLICATIONS

Most children outgrow allergies to milk, soy, and egg by five years of age, but allergies to peanuts, tree nuts, and shellfish tend to be lifelong.

Eosinophilia

Eosinophil production is stimulated by Th2 cells and by IL-3 and IL-5 under a variety of circumstances (see Table 3-2).

ALLERGY, IMMUNOLOGY, AND RHEUMATOLOGY

TABLE 3-2. Causes of Eosinophilia

CATEGORY	DISEASE
Allergic	Allergic rhinitis, eczema, asthma, drug allergy.
Infectious	Parasitic, mycobacterial, fungal.
Endocrine	Adrenal insufficiency.
Immune dysfunction	IBD, SLE, Churg-Strauss syndrome, Omenn syndrome, hyper-IgE syndrome.
Neoplastic	AML, ALL, lymphoma, mastocytoma.
Idiopathic	Hypereosinophilic syndrome, eosinophilic pneumonia, eosinophilic gastroenteritis.

TREATMENT

Steroids can be given if there is evidence of end-organ damage from eosinophils, but infectious etiologies must first be ruled out.

COMPLICATIONS

- The toxic effects of eosinophil granules on the heart can → **Löffler's endocarditis** (endomyocardial fibrosis).
- Pulmonary and CNS involvement can occur in idiopathic hypereosinophilic syndromes.

IMMUNOLOGY

Humoral Immunodeficiency

A group of disorders in which the ability of B cells to produce antibodies is impaired (see Table 3-3).

SYMPTOMS

- Infections begin after six months of age, when maternal IgG levels begin to wane.
- Infections tend to be recurrent and may become increasingly severe or respond poorly to antibiotics.
- Typical pathogens include pneumococcus, meningococcus, *Haemophilus influenzae*, *S. aureus*, *Pseudomonas*, *Mycoplasma*, and enterovirus.
- Typical infections include pneumonia, otitis, sinusitis, sepsis, and meningitis, including chronic enteroviral meningoencephalitis.

EXAM

Examination reveals absent tonsils in agammaglobulinemia.

IgG crosses the placenta and persists in the circulation, providing protection from infection for approximately six months.

TABLE 3-3. Humoral Immunodeficiencies

DISEASE	MECHANISM	LABS	CLINICAL MANIFESTATION
Bruton's agamma-globulinemia	Congenital absence of B cells. Most commonly X linked; due to absence of Bruton's tyrosine kinase.	Very low IgA, IgM, and IgG; vaccine responses are absent; **no B cells.**	**Pyogenic bacteria** and **enteroviral** infections after six months of age.
Common variable immunodeficiency (CVID)	An acquired disorder of antibody production whose mechanism is unknown.	Low IgA, IgG, or IgM; vaccine responses are absent; **B cells are present.**	Presents after two years of age with severe infections; associated with **autoimmune disease** and **lymphoma.**
IgA deficiency	Patients may have relatives with CVID. The mechanism is unknown.	**Isolated low IgA.**	Presents with minor infections or is asymptomatic; associated with spruelike disease and with anaphylaxis to IgA-containing blood products.
Transient hypogamma-globulinemia of infancy	Patients are slow to develop normal levels of antibody.	Low IgA, IgG, or IgM; vaccine responses are present.	Presents with minor infections or is asymptomatic; resolves by four years of age.

DIFFERENTIAL

- **Similar infections** seen with congenital or 2° asplenia and classic complement component deficiency.
- **Similar labs** may be seen with the following:
  - Immunoglobulin loss due to protein-losing enteropathy, nephrotic syndrome, or chylothorax.
  - X-linked hyper-IgM syndrome; Wiskott-Aldrich syndrome; ataxia-telangiectasia.

DIAGNOSIS

- Low or absent B cells (Bruton's agammaglobulinemia).
- Immunoglobulin levels (IgG, IgA, IgM) reveal the quantity of antibody.
- Vaccine titers reveal the quality of antibody.

TREATMENT

- Severe diseases such as agammaglobulinemia or CVID are treated with monthly immunoglobulin infusions.
- Milder disease such as IgA deficiency or transient hypogammaglobulinemia of infancy can first be managed with prophylactic antibiotics.

COMPLICATIONS

- Infectious complications, especially bronchiectasis.
- CVID is associated with lymphoma as well as with autoimmune conditions such as arthritis, hemolytic anemia, and vasculitis.

ALLERGY, IMMUNOLOGY, AND RHEUMATOLOGY

A five-month-old boy with no past history of infections is admitted to the hospital for respiratory distress accompanied by a CXR demonstrating bilateral interstitial pneumonia. The child is treated with ceftriaxone and erythromycin, but he continues to deteriorate and eventually requires intubation. Labs are as follows: WBC count 20.4 (30% PMNs, 60% lymphocytes), IgG 20 (200–1200), IgA 1 (8–90), and IgM 100 (10–90). Analysis of lymphocytes reveals 40% CD4 T cells, 20% CD8 T cells, and 30% B cells. Testing further reveals *Pneumocystis carinii* pneumonia (PCP). Which arm of the immune system is affected, and what is the likely treatment? More important than recognizing this entity as hyper-IgM syndrome is recognizing that the presence of an opportunistic infection (PCP) is characteristic of a combined immunodeficiency. In this case, T-cell and B-cell function are impaired despite a normal lymphocyte number. Unlike humoral immunodeficiencies, which can be treated with regular IVIG therapy, this disease must be treated with prophylactic antimicrobials as well. If sibling-matched bone marrow is available, a transplant can also be done.

In general, the severity of immunodeficiencies correlates with the degree of helper T-cell dysfunction.

> **DiGeorge syndrome—CATCH 22**
>
> **C**ardiac anomalies
> **A**bnormal facies
> **T**hymic hypoplasia
> **C**left palate
> **H**ypocalcemia
> **22**q11 deletion

Combined Immunodeficiency

A group of disorders of both cellular and humoral immunity resulting either from combined T- and B-cell dysfunction or from 1° T-cell dysfunction, impairing help for B cells.

SYMPTOMS

- Usually presents before six months of age with **failure to thrive (FTT)**.
- Typical pathogens are those that → **opportunistic infections,** including viral, bacterial, and fungal agents as well as nontuberculous mycobacteria and *Pneumocystis*.
- Typical infections include chronic **diarrhea,** recurrent pulmonary infections, **oral thrush,** gram-⊖ sepsis, and severe viral infections.

EXAM

Many combined immunodeficiencies have other syndromic features (see Table 3-4).

DIFFERENTIAL

HIV, chylothorax (can lose lymphocytes).

DIAGNOSIS

- Lymphocyte subsets include helper T cells (CD4), cytotoxic T cells (CD8), B cells (CD19), and NK cells (CD16 or CD56); see Table 3-5.
- Delayed-type hypersensitivity to *Candida* can assess T-cell function.
- Quantifying lymphocyte proliferation to mitogen or antigen can further assess T-cell function.
- Lack of T-cell help impairs antigen-specific antibody production → low vaccine titers.
- X-linked hyper-IgM syndrome specifically impairs the T-cell help that is required for isotype switching. Patients thus have low IgG and IgA with normal or ↑ IgM as well as PCP infection.

SYNDROME	COMMENTS
DiGeorge syndrome	A complete or partial T-cell deficiency due to **thymic hypoplasia.** Has variable association with conotruncal anomalies, dysmorphic face, cleft palate, and hypoparathyroidism; often associated with microdeletions on chromosome 22.
Wiskott-Aldrich syndrome	An X-linked triad of **eczema, thrombocytopenia,** and **severe infections.**
Ataxia-telangiectasia	A **DNA breakage repair deficiency** that affects T- and B-cell gene rearrangement. Symptoms include ataxia, telangiectasias, leukemia, lymphoma, and immunodeficiency.
NF-κB essential modifier (NEMO) mutations	Associated with ectodermal dysplasia, **conical teeth,** and mycobacterial infections.

TREATMENT

- Bone marrow transplantation as early as possible (induction therapy is too toxic for patients with DNA repair defects).
- Thymus transplantation for complete DiGeorge syndrome.
- IVIG replacement until transplantation.
- PCP prophylaxis.

Think severe combined immunodeficiency (SCID) when chromosome studies cannot be sent because of a lack of lymphocyte proliferation required for chromosome preparations.

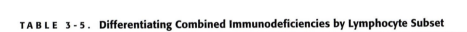

LYMPHOCYTE PHENOTYPE	IMMUNODEFICIENCY
T−, B−, NK−	**Adenosine deaminase (ADA) deficiency** → impaired lymphocyte development and survival owing to disruption of the purine salvage pathway. Purine nucleoside phosphorylase (PNP) deficiency is less severe. Reticular dysgenesis → failure of both lymphoid and myeloid lineage.
T−, B−, NK+	**Recombinase activating gene (RAG) deficiency** prevents proper re-arrangement of the T-cell and B-cell receptor genes.
T−, B+, NK variable	Mutations in certain cytokine signals, most notably the shared **cytokine receptor γ-chain** (X-linked SCID), → absent T cells and poorly functioning B cells. Patients with complete **DiGeorge syndrome** lack a thymus and thus do not develop T cells.

COMPLICATIONS

- Significant morbidity and mortality from infections; FTT; graft-versus-host disease due to nonirradiated blood transfusion.
- SCID is usually fatal in infancy or childhood.

Phagocyte Dysfunction

A group of disorders affecting neutrophil number or function (see Table 3-6).

SYMPTOMS

- Typical pathogens are bacteria (especially *S. aureus* and other catalase-⊕ organisms in chronic granulomatous disease [CGD]) and fungi.
- Typical infections include respiratory tract infections, stomatitis, and abscesses of the skin and internal organs.

EXAM

- Persistence of the umbilical stump is associated with leukocyte adhesion deficiency.
- Partial albinism is associated with Chédiak-Higashi syndrome.

DIFFERENTIAL

- Neutropenia:
  - Acquired disease 2° to ↓ production (e.g., cancer, viral suppression), sequestration, or destruction.
  - Glycogen storage disease type Ib.

TABLE 3-6. Overview of Common Neutrophil Disorders

DISEASE	MECHANISM	LABS	CLINICAL MANIFESTATION
Chronic granulomatous disease	Neutrophils lack **NADPH oxidase.**	Nitroblue tetrazolium test or rhodamine dye test.	Skin and organ abscesses with *S. aureus, Pseudomonas, Serratia,* and *Aspergillus;* noninfectious colitis.
Leukocyte adhesion deficiency	Neutrophils cannot migrate out of blood vessels.	High neutrophil count.	Abscesses without pus.
Chédiak-Higashi syndrome	Abnormal phagosome trafficking.	**Giant granules** in PMNs.	Partial **albinism;** lymphohistiocytic phase → death.
Cyclic neutropenia, congenital neutropenia (Kostmann's disease)	Low absolute neutrophil count (ANC); mechanisms are unclear.	Neutropenia in **cycles** of approximately three weeks.	Stomatitis, abscesses.
Shwachman-Diamond syndrome	Low ANC.	Neutropenia; fat malabsorption due to pancreatic insufficiency.	Respiratory infections, diarrhea, FTT, metaphyseal dysplasia.

- **Infections:**
  - Respiratory infections occur with humoral immunodeficiencies.
  - Abscesses occur with abnormal skin barrier function, as is seen with eczema or in drug abusers.

DIAGNOSIS

- CBC with smear can detect neutropenia or abnormal neutrophil granules.
- Nitroblue tetrazolium or rhodamine stains detect oxidative burst.

TREATMENT

- Neutropenia responds to G-CSF.
- Patients with CGD should receive antimicrobial prophylaxis (TMP-SMX [Bactrim], itraconazole); IFN-γ has demonstrated efficacy in preventing infections.
- Bone marrow transplantation.

COMPLICATIONS

Autoimmune colitis can develop in CGD; a hemophagocytic phase occurs in Chédiak-Higashi disease.

> A four-year-old girl with a history of glomerulonephritis develops pneumo-coccal meningitis. Labs are as follows: WBC count 15.1 (75% PMNs, 22% lymphocytes), IgG 1000, IgA 120, IgM 80, 75% CD3, 50% CD4, 25% CD8, and 15% B cells. These values are essentially normal, and you suspect a complement deficiency. Where in the complement cascade is the deficiency? In addition to an SLE-like illness (such as glomerulonephritis), deficiencies of any of the early components of the complement cascade are associated with infections due to encapsulated organisms (including pneumococcus). By contrast, children with deficiencies in the late complement components are more susceptible to meningococcus infections. Therefore, this is likely an early component deficiency that includes C1, C2, C3, C4, factor H, and factor I.

Complement Deficiency

Early complement components (C1–C4, factor I, factor H) participate in the clearance of immune complexes and opsonization. Late complement components (C5–C9) are primarily involved with lytic activity.

SYMPTOMS/EXAM

- **Deficiency of early components** (especially C3): Associated with infection with encapsulated bacteria.
- **Deficiency of late components:** Associated with *Neisseria* infections.

DIFFERENTIAL

- Infections associated with early complement components are similar to those associated with humoral immune deficiency.

Complement deficiencies are often associated with an autoimmune SLE-like condition as well as with infections.

- Low complement levels are seen with excessive consumption—e.g., SLE, poststreptococcal glomerulonephritis.

DIAGNOSIS

- CH50 is a functional assay that assesses the entire complement cascade.
- Levels of individual complement components can be measured.

TREATMENT

- Currently there is no treatment to replace missing complement components.
- Management is focused on treating infectious and autoimmune sequelae.

Miscellaneous Immunologic Disorders

- **Autoimmune polyglandular syndrome:** Includes multiple autoimmune **polyendocrinopathy** and **chronic mucocutaneous candidiasis**. Mutations in the AIRE gene limit T-cell tolerance to endocrine organs by limiting the expression of many antigens in the thymus.
- **Hyper-IgE syndrome (Job syndrome):** Associated with staphylococcal microabscesses, pneumonia with pneumatoceles, coarse facies, dermatitis, and markedly ↑ IgE.

X-linked immunodeficiencies include X-linked hyper-IgM syndrome, X-linked SCID, X-linked agammaglobulinemia, Wiskott-Aldrich syndrome, NEMO, and 75% of CGD cases.

RHEUMATOLOGY

Common Labs in Rheumatology

ACUTE-PHASE REACTANTS

- Include CRP, fibrinogen, α_1-antitrypsin, haptoglobin, and complement.
- When these are ↑, transferrin and albumin are correspondingly ↓.
- An ↑ ESR reflects ↑ sedimentation of RBCs in the presence of acute-phase reactants such as fibrinogen, which neutralize electrostatic repulsion between cells.
    - ESR is ↑ with many inflammatory conditions, such as infection, autoimmune disease, and malignancy
    - It is also ↑ with anemia, hypoalbuminemia, OCPs, and heparin therapy.

ANTINUCLEAR ANTIBODIES (ANAs)

- Detected by immunofluorescence against the nuclei of cultured cells.
- ⊕ in multiple autoimmune conditions (e.g., SLE, drug-induced lupus, mixed connective tissue disease, scleroderma, Sjögren syndrome, juvenile rheumatoid arthritis [JRA], autoimmune thyroid disease, autoimmune hepatitis) as well as in viral infections; also ⊕ in many normal individuals (see Table 3-7).
- Higher titers and persistent elevations are more likely to be associated with disease.

ANTIPHOSPHOLIPID ANTIBODIES

- Include antibodies to cardiolipin, a phospholipid, or to β_2-glycoprotein I, a phospholipid-binding protein.

TABLE 3-7. Antinuclear Antibodies Observed in Rheumatic Diseases

					FREQUENCY OF A ⊕ TEST			
ANTIBODY	**SLE**	**SJÖGREN'S SYNDROME**	**SYSTEMIC SCLEROSIS**	**CREST**	**POLYMYOSITIS/ DERMATOMYOSITIS**	**DRUG-INDUCED LUPUS**	**MIXED CONNECTIVE TISSUE DISEASE**	**JRA**
ANA	95–100	95	80–95	80–95	80–95	100	95	60
dsDNA	60							
Smith	10–30							
Histone						90		
RNP							90	
SSA (Ro)	15–40	60–90						
SSB (La)	5–20	60–70						
Scl-70			33	10–20				
Centromere				50–85				

- Can prolong phospholipid-dependent coagulation tests such as PT, PTT, and the dilute Russell viper venom test, which does not correct when mixed 1:1 with normal serum.
- Found in 40% of patients with SLE.
- Antiphospholipid syndrome is an association of antibodies with a tendency to form arterial and venous thrombosis or recurrent miscarriages.

RHEUMATOID FACTOR (RF)

- An antibody to the Fc portion of immunoglobulin.
- Can be seen in JRA, SLE, Sjögren syndrome, chronic infections (especially HCV), and acute viral infections as well as with malignancy.

ANTINEUTROPHIL CYTOPLASMIC ANTIBODIES

- p-ANCA (perinuclear pattern) is associated with many diseases, including microscopic polyangiitis, vasculitis, IBD, SLE, and JRA.
- c-ANCA (diffuse cytoplasmic pattern) directed at proteinase 3 is associated with Wegener's granulomatosis.

A ⊕ RF is rare in JRA but is more common in adult RA and adolescent JRA. Patients with RF-⊕ JRA have more aggressive, erosive arthritis.

p-ANCA is found in a **P**lethora of diseases. **c**-ANCA is found primarily in Wegener's, which involves **C**ough (lungs), **C**reatinine (kidneys), and **C**ongestion (sinuses).

Inflammatory conditions ↓ the viscosity of synovial fluid → stiffness with inactivity and cold. Symptoms improve with use and application of heat.

Arthritis differs from arthralgia because of the presence of objective findings.

Monoarticular hip pain is not a common presentation of JRA.

Juvenile Rheumatoid Arthritis (JRA)

Incidence is 10 in 100,000 annually.

SYMPTOMS

- Young children may simply avoid using certain joints; older children complain of stiffness and mild pain.
- Symptoms are typically worse in the morning or after periods of inactivity (gelling phenomenon); see Table 3-8.
- Pain is usually not as severe as in septic joint or rheumatic fever.

EXAM

- Arthritis requires exam findings such as swelling, tenderness, and warmth.
- Deformities such as ulnar deviation can be seen.
- Leg length discrepancy suggests chronic disease that → asymmetric growth.
- Other findings are specific to the type of JRA:
  - **Pauciarticular: Asymmetric** involvement of the ankle, knees, and elbows. Rarely affects the hips at presentation.
  - **Polyarticular: Symmetric** involvement of almost any joint, including the ankle, knee, elbow, wrist, hands, feet, temporomandibular joint, or cervical spine. Rarely affects the hips at presentation.
  - **Systemic:** Often there is no joint involvement at the time of presentation. May present with daily or twice-daily fever; a fleeting, macular pink ("salmon-colored") rash; and lymphadenopathy, hepatosplenomegaly, and pericarditis.

DIFFERENTIAL

The differential includes the following (see also Table 3-9):

- **Spondyloarthropathy** can mimic pauciarticular JRA.

TABLE 3-8. Pattern of Joint Pain by Etiology

ETIOLOGY	MORNING (BEFORE ACTIVITY)	EVENING (AFTER ACTIVITY)	OVERNIGHT
Inflammatory (JRA)	++	+	
Mechanical (overuse injury)		++	
Neuropathic (fibromyalgia)	++	++	
Infiltrative (cancer)	++	++	++

ALLERGY, IMMUNOLOGY, AND RHEUMATOLOGY

TABLE 3-9. Common Causes of Joint Pain by Pattern of Involvement

MIGRATORY	ADDITIVE	MONOARTICULAR
Acute rheumatic fever	JRA	Septic arthritis
Disseminated gonococcal infection	Spondyloarthropathy	Adjacent osteomyelitis
Leukemia	Connective tissue disease	Lyme disease
Henoch-Schönlein purpura		Pauciarticular JRA
IBD-associated arthritis		Spondyloarthropathy
		Avascular necrosis
		Slipped capital femoral epiphysis
		Overuse syndrome
		Trauma

Adapted, with permission, from Rudolph CD et al. *Rudolph's Pediatrics,* 21st ed. New York: McGraw Hill, 2002:833.

- **SLE** or **Kawasaki disease** can mimic systemic JRA.
- **Other:** Rheumatic fever, Henoch-Schönlein purpura, leukemia, Lyme disease.

DIAGNOSIS

- Diagnosed by the American College of Rheumatology criteria:
  - Age < 16 years.
  - Arthritis—swelling/effusion or at least two of the following: limited range of motion, pain on motion, tenderness, warmth.
  - Symptoms persist > 6 weeks.
  - Exclude other causes.
  - Subtype is defined by symptoms in the first six months.
    - Polyarticular involves ≥ 5 joints.
    - Pauciarticular involves 1–4 joints.
    - Systemic is associated with > 2 weeks of fever and organ involvement.
- Additional studies include the following:
  - ANA ⊕ (pauciarticular > polyarticular > systemic).
  - RF ⊕ in 10% of adolescent polyarticular disease at onset.
  - Patients with systemic onset can have low-grade macrophage activation syndrome with ↑ D-dimer, ferritin, and triglycerides and with coagulation studies that are consistent with DIC.

TREATMENT

- NSAIDs treat symptoms but will not prevent erosion.
- Sulfasalazine, methotrexate, TNF inhibitors.
- If only a few joints are involved, intra-articular steroids can be effective.

COMPLICATIONS

- Permanently limited range of motion, asymmetric bone growth, atlantoaxial subluxation, osteoporosis.
- Uveitis is more common in girls, patients < 6 years of age, and ANA-⊕ patients.
- Macrophage activation syndrome (systemic subtype) may be seen.

Beware of the patient with systemic JRA who develops thrombocytopenia, anemia, ↑ D-dimer, ↓ ESR, and high ferritin, as these findings suggest macrophage activation syndrome, also known as hemophagocytic lymphohistiocytosis.

ALLERGY, IMMUNOLOGY, AND RHEUMATOLOGY

Spondyloarthropathy

A group of RF-⊖, chronic, idiopathic arthritides that can involve the axial skeleton and tendons, including juvenile ankylosing spondylitis (JAS), psoriatic arthritis, and IBD-associated arthritis. Incidence is 10–100 in 100,000 annually. JAS is more common in boys.

SYMPTOMS/EXAM

- Joint symptoms mimic JRA but occasionally involve ↑ pain.
- Can present with enthesitis, or inflammation of the junction of tendon to bone (e.g., Achilles or patellar tendonitis), as well as with tenosynovitis of a single digit (sausage finger/toe).
- Psoriatic arthritis is suggested by nail pits and by a first-degree relative with psoriasis.
- IBD-associated arthritis may parallel GI symptoms or appear independently.
- Reactive arthritis follows a history of bacterial GI or GU infection and can occur with urethritis and conjunctivitis (Reiter syndrome).

DIFFERENTIAL

- Oligoarticular JRA.
- Hip joint pain must be distinguished from transient synovitis, avascular necrosis, and slipped capital femoral epiphysis.

DIAGNOSIS

- HLA-B27 (> 90% of JAS cases).
- ANA (50% of psoriatic arthritis cases).
- All are RF ⊖.
- JAS shows evidence of sacroiliac involvement on x-ray.

TREATMENT

Similar to that of JRA.

COMPLICATIONS

Ankylosis of the spine (JAS), acute painful uveitis, chronic uveitis (15% of psoriatic arthritis).

ALLERGY, IMMUNOLOGY, AND RHEUMATOLOGY

Systemic Lupus Erythematosus (SLE)

An episodic multisystem autoimmune disease of variable presentation that is mediated by deposition of immune complexes. Affects 0.5 in 100,000 children annually. Less common in Caucasians, males, and children < 8 years of age.

SYMPTOMS/EXAM

- **General: Fever,** fatigue, lymphadenopathy, weight loss, alopecia.
- **Skin: Malar rash,** discoid rash (rare), photosensitivity, livedo, vasculitic rash.
- **Musculoskeletal: Arthritis,** myositis, tendonitis, avascular necrosis.
- **Neurologic:** Headaches, seizures, psychosis, strokes, peripheral neuropathy.
- **GI:** Gut vasculitis, serositis, hepatitis, pancreatitis, pain.
- **Cardiac: Pericarditis,** myocarditis, Libman-Sacks valve lesions.
- **Pulmonary:** Pleuritis, restrictive lung disease, pulmonary hemorrhage.
- **Renal: Nephritis,** nephrotic syndrome, hypertension.
- **Hematologic: Lymphopenia, anemia,** thrombocytopenia, thrombosis.

DIFFERENTIAL

SLE is on the differential of many diseases because of its multisystem involvement. More commonly in the differential are fever of unknown origin (FUO), leukemia, autoimmune hepatitis, and parvovirus infection.

DIAGNOSIS

- Lupus is diagnosed clinically by the fulfillment of 4 of the 11 criteria listed in Table 3-10.
- ANA is sensitive but not specific.
- Anti-Smith and anti-dsDNA are specific but not sensitive.
- Complement levels may ↓ and dsDNA titers may ↑ with disease activity.
- Lymphocyte count is low and IgG level high.
- Antihistone antibody is seen in drug-induced lupus.

Unlike JRA, the arthritis associated with SLE is not erosive.

ALLERGY, IMMUNOLOGY, AND RHEUMATOLOGY

TABLE 3-10. Diagnostic Criteria for SLE[a]

CRITERIA	COMMENTS
Skin criteria (3):	
1. Malar rash	Erythematous rash sparing the nasolabial folds.
2. Discoid rash	Erythematous rash with adherent scale and follicular plugging that heals with atrophic scarring.
3. Photosensitivity	
Clinical criteria (4):	
4. Oral or nasal ulcers	Usually painless and occurring on the hard palate.
5. Arthritis	Nonerosive, affecting > 2 joints.
6. Serositis	Pleural or pericardial effusion, rub, pleuritic pain, or suggestive ECG.
7. Neurologic disorders	Psychosis or seizure without other explanation.
Lab criteria (4):	
8. Cytopenia	Hemolytic anemia, or WBC < 4000 on two occasions, or lymphocyte count < 1500 on two occasions, or platelet count < 100,000 without other known cause.
9. Urine abnormality	Cellular casts or proteinuria (> 0.5 g/day or 3+).
10. Immune labs	Anti-dsDNA, anti-Smith, or antiphospholipid (anticardiolipin, ⊕ lupus anticoagulant, or false-⊕ syphilis testing).
11. ANA	

[a] Patients must satisfy 4 of 11 of these criteria.

SLE diagnostic criteria—RASH ON MAIDS

Renal
ANA
Serositis
Hematologic abnormalities
Oral ulcers
Neurologic disorders
Malar rash
Arthritis
Immune labs
Discoid rash
Sun sensitivity

TREATMENT

- Sunscreen and hydroxychloroquine to prevent flares.
- Steroids are the mainstay of therapy and can work acutely as well as chronically.
- Azathioprine can be used to allow for the reduction of chronic steroid dosages.
- Diffuse proliferative glomerulonephritis (stage IV) and CNS involvement are treated aggressively with cyclophosphamide.

COMPLICATIONS

- **Infections** (patients have hyposplenism and are usually receiving immune suppression).
- End-stage **renal disease**, pulmonary disease, MI.
- Chronic steroid use can → acne, skin atrophy, cushingoid facies, weight gain, headache, pseudotumor cerebri, hypertension, gastritis/ulcers, adrenal suppression, glucose intolerance, osteoporosis, and immunosuppression.

Scleroderma

An autoimmune disease characterized by endothelial damage → fibrosis of the dermis and variable systemic involvement. Rare in childhood.

SYMPTOMS/EXAM

- Skin lesions appear atrophic, shiny, or bound down.
- Other symptoms are as follows:
  - **Systemic sclerosis:** A diffuse sclerosis that begins distally with subcutaneous loss → tapered fingers, joint contractures, and puckered mouth. Common systemic signs include pulmonary hypertension, abnormal gut motility, renal artery disease, and Raynaud's phenomenon. Nail bed capillary changes similar to those of dermatomyositis or SLE may be seen.
  - **Limited scleroderma:** Also known as CREST syndrome; includes **C**alcinosis, **R**aynaud's phenomenon, **E**sophageal dysfunction, **S**cleroderma limited to the extremities and face, and **T**elangiectasias.
  - **Morphea:** Well-demarcated skin lesions without organ involvement that can involve a linear area on the forehead (coup de sabre) or part or all of a limb.

DIFFERENTIAL

1° Raynaud's phenomenon (not associated with systemic disease), SLE, graft-versus-host disease.

DIAGNOSIS

- ANA is ⊕.
- Scl-70 or anticentromere antibodies are seen in systemic forms (see Table 3-11).
- Obtain PFTs with DL_{CO} to look for pulmonary fibrosis.
- Esophagography to evaluate for dysmotility; echocardiography to look for pulmonary hypertension.

Patients with systemic scleroderma often die of pulmonary hypertension or renal disease.

TREATMENT

Treatment is outlined in Table 3-11.

TABLE 3-11. Symptomatic Treatment of Systemic Sclerosis

ORGAN	COMPLICATION	TREATMENT
Kidney	Renal crisis (malignant hypertension, renal failure, and microangiopathic hemolytic anemia).	ACEIs.
Lung	Interstitial pneumonitis, interstitial fibrosis.	Corticosteroids,[a] immunosuppressants.
Heart	Myocarditis, myocardial fibrosis, heart failure, pericardial effusions, conduction system disease.	Corticosteroids,[a] immunosuppressants, CHF therapy, pacemakers.
GI	Delayed gastric emptying, intestinal malabsorption, bacterial overgrowth.	Frequent small meals, promotility agents, antibiotics.

[a] Corticosteroids are usually avoided in scleroderma (unless severe organ-related disease leaves little other choice) because they may precipitate renal crisis.

> An ill-appearing four-year-old boy presents with one day of fever and a rash associated with fatigue, abdominal pain, diarrhea, and edema that is most notable on the hands and feet. The rash consists of petechiae over areas of pressure and appears predominantly on the buttocks and legs. Labs are as follows: WBC count 9.6, hematocrit 28%, platelets 80,000, Na 134, K 4.5, Cl 102, HCO_3 20, BUN 42, and creatinine 2.5. UA is 1.018 with 2+ protein and 1+ blood and is otherwise normal by dipstick. What is the diagnosis? Hemolytic-uremic syndrome (HUS). While many features of HUS are similar to Henoch-Schönlein purpura (e.g., abdominal pain, renal disease, petechiae, and edema), the low platelet count seen here is more suggestive of HUS (see the Renal System chapter).

Tetrad of Henoch-Schönlein purpura—NAPA

Nephritis
Arthritis
Purpura
Abdominal pain

Henoch-Schönlein Purpura

A **leukocytoclastic vasculitis** that affects small blood vessels and → a classic tetrad of palpable purpura, arthritis, abdominal pain, and glomerulonephritis. The most common vasculitis, it has an incidence of 13 in 100,000 annually. The peak age at onset is 2–8 years of age, and the male-to-female ratio is 2:1.

SYMPTOMS

- Antecedent viral illness.
- Fever and malaise.
- Abdominal colic, frequently with occult blood (66% of patients; 10% at onset).

EXAM

- Examination reveals **palpable purpura** in dependent areas (100% of patients; 50% at onset); see Figure 3-1.
- Abdominal pain may precede rash and may present as an **acute abdomen.**
- Other findings are as follows:
    - Arthritis, commonly of the knees and ankles and occasionally migratory (66% of patients; 25% at onset).
    - Edema of the dorsum of hands, feet, scalp, and scrotum.
    - Hypertension resulting from renal disease.

DIFFERENTIAL

Meningococcemia or Rocky Mountain spotted fever, HUS, JRA, rheumatic fever, sepsis, septic arthritis.

DIAGNOSIS

- Normal platelet count.
- ↑ ESR or CRP; ↑ IgA.
- Urine must be checked frequently for signs of nephritis.
- Renal findings are similar to IgA nephropathy.

TREATMENT

- Pain control.
- IV hydration may be needed along with IV nutrition if severe.
- Although controversial, steroids may help with abdominal pain or edema.
- Cyclophosphamide and possibly steroids for severe renal disease.

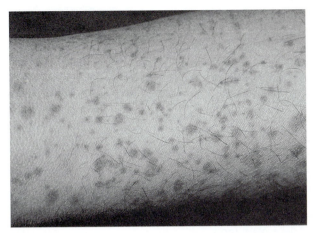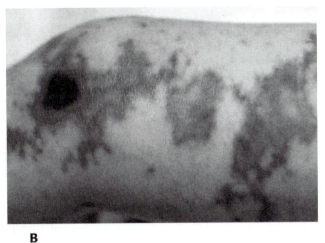

A   **B**

FIGURE 3-1. Henoch-Schönlein purpura (A) and meningococcemia (B).

The appearance of Henoch-Schönlein purpura, while similar to that of meningococcemia, can be distinguished because in meningococcemia purpura is more extensive, necrosis may be present, and patients appear ill. (A: Reproduced, with permission, from Rudolph CD et al. *Rudolph's Pediatrics*, 21st ed. New York: McGraw Hill, 2003: Color Plate 12; B: Reproduced, with permission, from Wolff K, Johnson RA, Suurmond D. *Fitzpatrick's Color Atlas & Synopsis of Clinical Dermatology*, 5th ed. New York: McGraw-Hill, 2005:643.) (Also see Color Insert.)

COMPLICATIONS

- In the acute phase, intussusception (usually **ileoileal**), perforation, and GI bleeding may occur.
- In some patients, the rash may episodically recur for > 1 year.
- In the chronic phase, severe renal disease occurs in 1–2% of patients.

A six-month-old Asian boy adopted from China at one month of age has had a fever up to 39.4°C for the past eight days with slight diarrhea, bilateral conjunctivitis, irritability, morbilliform rash, and erythema at the site of a prior BCG inoculation. His examination reveals tachycardia without murmur or gallop. Labs are as follows: WBC count 15.3 with neutrophil predominance, hematocrit 29%, platelets 510,000, AST 45, ALT 62, albumin 2.9, and ESR 68. Blood culture from two days before is ⊖, and a urine culture from the same time is ⊖ despite 20 WBCs/hpf on microscopy from a bag specimen. What is the next test you would order? This patient most likely has Kawasaki disease. Although he does not meet the full diagnostic criteria, the patient's ethnicity, his erythema at the BCG site, and his labs all suggest this diagnosis. Viral infection is also a possibility, but given the high risk of aneurysm in infants, an echocardiogram should be done to search for early evidence of coronary changes.

Kawasaki Disease

A vasculitis of small and medium-sized blood vessels. Its incidence among Caucasian children < 5 years of age is 10 in 100,000 annually but is 10-fold higher among Asians. More common in males than in females.

Symptoms/Exam

- Diagnostic criteria consist of fever for ≥ 5 days plus four out of five of the following:
  - Rash (bullous and vesicular lesions are atypical).
  - Conjunctival injection without exudates (usually spares the limbus).
  - Red or cracked lips, strawberry tongue, and diffuse erythema. Exudates and ulceration are uncommon.
  - Lymphadenopathy > 1.5 cm.
  - Hand and/or foot edema, erythema, or desquamation (desquamation occurs after 2–3 weeks).
- Note that the criteria above were defined before the recognition of coronary artery dilatation, and many patients develop aneurysms without ever meeting the full criteria ("atypical" or "incomplete" Kawasaki). This is especially true of children < 1 year of age.
- Other findings include the following:
  - **Heart:** Coronary artery aneurysm, myocarditis, CHF.
  - **GI:** Abdominal pain, vomiting, diarrhea, hydrops of the gallbladder.
  - **Joints:** Arthritis.
  - **CNS:** Irritability.
  - **Eyes:** Anterior uveitis.
  - **Skin:** Erythema at BCG site or periumbilical erythema (Sundel sign).

> **Kawasaki criteria—FEAR ME**
>
> **F**ever plus four of the following five:
> **E**ye injection
> **A**denopathy
> **R**ash
> **M**ucous membrane changes
> **E**xtremity changes

Differential

Scarlet fever, viral infection (especially adenovirus and EBV), toxic shock syndrome, Stevens-Johnson syndrome.

Diagnosis

- See the diagnostic criteria above.
- Lab findings include the following:
  - ↑ ESR and/or CRP.
  - ↑ WBC count with PMN predominance.
  - ↑ platelets (generally after the first week).
  - Anemia, sterile pyuria, low albumin.
  - ↑ ALT; a cholestatic picture with ↑ alkaline phosphatase, bilirubin, and GGT may also be seen.
  - CSF pleocytosis.

Treatment

- IVIG, aspirin.
- Patients should be followed by cardiology and may need serial echocardiography, depending on the presence and degree of coronary aneurysms. The duration of aspirin therapy usually depends on echocardiographic findings.

Complications

MI can occur acutely or up to years later as a result of coronary artery aneurysms and thrombosis.

Children < 1 year of age tend to present with less than full criteria and have a higher risk of coronary artery aneurysm.

Dermatomyositis

An inflammatory condition affecting the blood vessels that feed the muscle and skin. Incidence is 1 in 300,000, with females affected more often than males. Average age of onset is six years of age.

SYMPTOMS/EXAM

- Presents with proximal muscle weakness, usually of insidious onset (patients cannot climb stairs or comb hair).
- Other symptoms and signs are as follows:
  - **Gottron's papules: Pink, thickened skin** over the **PIP and MCP joints** and occasionally over the **knees and elbows** (see Figure 3-2).
  - **Heliotrope rash: Violaceous hue** to the **periorbital area.**
  - **Malar and body rash, especially in sun-exposed areas.**
  - Nail bed telangiectasia; abdominal pain in the presence of gut vasculitis.

DIFFERENTIAL

- CNS disease (usually accompanied by other cognitive or higher brain dysfunction).
- Peripheral neuropathy (usually distal weakness or random and asymmetric neuropathy).
- Myasthenia gravis (worsens with use; ocular involvement).
- Myopathies may be due to influenza, overuse, or muscular dystrophy, or they may be metabolic or drug induced.
- SLE.

DIAGNOSIS

- ↑ muscle enzymes (CK, aldolase, AST, LDH).
- ↑ von Willebrand's factor antigen (seen in two-thirds of patients) suggests endothelial damage.
- ANA is ⊕ in 60% of patients.
- MRI of the thighs can show enhancement of muscle and skin.
- ECG to rule out cardiac involvement; modified barium swallow to rule out risk of aspiration; stool guaiac to rule out gut vasculitis.

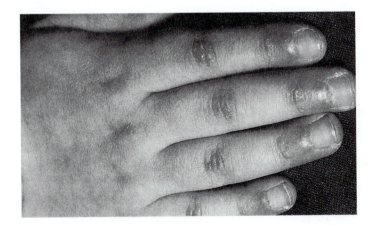

FIGURE 3-2. Gottron's papules.

Erythematous papules are seen overlying the knuckles. (Reproduced, with permission, from Rudolph CD et al. *Rudolph's Pediatrics*, 21st ed. New York: McGraw Hill, 2002, Color Plate 11.) (Also see Color Insert.)

- **Nonpharmacologic:** Physical therapy, sunscreen.
- **Pharmacologic:** IV and/or oral steroids, methotrexate, cyclophosphamide, cyclosporine.
- Overall prognosis has improved with available treatments; mortality is now roughly 3%.

COMPLICATIONS

- **Calcinosis:** Calcium deposits in the muscle that serve as a nidus for infection.
- Aspiration pneumonia due to bulbar weakness.
- Medication side effects.
- Cardiac involvement can → conduction delay and dysrhythmia.
- Intestinal ischemia can result from gut vasculitis.
- Respiratory muscle weakness and restrictive lung disease can occur.

Miscellaneous Disorders

SJÖGREN'S SYNDROME

- **Sx/Exam:** Presents with dry eyes, dry mouth, and recurrent parotitis.
- **Dx:** ↑ ANA, anti-Ro, anti-La, RF, and IgG.
- **Complications:** Associated with an ↑ risk of JRA, SLE, scleroderma, thyroid disease, polyarteritis nodosa, and lymphoma.

SARCOIDOSIS

- A disease characterized by infiltration of multiple tissues with noncaseating granulomas.
- **Sx/Exam:** Presents with fever, lymphadenopathy, weight loss, hepatosplenomegaly, uveitis, pulmonary infiltrates, cardiac involvement, and CNS disease.
- **Dx:** ↑ ESR, CRP, and angiotensin-converting enzyme; hypercalcemia.

> A three-day-old baby boy in the NICU has developed an erythematous rash after starting phototherapy. He was born at term, and his postnatal course was notable for a ⊖ sepsis workup because of thrombocytopenia. He has also had persistent bradycardia since birth, and his ECG shows evidence of congenital heart block. What lab test should be obtained? This baby has neonatal lupus, which is associated with the presence of SSA (anti-Ro) or SSB (anti-La).

NEONATAL LUPUS

- Caused by transfer to the fetus of anti-Ro (SSA) or anti-La (SSB) from a mother with either SLE or Sjögren syndrome.
- **Sx/Exam:** Presents with rash, thrombocytopenia, neutropenia, hepatitis, and congenital heart block.

WEGENER'S GRANULOMATOSIS

- **Sx/Exam:**
  - Small-vessel vasculitis → the triad of **sinus, lung,** and **kidney disease.**
  - Other findings include saddle-nose deformity, fever, rash, subglottic stenosis, proptosis, and pericardial and neural involvement.
- **Dx:** c-ANCA ⊕.

TAKAYASU'S ARTERITIS

- A large-vessel vasculitis affecting the aorta and its branches.
- **Sx/Exam:** Fever, ↓ pulses, claudication, renal vascular disease, strokes, CHF.

FAMILIAL MEDITERRANEAN FEVER

- **Sx/Exam:**
  - Regular fevers, abdominal pain, occasional pericarditis, pleuritis, and arthritis.
  - Long-standing inflammation → amyloidosis.
- **Tx:** Treat with prophylactic colchicine.

BEHÇET'S DISEASE

- **Sx/Exam:** Oral ulcers, genital ulcers, eye disease (uveitis, retinal vasculitis).
- **Dx:** **Pathergy** test (pustules form at needle stick sites).

Uveitis is seen in a number of rheumatologic conditions, including SLE, JRA, spondyloarthropathy, Kawasaki disease, sarcoid, and Behçet's disease. A slit-lamp exam is needed to make the diagnosis.

ALLERGY, IMMUNOLOGY, AND RHEUMATOLOGY

CHAPTER 4

Cardiology

David Harrild, MD, PhD
Nancy Kim, MD
reviewed by Clifford Chin, MD

A four-year-old girl presents for well-child care. She has been growing on the 25th percentile for height and weight and developing normally. On examination, you note that she has a quiet precordium, a regular rate, and normal S1 and S2 with a 2/6 systolic ejection murmur that is louder when the patient is supine. There is no radiation of the murmur to the neck, axillae, or back. What is the next step in management? Reassure the parent that the murmur is innocent and observe the patient.

EVALUATION OF A MURMUR

More than 80% of children have an innocent murmur at some point during childhood. Most of these murmurs are accentuated during high-output states (e.g., fever, anemia, dehydration). The most important point in evaluating a murmur is to distinguish those that are **innocent** or physiologic from those that are **pathologic**. The types and presentations of murmur are listed in Table 4-1.

SYMPTOMS/EXAM

Assess the following:

- **Intensity:** Grades 1–6 (barely audible to audible with stethoscope off the chest).
- **Quality:** Harsh, blowing, vibratory, high pitched, low pitched, ejection, regurgitant, and the like.
- **Timing:** Systolic, diastolic, continuous.
- **Location:** Left upper sternal border, right upper sternal border, left lower sternal border, apex (see Table 4-1).
- **Radiation:** Neck, back, axillae.

DIAGNOSIS

Think pathologic murmur if the patient is symptomatic or if the murmur is loud, is diastolic, or has associated clicks or gallops.

Clues that a murmur is pathologic include the following:

- The patient has a syndrome with a high incidence of heart defects (e.g., Down, Turner, Marfan, Williams, and Noonan syndromes).
- The patient is symptomatic (e.g., presents with failure to thrive, excessive sweating, tachypnea).
- The patient is cyanotic.
- The murmur is grade 3/6 or louder.
- The murmur is heard in diastole.
- Other abnormal sounds are heard on exam (e.g., clicks or gallops).
- CXR or ECG is abnormal.

TREATMENT

- Once the diagnosis of a pathologic murmur is made, the patient should be referred to a pediatric cardiologist.
- If the patient is asymptomatic with normal growth parameters and normal CXR and ECG, do nothing and observe.

TABLE 4-1. Types of Murmurs Based on Location of Loudest Intensity

LOCATION/DIAGNOSIS	UNIQUE FEATURES
Right upper sternal border	
Venous hum	Continuous; disappears when the jugular vein is compressed, when the patient's head is turned, or when the patient is supine; benign.
Aortic stenosis	Systolic ejection quality; radiates to the neck; presents with thrill in the suprasternal notch; often associated with a valve click.
Left upper sternal border	
Peripheral pulmonary stenosis	Systolic ejection quality; usually seen in infants; often louder in the axillae than over the precordium; benign.
Pulmonary stenosis	Systolic ejection quality; radiates to the back and axillae; may be associated with a valve click.
PDA	Continuous; **"machinery"** quality; bounding pulses.
ASD	Systolic; fixed, split S2.
Coarctation of the aorta	Systolic; radiation to the back; weak, delayed femoral pulses.
Left lower sternal border	
Still's murmur	**"Vibratory"** systolic ejection quality; no radiation; louder when the patient is supine; benign.
VSD	Holosystolic; harsh quality; often radiates all over the precordium; often louder as the defect gets smaller.
Hypertrophic obstructive cardiomyopathy	Systolic ejection quality; gets louder when the patient is upright; often radiates to the apex; may be heard in patients who have chest pain with activity.
Apex	
Mitral regurgitation	Holosystolic, decrescendo, **"cooing dove"** quality.

You are about to discharge a term well infant home after an uncomplicated two-day hospitalization. On your discharge exam, you notice that the baby's skin has a mottled appearance; she appears to be breathing quickly, and you are having difficulty feeling femoral pulses. You hear no murmur on exam. What is the most likely etiology of these findings? Concerned that this baby has a left-sided obstructive lesion known as hypoplastic left heart, you immediately call for the administration of prostaglandins.

PRESENTATIONS OF CONGENITAL HEART DISEASE IN INFANCY

Most common structural cardiac lesions become manifest in infancy. Their presentations can be broadly classified into three categories: shock, tachypnea, and cyanosis. Some lesions include elements from multiple categories. Understanding the pathophysiology of these lesions is key to understanding their presentations.

CARDIOLOGY

Shock

Cardiogenic shock is a condition in which the supply of O_2 is inadequate to satisfy the metabolic demands of the vital organs. In the setting of left-sided obstructive heart lesions, in which systemic blood flow traverses the ductus arteriosus, it often occurs at the time of its closure. This class of lesions represent an **early** cause of CHF (see Table 4-2).

Left-sided obstructive heart lesions may present with respiratory distress as a consequence of pulmonary edema from blood flow backing up into the lungs.

SYMPTOMS/EXAM

- Poor perfusion → pallor, metabolic acidosis, hypotension, and eventual obtundation.
- CXR reveals cardiomegaly.

DIFFERENTIAL

Shock results from lesions that → **left-sided obstruction to blood flow.** These include coarctation of the aorta, severe aortic stenosis, hypoplastic left heart, interrupted aortic arch, and total anomalous pulmonary venous return with obstruction.

TREATMENT

- **Use prostaglandins (PGE)!**
  - Keep the ductus arteriosus open and preserve systemic circulation.
  - In coarctation of the aorta, opening the duct also helps relieve the coarctation.
- **Keep pulmonary vascular resistance high:**
  - Minimize "steal" of systemic flow to pulmonary circulation.
  - **Avoid supplemental O_2** (acts as a pulmonary vasodilator).
  - Even $FiO_2 < 21\%$ may be tried.
  - Can hypoventilate; ↑ pCO_2 → acidosis → ↑ pulmonary vascular resistance.
- Consider inotropes to improve BP.

Tachypnea

Caused by heart lesions that significantly ↑ blood flow through the lungs, such as defects with left-to-right shunting or admixture (with free bidirectional shunting), which ↑ pulmonary flow. This → pulmonary venous congestion, which in turn → pulmonary edema and the observed tachypnea. Groups 1 and 2 in Figure 4-1 show lesions commonly associated with this finding.

TABLE 4-2. Typical Ages at Presentation of Lesions Leading to CHF

LESION	AGE AT PRESENTATION
Critical aortic stenosis/hypoplastic left heart syndrome	1–2 weeks
AV canal defect	1–2 months
VSD/PDA	6–8 weeks
ASD	Adult or never

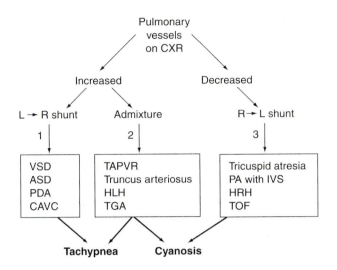

FIGURE 4-1. Classification system for congenital heart disease lesions based on CXR findings and associated symptomatology.

Lesions in group 1 present with tachypnea alone, group 2 with both tachypnea and cyanosis, and group 3 with cyanosis alone. CAVC = complete AV canal; TAPVR = total anomalous pulmonary venous return; HLH = hypoplastic left heart; TGA = transposition of the great arteries; PA with IVS = pulmonary atresia with intact ventricular septum; HRH = hypoplastic right heart; TOF = tetralogy of Fallot.

COMPLICATIONS

- Pulmonary vascular overcirculation can → CHF. This CHF occurs **late** in relation to the left-sided obstructive lesions (see Table 4-2).
- Long-term pulmonary overcirculation can → pulmonary hypertension and to reversal of the shunt → cyanosis. Referred to as **Eisenmenger syndrome.**

Cyanosis

Present when there is at least 5 g/dL of reduced hemoglobin. More readily apparent with higher hemoglobin, and most reliably detected in the mucous membranes, the tongue, and the lips. Cyanosis in CHF results from either pure right-to-left shunting or admixture lesions. Groups 2 and 3 in Figure 4-1 identify a number of cyanotic heart lesions.

DIFFERENTIAL

Acrocyanosis is a benign, self-limited condition that has a sudden onset and resolves without distress. It may be accompanied by cutis marmorata (a lacy, reddish, mottled appearance of the extremities) but is not associated with arterial desaturation.

TREATMENT

PGE may be used to preserve pulmonary blood flow by keeping the ductus arteriosus open.

COMPLICATIONS

- **Stroke:** Results from polycythemia that occurs as a reaction to the cyanosis. Exacerbated by **iron deficiency.** Microcytosis → poorly deformable cell membranes.

- **Cerebral abscess:** Right-to-left shunting gives microemboli direct access to the cerebral circulation.
- **Developmental delay and poor school performance:** Occurs more often in children with cyanosis than in those with acyanotic heart disease. May be related to the degree and duration of preoperative hypoxia or to the duration of intraoperative circulatory arrest.

Diagnostic Tools

- **Pre- and postductal O$_2$ saturations (see Figure 4-2):** The requirements for a difference in pre- and postductal saturations are as follows:
    - Right-to-left flow across the PDA caused by a R > L pressure difference.
    - Different aortic and pulmonary arterial saturations—e.g., **not** admixture lesions such as total anomalous pulmonary venous return, single ventricle.
- **Hyperoxia test:** Repeat ABG on 100% Fio$_2$. If Pao$_2$ > 100 mmHg or ↑ by > 30 mmHg, cardiac disease is less likely. Use Pao$_2$, not O$_2$ saturation, as the indicator.
- **ECG:** Provides information about rhythm and, grossly, ventricular size. Examine both the axis and the magnitude of the deflections. Remember that **right-axis deviation is normal for a neonate.**
- **CXR:** The appearance of the vasculature on CXR provides information about pulmonary blood flow and helps classify the lesion (see Figure 4-1). The classic radiographic descriptors of a number of congenital cardiac lesions are summarized in Table 4-3.
- **Echocardiogram:** The **gold standard** of diagnosis, as well as a noninvasive means of assessing the cardiac anatomy, pressure gradients across any stenotic valves, and the overall function of the heart.
- **MRI:** An increasing number of centers are using MRI as an alternative to echocardiography to image the cardiac anatomy with high resolution.

SPECIFIC LESIONS IN CONGENITAL HEART DISEASE

The specific defects that comprise congenital heart disease may be broadly classified into three categories:

- Those that → some degree of **cyanosis**, including **right-to-left shunting lesions** and **admixture defects.**
- **Left-to-right shunting lesions** → pulmonary overcirculation and tachypnea.
- **Left-sided obstructive lesions**, which may → **hypotension and/or cyanosis** due to pulmonary edema.

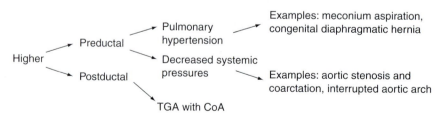

FIGURE 4-2. Classification scheme for cardiac lesions based on a comparison of pre- and postductal saturations.

TABLE 4-3. Radiographic Appearances of Common Congenital Heart Lesions

LESION	APPEARANCE
Tetralogy of Fallot	Boot-shaped heart.
Transposition of the great arteries	"Egg on a string."
Coarctation of the aorta	"3" sign.
Total anomalous pulmonary venous return	"Snowman" sign.

Heart Defects Leading to Cyanosis

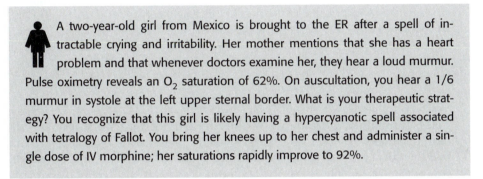

A two-year-old girl from Mexico is brought to the ER after a spell of intractable crying and irritability. Her mother mentions that she has a heart problem and that whenever doctors examine her, they hear a loud murmur. Pulse oximetry reveals an O_2 saturation of 62%. On auscultation, you hear a 1/6 murmur in systole at the left upper sternal border. What is your therapeutic strategy? You recognize that this girl is likely having a hypercyanotic spell associated with tetralogy of Fallot. You bring her knees up to her chest and administer a single dose of IV morphine; her saturations rapidly improve to 92%.

RIGHT-TO-LEFT SHUNTING LESIONS

- **Tetralogy of Fallot:**
  - Includes VSD, pulmonary stenosis, overriding aorta, and RVH (see Figure 4-3).
  - **Sx/Exam:** Blood flow through a stenotic pulmonary valve produces a loud pulmonary stenosis murmur; a VSD (holosystolic) murmur may also be heard. A variable degree of cyanosis is present depending on the amount of right-to-left shunting.
  - **Tx/Complications:** Surgical repair often involves placement of a transannular patch across the pulmonary valve → valvular incompetence and right heart dilation.
- **Tricuspid atresia/hypoplastic right heart:** Complete or partial agenesis of the right ventricular cavity, in which the left ventricle provides pulmonary blood flow through the ductus arteriosus.
- **Pulmonary atresia with intact ventricular septum:** Pulmonary blood flow is provided by the left ventricle via the ductus. Coronary sinusoids decompress a hypertensive right ventricle. On exam, S2 is single, and there is no murmur.

ADMIXTURE LESIONS

- **Transposition of the great arteries:** The systemic and pulmonary circulations operate in parallel, as the left ventricle is connected to the pulmonary artery and the right ventricle is attached to the aorta (see Figure 4-4). Examination reveals a single S2 and no murmur.

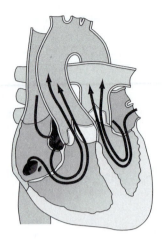

FIGURE 4-3. Tetralogy of Fallot.

Four anatomical findings comprise the tetralogy of Fallot: pulmonary stenosis, a VSD, RVH, and an overriding aorta. The circulatory flow patterns created by this constellation of features are indicated by the heavy black arrows. (Reproduced, with permission, from Kasper DL et al. *Harrison's Principles of Internal Medicine*, 16th ed. New York: McGraw-Hill, 2005:1388.)

- **Total anomalous pulmonary venous return without obstruction:** Pulmonary venous return is to the right atrium, and an ASD must be present to allow for left atrial filling (see Figure 4-5). Volume loading of the right ventricle → a widely fixed, split S2 and ↑ precordial activity. Atrial septostomy may be performed to decompress the right atrium if a restrictive ASD is present.
- **Truncus arteriosus:** A single arterial trunk arises from the ventricles and divides into the aorta and pulmonary arteries. The condition → CHF. Presents with systolic murmur from VSD (always present) located under the

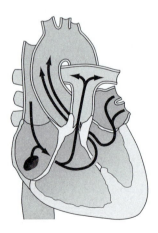

FIGURE 4-4. Transposition of the great arteries.

In this condition, the systemic and pulmonary circulations operate in a parallel fashion. Not shown is the obligatory mixing required for survival occurring at an ASD, VSD, or PDA. (Reproduced, with permission, from Kasper DL et al. *Harrison's Principles of Internal Medicine*, 16th ed. New York: McGraw-Hill, 2005:1388.)

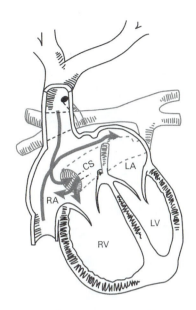

FIGURE 4-5. **Total anomalous pulmonary venous return.**

In this condition, left-sided (oxygenated) blood is returned to the right-sided circulation, creating a mixing lesion that requires an ASD to allow for left atrial filling. In this figure, the pulmonary venous return is to the right atrium by way of the coronary sinus. (Reproduced, with permission, from Fuster V et al. *Hurst's the Heart*, 11th ed. New York: McGraw-Hill, 2004, Fig. 73-34 B.)

truncal valve, as well as with wide pulse pressure from systemic diastolic runoff into the pulmonary circulation.

- **Double-outlet right ventricle:** Both great arteries arise from the right ventricle. Pulmonary overcirculation results unless significant pulmonary stenosis is present.
- **Hypoplastic left heart:** See the discussion below on left-sided obstructive lesions.

Left-to-Right Shunting Lesions

VENTRICULAR SEPTAL DEFECT (VSD)

- Figure 4-6 illustrates the mechanism of a VSD.
- **Sx/Exam:**
  - Presents with tachypnea and sweating with feedings; poor weight gain beginning at 2–3 months of age; and hepatomegaly.
  - 1° murmur is holosystolic. A diastolic rumble may also be heard from ↑ flow across the mitral valve.
- **Tx:**
  - **Medical:** Diuretics +/− digoxin.
  - **Surgical:** Surgery is indicated if significant pulmonary overcirculation results or if growth failure is present despite medical management.

A hypercyanotic (or Tet) spell is characterized by a sudden marked ↑ in right-to-left flow that is associated with deep cyanosis and lessening of the pulmonary stenosis murmur. Treatment is based on ↓ pulmonary vascular resistance and ↑ systemic vascular resistance (e.g., calm the patient; perform knee-to-chest maneuvers; administer morphine, O_2 and fluid bolus; consider phenylephrine).

A fixed, split S2 is associated with any cardiac defect that → ↑ pulmonary blood flow.

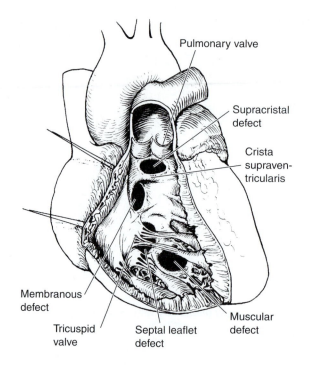

FIGURE 4-6. Ventricular septal defect.

A VSD results in a left-to-right shunt that may occur anatomically at any of a number of distinct sites. (Reproduced, with permission, from Doherty GM, Way LW [eds]. *Current Surgical Diagnosis & Treatment,* 12th ed. New York: McGraw-Hill, 2006, Fig 19-29.)

ATRIAL SEPTAL DEFECT (ASD)

▪ A **fixed, split S2** is the **hallmark finding.**
▪ An ejection murmur may also be heard at the left upper sternal border from ↑ pulmonary flow.
▪ A diastolic rumble of relative tricuspid stenosis may be heard as well.

PATENT DUCTUS ARTERIOSUS (PDA)

▪ Persistence of the PDA beyond approximately one week of life is considered abnormal.
▪ **Sx/Exam:** Presents with bounding pulses from the aorta → pulmonary artery diastolic runoff, continuous machinery murmur, and a hyperdynamic precordium.
▪ **Tx:**
  ▪ In the premature infant, try indomethacin.
  ▪ If the PDA persists, surgical closure in the OR or device closure in the catheterization laboratory is indicated.
▪ **Complications:** Respiratory distress; left ventricular dysfunction from ↓ coronary perfusion or volume overload.

Atrioventricular Canal Defect

- Incorporates both an ASD and a VSD, and may have abnormalities of the AV valves. Also called *endocardial cushion defect.*
- **Exam/Tx:** Similar to that of a VSD. Commonly associated with trisomy 21.

Left-Sided Obstructive Lesions

Inflow Obstruction

Total anomalous pulmonary venous return with obstruction presents as follows:

- Pulmonary venous return is anomalous to the right heart, as above, but is also **obstructed,** → dramatically ↑ pulmonary vascular resistance and marked pulmonary edema.
- Emergent surgery must be performed to relieve the obstruction.

Outflow Obstruction

- **Aortic stenosis:** Presents with an ejection click and a murmur at the right upper sternal border, together with a palpable thrill in the suprasternal notch.
- **Coarctation of the aorta:** Presents with weak or absent lower extremity pulses and upper > lower BP. If the PDA is open, ↓ postductal saturation may be seen from right-to-left ductal flow.
- **Interrupted aortic arch:** The presentation is the same as that of coarctation, but lower extremity circulation is entirely duct dependent and is right to left.
- **Hypoplastic left heart:** In this condition, the right ventricle serves as the single ventricle for both pulmonary and systemic blood flow. The latter flows right to left across the ductus arteriosus. On exam, no murmur is heard. Presents with a loud, single S2 and a hyperactive precordium. Desaturation is seen but with minimal cyanosis unless restrictive ASD → pulmonary edema. Treatment is a surgical repair with three stages:
  - **Norwood procedure:** Division of the main pulmonary artery and anastomosis of the proximal portion to the ascending aorta; atrial septectomy; and modified Blalock-Taussig shunt (conduit between the subclavian artery and pulmonary artery). The right ventricle provides both systemic and pulmonary blood flow.
  - **Bidirectional Glenn procedure:** Takedown of the Blalock-Taussig shunt followed by SVC → pulmonary artery anastomosis; pulmonary blood flow comes only from the SVC. IVC (deoxygenated) blood mixes with pulmonary venous return in the atria.
  - **Fontan procedure:** Inclusion of the IVC to the above anastomosis; the entire venous return then flows passively through the lungs, and mixing of saturated/desaturated blood is eliminated.

A two-month-old girl presents for well-child care. Her mother tells you that she tires easily and sweats profusely during feeds. On exam, you note that the child has not gained any weight since she was one month old and that she is tachypneic with subcostal retractions. She has a 3/6 holosystolic murmur at the left lower sternal border that radiates all over the precordium as well as a diastolic rumble. The liver edge is palpable 4 cm below the right costal margin. You make the diagnosis of a VSD with CHF. Why is she presenting with symptoms now? The pulmonary vascular resistance starts to fall at the time of birth but typically does not become low enough to → symptoms of CHF from excessive pulmonary blood flow until 6–8 weeks of age.

CONGESTIVE HEART FAILURE (CHF)

SYMPTOMS/EXAM

The symptoms of CHF in infants and children are often **nonspecific**, ranging from poor feeding and excessive sweating to abdominal pain and cough. Cardiomegaly with ↑ pulmonary vascular markings on CXR is nearly a prerequisite. Table 4-4 summarizes common signs and symptoms along with most likely diagnoses by age group.

DIAGNOSIS/TREATMENT

- Diagnose and treat the underlying cause (e.g., surgical VSD closure).
- O_2 for patients with respiratory distress.
- Treat exacerbating factors (e.g., fever, anemia, infection, arrhythmia, hypertension).
- **Diuretics** are first-line medication for patients with pulmonary congestion.
- Digoxin for stable outpatients; inotropic agents for severe CHF (e.g., dopamine, epinephrine, milrinone, dobutamine).
- Afterload reduction (e.g., hydralazine, ACEIs, nitroglycerin).

TABLE 4-4. **Presentation and Differential Diagnosis of CHF by Age**

AGE	PRESENTATION	DIFFERENTIAL DIAGNOSIS
First month	Tachycardia, tachypnea, hepatomegaly.	Hypoplastic left heart syndrome, transposition of the great arteries, total anomalous pulmonary venous return, systemic AV fistula, critical aortic/pulmonary stenosis, coarctation of the aorta.
Four weeks to four months	Poor feeding, tachypnea, failure to thrive, sweating, hepatomegaly.	Large left-to-right shunts (VSD, PDA, atrioventricular canal), SVT.
Children	Abdominal pain +/− vomiting, cough, wheezing, and shortness of breath, especially with exertion. Orthopnea, easy fatigability, puffy eyelids, swollen feet, tachycardia, gallop rhythm.	Viral myocarditis, acute rheumatic fever, dilated cardiomyopathy.

Kawasaki Disease

A multisystem vasculitis with multiple manifestations. Occurs primarily in young children (80% of patients are < 4 years of age and 50% < 2 years of age). Refer to the Rheumatology section for diagnostic criteria and other associated findings.

SYMPTOMS/EXAM

Cardiac manifestations are as follows:

- Pericardial effusion and pericarditis.
- Myocarditis and endocarditis usually resolve when the fever resolves.
- **Coronary artery aneurysms:**
  - Seen by echocardiogram in 20–25% of patients who do not receive treatment within 10 days of onset of fever.
  - The risk of coronary aneurysms is higher in males, infants < 12 months of age, children > 8 years of age, patients whose fever lasts > 10 days, anemic patients (hemoglobin < 10 g/dL), and those with thrombocytopenia and persistent fever following treatment.
  - Aneurysms typically occur 1–4 weeks after the onset of illness and rarely occur > 6 weeks after onset.
  - Coronary artery dimensions often return to baseline within 6–8 weeks of disease onset. Roughly half of nongiant aneurysms regress to normal size within 1–2 years.
  - Giant coronary aneurysms (≥ 8 mm) are likely to be associated with long-term complications.
  - Coronary artery stenosis can occur as a late complication as aneurysms regress.

TREATMENT

- Includes **IVIG** and high-dose **aspirin** in the acute phase followed by low-dose aspirin after resolution of fever for at least 6–8 weeks or until coronary ectasia resolves (whichever is later).
- **Serial echocardiograms** at the time of diagnosis and at 6–8 weeks and 6–12 months after diagnosis. Echocardiograms should be done at shorter intervals in the presence of coronary abnormalities, left ventricular dysfunction, or valvar regurgitation.

COMPLICATIONS

- The U.S. case fatality rate is < 0.01%.
- Large coronary aneurysms rarely rupture.
- Most fatalities occur within six weeks of symptom onset.

The principal cause of death in Kawasaki disease is MI from coronary occlusion resulting from thrombosis or progressive stenosis.

Acute Rheumatic Fever

Uncommon in the United States; thought to be a late sequela of group A streptococcal infection of the **throat** (but not of the skin).

SYMPTOMS/EXAM

Criteria for the diagnosis of acute rheumatic fever are as follows (see the mnemonic **JONES PEACE**):

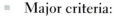

Jones criteria for acute rheumatic fever—J❤NES PEACE

Major criteria:
Joints
❤ Pancarditis
Nodules
Erythema marginatum
Sydenham chorea
Minor criteria:
PR interval prolonged
ESR ↑
Arthralgias
CRP ↑
Elevated temperature (fever)

Acute rheumatic fever most commonly affects the mitral valve, followed by the aortic valve.

All patients with cardiomyopathy may become candidates for heart transplantation when medical management fails.

- **Major criteria:**
  - Joints: Migratory arthritis, usually of the large joints.
  - ❤ pancarditis:
    - Tachycardia out of proportion to the amount of fever is a sign of myocarditis.
    - New-onset murmur (of mitral or aortic insufficiency) is a sign of valvulitis. The mitral valve is most commonly affected, followed by the aortic valve.
    - Friction rub and pericardial effusion are signs of pericarditis.
    - Other exam findings include chest pain, gallop rhythm, and distant heart sounds.
  - Subcutaneous **N**odules: Hard, painless, mobile nodules usually found symmetrically over the extensor surfaces.
  - Erythema marginatum: A nonpruritic, evanescent, serpiginous or annular rash found primarily on the trunk (**never** on the face).
  - Sydenham chorea: More common in girls; begins with emotional lability and personality changes that are later replaced by the characteristic spontaneous, purposeless movements.
- **Minor criteria:**
  - PR interval prolonged.
  - ESR ↑.
  - Arthralgias rather than arthritis (no swelling, warmth, or redness).
  - CRP ↑.
  - Elevated temperature (fever ≥ 39°C).

DIAGNOSIS

Evidence of recent streptococcal disease (scarlet fever, ⊕ culture or ASO titer) *and* two major or one major and two minor criteria.

TREATMENT

- **Benzathine penicillin G IM** to eradicate streptococci.
- Anti-inflammatory therapy with salicylates and/or steroids depending on the severity of joint and cardiac involvement. Salicylates usually have a dramatic effect on the arthritis.
- Treat CHF.
- Treat chorea by ↓ physical and emotional stress. Medications used include phenobarbital, haloperidol, valproic acid, and diazepam.

PREVENTION

- **1° prevention:** Treat streptococcal pharyngitis with an appropriate antibiotic course.
- **2° prevention:** Treat patients with a history of rheumatic fever with prophylactic antibiotics (benzathine penicillin G IM vs. oral penicillin V).

Cardiomyopathy

A 1° disease of the heart muscle → impaired function. The three general types are dilated, hypertrophic, and restrictive; each has distinct anatomic and functional features (see Table 4-5).

TABLE 4-5. Dilated, Hypertrophic, and Restrictive Cardiomyopathies

FEATURES	DILATED	HYPERTROPHIC	RESTRICTIVE
Pathophysiology	Extensive areas of degeneration and necrosis → dilation of the chambers and weakened systolic contractile function; can have thrombus formation in the ventricles.	Asymmetric septal hypertrophy → dynamic intracavitary obstruction during systole and abnormal stiffness of the left ventricle during diastole.	The least common of the three types. Excessively stiff ventricles → abnormal diastolic filling and atrial enlargement with preserved systolic function.
History and physical exam	Signs and symptoms of CHF; displaced PMI; S3 gallop; mitral regurgitation murmur.	⊕ family history in 30–60% of cases; left ventricular lift; possible late systolic ejection murmur at the apex.	Exercise intolerance; gallop rhythm; mitral regurgitation murmur.
Diagnostic studies	**ECG:** LVH; ST-T changes. **Echo:** Left and right ventricular dilation; ↓ ejection fraction.	**ECG:** LVH; deep Q waves. **Echo:** Usually diagnostic, showing septal hypertrophy.	**ECG:** Biatrial enlargement. **Echo:** Biatrial enlargement; normal left ventricle size and ejection fraction.
Natural history	Progressive deterioration; death from CHF, sudden arrhythmia, or massive embolization of thrombus.	Associated with a 4–6% incidence of sudden death per year; dilated cardiomyopathy may develop later.	Poor prognosis, with a 45–50% two-year survival from diagnosis.
Treatment	Treatment of CHF (diuretics, ACEIs, β-blockers); anticoagulation; antiarrhythmic medications +/– an implantable cardiac defibrillator (ICD).	Activity restriction; β-blockers or calcium channel blockers to improve diastolic filling; antiarrhythmic medications +/– an ICD.	Diuretics; anticoagulation.

Myocarditis

An inflammatory disorder of the myocardium with necrosis of the myocytes and associated inflammatory infiltrate. Viruses, particularly **adenovirus and enterovirus** (e.g., coxsackievirus) infections, are the most common causes in North America. Many other viruses can → myocarditis, including CMV, echovirus, EBV, HIV, varicella, and influenza. Immune-mediated diseases such as the collagen vascular diseases, acute rheumatic fever, and Kawasaki disease can also → myocarditis.

SYMPTOMS/EXAM

- In severe cases, patients often present with acute signs and symptoms of heart failure (e.g., tachycardia, S3 gallop, diminished heart sounds, hepatomegaly).

Endomyocardial biopsy is the gold standard for diagnosis and classification of myocarditis.

- Infants and young children may present with a chief complaint of anorexia, vomiting, and lethargy.
- Chest pain may be the initial presentation for older children, adolescents, and adults.

DIAGNOSIS

- Cardiomegaly may be present on CXR.
- Echocardiogram may show left ventricular dysfunction and chamber enlargement.

TREATMENT

- Bed rest is recommended during the acute phase of the illness.
- Symptoms of heart failure should be treated with diuretics, afterload reduction, and inotropic agents.
- Treatment with immunosuppressive and immunomodulatory agents (e.g., IVIG, prednisone, azathioprine, cyclosporine) is still controversial.

COMPLICATIONS

Most patients will recover completely, but some will develop a dilated cardiomyopathy.

Pericarditis

Causes of pericarditis—CARDIAC RIND

Collagen vascular disease
Aortic aneurysm
Radiation
Drugs (e.g.,hydralazine)
Infections
Acute renal failure
Cardiac infarction
Rheumatic fever
Injury
Neoplasms
Dressler syndrome

Many of the same viruses that → myocarditis can also → pericarditis. Bacteria (purulent pericarditis), *Mycobacterium tuberculosis*, rheumatic fever, Kawasaki disease, uremia, and the collagen vascular diseases are other etiologies (see the mnemonic **CARDIAC RIND**). Inflammation of the pericardium → a pericardial effusion and thickening of the pericardial membranes.

SYMPTOMS/EXAM

- Fever and chest pain are the most common presenting complaints. **The chest pain is usually dull and may be positional with relief when leaning forward.**
- Pericardial friction rub is almost always present.
- If a pericardial effusion accumulates, there may be signs of cardiac tamponade (e.g., distant heart sounds, tachycardia, pulsus paradoxus).

Pulsus paradoxus is pathognomonic for pericardial tamponade. Pulsus paradoxus is present when there is more than a 12-mmHg difference between the pressure at which the first Korotkoff sound is heard during expiration and when it is heard during inspiration.

DIAGNOSIS

- **ECG: Low-voltage QRS complexes and ST-segment elevation** (see Figure 4-7) **followed by T-wave inversion are the characteristic findings.**
- **CXR:** Water bottle–shaped heart is characteristic of a large effusion.
- **Echocardiogram:** Diagnostic for pericardial effusion and can be helpful in evaluating for cardiac tamponade.

TREATMENT

- Pericardiocentesis is diagnostic and therapeutic.
- Aspirin and corticosteroids are often used for their anti-inflammatory effects in nonpurulent pericarditis.
- Specific treatment of any underlying etiology that is identified should also be undertaken.

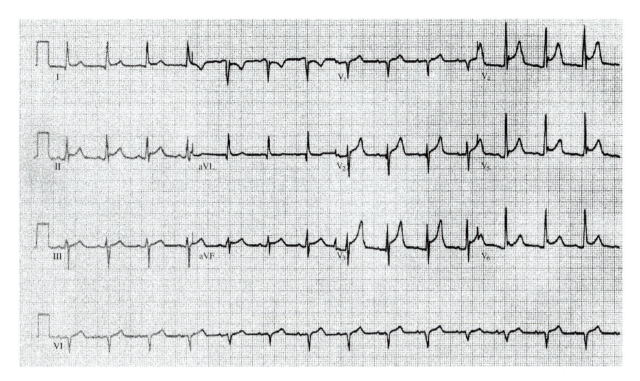

FIGURE 4-7. ECG in early pericarditis showing ST-segment elevation and upright T waves.

(Reproduced, with permission, from Crawford MH. *Current Diagnosis & Treatment in Cardiology*, 2nd ed. New York: McGraw-Hill, 2003, Fig. 17-1.)

Infective Endocarditis

Two factors are important in the pathogenesis of infective endocarditis: (1) the presence of a structural abnormality of the heart → turbulent blood flow with a pressure gradient; and (2) bacteremia.

SYMPTOMS/EXAM

- Insidious onset with fever, malaise, and pallor is common.
- **New-onset murmur** is universal.
- Splenomegaly is common.
- Skin manifestations include petechiae, Osler's nodes (tender red nodes on the ends of fingers), Janeway lesions (painless hemorrhagic areas on the palms or soles), and splinter hemorrhages under the nails.
- Evidence of emboli to other organs is common—e.g., pulmonary emboli, seizures, hemiparesis, hematuria, Roth's spots (retinal hemorrhages).
- Carious teeth or periodontal or gingival disease is frequently present.

Viridans streptococci, enterococci, and S. aureus *are responsible for > 90% of cases of infective endocarditis.*

DIAGNOSIS

- Labs and studies include the following:
  - Serial blood cultures (at least two sets 12 hours apart).
  - **CBC:** Often shows anemia and leukocytosis with left shift.

CARDIOLOGY

- **ESR:** Almost always ↑ unless the patient is polycythemic.
- **UA:** Detects hematuria in 30% of patients.
- **Echocardiogram:** May demonstrate vegetations, although a ⊖ echo does not rule out the diagnosis.
- **Duke criteria:** Two major, one major and three minor, or five minor criteria are needed for diagnosis.
  - **Major criteria:**
    - ⊕ blood cultures (two separate cultures 12 hours apart).
    - An oscillating mass depicted on echocardiogram.
    - A periannular abscess depicted on echocardiogram.
    - Partial dehiscence of a prosthetic valve.
    - A new valvular regurgitant jet depicted on echocardiogram.
  - **Minor criteria:**
    - A history of IV drug use.
    - A history of congenital heart disease.
    - Fever > 38.4°C.
    - Arterial emboli.
    - Intracranial hemorrhage.
    - Conjunctival hemorrhage.
    - Janeway lesions.
    - Glomerulonephritis.
    - Osler's nodes.
    - Roth's spots.
    - ⊕ RF.
    - ⊕ blood cultures but not meeting the above criteria.

A ⊖ echo does not rule out endocarditis.

TREATMENT

- Administer a prolonged course of parenteral antibiotics (usually 4–6 weeks) to eradicate bacteria from the vegetations.
- Absolute indications for surgery include cardiac failure, valve obstruction, definitive perivalvular abscess, noncandidal fungal infection, and pseudomonal infection.

Maintenance of good oral hygiene is more important than antibiotic prophylaxis in the prevention of infective endocarditis.

PREVENTION

Antibiotic prophylaxis is recommended for patients with most kinds of congenital heart disease for any potentially bacteremia-causing procedure. The American Heart Association publishes recommendations that vary depending on the type of procedure that is anticipated (see Tables 4-6 and 4-7).

ARRHYTHMIAS

As in adults, pediatric patients may also present with abnormal heart rhythms, though much less frequently. Such disturbances are much more common in children who have had surgery for congenital heart disease. Arrhythmias may be broadly subclassified as tachycardias (too fast), bradycardias (too slow), and other abnormal rhythms.

TABLE 4-6. Cardiac Conditions and Prophylaxis Recommendations

RISK CATEGORY	CONDITION	DENTAL, ORAL, RESPIRATORY, AND ESOPHAGEAL PROCEDURES	GI AND GU PROCEDURES
High risk	Prosthetic cardiac valves, previous endocarditis, complex cyanotic congenital heart disease, surgically constructed systemic-pulmonary shunts or conduits.	Amoxicillin PO or ampicillin IV/IM. **Penicillin allergic:** Clindamycin PO/IV or cephalexin PO or cefazolin IV/IM or azithromycin PO.	Ampicillin q 6 h × 2 doses + gentamicin × 1 dose. **Penicillin allergic:** Vancomycin + gentamicin × 1 dose each.
Moderate risk	Congenital heart disease is not listed as high or as a negligible risk. Includes acquired valvular dysfunction, hypertrophic cardiomyopathy, and mitral valve prolapse with mitral regurgitation.	Amoxicillin PO one hour before or ampicillin IV/IM within 30 minutes of the procedure. **Penicillin allergic:** Clindamycin PO/IV or cephalexin PO or cefazolin IV/IM or azithromycin PO.	Amoxicillin PO or ampicillin IV/IM × 1 dose. **Penicillin allergic:** Vancomycin IV × 1 dose.
Negligible risk	Isolated secundum ASD; surgical repair of ASD, VSD, or PDA (without residua beyond six months); mitral valve prolapse without mitral regurgitation; innocent heart murmur; previous Kawasaki disease; pacemaker implant.	Prophylaxis not recommended.	Prophylaxis not recommended.

Tachycardia

A seven-year-old boy is brought into the ER complaining of "a funny feeling in his chest" and some difficulty catching his breath. The EMTs report that his heart rate on the monitor is 240 and that the QRS is narrow without obvious P waves. He has strong and symmetric pulses and a BP of 105/65. Two IV lines have been placed in the field. What is your immediate course of action? Realizing that he is in SVT, you administer adenosine 0.1 mg/kg × 1 by rapid push with a saline flush. His rhythm normalizes immediately to sinus at a rate of 120.

SUPRAVENTRICULAR TACHYCARDIA (SVT)

SVT is a term used for a class of narrow-complex tachycardias that are not primarily ventricular in origin. These rhythms may be broadly subclassified as ei-

TABLE 4-7. Recommendations for Endocarditis Prophylaxis by Procedure

PROCEDURE TYPE	RECOMMENDED	RECOMMENDED FOR HIGH RISK, OPTIONAL FOR MODERATE RISK	OPTIONAL FOR HIGH RISK	NOT RECOMMENDED
Dental	Extractions, periodontal implants, endodontic procedures.			
Respiratory	Tonsillectomy; procedures involving respiratory mucosa; rigid bronchoscopy.			Endotracheal intubation; flexible bronchoscopy; tympanostomy tube insertion.
GI		Sclerotherapy; esophageal stricture dilation; endoscopic retrograde cholangiography; biliary tract surgery; procedures involving intestinal mucosa.	Transesophageal echocardiography; endoscopy +/− biopsy.	
GU	Prostatic surgery; cystoscopy; urethral dilation.		Vaginal hysterectomy; vaginal delivery.	Cesarean section.
Other				Urethral catheterization; cardiac catheterization; pacemaker implantation; circumcision.

ther **reentrant** or **automatic.** Reentrant SVT includes **AV nodal reentrant tachycardia** (AVNRT), in which the accessory pathway is within the AV node, and **AV reentrant tachycardia** (AVRT), in which the pathway lies outside of the node. Automatic SVT usually involves an ectopic atrial focus that overtakes the sinoatrial node as the heart's intrinsic pacemaker.

- Reentrant SVT:
    - **Dx:** ECG shows narrow-complex tachycardia with an HR of 220–270. In **AVNRT,** P waves are usually hidden within the QRS complex. In **AVRT,** P waves usually follow the QRS complex and fall within the ST segments.
    - **Tx:** If the patient is hemodynamically unstable, treat with immediate cardioversion. Otherwise, attempt to block the reentrant circuit at the AV node. **Vagal maneuvers** include application of an ice bag to the face and Valsalva; **pharmacologic** treatment includes adenosine (→ transient complete AV block; very safe, but should be done with DC cardioversion if available).

An example of an AVRT is Wolff-Parkinson-White syndrome (see Figure 4-8), which is characterized by the presence of an accessory pathway that creates a delta wave with a short PR on ECG.

CARDIOLOGY

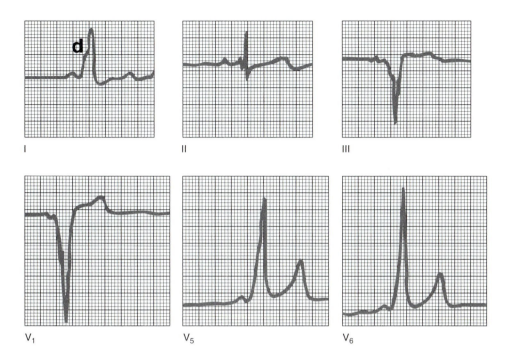

FIGURE 4-8. Examples of ECG tracings in the frontal and precordial leads in a patient with Wolff-Parkinson-White syndrome.

Note the presence of the delta wave (the slurred upstroke of the QRS indicated by the letter *d*) and the short PR interval. (Reproduced, with permission, from Kasper DL et al. *Harrison's Principles of Internal Medicine*, 16th ed. New York: McGraw-Hill, 2005:1350.)

- **Long-term management:** Often involves identification and ablation of the accessory pathway in the electrophysiology laboratory. Alternatively, AVNRT may be managed medically with digoxin, β-blockers, or verapamil **(not in infants)**.
- **Automatic SVT:** Includes ectopic atrial tachycardia. On ECG, the P-wave axis is often abnormal. In contrast with reentrant SVT, heart rate changes are gradual rather than sudden. Treatment may be pharmacologic (β-blockers, class IC or III agents) or electrophysiologic (e.g., radiofrequency ablation of the ectopic focus).

ATRIAL FIBRILLATION

- An irregularly irregular rhythm that is common among the elderly; in pediatrics, it is almost always associated with structural heart disease.
- **Dx:** On ECG, QRS is narrow complex, no P waves are identifiable, and the baseline is wavering (see Figure 4-9A).
- **Tx:**
  - Acute cardioversion may be electrical (DC cardioversion) or pharmacologic (class I and III agents).
  - Long-term control of ventricular rate with digoxin.

Avoid the use of calcium channel blockers in infants in light of the risks of bradycardia and depressed cardiac function.

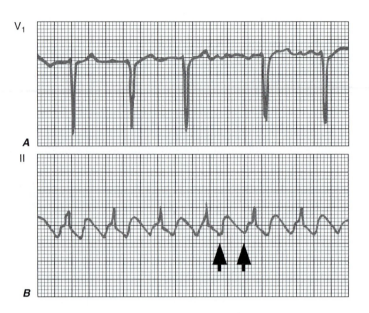

FIGURE 4-9. **Atrial fibrillation and atrial flutter.**

The top tracing (A) shows the wavering baseline that is characteristic of atrial fibrillation, with variable ventricular response. The bottom tracing (B) shows the sawtooth pattern of atrial flutter with 2:1 AV block. (Reproduced, with permission, from Kasper DL et al. *Harrison's Principles of Internal Medicine*, 16th ed. New York: McGraw-Hill, 2005:1345.)

ATRIAL FLUTTER

- An intra-atrial reentrant circuit in which the atrial rate is fixed but the ventricular rate is variable depending on the degree of AV block.
- **Dx:** Sawtooth P waves are seen on ECG (see Figure 4-9B).
- **Tx:** Pharmacologic therapy is similar to that for atrial fibrillation; in addition, radiofrequency ablation may be used to disrupt the flutter pathway in the electrophysiology laboratory.

VENTRICULAR TACHYCARDIA

Always assume that a wide-complex tachycardia is ventricular tachycardia until proven otherwise!

- A reentrant arrhythmia in which the circuit pathway is confined to the ventricular myocardium. Ventricular tachycardia is surprisingly well tolerated in children, especially infants, and can represent a stable hemodynamic rhythm.
- **Dx:** ECG reveals wide-complex tachycardia that may be monomorphic (a single QRS shape) or polymorphic (varying QRS shapes) (see Figure 4-10B).
- **Tx:**
  - **Acute:** Treat in accordance with the Pediatric Advanced Life Support (PALS) protocol.
    - If unstable, immediate DC cardioversion.
    - Pharmacologic conversion with lidocaine, procainamide, or amiodarone.
  - **Chronic:** β-blockers or class I or III antiarrhythmics, or placement of an automatic implantable cardiac defibrillator (AICD).

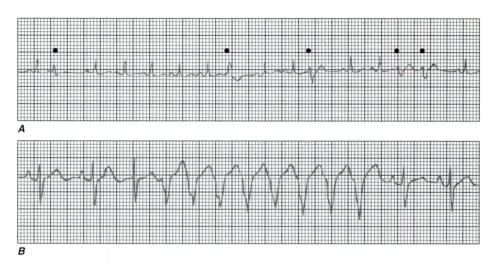

A

B

FIGURE 4-10. Ventricular premature beats and ventricular tachycardia.

In the top tracing (A), the solid black dots indicate the premature QRS complexes known as ventricular premature beats. Note their wide nature and changing morphology. The bottom tracing (B) shows a run of ventricular tachycardia followed by two beats of normal sinus rhythm. (Reproduced, with permission, from Kasper DL et al. *Harrison's Principles of Internal Medicine*, 16th ed. New York: McGraw-Hill, 2005:1343.)

Bradycardia

ATRIOVENTRICULAR (AV) BLOCK

- **First degree:** Long PR interval of fixed duration; every P wave is followed by a QRS.
- **Second degree:**
  - **Mobitz I (Wenckebach):** Characterized by a gradual ↑ in PR interval (see Figure 4-11) until eventual block of the atrial impulse. This is a benign condition that can be seen in healthy adolescents and athletes.
  - **Mobitz II:** Rare; AV block is occasional and unpredictable. Can progress to third-degree block.
- **Third degree:** Complete heart block in which the atria and ventricles operate independently (see Figure 4-12).
- **Treatment:** Placement of an artificial pacemaker.

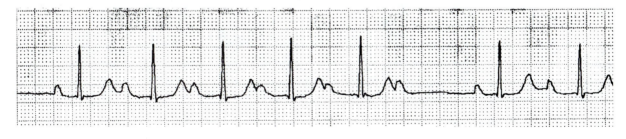

FIGURE 4-11. Mobitz I second-degree heart block.

Note the progressive widening of the PR interval characteristic of Wenckebach periodicity. (Reproduced, with permission, from Fuster V et al. *Hurst's the Heart*, 11th ed. New York: McGraw-Hill, 2004, Fig. 32-6.)

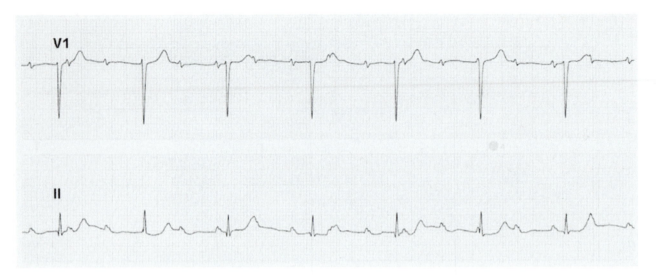

FIGURE 4-12. Third-degree AV block.

The atrial P wave and ventricular QRS complexes march out at a rate completely independent of one another. (Reproduced, with permission, from Fuster V et al. *Hurst's the Heart*, 11th ed. New York: McGraw-Hill, 2004, Fig. 32-9.)

SICK SINUS SYNDROME

1° dysfunction of the sinoatrial node that is usually found in combination with heterotaxy syndromes.

Other Abnormal Rhythms

ATRIAL PREMATURE BEAT

Atrial premature beats are a common "cause of pauses."

- Also known as premature atrial contraction.
- **Dx:** Depending on the degree of prematurity of the early atrial beat, conduction may **block** (presenting as a pause in an otherwise normal rhythm), **proceed aberrantly** (→ a wide-complex QRS), or **proceed normally** (→ a narrow-complex QRS) (see Figure 4-13).

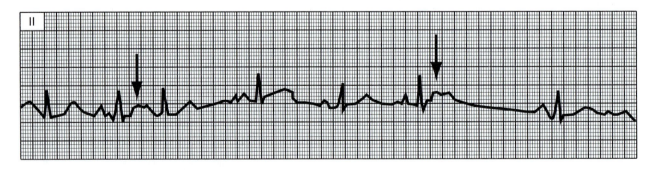

FIGURE 4-13. Atrial premature beat.

The solid arrows highlight the atrial premature beats in this strip. The first P wave is conducted with a narrow-complex QRS; the second is blocked and leads to an incomplete compensatory pause. (Reproduced, with permission, from Goldschlager N, Goldman MJ. *Principles of Clinical Electrocardiography*, 13th ed. Appleton & Lange, 1989. Copyright © 2006 The McGraw-Hill Companies, Inc.)

VENTRICULAR PREMATURE BEAT

- Also called premature ventricular contraction.
- **Dx:** Bizarre, wide-complex QRS complexes on ECG associated with pause in rhythm (see Figure 4-10A).
- **Complications:** Rare; generally a benign condition.

LONG QT SYNDROME

- A familial condition with both autosomal-dominant and autosomal-recessive forms (referred to as Romano-Ward syndrome and Jervell and Lange-Nielsen syndrome, respectively). The latter form is associated with deafness.
- Other causes include medication use and electrolyte abnormalities.
- **Dx:** $QT/\sqrt{RR} > 0.46$ (upper limit of normal—440 msec).
- **Complications:** Conversion of the rhythm into torsades de pointes, a polymorphic ventricular tachycardia that is associated with sudden death.

TREATMENT

- **Pharmacologic:** β-blockers.
- **Interventional:** Placement of a pacemaker or an ICD prevents bradycardia associated with conversion to torsades and provides shock to convert to normal sinus rhythm if necessary.

CHEST PAIN

A common complaint in children and adolescents. The etiology is **benign in most cases.** A pulmonary cause of chest pain (e.g., pneumonia, asthma) is more common in younger children, while psychogenic causes are more likely in adolescents. The top three causes in children (accounting for 45–65% of cases) are costochondritis, musculoskeletal pain from trauma or muscle strain, and pulmonary conditions associated with cough (see Table 4-8).

Children with heart disease rarely present with chest pain.

SYMPTOMS

- **Description of chest pain:** Should include time course, duration, quality, location, radiation, and severity.
  - Chronic chest pain is less likely to be caused by a serious underlying condition.
  - Acute pain is more likely to be caused by a medical condition.
  - Ischemic cardiac pain is often described as squeezing, pressure, or chest fullness.
  - Pain from aortic root dissection is a severe tearing sensation with radiation to the back.
  - Localized pain is more likely to originate from the chest wall or pleura.
  - Radiation of the pain is associated with uncommon causes of chest pain in children.
- **Associated symptoms:**
  - Fever suggests infection (e.g., pneumonia, myocarditis, Kawasaki disease).
  - Vomiting or painful swallowing suggests GI disease such as GERD or esophagitis.
  - Other somatic complaints (e.g., headache, abdominal pain) commonly occur in children with psychogenic chest pain.
  - **Syncope or palpitations suggest a cardiac disorder.**

Myocardial ischemic pain radiates to the left jaw and arm; acute cholecystitis pain to the right shoulder; aortic root dissection to the back; and pericarditis pain to the left shoulder.

TABLE 4-8. Causes of Chest Pain in Children

CAUSE	RELATIVE FREQUENCY (%)	DISTINGUISHING FEATURES	SPECIFIC TREATMENT
Idiopathic	20–45	Normal physical exam.	Reassurance and follow-up.
Chest wall trauma or muscle strain	~ 20	History of trauma or vigorous exercise; tenderness on palpation.	Analgesics, rest.
Costochondritis	10–22	Reproducible tenderness on palpation of the costochondral junction; often unilateral (L > R).	Analgesics, reassurance.
Respiratory disorders (e.g., pneumonia, asthma, bronchitis)	15–20	Pain tends to be pleuritic and is usually associated with coughing; may also be caused by pleural effusion or pneumothorax.	Antibiotics for infections; bronchodilators for reactive airways.
Psychogenic	~ 10	More common in adolescents; most have other somatic complaints (e.g., headache, abdominal pain); associated with a history of a stressful life event.	Reassurance and follow-up; may need additional counseling.
GI	4–7	Onset and relief of pain are associated with eating; associated with a history of foreign body or caustic ingestion.	Treatment of GERD or esophagitis.
Heart disease	1–6	More likely if chest pain is recurrent and occurs with exertion; almost always have abnormal cardiac exam. Specific conditions include left ventricular outflow tract obstruction, aortic dissection, coronary anomalies, arrhythmias, and myocarditis.	Referral to a cardiologist for treatment of the underlying etiology.
Breast	< 5	Mastalgia, fibrocystic disease, pregnancy; males with gynecomastia may present with pain.	Analgesics.
Acute chest syndrome	~ 2	Serious and potentially fatal in patients with sickle cell disease; characterized by new pulmonary infiltrate, fever, tachypnea, and cough.	O_2, antibiotics, fluids.
Precordial catch (Texidor's twinge)	Uncommon	Brief episodes of sharp, localized pain; associated with bending or slouching.	Relieved by straightening and shallow breathing.
Pneumothorax or pneumomediastinum	Rare	Higher likelihood in children with asthma, cystic fibrosis, or Marfan.	O_2.
Pulmonary embolism	Rare	Major risk factors include OCP use, pregnancy termination, immobility, and hypercoagulable states; presents with pleuritic chest pain associated with fever, cough, and hemoptysis.	O_2, anticoagulation.

- **Precipitating events:**
  - Chest pain with exertion often has a cardiac or respiratory cause.
  - Pain that worsens with swallowing is likely esophageal in origin.
- **Past medical history:** Look for a history of asthma, Kawasaki disease, sickle cell anemia, and the like.
- **Family history:**
  - Marfan, Turner, and Ehlers-Danlos syndromes predispose to aortic root dissection.
  - Hypertrophic cardiomyopathy may present with exertional chest pain.

EXAM

- Musculoskeletal pain is often **reproducible on palpation** of the chest.
- Diminished breath sounds or wheezing on auscultation may indicate pneumonia or asthma, respectively.
- A murmur, abnormal heart sounds, or an abnormal pulse or BP is suggestive of a cardiac cause of chest pain.
  - Signs of left ventricular outflow tract obstruction include a systolic ejection murmur at the right upper sternal border.
  - Coarctation of the aorta is associated with hypertension in the arms and a differential in BPs between the arms and legs.
  - A pericardial effusion may → a friction rub or distant heart sounds, depending on the size of the effusion.
  - Muffled heart sounds with a gallop rhythm and a murmur of mitral regurgitation are signs of myocarditis.

DIAGNOSIS

- Most patients have a normal physical exam or findings consistent with musculoskeletal pain and do not require further diagnostic studies.
- **CXR:** Helpful in the diagnosis of pneumonia, pleural effusion, or pneumothorax/pneumomediastinum. Cardiomegaly may be noted on CXR in patients with myocarditis, left ventricular outflow tract obstruction, or pericardial effusion.
- **ECG:** May be helpful in the diagnosis of a cardiac origin of chest pain.
  - An arrhythmia may be detected in a patient with associated palpitations.
  - Patients with left ventricular outflow tract obstruction may have evidence of left ventricular hypertrophy.
  - Generalized ST-segment elevation may be seen in patients with pericarditis.
- **Echocardiography:** Can establish a cardiac diagnosis and help assess the severity of disease.
  - Can assess the severity and location of left ventricular outflow tract obstruction.
  - Can assess the size of pericardial effusion, identify coronary artery anomalies, and diagnose aortic root dissection.

TREATMENT

- Underlying disorders should be treated appropriately.
- Musculoskeletal pain typically responds to analgesics and rest.
- Patients with GI complaints should be referred to a gastroenterologist.
- Patients with known heart disease or chest pain with exertion, syncope, or palpitations should be referred to a cardiologist.
- Provide reassurance that the etiology is usually benign in children. Patients with psychogenic chest pain may require additional counseling.
- Follow-up should be provided until symptoms resolve.

Defined as an abrupt loss of consciousness and postural tone that reverses spontaneously. The exact incidence of pediatric syncope is unknown, but it appears to be common; by young adulthood, 15–25% of children have experienced at least one syncopal episode. As with murmurs and chest pain in children, syncope often has a benign etiology. However, it is important to distinguish children with syncope of a benign etiology from those with serious underlying pathology. Causes include the following:

- **Circulatory:** Vasovagal syncope (also called vasodepressor, neurocardiogenic, or common syncope); orthostatic hypotension.
- **Cardiac:**
  - Severe obstructive lesions (e.g., aortic stenosis, pulmonary stenosis, hypertrophic cardiomyopathy, pulmonary hypertension).
  - Myocardial dysfunction (e.g., congenital coronary anomalies, Kawasaki disease).
  - Arrhythmias, including long QT syndrome.
- **Metabolic:** Hypoglycemia, hyperventilation syndrome, hypoxia.
- **Neuropsychological:** Epilepsy, brain tumor, migraine, hysteria, nonconvulsive seizures.

The three most common causes of syncope in children are vasovagal syncope, orthostatic hypotension, and hyperventilation syncope.

SYMPTOMS/EXAM

- **Vasovagal syncope:** Characterized by a prodrome (dizziness, lightheadedness, pallor, nausea, diaphoresis, hyperventilation) followed by loss of consciousness; often associated with anxiety, the sight of blood, fasting, crowded places, and prolonged and motionless standing.
- **Orthostatic hypotension:** Patients experience only lightheadedness prior to syncope.
  - Prolonged bed rest, prolonged standing, and dehydration can precipitate orthostatic hypotension.
  - **A drop of 10–15 mmHg in systolic BP when measured from supine to standing is highly suggestive of orthostasis.**
- **Micturition syncope:** A rare form of orthostatic hypotension in which rapid bladder decompression → ↓ peripheral vascular resistance and postural hypotension.
- **Cardiac causes of syncope:** Should be suspected when syncope occurs in a recumbent position, is provoked by exercise, is associated with chest pain, or occurs in a patient with a family history of sudden death.
- **Seizure-related syncope:** A patient with loss of consciousness due to seizure activity may have incontinence, tonic-clonic motion, and postictal confusion.
- **Psychogenic syncope:** Rarely occurs before 10 years of age; is not associated with injury, and almost always occurs in front of an audience.
- **Hyperventilation syncope:** Can be reproduced in the office by having the patient hyperventilate.

Syncope from arrhythmias in children with structurally normal hearts is rare except in those with long QT syndrome, Wolff-Parkinson-White syndrome, and arrhythmogenic right ventricular dysplasia.

DIAGNOSIS

For typical vasovagal and orthostatic syncope, further diagnostic evaluation is generally not indicated. Further investigative studies are indicated when syncope is exercise induced, preceded by chest pain, associated with abnormal findings on physical exam, or associated with a family history of unexplained death. Studies include the following:

- **ECG:** A prolonged corrected QT interval is suggestive of long QT syndrome; delta waves with a short PR interval are diagnostic for Wolff-Parkinson-White syndrome.
- **Holter monitoring:** Can help document a causal relationship between symptoms and arrhythmias.
- **Echocardiogram:** Can diagnose hypertrophic cardiomyopathy and evaluate the severity of obstructive lesions that may → syncope.
- **EEG:** Can help distinguish seizure activity from syncope of a circulatory etiology.
- **CT or MRI of the brain.**
- **Tilt-table testing:** Used to diagnose vasovagal syncope, but the overall reproducibility of results is low (about 60%), making it difficult to interpret the results of a single test.

TREATMENT

- With vasovagal syncope, maintaining a supine position until symptoms resolve is usually all that is necessary. Fludrocortisone and metoprolol have been reported to be successful in the prevention of syncopal episodes in patients with vasovagal syncope.
- Patients with orthostatic hypotension should be counseled to move to an upright position slowly and to stay well hydrated.
- Patients with abnormal neurologic findings should be referred to a neurologist for further evaluation and management.
- Patients with documented arrhythmias, cardiomyopathy, or obstructive heart lesions should be referred to a cardiologist for specific treatment.
- Patients with long QT syndrome are at significant risk for sudden death and are often treated with β-blockade and/or implantation of an AICD.
- Patients with hypertrophic cardiomyopathy are also at significant risk for sudden death even after surgical relief of left ventricular outflow tract obstruction and are also often treated with β-blockade and/or implantation of an AICD.
- Patients with reentrant tachyarrhythmias (e.g., those with Wolff-Parkinson-White syndrome and/or SVT) can be treated medically or with ablation of their accessory pathways.

SPECIAL TOPICS

The Athlete's Heart

Sudden death in the young athlete has an estimated prevalence of between 1:100,000 and 1:300,000. Most athletes who die suddenly have no symptoms, and the cardiovascular conditions that predispose them to sudden death are rare and difficult to detect. The risk of sudden death is much higher in males than in females. Cardiovascular conditions → sudden death in young athletes include hypertrophic cardiomyopathy, coronary artery anomalies, myocarditis, aortic rupture, and arrhythmogenic right ventricular dysplasia.

SYMPTOMS/EXAM

- Factors that are important to elicit during a pre-participation physical exam include a history of hypertension, syncope, near-syncope, angina, chest pain, or palpitations during exercise.

- Also look for a family history of cardiovascular disease, sudden death, hypertrophic cardiomyopathy, dilated cardiomyopathy, long QT syndrome, Marfan syndrome, or significant arrhythmia.
- Children with hypertrophic cardiomyopathy or coronary artery anomalies may report a history of syncope or anginal chest pain.
- Highly competitive and well-conditioned adolescent athletes may have a resting bradycardia of 40–50 bpm. If the remainder of the history and physical is normal, no further testing is necessary.
- If cardiovascular abnormalities are identified or suspected on the history and physical, the athlete should be restricted from activity pending evaluation by a cardiologist.

Infants of women with SLE, especially women with $\oplus$ anti-Ro and anti-La antibody titers, are at risk for congenital complete heart block.

Syndromes Associated with Heart Lesions

Table 4-9 summarizes genetic syndromes with a high incidence of congenital heart disease.

TABLE 4-9. Genetic Syndromes Associated with Congenital Heart Disease[a]

SYNDROME	GENETIC DEFECT	INCIDENCE OF DISEASE (%)	SPECIFIC HEART LESION
Down	Trisomy 21	40–50	Endocardial cushion defect (~ 60% of congenital heart disease), VSD, ASD, PDA, tetralogy of Fallot.
Edwards	Trisomy 18	~ 90	VSD and PDA (most common), ASD.
Patau	Trisomy 13	~ 80	VSD (most common), PDA, ASD, transposition of the great arteries.
DiGeorge/ velocardiofacial	22q11 deletion	80	Tetralogy of Fallot, truncus arteriosus, interrupted aortic arch.
Turner	Monosomy X	20	Coarctation of the aorta (~ 50% if congenital heart disease), valvular aortic stenosis, hypoplastic left heart syndrome.
Noonan	AD, 12q deletion	~ 66	Valvular pulmonary stenosis (~ 50% of congenital heart disease), hypertrophic cardiomyopathy.
Tuberous sclerosis	AD, 9 and 16 mutations	47–67	Cardiac rhabdomyomas, Wolff-Parkinson-White syndrome.
Holt-Oram	AD, 12q mutation	90	Secundum ASD (most common), VSD, heart block.
Alagille	AD, 20p microdeletion	90–97	Valvular and branch pulmonary stenosis (67%), tetralogy of Fallot (7–16%).
Smith-Lemli-Opitz	AR, 11q mutation	38	Endocardial cushion defect, anomalous pulmonary venous drainage.

Syndrome	Genetic Defect	Incidence of Disease (%)	Specific Heart Lesion
Ellis–van Creveld	AR	50	Primum ASD; the common atrium is most common.
Pompe	AR, 17q mutation	100	Hypertrophic cardiomyopathy.
Hurler/ mucopolysaccharidosis	AR, 4p mutation	100	Mitral regurgitation, aortic insufficiency, myocardial hypertrophy, cardiomyopathy, CAD, sudden death.
Williams	AD, 7q microdeletion	75	Supravalvular aortic stenosis (> 50%), valvular and branch pulmonary stenosis.
Marfan	AD, fibrillin gene mutation	80–100	Dilation and dissection of the ascending aorta, mitral valve prolapse.
Duchenne	XR, dystrophin gene mutation	100 by age 18	Dilated cardiomyopathy.
CHARGE	AD, chromodomain 7 mutation	65–75	Tetralogy of Fallot, aortic arch anomalies.
VACTERL/VATER	Unknown	Unknown	VSD, tetralogy of Fallot, ASD, PDA.

[a]AD = autosomal dominant; AR = autosomal recessive; CHARGE = coloboma, heart defects, atresia of the choanae, retardation of growth and development, genital and urinary abnormalities, ear abnormalities and/or hearing loss; VACTERL = vertebral anomalies, anal atresia, cardiac abnormalities, tracheoesophageal fistula, renal agenesis, limb defects; VATER = vertebral defects, anal atresia, tracheoesophageal fistula with esophageal atresia, radial dysplasia; XR = X-linked recessive.

Systemic Conditions Affecting the Heart

Table 4-10 summarizes cardiac manifestations of systemic conditions that affect the heart.

TABLE 4-10. Systemic Conditions Affecting the Heart

Condition	Cardiac Manifestation
Hyperthyroidism	Tachycardia, high-output heart failure, systemic hypertension.
Hypothyroidism	Bradycardia, pericardial effusion, low-voltage ECG.
Juvenile rheumatoid arthritis	Pericarditis; rarely, myocarditis.
SLE	Occur in roughly 40% of cases; pericarditis and pericardial effusion are most common. May also include Libman-Sacks endocarditis and **congenital complete heart block in infants of women with SLE.**
Scleroderma	Pulmonary hypertension, myocardial fibrosis, cardiomyopathy.
Lyme disease	Arrhythmias, myocarditis.
Anemia (iron deficiency, thalassemia, sickle cell)	High-output heart failure.
Iron overload (hemochromatosis, chronic transfusion therapy)	Cardiomyopathy from iron deposition in the myocardium.

CHAPTER 5

Dermatology

Julie Bokser, MD
reviewed by Anna L. Bruckner, MD

DERMATOLOGY DEFINITIONS

Definitions of commonly used terms in dermatology are as follows:

- **1° lesions:** Lesions that are caused by a 1° disease process (see Table 5-1).
- **2° lesions:** Lesions that are the result of factors such as rubbing, itching, infection, and the environment (see Table 5-2).

> In the newborn nursery, you are asked to evaluate a term male baby with scattered pustules that easily rupture. In addition to the pustules, you notice scales and pigmented macules at the sites of resolving pustules in this otherwise healthy infant. What will visualization of pustule contents most likely reveal? PMNs.

DERMATOSES IN THE NEWBORN

Table 5-3 outlines common etiologies of dermatologic disease in the newborn.

DIAPER DERMATITIS

- An inflammatory disorder affecting the skin of the lower abdomen, genitalia, buttocks, and thighs in infants and toddlers.

TABLE 5-1. Differential of 1° Dermatologic Lesions

1° LESION	DESCRIPTION
Macule	Flat, circumscribed change in skin coloration < 1 cm in diameter.
Patch	Flat, circumscribed change in skin coloration > 1 cm in diameter.
Papule	Raised, solid superficial lesion < 5 mm in diameter.
Plaque	Raised, solid superficial lesion > 5 mm in diameter.
Nodule	Raised, solid lesion arising from deeper underlying tissue < 2 cm in diameter.
Tumor	Raised, solid lesion arising from deeper underlying tissue > 2 cm in diameter.
Vesicle	Raised, fluid-filled superficial lesion < 5 mm in diameter.
Bulla	Raised, fluid-filled superficial lesion > 5 mm in diameter.
Pustule	Pus-filled superficial lesion.
Abscess	Pus-filled lesion arising from underlying tissue.
Wheal	Evanescent, raised, round or flat-topped lesion caused by edema.

TABLE 5-2. Differential of 2° Dermatologic Lesions

2° LESION	DESCRIPTION
Scale	Accumulation of dead epidermal cells (stratum corneum).
Crust	Dried exudates (blood, pus, serum) on the skin surface.
Lichenification	Thickened epidermis with accentuation of normal skin markings.
Erosion	Loss of epidermal layer only; heals without scar formation.
Ulcer	Loss of the epidermis and a portion of the dermis; heals with scar formation.
Atrophy	Thinning of the epidermis or dermis.
Excoriation	Linear disruption of the epidermis produced by scratching.
Fissure	Linear crack extending into the dermis.
Scar	Fibrous tissue formed in the place of normal skin.

TABLE 5-3. Sources of Blisters and Pustules in the Newborn

	EPIDEMIOLOGY	EXAM	DIAGNOSIS	TREATMENT
Erythema toxicum neonatorum	Affects 30–70% of all babies; appears in the first 24 hours to two weeks of life.	Presents with 1- to 2-mm, yellow/white papulovesicles surrounded by erythema on the trunk, arms, and legs.	Wright's stain of vesicle contents reveals eosinophils.	None.
Transient neonatal pustular melanosis	Occurs in black infants more often than white infants (4.4% vs. 0.2%); presents at birth.	Superficial pustules and pigmented macules on the upper body.	Lesions contain PMNs with no organisms.	None.
Miliaria (crystallina and rubra)	Incidence is greatest in the first few weeks of life because of immaturity of the eccrine glands and retained sweat.	Occurs in intertriginous or other occluded areas. ■ **Crystallina:** 1- to 2-mm, easily ruptured vesicles with the appearance of "drops of water" on the skin. ■ **Rubra:** Erythematous papulovesicular lesions on the head, neck, face, scalp, and trunk.	Improves with reduction of ambient temperature or fever.	Prevent excessive sweating and occlusion.

TABLE 5-3. Sources of Blisters and Pustules in the Newborn (continued)

	EPIDEMIOLOGY	EXAM	DIAGNOSIS	TREATMENT
Neonatal acne	Affects 20% of newborns in the first six months of life.	Presents with 1- to 3-mm papules and pustules on the face and trunk.	Looks like adolescent acne.	To prevent scarring in severe cases, consider low-pH soaps or 5% benzoyl peroxide wash.
Milia	Affects 40% of newborns.	Presents with 1- to 2-mm whitish papules (epidermal inclusion cysts) on the face or in the mouth (Epstein's pearls).		None.
Acropustulosis of infancy	Affects < 1% of the population (blacks more than whites) during the first year of life.	Recurrent crops (every 2–4 weeks) of severely pruritic, 1- to 3-mm vesiculopustular lesions on the hands and feet (see Figure 5-1).	Eosinophilia on CBC; Gram stain/Tzanck smear show PMNs. The differential includes scabies and HSV.	Antihistamines and low-potency topical steroids.
Sucking blister	Incidence is 1 in 250 births.	Bullae on the thumb, index finger, dorsum of hand, or wrist.		None.
Sebaceous gland hyperplasia		Multiple, tiny yellow papules on the nose and cheeks due to maternal androgen stimulation.		None.
Neonatal HSV	See the discussion of congenital infections.			
Incontinentia pigmenti	A rare, X-linked dominant disorder; lethal in males.	Erythematous, linear streaks and plaques of vesicles on the limbs and trunk.	Eosinophil-filled intraepidermal vesicles. The differential includes bullous impetigo, HSV, and mastocytosis.	Ocular and CNS involvement must be ruled out.
Epidermolysis bullosa	Rare; genetic inheritance pattern based on type (simplex, junctional, dystrophic).	Large blisters and erosions that arise in areas of minor trauma to the skin.		Manage in an NICU familiar with epidermolysis bullosa.

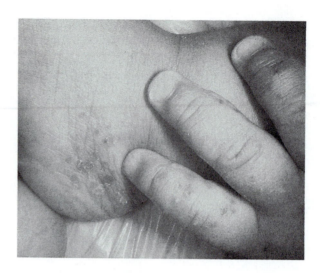

FIGURE 5-1. Acropustulosis of infancy.

(Reproduced, with permission, from Weinberg S et al. *Color Atlas of Pediatric Dermatology*, 3rd ed. New York: McGraw-Hill, 1998:4.) (Also see Color Insert.)

- Etiologies include wetness; impervious diapers; ↑ pH due to liberation of urea → acute irritation; and superinfection with *Candida* and bacteria (a common cause).
- **Sx/Exam:** Affects "convex" areas of skin; spares intertriginous areas.
- **Ddx:** See Table 5-4.
- **Tx:** Avoidance of irritants, frequent diaper changes, barrier creams.

A two-month-old infant presents to your clinic with a recalcitrant diaper rash that you had suspected was seborrheic dermatitis. On examination, you notice a scaly, erythematous eruption with petechiae on the scalp, neck folds, axillae, and diaper area, accompanied by hepatosplenomegaly. What test will confirm the diagnosis? Skin biopsy for CD1a and S-100.

TABLE 5-4. Differential Diagnosis of Diaper Dermatitis

DISORDER	SYMPTOMS/EXAM	DIAGNOSIS	TREATMENT
Seborrheic dermatitis	Greasy scaling over red, inflamed skin.	Clinical diagnosis. Consider if there is scalp dermatitis.	Short-term topical corticosteroids.
Candidiasis	Beefy-red erythema on the buttocks, lower abdomen, and thighs with pinpoint pustulovesicular satellite lesions involving the intertriginous areas. Often seen in association with oral thrush and maternal candidal nipple infection.	Consider in any rash that does not improve with usual measures or that develops following antibiotic usage. Diagnosis can be confirmed with KOH prep.	Topical antifungal cream.

TABLE 5-4. Differential Diagnosis of Diaper Dermatitis *(continued)*

DISORDER	SYMPTOMS/EXAM	DIAGNOSIS	TREATMENT
Psoriasis	Red, well-marginated plaques with silvery scale on the trunk, face, and scalp; concomitant nail involvement (see Figure 5-2). Patients often have a ⊕ family history.	Consider with persistent rashes that do not respond to therapy.	Low-potency topical steroids.
Congenital syphilis	Development of reddish-brown macules, papules, and bullae in the groin area with associated involvement of the palms and soles. Associated hepatosplenomegaly and anemia.	See discussion below.	See discussion below.
Langerhans cell histiocytosis	Severe and chronic, hemorrhagic, seborrhea-like eruption in the diaper area (see Figure 5-3).	Histiocytic infiltrate on cutaneous biopsy; ⊕ staining for S-100 and CD1a.	Chemotherapy is indicated for children with multisystem disease.
Acrodermatitis enteropathica	An autosomal-recessive condition involving GI malabsorption of zinc; mimics severe candidal diaper dermatitis or psoriasis (see Figure 5-4). May be accompanied by vesiculobullous eruptions of the perioral area, fingers, and toes as well as by alopecia and diarrhea.	Plasma zinc levels are low; skin biopsy shows parakeratosis of the stratum corneum and intracellular edema.	Lifetime zinc supplementation.
Staphylococcal pustulosis	Thin-walled pustules on an erythematous base that easily rupture, producing surrounding scale.	Clinical diagnosis. Gram stain and/or bacterial culture of unroofed pustule will reveal gram-⊕ cocci in clusters.	Antistaphylococcal topical or oral antiobiotics depending on severity.
Perianal streptococcus	A bright red, sharply demarcated perianal rash caused by group A β-hemolytic streptococci. Symptoms may include itching, pain, and blood-streaked stools. Occurs primarily in children six months to ten years of age.	⊕ rapid group A streptococcal test or culture.	Penicillin.

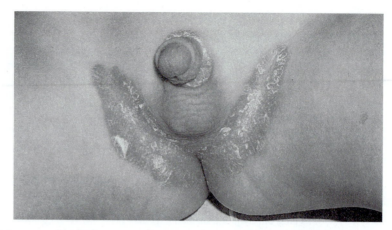

FIGURE 5-2. Psoriasis.

(Reproduced, with permission, from Weinberg S et al. *Color Atlas of Pediatric Dermatology*, 3rd ed. New York: McGraw-Hill, 1998:91.) (Also see Color Insert.)

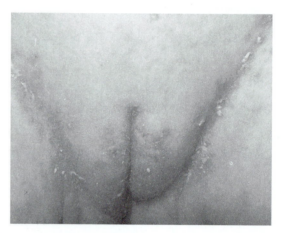

FIGURE 5-3. Langerhans cell histiocytosis.

(Reproduced, with permission, from Weinberg S et al. *Color Atlas of Pediatric Dermatology*, 3rd ed. New York: McGraw-Hill, 1998:214.) (Also see Color Insert.)

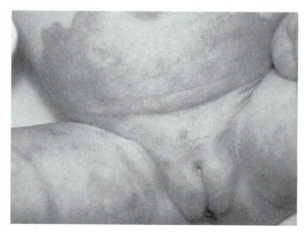

FIGURE 5-4. Acrodermatitis enteropathica.

(Reproduced, with permission, from Weinberg S et al. *Color Atlas of Pediatric Dermatology*, 3rd ed. New York: McGraw-Hill, 1998:106.) (Also see Color Insert.)

Table 5-5 outlines some common congenital infections with dermatologic manifestations.

TABLE 5-5. Congenital Infections with Dermatologic Features

	EPIDEMIOLOGY	CLINICAL MANIFESTATIONS	CUTANEOUS FEATURES	DIAGNOSIS	TREATMENT/ PROGNOSIS
Congenital rubella	Occurs following maternal rubella infection during the first 20 weeks of pregnancy.	Presents with the triad of congenital cataracts, deafness, and congenital heart malformations. Intrauterine growth retardation (IUGR) is also seen.	Thrombocytopenic purpura; 2- to 8-mm bluish-red macules ("blueberry muffin" lesions—dermal erythropoiesis) are noted within the first day of life on the head, neck, trunk, and extremities.		Failure to thrive; 20–30% mortality within the first year of life.
Congenital toxo-plasmosis	Incidence in the United States is 2 in 1000 live births.	Stillbirth or premature delivery. Chorioretinitis (80–90%). Also presents with malaise, vomiting, diarrhea, jaundice, hepatosplenomegaly, pneumonitis, and cataracts.	Rubella-like rash with ecchymoses/ purpura sparing the face, palms, and soles; blueberry muffin lesions.	Demonstration of organism in CSF or on tissue biopsy.	Treat with pyrimethamine + sulfadiazine + folinic acid + prednisone. Prognosis is poor when symptoms present at birth. Survivors have chorioretinitis, blindness, hydrocephalus, and mental retardation.
Herpes neonatorum	Affects 1500–2000 infants annually in the United States, 80% with HSV-2. A high risk of transmission (40–50%) is found after vaginal delivery in mothers with a 1° genital outbreak.	Disseminated, local, or asymptomatic infections (see Figure 5-5).	Some 70% of infants with neonatal HSV will have skin lesions (vesicles); if left untreated, 70% of these will progress to systemic infection.		Treat with IV acyclovir. Untreated infections are associated with a 60% mortality rate. Some 50% of survivors have significant ocular or neurologic sequelae.

TABLE 5-5. Congenital Infections with Dermatologic Features *(continued)*

	EPIDEMIOLOGY	CLINICAL MANIFESTATIONS	CUTANEOUS FEATURES	DIAGNOSIS	TREATMENT/ PROGNOSIS
Syphilis	Incidence is ↑.	**Early congenital syphilis (before age 2):** Anemia, fever, wasting, hepatosplenomegaly, lymphadenopathy, snuffles, rash. **Late congenital syphilis (after age 2):** Interstitial keratitis, Hutchinson's incisors, CN VIII deafness.	Cutaneous lesions are seen in 30–50% of affected infants. Slow onset of large, round maculopapular lesions like those of 2° syphilis in teens and adults, lasting 1–3 months. Lesions are most pronounced on the face, dorsal surface of the trunk, legs, diaper area, palms, and soles. Mucous membrane patches (extremely infectious); diffuse desquamation.	Darkfield microscopy of specimens from skin lesions or placenta. RPR or VDRL. CSF VDRL. FTA-ABS. Long bone radiographs.	Treat with penicillin × 10–21 days. 25% will die in utero; if left untreated, 30% will die shortly after birth.
CMV	Maternal CMV infection affects 3–6% of pregnant women; 1 in 3000 exposed infants will develop symptomatic CMV disease. Some 90% of congenital CMV infections are asymptomatic; the remaining 10% present with mild to severe disease.	Lethargy, early jaundice, hepatospleno-megaly, anemia, thrombocytopenia, pneumonia, seizures, chorioretinitis, periventricular calcifications.	Petechiae and purpura; generalized maculopapular rash; blueberry muffin rash.	Recovery of virus from urine, serum, or CSF; anti-CMV IgM.	Most symptomatic cases are fatal in the first two months of life; survivors have severe neurologic sequelae. Roughly 5–15% of asymptomatic infections → late-onset hearing loss, chorioretinitis, and mental retardation.

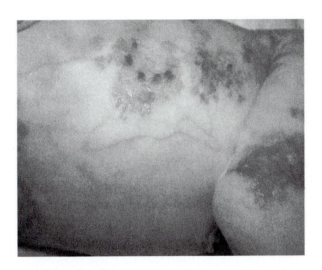

FIGURE 5-5. Herpes neonatorum.

(Reproduced, with permission, from Weinberg S et al. *Color Atlas of Pediatric Dermatology*, 3rd ed. New York: McGraw-Hill, 1998:37.) (Also see Color Insert.)

INFECTIOUS RASHES

Bacterial Infections

IMPETIGO

Divided into bullous and nonbullous types.

- **Nonbullous:**
    - A bacterial infection of the epidermis caused by *S. aureus* and group A streptococci.
    - Often preceded by local trauma (insect bites or nose picking); contagious and spread by direct contact (e.g., scratching).
- **Bullous:** A bacterial infection of the epidermis caused by epidermolytic, toxin-producing *S. aureus*.

SYMPTOMS/EXAM

- **Nonbullous impetigo:** Superficial vesicles and pustules with typical honey-colored crust.
- **Bullous impetigo:** Flaccid vesicles and bullae up to 3 cm in diameter (see Figure 5-6).

TREATMENT

- **Mild cases:** Topical mupirocin.
- **Moderate to severe cases:** Systemic antibiotics.

CELLULITIS

- Infection of the deep dermis and subcutaneous fat; caused by group A streptococcus and *S. aureus*.
- **Sx/Exam:**
    - Often preceded by local skin injury.
    - Presents with an area of erythema, warmth, and tenderness that is not well circumscribed.

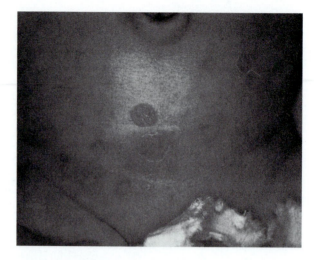

FIGURE 5-6. Bullous impetigo.

(Reproduced, with permission, from Weinberg S et al. *Color Atlas of Pediatric Dermatology*, 3rd ed. New York: McGraw-Hill, 1998:14.) (Also see Color Insert.)

- **Tx:** Systemic antibiotics; consider community-acquired methicillin-resistant *S. aureus* (MRSA) if no improvement is seen.
- **Complications:** MRSA, lymphangitis, necrotizing fasciitis.

ERYSIPELAS

- A bacterial infection of the dermis caused by group A streptococcus and *S. aureus*.
- **Sx/Exam:** Well-circumscribed, raised, indurated, erythematous lesions that most often affect the face or legs.
- **Tx:** Apply saline wet dressings to ulcerated areas; antibiotic therapy with penicillin or a macrolide (if penicillin allergic) is indicated.

ERYTHEMA CHRONICUM MIGRANS

- A skin manifestation of Lyme disease caused by *Borrelia burgdorferi* and transmitted via tick bite.
- **Sx/Exam:**
  - Begins as an erythematous papule at the site of the bite.
  - Evolves into an annular, erythematous rash (up to 20 cm in size) with an area of central clearing (see Figure 5-7).
- **Tx:** Systemic antibiotics.

Toxin-Related Rashes

SCARLET FEVER

- A clinical syndrome caused by group A streptococcus and characterized by a toxin-mediated rash.
- **Sx/Exam:**
  - Presents with fever, exudative pharyngitis and palatal petechiae, strawberry tongue (prominent papillae), and lymphadenopathy.
  - Pastia lines (petechiae in skin folds) are also seen.

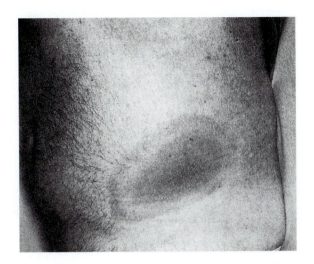

FIGURE 5-7. Erythema chronicum migrans.

(Reproduced, with permission, from Weinberg S et al. *Color Atlas of Pediatric Dermatology*, 3rd ed. New York: McGraw-Hill, 1998:25.) (Also see Color Insert.)

- Skin infection takes the form of a classic fine maculopapular rash with an erythematous background ("sandpaper rash").
- **Ddx:** Kawasaki disease, viral exanthem, drug eruption.
- **Dx:** Clinical; obtain throat culture.
- **Tx:** Penicillin IM or PO.
- **Complications:** Acute rheumatic fever, poststreptococcal glomerulonephritis.

STAPHYLOCOCCAL SCALDED SKIN SYNDROME

- Caused by exfoliative toxin-producing S. *aureus.*
- **Sx/Exam:**
  - Often begins as a 1° skin infection (impetigo) or as nasopharyngitis/conjunctivitis.
  - Fever and malaise are also seen.
  - Skin infection is characterized by a tender, sunburn-like rash that becomes scarlatiniform, followed by widespread blistering and peeling of the skin (see Figure 5-8).
  - One to three days after the appearance of the rash, easily ruptured bullous lesions develop.
  - Gentle traction of the skin causes the epidermis to separate from the dermis, leaving raw and red skin underneath (Nikolsky's sign).
- **Ddx:** Scarlet fever, toxic epidermal necrolysis.
- **Dx:** Clinical (fluid in bullae is sterile); consider blood culture.
- **Tx:**
  - Give a first-generation cephalosporin (e.g., cephalexin).
  - Apply emollient or bacitracin to ruptured bullae.
  - In most cases, resolution occurs in 10–14 days without scarring.
  - With extensive loss of epidermis, one may see FEN imbalances, infection, and problems with temperature regulation (e.g., severe burn).

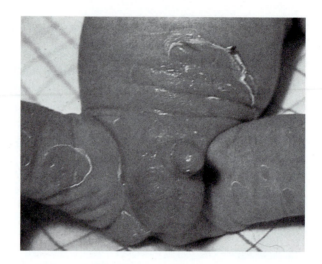

FIGURE 5-8. **Staphylococcal scalded skin syndrome.**

(Reproduced, with permission, from Weinberg S et al. *Color Atlas of Pediatric Dermatology*, 3rd ed. New York: McGraw-Hill, 1998:16.) (Also see Color Insert.)

Fungal Infections

TINEA INFECTIONS (DERMATOPHYTOSES)

A group of cutaneous fungal infections caused primarily by *Trichophyton tonsurans* and *Microsporum canis*. Spread in the pediatric population by immunocompetent children in day care centers and elementary schools as well as by children with immunodeficiencies. Subtypes are as follows:

- **Tinea capitis:** A fungal infection of the scalp characterized by scaling and patchy alopecia, broken hairs, and cervical/occipital lymphadenopathy. May present with a boggy, indurated, tender inflammatory mass (kerion) +/− a purulent discharge due to hypersensitivity reaction.
- **Tinea pedis ("athlete's foot"):** Affects the instep or the entire weight-bearing surface. The differential includes foot eczema and shoe dermatitis (a red, scaly vesicular rash on the dorsa of the toes and the distal third of the foot).
- **Tinea corporis:** A superficial infection of nonhairy skin marked by annular, well-demarcated, scaly patches with central clearing and a scaly papulovesicular border. The differential includes pityriasis rosea, nummular eczema, psoriasis, granuloma annulare (see Figure 5-9), and fixed drug eruption.
- **Tinea manus:** Ringworm infection of the hand.
- **Tinea cruris ("jock itch"):** Superficial infection of the groin and thighs. The differential includes erythrasma, a chronic superficial dermatosis of the crural area caused by *Corynebacterium minutissimum* that is diagnosed by a coral-red immunofluorescence seen under Wood's light.
- **Onychomycosis:** Chronic fungal infection of the fingernails or toenails.
- **Tinea versicolor:** Multiple hypopigmented or hyperpigmented scaling, oval, macular lesions over the trunk and proximal arms (see Figure 5-10). The differential includes pityriasis alba.

DIAGNOSIS

- Diagnosis is largely clinical.
- KOH prep reveals budding hyphae; short hyphae and yeast (yielding a "spaghetti and meatballs" appearance) are found in tinea versicolor.

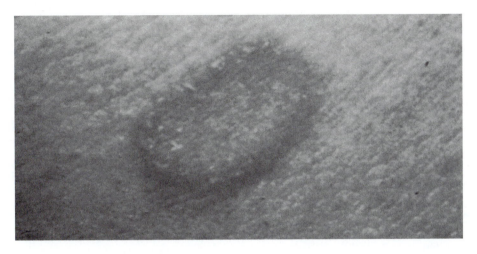

FIGURE 5-9. Tinea corporis.

(Reproduced, with permission, from Knoop K. *Emergency Atlas of Medicine*, 2nd ed. New York: McGraw-Hill, 2002, Fig. 13.26.) (Also see Color Insert.)

- Fungal culture.
- Fluorescence of infected hair by Wood's light (except *Trichophyton tonsurans*).

TREATMENT

- **Tinea corporis/pedis/manus/cruris:** Topical antifungals (imidazoles and terbinafine).
- **Tinea capitis:** Long-term systemic antifungals.
  - **First-line treatment:** Griseofulvin.
  - **Alternatives:** Azoles, terbinafine.
  - **Adjunctive therapy:** Selenium sulfide shampoo to minimize spread.
- **Onychomycosis:** Long-term systemic antifungals.
  - **First-line treatment:** Terbinafine.
  - **Alternatives:** Azoles.
- **Tinea versicolor:** Selenium sulfide shampoo.

Griseofulvin should be given with milk or fatty food to ↑ absorption.

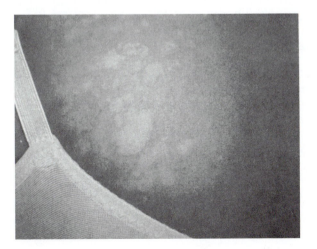

FIGURE 5-10. Tinea versicolor.

(Reproduced, with permission, from Weinberg S et al. *Color Atlas of Pediatric Dermatology*, 3rd ed. New York: McGraw-Hill, 1998:55, Fig. 178.) (Also see Color Insert.)

CANDIDIASIS

An acute or chronic infection of the skin and mucous membranes caused by proliferation of *Candida albicans* (normal flora) as a result of an alteration in host defense. Manifestations include the following:

- **Oral candidiasis** (thrush).
- **Cutaneous candidiasis:** Affects intertriginous areas, including the groin, perineum, and intergluteal and inframammary folds. The differential includes psoriasis.
- **Vulvovaginitis:** Presents with pruritus, erythematous and edematous labia, and leukorrhea.

DIAGNOSIS

- Diagnosis is largely clinical.
- Consider KOH prep or fungal culture.

TREATMENT

Topical antifungal preparations.

Cutaneous Viral Infections

WARTS

- Caused by the human papillomavirus (HPV). Subtypes include verruca vulgaris (common wart), verruca plana (flat wart), verruca plantaris (plantar wart), and condylomata acuminata (genital warts).
- **Dx:** Clinical.
- **Tx:**
  - Some 50–66% of cases resolve spontaneously within two years.
  - Treatment options include salicylic acid, cryotherapy, duct tape occlusion, and imiquimod.

MOLLUSCUM CONTAGIOSUM

A molluscipoxvirus infection of the skin and mucous membranes that is common among healthy toddlers and children.

SYMPTOMS/EXAM

- Presents with umbilicated papules, often with involvement of the trunk and face (see Figure 5-11).
- Numerous lesions are seen in immunocompromised children and teens.

DIFFERENTIAL

Warts.

DIAGNOSIS

Clinical.

TREATMENT

- None, or the same as that for warts (e.g., imiquimod, cantharidin).
- Spontaneous resolution is seen in immunocompetent patients.

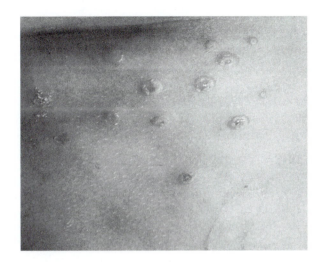

FIGURE 5-11. Molluscum contagiosum.

(Reproduced, with permission, from Weinberg S et al. *Color Atlas of Pediatric Dermatology*, 3rd ed. New York: McGraw-Hill, 1998:34.) (Also see Color Insert.)

Viral Exanthems

Defined as rashes associated with particular viruses (see Table 5-6). Caused by a direct or immunologic reaction of the skin to viremia.

Scabies

A contagious infection caused by infestation by the mite *Sarcoptes scabiei*.

Symptoms/Exam

- Classic burrows; papules, vesicles, pustules.
- **Infants:** Lesions appear on the trunk, palms, soles, and face.
- **Older children:** Lesions are found in flexural areas and on the wrists, axillae, trunk, and breasts.

Differential

Atopic dermatitis, dyshidrotic eczema, contact dermatitis, impetigo, insect bites, infantile acropustulosis.

Diagnosis

Microscopic evaluation of scrapings from burrows under mineral oil or KOH.

Treatment

- Give 5% permethrin cream or oral ivermectin.
- The entire family and close contacts must be treated.
- Consider precipitated sulfur in petrolatum for very young infants or pregnant women.

All close contacts and family members of children with scabies should also be empirically treated.

TABLE 5-6. Common Viral Exanthems

Virus	Epidemiology	Associated Symptoms	Rash	Diagnosis	Treatment	Complications
Varicella	Some 50% of infections occur before age five; has a two- to three-week incubation.	Fever, malaise, headache.	Affects the trunk and then the extremities; evolves from papules to vesicles and then to crusts. "Dewdrops on a rose petal" appearance; pruritic.	Viral culture, Tzanck smear.	Supportive.	Bacterial superinfection.
Parvovirus B19	Common in the spring; affects school-age children; has a 4- to 21-day incubation.	Fever and malaise.	"Slapped cheek" appearance; abrupt onset of facial erythema with a diffuse maculopapular rash over the body.	Clinical; serology to confirm.	Supportive; in cases of aplastic anemia, give transfusions and IVIG.	Aplastic anemia, fetal hydrops, fetal demise.
HHV-6/7 (roseola)	Affects newborns to children three years of age.	High fever precedes rash; coryza.	Rose-colored macules < 5 mm.		Supportive.	None.
Measles (rubeola)	Epidemics occur in the unimmunized; has an 8- to 12-day incubation.	Cough, coryza, conjunctivitis, fever.	Erythematous, blanching macules starting on the forehead and moving down the body.	Serology.	Supportive.	Pneumonia, encephalitis.
Rubella	Primarily affects teens; has a two- to three-week incubation.	Tender lymphadenopathy.	First affects the face, followed by the trunk and then the extremities; evolves from macules to pinpoint papules. Clearing occurs in about three days.	Serology.	Supportive.	Polyarthritis, fetal infection → congenital malformations.

TABLE 5-6. Common Viral Exanthems *(continued)*

VIRUS	EPIDEMIOLOGY	ASSOCIATED SYMPTOMS	RASH	DIAGNOSIS	TREATMENT	COMPLICATIONS
Coxsackievirus (hand-foot-and-mouth disease)	Affects toddlers.	Fever, sore throat.	Painful oral mucosal ulcers; 5-mm vesicles on the palms, soles, and perianal area.		Supportive.	Rare.

ECZEMATOUS ERUPTIONS

Inflammatory eruptions characterized by redness, papules, vesicles, edema, oozing, crusting, and itching.

Atopic Dermatitis

A chronic and relapsing condition that exhibits a genetic predisposition. Associated with the following:

- An abnormal skin barrier.
- An aberrant immune response.
- Abnormal innate immunity (*S. aureus* commonly colonizes the skin of patients with atopic dermatitis).
- A predisposition to pruritus, which → scratching, skin trauma, and irritation and then to the classic findings of atopic dermatitis.
- A self-perpetuating cycle of itching/scratching/rash/itching.
- Although the role of allergens is controversial, food sensitivity has been shown to aggravate dermatitis in some individuals.
- Some 75% of patients improve by puberty; 25% have persistent atopic dermatitis during adult life.

Atopic dermatitis is often described as "the itch that rashes."

SYMPTOMS/EXAM

Presentation varies with age and subtype:

- **Infantile atopic dermatitis:**
    - **Location:** Cheeks, forehead, trunk, extremities (**spares the diaper area**).
    - **Appearance:** Papules, vesicles; oozing, crusting.
- **Childhood atopic dermatitis:**
    - **Location:** Wrists, ankles, antecubital and popliteal fossae.
    - **Symptoms:** Severe pruritus.
    - **Appearance:** Dry, scaly patches with lichenification that are prone to superinfection.
- **Adolescent/adult atopic dermatitis:**
    - **Location:** Flexor folds, face and neck, upper arms and back, dorsa of the hands and feet.
    - **Appearance:** Confluent papules and large lichenified plaques that are prone to superinfection.

Keratosis pilaris presents with spiny follicular papules and is often seen with atopic dermatitis.

- **Nummular eczema:**
  - **Location:** Extensor surfaces of the hands, arms, and legs.
  - **Appearance:** Round, ≥ 1-cm lesions of grouped papules and lichenified plaques.

DIFFERENTIAL

Seborrheic dermatitis, contact dermatitis, psoriasis, scabies, histiocytosis, Wiskott-Aldrich syndrome.

DIAGNOSIS

Clinical (itching, typical morphology and distribution, course, ⊕ family history).

TREATMENT

- Hydration with limited bathing and generous use of emollients.
- Avoidance of allergens.
- Low- to moderate-potency topical corticosteroids for red, inflamed, rough, or lichenified areas (side effects include atrophy, striae, rosacea, and telangiectasia).
- Antihistamines for itching.
- Calcineurin inhibitors (tacrolimus, pimecrolimus).
- Antistaphylococcal antibiotics if superinfection is a concern.

COMPLICATIONS

- **Superinfection with staphylococcus and β-hemolytic streptococci:** Consider with a flare of chronic atopic dermatitis or failed response to treatment.
- **Eczema herpeticum:** A vesicular eruption due to HSV in atopic individuals.

Seborrheic Dermatitis

The etiology is not well understood; *Pityrosporum ovale* may play a role in its development.

SYMPTOMS/EXAM

- Begins during the first three months of life with **nonpruritic,** scaly dermatitis over the scalp (cradle cap) as well as on the forehead, ears, eyebrows, and neck and other parts of the body.
- Presents as salmon-colored, greasy scales with associated redness and weeping on the scalp and face as well as in flexural and intertriginous areas; scaly oval lesions are seen on other parts of the body, including the trunk, umbilicus, and groin.
- No stigmata of atopy (no evidence of dry skin or itching).

DIFFERENTIAL

Atopic dermatitis, psoriasis, Langerhans cell histiocytosis, acrodermatitis enteropathica.

DIAGNOSIS

Clinical. Consider biopsy if histiocytosis is a concern.

TREATMENT

- **Cradle cap:** Antiseborrheic shampoos; removal of scale with mineral oil and a soft brush.
- **Persistent or itchy lesions:** Topical corticosteroids.
- Prognosis is good, with resolution occurring in most cases by 8–12 months of age.

Pityriasis Alba

- A mild inflammation with postinflammatory hypopigmentation that most often appears following sun exposure.
- **Sx/Exam:** Discrete, hypopigmented patches on the face, neck, upper trunk, and proximal extremities of children and young adults.
- **Ddx:** Tinea corporis, tinea versicolor, vitiligo, postinflammatory hypopigmentation.
- **Dx:** Clinical.
- **Tx:** Hydration and topical corticosteroids; repigmentation occurs within several weeks.

Allergic Contact Dermatitis

Caused by a type IV (delayed hypersensitivity) immunologic response. Common allergens include hospital ID bands, jewelry (nickel), neomycin, cosmetics, poison ivy, and adhesive tape.

SYMPTOMS/EXAM

- Acute erythema; edema; papules, vesicles, bullae.
- Oozing with sharp demarcation between involved and noninvolved skin.
- Occurs where skin has direct contact with an allergen.
- Rhus dermatitis (poison ivy) appears 1–3 days after contact with the sensitizing oleoresin and persists for 1–3 weeks.

DIFFERENTIAL

Atopic dermatitis, irritant dermatitis.

DIAGNOSIS

Patch testing.

TREATMENT

- Allergen avoidance; thorough washing after exposure.
- Cool compresses.
- Calamine lotion and oral antihistamines.
- Topical corticosteroids.
- For severe cases, consider a short course of systemic corticosteroids.

A 10-year-old girl is brought to your office for evaluation of a recurrent rash on her ankle. Her mother says that this rash appears in association with respiratory infections, adding that it always occurs in the same location and resolves between these illnesses. On examination, you see a large, reddish-purple, well-demarcated edematous plaque with a small bulla over the dorsum of her ankle. What is the most likely diagnosis? Fixed drug eruption.

Fixed Drug Eruption

- Results from exposure to particular drugs (e.g., phenolphthalein, penicillin, tetracycline, pseudoephedrine). The etiology is unknown.
- **Sx/Exam:** Well-demarcated, localized, erythematous round patches or bullae that recur at the same sites with subsequent exposure to the offending substance; heal with desquamation and hyperpigmentation. Residual hyperpigmentation may persist for months.
- **Tx:** Drug avoidance.

PAPULOSQUAMOUS ERUPTIONS

A 10-year-old boy presents for evaluation of a new rash. Physical examination reveals erythematous plaques with thick silvery scale on his elbows and scalp. What is the most appropriate initial therapy for this patient? Topical steroid.

Psoriasis

The etiology of psoriasis is unknown, but it may have a genetic component.

The Auspitz sign consists of slow, pinpoint bleeding after the physical removal of a psoriasis scale.

SYMPTOMS/EXAM

Presents as a symmetric inflammatory distribution of thick, erythematous patches with silvery scale that shows a predilection for the scalp and the extensor surfaces of the extremities (see Figure 5-12). Patches have a "pasted-on" appearance. Roughly 50% of cases present with pitting of the nails and onycholysis. Subtypes are as follows:

- **Guttate psoriasis:** Presents with droplet-sized lesions on the trunk and proximal extremities. A common form in children.
- **Pustular psoriasis:** Pustules on a background of redness and swelling.
- **Erythrodermic psoriasis:** Generalized scaling and inflammatory plaques.

DIAGNOSIS

Clinical history exam. Differentiate from tinea and 2° syphilis.

TREATMENT

Topical steroids, retinoids, or vitamin D analogs if localized; light therapy or immunosuppressives and anti-TNF drugs if severe.

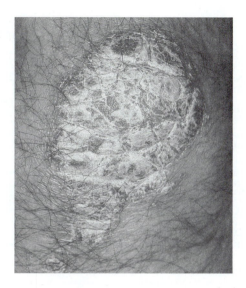

FIGURE 5-12. Psoriasis vulgaris (elbow).

(Reproduced, with permission, from Wolff K, Johnson RA, Suurmond D. *Fitzpatrick's Color Atlas & Synopsis of Clinical Dermatology*, 5th ed. New York: McGraw-Hill, 2005:57.)

In urgent care, you evaluate a 14-year-old girl who comes to the office complaining of an itchy rash. The rash began roughly two weeks ago as a large itchy patch on the chest, and it has since spread. On physical examination, you see numerous orange-pink macules and papules with a rim of scale clustered on the trunk, axillae, and proximal extremities. What is the most likely diagnosis? Pityriasis rosea.

Pityriasis Rosea

- May be associated with viral infection or drugs.
- Sx/Exam:
  - **"Herald patch"**: Initially presents as a 2- to 6-cm, oval/round, salmon-colored plaque with a scaly border appearing on the trunk or a proximal extremity.
  - Days to weeks later, smaller papules appear along skin cleavage lines in a **"Christmas tree"** pattern (see Figure 5-13).
- **Ddx:** Tinea corporis, 2° syphilis, guttate psoriasis, nummular eczema, lichen planus, drug reaction.
- **Dx:** Clinical. Consider evaluation to rule out tinea and 2° syphilis.
- **Tx:**
  - Treatment is symptomatic. Consider antihistamines for pruritus.
  - Resolution occurs over 2–4 months.

Testing for syphilis is recommended for any sexually active individual with pityriasis rosea.

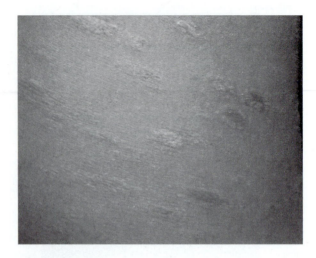

FIGURE 5-13. Pityriasis rosea.

Note the "Christmas tree" pattern of distribution. (Reproduced, with permission, from Weinberg S et al. *Color Atlas of Pediatric Dermatology*, 3rd ed. New York: McGraw-Hill, 1998:94.) (Also see Color Insert.)

Papular Acrodermatitis of Childhood (Gianotti-Crosti Syndrome)

- A distinct viral exanthem caused primarily by EBV, CMV, and HBV.
- Sx/Exam:
  - Flat-topped, pale pink papules appearing in crops over the face, buttocks, extremities, palms, and soles (spares the trunk); persist for weeks.
  - Associated constitutional symptoms and acute hepatitis are also seen.
- Dx: Clinical.
- Tx: None; resolves over 1–2 months.

Lichen Striatus

- Affects children 5–10 years of age; found more frequently in girls than in boys. The etiology is unknown.
- Sx/Exam: Presents as a linear band of discrete, confluent, flesh-colored, lichenoid papules that appear suddenly on an extremity.
- Ddx: Lichen planus, psoriasis, tinea corporis, epidermal nevus.
- Dx: Clinical.
- Tx: Spontaneous resolution occurs in 3–12 months. Consider topical corticosteroids if treatment is desired.

VASCULAR DISORDERS

Pyogenic Granuloma

- A common acquired vascular lesion whose etiology may be an exaggerated healing response.
- Sx/Exam:
  - Presents with an abrupt-onset, 5-mm to 2-cm solitary lesion appearing on areas subject to trauma (e.g., the hands, forearms, face).
  - The lesion is a bright red to reddish-brown, soft or moderately firm, raised, pedunculated nodule that bleeds easily (see Figure 5-14).
- Tx: Surgical removal or laser ablation. Unlikely to resolve without treatment.

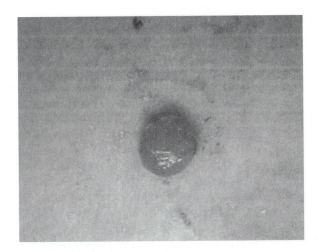

FIGURE 5-14. Pyogenic granuloma.

(Reproduced, with permission, from Weinberg S et al. *Color Atlas of Pediatric Dermatology*, 3rd ed. New York: McGraw-Hill, 1998:204.) (Also see Color Insert.)

Vascular Nevi

The largest group of anomalies in infancy and childhood, occurring in up to 40% of newborns; have a developmental origin. Include the following:

- **Superficial hemangiomas:**
  - Proliferating vascular endothelium.
  - Occur in 2.6% of all newborns and in 8–12% of Caucasian infants by one year of age.
  - Appear during the first month of life as small, well-demarcated telangiectatic macules that become vascularized and grow into raised red lobulated tumors with a strawberry-like appearance.
  - Rapid growth is seen during the first six months of life, with peak size at one year and gradual involution occurring over subsequent years (50% complete involution by five years of age; 90% by nine years of age).
- **Deep hemangiomas:**
  - Proliferating vascular endothelium arising within the dermis and subcutaneous tissues with little penetration of overlying skin.
  - Present at birth; grow into bluish-red masses with indistinct borders.
  - The natural history of deep hemangiomas parallels that of superficial hemangiomas, but the former are more likely to involute with abnormal-appearing skin.
- **PHACE syndrome:** Posterior fossa malformations, large facial Hemangiomas, Arterial anomalies, Coarctation of the aorta and other cardiac defects, Eye abnormalities.
- **Kasabach-Merritt syndrome:** Association of vascular tumor with consumption coagulopathy and thrombocytopenia due to platelet sequestration. Seen with kaposiform hemangioendotheliomas and tufted angiomas, not with common hemangiomas. Most likely to occur in the first few months of life.
- **Salmon patches (nevus simplex, "stork bite"):**
  - Occur in 30–40% of newborns.
  - Represent persistent fetal circulation.
  - Present as flat pink macular lesions on the nape of neck, glabella, forehead, upper eyelids, and nasolabial area.
  - Most resolve over time, although lesions on the neck tend to persist.

- **Port-wine stains:**
  - Congenital vascular malformations composed of mature dilated capillary-like vessels without proliferation.
  - Occur in 0.3–0.5% of all newborns.
  - Present as reddish-purple, flat patches that most commonly involve the face.
  - Present at birth; grow in proportion to the child and persist throughout life.
  - When located in the distribution of the ophthalmic branch (V_1) of the trigeminal nerve, carries an ↑ risk of ocular or intracranial abnormalities (Sturge-Weber syndrome).
- **Klippel-Trenaunay syndrome:** A vascular malformation characterized by an extensive port-wine stain involving a limb, underlying venous varicosities, soft tissue hypertrophy, and bone overgrowth.

DIAGNOSIS

Clinical.

TREATMENT

- **Hemangiomas:**
  - Most cases require no therapy.
  - Give prednisone (2–3 mg/kg) for hemangiomas that threaten vital structures (eyes, nares, ears, pharynx, larynx).
- **Port-wine stains:** Consider laser therapy.

CUTANEOUS TUMORS

Congenital Melanocytic Nevus

- Congenital proliferations of melanocytic nevus cells. Although most cases present at birth, some appear before 18 months of age. Associated with an ↑ risk of malignancy.
- Smaller lesions are associated with a lower risk of malignancy (1% lifetime risk for lesions < 1.5 cm).
- Risk is 5–10% with giant nevi (> 20 cm in diameter).

SYMPTOMS/EXAM

- Lesions may be flat, elevated, verrucous, or nodular and may be brown, blue, or black, appearing on the posterior trunk, head, and extremities.
- Some 30% of those on the posterior trunk are associated with leptomeningeal involvement.

DIAGNOSIS/TREATMENT

- Close clinical follow-up or excision.
  - For small nevi, consider size, location, the potential for scarring, and the overall risk of melanoma.
  - For giant nevi, repair with tissue expanders or grafting (often needed).
- Obtain an MRI of the brain and spinal cord for giant nevi overlying the head or spine to evaluate for neurocutaneous melanosis.

Acquired Melanocytic Nevus

- Acquired proliferations of melanocytes arising from the epidermal-dermal junction or the upper dermis. Lesions appear after 18 months of age, with the mean number by adulthood 25–35.
- Sx/Exam:
  - **Junctional nevi (90%):** Flat, nonpalpable brown lesions.
  - **Compound nevi:** Elevated pigmented lesions.
  - **Intradermal nevi:** Skin-colored, elevated lesions.
- Tx: Biopsy/removal if malignant transformation is a concern.

Melanoma

- Represents 1–3% of all pediatric malignancies. Risk factors include a ⊕ family history, xeroderma pigmentosum, fair complexion, excessive sun exposure, and immunosuppression. Associated with a 40% mortality rate.
- Sx/Exam: Red flags are as follows:
  - Asymmetry
  - Border irregularity
  - Color changes
  - Diameter > 6 mm
  - Enlarging

> **Melanoma red flags—ABCDE**
>
> **A**symmetry
> **B**order irregularity
> **C**olor changes
> **D**iameter > 6 mm
> **E**nlarging

Halo Nevus

- Sx/Exam: Development of a zone of depigmentation (halo) around a nevus with subsequent disappearance of the nevus over months (see Figure 5-15).
- Tx: Normally no treatment is necessary. A yearly skin exam is recommended for those with halo nevi to make sure there are no atypical moles or signs of malignant melanoma.

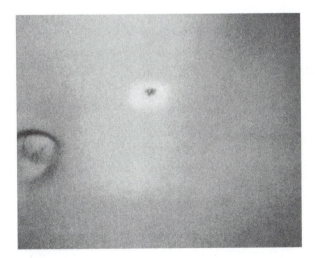

FIGURE 5-15. Halo nevus.

(Reproduced, with permission, from Weinberg S et al. *Color Atlas of Pediatric Dermatology*, 3rd ed. New York: McGraw-Hill, 1998:225.) (Also see Color Insert.)

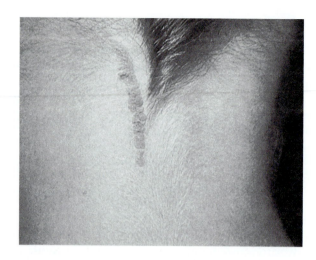

FIGURE 5-16. **Epidermal nevus.**

(Reproduced, with permission, from Weinberg S et al. *Color Atlas of Pediatric Dermatology*, 3rd ed. New York: McGraw-Hill, 1998:136.) (Also see Color Insert.)

Epidermal Nevus

- A hamartomatous lesion characterized by hyperplasia of the epidermis. The lesion is visible at birth or develops within the first years of life.
- **Sx/Exam:** A discolored, slightly scaly patch that becomes linear, verrucous, and hyperpigmented (see Figure 5-16).
- **Tx:** Consider full excision (often difficult) for symptomatic or cosmetic reasons.

Nevus Sebaceus (of Jadassohn)

- Carries a small risk of malignant transformation after puberty (basal cell carcinoma).
- **Sx/Exam:**
    - Presents as a well-demarcated, linear, hairless orange plaque occurring on the head and neck of infants.
    - During puberty, lesions become verrucous and nodular.
- **Tx:** Total excision before adolescence.

Mongolian Spots

- Benign collections of spindle-shaped melanocytes deep in the dermis. Result from arrest during migration from the neural crest to the epidermis. Common in darker-pigmented infants.
- **Sx/Exam:**
    - Slate-gray/blue macules over the lumbosacral areas and buttocks.
    - Present at birth but fade over the first two years of life.
- **Tx:** None.

Erythema Multiforme (EM)

An uncommon, acute, often recurrent inflammatory disease that commonly affects young males 18–30 years of age. Etiologies are as follows:

- **Sporadic EM:** HSV (60%), other infections.
- **Recurrent EM:** Recurrent HSV.

SYMPTOMS/EXAM

- Abrupt onset of dusky-red, round papules appearing in a symmetric pattern over the extensor aspects of the extremities (see Figure 5-17).
- Expands over 1–2 days into classic 1- to 3-cm "target" or "iris" lesions with an erythematous outer border, an inner pale zone, and a dusky, necrotic center.
- Individual lesions resolve in 1–2 weeks.
- Isolated oral lesions are seen in 70% of cases.

DIFFERENTIAL

- **Stevens-Johnson syndrome:** Skin and mucosal involvement are much more severe.
- **Urticaria:** Lesions migrate (vs. EM lesions, which persist for > 24 hours).
- HSV, other bullous disorders.

DIAGNOSIS

Clinical; consider DFA to rule out HSV.

TREATMENT

- Supportive; give emollients and antihistamines for itching.
- Corticosteroids have no proven benefit.
- Prophylactic oral acyclovir to prevent recurrences of HSV-associated EM.

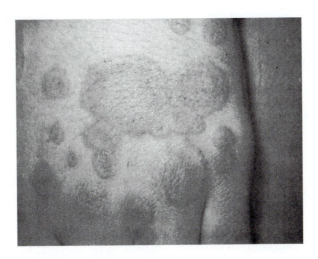

FIGURE 5-17. Erythema multiforme.

(Reproduced, with permission, from Weinberg S et al. *Color Atlas of Pediatric Dermatology*, 3rd ed. New York: McGraw-Hill, 1998:141.) (Also see Color Insert.)

Stevens-Johnson Syndrome

A severe vesiculobullous disease of the skin, mouth, eyes, and genitals that occurs primarily in children and young adults. Etiologies include drugs (anticonvulsants, sulfonamides, NSAIDs) and infections (*Mycoplasma pneumoniae*).

SYMPTOMS/EXAM

- Preceding symptoms of URI/pneumonia; fever.
- **Skin lesions:** Flat target lesions or purpuric macules over the trunk, palms, and soles, typically involving < 30% of the body.
- **Mucosal lesions:** Blisters and erosions of the conjunctivae and mucous membranes of the nares, mouth, anorectal junction, vaginal region, and urethral meatus.
- **Ocular symptoms:** Corneal ulcerations.

DIAGNOSIS

Consider skin biopsy if atypical.

TREATMENT

- **Supportive/symptomatic:** Antihistamines, anesthetic mouthwashes, analgesia, nutritional support.
- Consultation with an ophthalmologist.
- Antibiotics in the presence of a 2° infection.
- If uncomplicated, resolution can be expected in 4–6 weeks.

COMPLICATIONS

- Conjunctival scarring, uveitis, hematuria, bacterial superinfection, sepsis, urethral strictures.
- Associated with a 1–5% mortality rate.

Toxic Epidermal Necrolysis

Confluent areas of full-thickness loss of epidermis (> 30% BSA) with a high mortality rate. Has an incidence of 1.3 cases in a million annually; associated with a 35–50% mortality rate. Caused by drugs (antibiotics, anticonvulsants, NSAIDs).

SYMPTOMS/EXAM

- **Prodrome:** Fever; flulike symptoms.
- **Skin:** Diffuse, hot, painful erythema; ⊕ Nikolsky's sign (with slight thumb pressure, the skin wrinkles and slides laterally, separating from the dermis).
- **Mucous membranes:** Painful blistering and erosions of the oropharynx and vaginal mucosa.
- **Eyes:** Purulent conjunctivitis and painful ulceration.
- **Respiratory tract:** Dyspnea, hypoxemia, ↑ bronchial secretions, respiratory decompensation requiring ventilatory support.
- **Infection:** Sepsis and gram-⊖ pneumonia.
- Fluid and electrolyte loss.
- **Renal:** Hematuria, proteinuria, ↑ creatinine.

DIFFERENTIAL

Staphylococcal scalded skin syndrome; acute graft-versus-host disease following bone marrow transplantation.

DIAGNOSIS

Clinical; consider skin biopsy.

TREATMENT

- Discontinue the causative agent.
- Supportive care (as with severe burns).
- Consider IVIG, corticosteroids.

CAUSES OF HAIR LOSS IN CHILDREN

Alopecia Areata

- An autoimmune process affecting the hair follicles.
- **Sx:** Sudden onset of round, hairless patches, most often on the scalp, that are not associated with visible inflammation.
- **Exam:** Absent hair follicles; no erythema, scale, papules, or crust.
- **Ddx:** Tinea capitis, telogen effluvium, traction alopecia.
- **Dx:** Clinical.
- **Tx:** Topical corticosteroids. Most patients have regrowth of hair within 1–2 years; younger children have a more guarded prognosis than do adolescents and adults.

Telogen Effluvium

- Regression of hair follicles to a resting or telogen state in response to stress.
- **Sx:** Diffuse hair loss that is often evident only to the patient and family.
- **Exam:** Subtle diffuse hair loss is seen.
- **Dx:** Clinical.
- **Tx:** None. The disorder is self-limited; regrowth of hair takes place 3–5 months after resolution of the stressor.

Traction Alopecia

- Results from hairstyles that place too much tension on the hair follicles.
- **Sx:** Focal hair loss.
- **Exam:** Linear distribution of hair loss at the hairline or part line; noninflammatory.
- **Dx:** Clinical.
- **Tx:** Change to a looser hairstyle.

Trichotillomania

- Defined as conscious or unconscious pulling out of one's own hair.
- **Sx:** Irregular hair loss.
- **Exam:** Patches of incomplete hair loss with short broken hairs of various lengths; may involve the scalp, eyebrows, and eyelashes.
- **Dx:** Clinical.
- **Tx:** None. For refractory cases, consider psychiatric evaluation.

A four-year-old boy presents with patchy hair loss and scaly scalp. Physical examination reveals patches of scale and crust with broken hairs. A presumptive diagnosis of tinea capitis is made, and griseofulvin is prescribed. Two days later, the patient presents with a pruritic papular rash appearing primarily on the face, neck, and trunk. What is the most appropriate next step? Recommend topical steroids.

Tinea Capitis

- *Trichophyton tonsurans* accounts for > 90% of cases. The majority of children affected are 1–10 years of age (black > Hispanic > Caucasian).
- **Sx:** Presents with round patches of hair loss (partial or complete), scaling over the scalp, pruritus, and inflammatory masses (kerion).
- **Exam:**
  - The classic presentation consists of one or more areas of alopecia with inflammation and erythema.
  - May include a boggy, tender, erythematous, and edematous plaque (kerion) or pustules with crust and scale.
  - May be accompanied by a papular morbilliform rash (id reaction).
- **Dx:** ⊕ KOH prep, fungal culture.
- **Tx:** Oral therapy with griseofulvin × 6–12 weeks; adjunctive therapy with sporicidal shampoo (selenium sulfide 2.5%) to ↓ contagiousness.

CUTANEOUS MANIFESTATIONS OF SYSTEMIC DISEASE

Table 5-7 outlines common systemic diseases with dermatologic manifestations.

A six-year-old boy is referred to you for evaluation of café-au-lait macules. On exam, you notice three tan macules, each measuring 5 mm. The remainder of his physical exam is normal. What is the most appropriate next step? Reassure the parents.

MISCELLANEOUS

Urticaria

May be localized or generalized as well as acute or chronic. Etiologies include the following:

- Extravasation of fluid from capillaries and small venules due to ↑ permeability.
- Immunologic or nonimmunologic mast cell degranulation (infection; allergic reaction from drugs, foods, insect bites, contact allergens).

SYMPTOMS/EXAM

- Presents with a center of edema with a halo of erythema accompanied by peripheral extension and coalescence.

- Intensely pruritic.
- **Acute:** < 6 weeks.
- **Chronic:** > 6 weeks.

DIFFERENTIAL

- Mastocytosis, EM.
- **Papular urticaria:** Red, firm, urticarial papules with central puncta due to hypersensitivity to insect bites; lesions persist for several weeks.

TREATMENT

Elimination of the etiologic agent; symptomatic treatment with antihistamines.

Serum Sickness–Like Reaction

- A drug reaction mimicking serum sickness and characterized by urticaria, fever, lymphadenopathy, splenomegaly, and arthritis; immune complexes are absent. Drugs involved include cefaclor and penicillin.
- **Sx/Exam:** Urticaria (90%).
- **Tx:** Antihistamines and analgesics.

TABLE 5-7. Cutaneous Manifestations of Systemic Disease

Tuberous sclerosis	**Ash leaf macules:** Oval, hypopigmented lesions best visualized with Wood's light. **Sebaceous adenomas** (see Figure 5-18): Tiny red nodules over the nose and cheeks (resemble acne). **Shagreen patch:** A rough, raised lesion with orange-peel texture in the lumbosacral region. Subungual/periungual fibromas.
Sturge-Weber disease	Port-wine stain (nevus flammeus) involving the distribution of the ophthalmic division of the trigeminal nerve.
Neurofibromatosis (NF)	**Café-au-lait macules** (see Figure 5-19): Large, oval, light brown macules (found in 10–20% of the normal population). A presumptive diagnosis of NF should be made in the presence of > 6 lesions > 5 mm in diameter. Axillary or inguinal freckling. ≥ 2 **Lisch nodules:** Hamartomas of the iris. ≥ 2 **neurofibromas:** Small rubbery papules; frequently involve skin and appear during adolescence. **Plexiform neurofibroma:** Evident at birth; often located in the orbital or temporal region of the face.
Wiskott-Aldrich syndrome	Eczematous dermatitis.
Ataxia-telangiectasia	Telangiectasias of the bulbar conjunctiva (see Figure 5-20), neck, upper chest, face, and pinna (first appear at 3–6 years of age). Large café-au-lait macules; eczematous or seborrheic dermatitis.
Xeroderma pigmentosum	Freckling, telangiectasias, cutaneous malignancies.
Histiocytosis	Seborrhea-like eruption of the diaper area or scalp with petechiae/small hemorrhages.

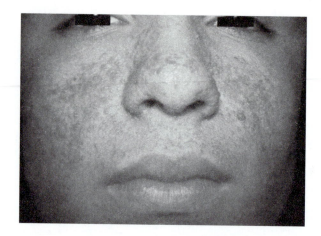

FIGURE 5-18. **Sebaceous adenomas.**

(Reproduced, with permission, from Weinberg S et al. *Color Atlas of Pediatric Dermatology*, 3rd ed. New York: McGraw-Hill, 1998:124.) (Also see Color Insert.)

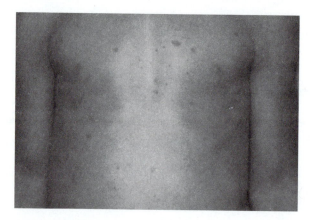

FIGURE 5-19. **Café-au-lait macules.**

(Reproduced, with permission, from Weinberg S et al. *Color Atlas of Pediatric Dermatology*, 3rd ed. New York: McGraw-Hill, 1998:122.) (Also see Color Insert.)

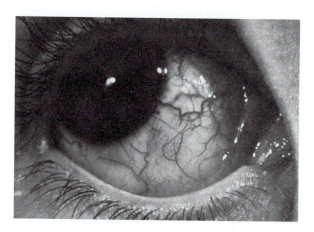

FIGURE 5-20. **Telangiectasias of the bulbar conjunctiva.**

(Reproduced, with permission, from Weinberg S et al. *Color Atlas of Pediatric Dermatology*, 3rd ed. New York: McGraw-Hill, 1998:117.) (Also see Color Insert.)

Mastocytosis

- Accumulation of mast cells in the skin and/or other organs. Some 75% of cases have an onset before two years of age. The etiology is unknown. The prognosis is good if onset occurs during childhood.
- Sx/Exam:
    - More than 90% have a $\oplus$ Darier's sign—localized urticaria after gentle irritation due to degranulation of mast cells.
    - **Solitary mastocytoma:** A localized, 1- to 5-cm flesh-colored nodule on the arms/neck/trunk; spontaneous resolution occurs by age 10.
    - **Urticaria pigmentosa:** Multiple hyperpigmented macules and papules on the trunk (see Figure 5-21). Onset is in the first year of life; 75% of cases have spontaneous resolution by adulthood. Occasional systemic involvement is seen.

Ichthyosis

- Hereditary skin disorders characterized by excessive scale.
- Sx/Exam:
    - **Ichthyosis vulgaris:** Fine scale; deep markings of the palms and soles (see Figure 5-22). The most common form of ichthyosis.
    - **X-linked ichthyosis:** Large, brown scale; occurs in males.
- Tx: Ammonium lactate 12% to restore hydration and control scale.

Acne Vulgaris

- A disorder of the pilosebaceous unit that primarily affects adolescents and young adults. Due to ↑ sebum production, obstruction of follicles with subsequent proliferation of *Propionibacterium acnes*, and inflammatory response.
- Sx/Exam:
    - **Open comedones:** Blackheads.
    - **Closed comedones:** Whiteheads.
    - **Inflammatory acne:** Pustules.

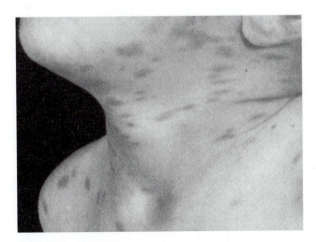

FIGURE 5-21. Urticaria pigmentosa.

(Reproduced, with permission, from Weinberg S et al. *Color Atlas of Pediatric Dermatology*, 3rd ed. New York: McGraw-Hill, 1998:186.) (Also see Color Insert.)

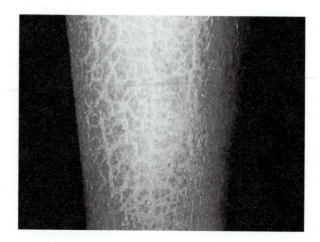

FIGURE 5-22. Ichthyosis vulgaris.

(Reproduced, with permission, from Weinberg S et al. *Color Atlas of Pediatric Dermatology,* 3rd ed. New York: McGraw-Hill, 1998:128.) (Also see Color Insert.)

- **Tx:**
  - **Comedones:** Topical retinoid or azelaic acid.
  - **Superficial pustules and papules:** Benzoyl peroxide or topical antibiotics.
  - **Deep pustules and papules:** Oral antibiotics.
  - Lesions start as papules that then undergo central involution and peripheral extension to form rings 1–5 cm in diameter with clear centers and elevated borders.
  - **Nodular acne:** Isotretinoin.
  - Consider OCPs for females.

> A four-year-old girl visits a clinic for a well-child checkup. Her mother's only concern is a persistent rash on her daughter's hand that was initially diagnosed as ringworm but has not improved with OTC antifungal therapy. You notice a single, 1.5-cm, flesh-colored circular plaque with a thickened, raised rim of small papules on the dorsum of her hand. What is the most likely diagnosis? Granuloma annulare.

Granuloma Annulare

- **Sx/Exam:**
  - Presents with papules grouped in a ringlike distribution on the lateral or dorsal surfaces of the hands or feet.
  - Lesions start as papules that then undergo central involutionand peripheral extension to form rings 1–5 cm in diameter with clear centers and elevated borders.
  - No scale is present.
- **Ddx:** Tinea.
- **Tx:** Spontaneous resolution; no treatment is necessary.

Emergency and Critical Care Medicine

Karin Salim, MD
reviewed by Anil Sapru, MD

A two-year-old girl is rushed into the ER in her mother's arms. As the nurses transfer her to the gurney, her mother exclaims, "She was eating a hot dog and started choking and then stopped breathing." The child is cyanotic and apneic. What is your next step? What equipment will you need? By following ABCs (airway, breathing, circulation) plus monitors, you successfully use a Macintosh laryngoscope and a Magill forceps to directly visualize and remove a piece of hot dog obstructing the patient's trachea.

Airway obstruction is the leading cause of pediatric cardiopulmonary arrest.

Airway

- Establish an airway using a head-tilt/chin-lift maneuver and rule out airway obstruction. A jaw-thrust maneuver should be performed and cervical spine stability maintained if cervical spine injury is suspected.
- **Assisted airway options** are as follows:
    - **Oral airway:** Poorly tolerated in conscious patients with gag reflex.
    - **Nasopharyngeal airway:** May be tolerated in conscious patients.
    - **Laryngeal mask airway:** Aspiration will not be prevented, but allows for assisted ventilation.
    - **Endotracheal intubation.**
- Devices with which to improve oxygenation include the following:
    - **Nasal cannulae:** May be poorly tolerated in toddlers; delivers an O_2 concentration of only 25–30%.
    - **Oxygen hood or tent:** Better tolerated by toddlers; able to deliver up to 50% O_2 concentration.
    - **Simple face mask:** Delivers up to 40% O_2.
    - **Nonrebreather face mask:** Capable of delivering 80–100% O_2.
- **Intubation:**
    - Use a straight (Miller) or curved (Macintosh) laryngoscope blade.
    - Suction with a large-diameter catheter should be available.
    - Verify endotracheal tube placement by utilizing **end-tidal CO_2 detection** (absent if no pulmonary circulation), chest rise, auscultation, and CXR.

Estimate the uncuffed endotracheal tube internal-diameter size with the equation (age + 16)/4.

Bradycardia is defined as a heart rate < 60 bpm in a child and < 100 bpm in a newborn.

Breathing

- Bag-mask ventilation should be initiated when appropriate respiration is not occurring.
- The stomach should be decompressed with an orogastric or NG tube.

Circulation

- Evaluate the heart rate.
- Assess the quality of perfusion by evaluating pulses and capillary refill (carotid in children and adults; brachial or femoral in infants and the newborn).
- Determine the blood pressure (BP).
- If pulseless or bradycardic with poor systemic perfusion, initiate chest compression (see Table 6-1).

Hypotension is defined as:

- *Neonates: SBP < 60*
- *Infants: SBP < 70*
- *One year of age and beyond:*

  SBP < [70 + (2 × age)]

- Fluid resuscitation should not be delayed.
- Central venous access should be attempted if the child is > 8 years of age or intraosseous placement is unsuccessful.
- An initial volume of 20 mL/kg is given over 5–15 minutes. Additional boluses may be needed if there is no improvement. Consider additional pharmacologic agents as well. Be cautious with fluid replacement if a cardiac etiology is suspected.

Intraosseous access should be utilized if peripheral IV attempts are unsuccessful after 90 seconds.

Pediatric Advanced Life Support (PALS) Algorithms

Algorithms for advanced life support in pediatric patients are as follows:

- **Pulseless arrest** (see Figure 6-1): Support ABCs and consider potential causes. Remember the possible causes using the mnemonic **4 H's and 4 T's.**
- **Bradycardia** (see Figure 6-2): Evaluate the patient for degree of cardiorespiratory compromise and consider possible etiologies using the mnemonic **5 H's and a T.** If perfusion is adequate despite the heart rate, continue supportive measures while performing an evaluation and making appropriate interventions. If the patient shows compromise such as hypotension, respiratory distress, altered mental status, or poor perfusion, additional pharmacologic intervention is warranted.
- **Tachycardia** (see Figure 6-3): Perfusion should be assessed during the ABCs of resuscitation; obtain an ECG. Etiologies include **5 HTP.**
    - A widened QRS suggests VT, whereas a narrow QRS is likely sinus tachycardia or supraventricular tachycardia (SVT).
    - Sinus tachycardia can be distinguished from SVT by the rate and rhythm, although both are characterized by a narrow QRS. In sinus tachycardia, the rate varies with activity and rarely exceeds 220 bpm in an infant or 180 bpm in a child. In contrast, SVT does not show variability in heart rate; the rate exceeds the limits seen in sinus tachycardia; and p waves are absent.

Causes of pulseless arrest—4 H's and 4 T's

Hypoxemia
Hypovolemia
Hypothermia
Hyper- or **H**ypokalemia
Tension pneumothorax
Toxins
Thromboembolism
Tamponade

TABLE 6-1. Guidelines for Basic Life Support

	NEWBORN	INFANTS (< 1 YEAR)	CHILDREN (1–8 YEARS)	OLDER CHILDREN (> 8 YEARS)
Anatomic landmark	A finger width below the intermammary line.	A finger width below the intermammary line.	Lower half of the sternum.	Lower half of the sternum.
Method	2–3 fingers or two thumbs around the chest.	2–3 fingers or two thumbs around the chest.	Heel of a hand.	Heel of a hand.
Depth	One-third to one-half of chest depth or 0.5–1.0 inch.	One-third to one-half of chest depth or 0.5–1.0 inch.	One-third to one-half of chest depth or 0.5–1.0 inch.	One-third to one-half of chest depth or 1.5–2 inches.
Compression rate	120/min	100/min	100/min	100/min
Compressions to breaths	15:2	15:2	15:2	15:2

Causes of severe bradycardia—5 H's and a T

Head injury
Hypoxemia
Hypothermia
Heart block
Heart transplant
Toxins

Causes of severe tachycardia—5 HTP

Head injury
Hypoxemia
Hyperthermia
Heart block
Heart transplant
Toxins
Pain

Drugs that may be given via endotracheal tube—LEAN

Lidocaine
Epinephrine
Atropine
Naloxone

Taken together, unintentional and intentional injuries are responsible for more childhood morbidity and mortality than all other disease states combined.

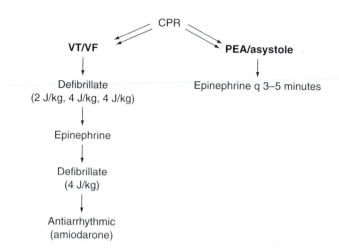

FIGURE 6-1. **Algorithm for the treatment of pulseless arrest.**

Rapid-Sequence Intubation (RSI)

- Defined as rapid induction of anesthesia to facilitate intubation by rendering the patient unconscious and providing muscle relaxation. Forceful bag-mask ventilation is minimized to prevent abdominal distention and aspiration of gastric contents.
- Careful and appropriate use of sedatives/analgesics involves an understanding of the pharmacologic properties and side effects of such drugs (see Table 6-2).
- Paralytics include depolarizing agents such as succinylcholine (a fast-acting agent, but can raise ICP and cause hyperkalemia) and nondepolarizing agents such as rocuronium and vecuronium.

TRAUMA

Prevention

- Head injury accounts for the most pediatric deaths and is the principal determinant of outcome in trauma survivors.

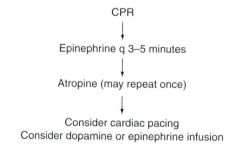

FIGURE 6-2. **Algorithm for the treatment of bradycardia with cardiorespiratory compromise.**

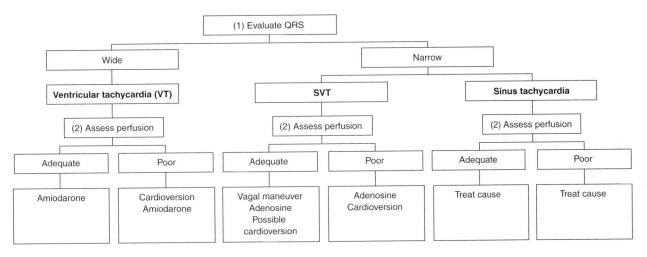

FIGURE 6-3. Algorithm for the treatment of tachycardia.

- The most frequent mechanism for injury is blunt rather than penetrating trauma.

1° Survey or Resuscitation Phase

Follow the basic **ABCDEs** of resuscitation with attention to issues that may arise 2° to trauma:

Motor vehicle accidents are the leading cause of injury-related mortality in all pediatric age groups.

- **Airway** should include cervical spine stabilization.
- **Breathing** must include assessment for life-threatening injuries such as hemo- or pneumothorax, flail chest, or CNS derangement.
- **Circulation** may require additional IV access, and any external hemorrhage should be controlled with direct pressure. Life-threatening injuries

TABLE 6-2. Sedatives and Analgesics Used in RSI

DRUG	CV	ICP	PROS	CONS
Benzodiazepines	May ↓ BP	—	Anticonvulsant, amnestic.	Respiratory depression.
Etomidate	—	↓	Anticonvulsant.	Nausea/vomiting, no analgesia, myoclonic movements, possible adrenal suppression.
Ketamine	—	↑	**Bronchodilator,** amnestic, analgesic; preserves spontaneous respirations.	↑ secretions, laryngospasm, emergence reaction.
Thiopental	↓ BP	↓	Anticonvulsant; blunts sympathetic response to intubation.	BP effect, **histamine release (bronchospasm),** respiratory depression.
Propofol	↓ BP	↓	Anticonvulsant, amnestic.	Hypotension.
Narcotics	May ↓ BP	Variable	Analgesia, reversible.	Chest wall rigidity (fentanyl), respiratory depression.

such as cardiac tamponade or massive internal hemorrhage must be considered.

- **Disability** necessitates a focused neurologic exam that includes assessment of pupil size and reactivity as well as level of consciousness.
- **Exposure** means removing a patient's clothing while still maintaining a normal temperature.

2° Survey or Thorough Examination Phase

- **Head:** Perform a "HEADS" exam for **H**emotympanum, **E**xternal wounds, **A**bnormal discharge (CNS leak), **D**ental injuries, or **S**kull fracture.
- **Spine:** No patient should be cleared unless the neurologic exam is normal, there are no distracting injuries, and imaging is normal.
    - Spinal cord injury without radiographic abnormality (SCIWORA) is unique to pediatrics and accounts for up to 20% of all pediatric spinal cord injuries.
    - Because a younger patient's vertebral column is not completely calcified, it can transiently deform and allow stretching of the cord or nerve without any radiographic abnormality.
    - The clinical clue is a child with a clear neurologic defect that has changed or resolved upon reassessment.
- **Thorax:** Rib fractures, pneumothorax, hemothorax, diaphragmatic rupture, or pulmonary contusion can occur. Definitive imaging may be necessary. Associated with high morbidity and mortality.
- **Abdomen:** CT scan is the diagnostic modality of choice (vs. peritoneal lavage). A fall across handlebars can lead to gastric injuries or duodenal hematoma. Splenic and hepatic injuries are also relatively common in children, but management is conservative in the stable patient given the postsplenectomy risks in this age group.
- **Pelvis:** Evaluate for instability or crepitus. A urinary catheter should not be placed if a pelvic fracture is suspected.
- **GU:** Defer placing a urinary catheter if urethral transection is suspected, which may be the case with a pelvic fracture. Blood at the external meatus requires additional studies before any manipulation of the urethra is initiated. Consider renal damage for injuries to the flank or back.
- **Extremities:** A careful evaluation of all extremities must be conducted, including assessment of pulses and sensation. Imaging must be reviewed for subtle growth plate disruption.
    - Pain out of proportion to injury raises suspicion of **compartment syndrome.**
    - Early findings include pain with palpation and ↑ pain with passive movement. Muscle weakness and/or ↓ sensation are late findings. Pulses are often palpable unless there is an associated vascular disruption.
- **Neurologic:** Traumatic brain injury is classified by the Glasgow Coma Scale (GCS) as mild (GCS 13–15), moderate (GCS 8–12), or severe (GCS 3–7); see Table 6-3. Intubation is generally indicated when the GCS is < 8. If the patient is unconscious, preverbal, or intubated, the motor response value is the most important for prognosis.

TABLE 6-3. Glasgow Coma Scale Scoring

	INFANT	CHILD	SCORE
Eye opening	Spontaneous	Spontaneous	4
	To verbal stimuli	To verbal stimuli	3
	To pain only	To pain only	2
	No response	No response	1
Verbal response	Coos and babbles	Appropriate	5
	Irritable cry	Confused	4
	Cries to pain	Inappropriate words	3
	Moans to pain	Incomprehensible sounds	2
	No response	No response	1
Motor response	Spontaneous movement	Obeys commands	6
	Withdraws to touch	Localizes pain	5
	Withdraws to pain	Withdraws to pain	4
	Flexion response to pain	Flexion response to pain	3
	Extensor response to pain	Extensor response to pain	2
	No response	No response	1

EMERGENCY AND CRITICAL CARE MEDICINE

Poison control consultation is recommended for all poisonings. Providing parents with the Poison Control phone number at well-child visits can speed appropriate management.

ACUTE POISONINGS AND INGESTIONS

Management Options

See Table 6-4. Use caution with any GI decontaminant in a patient with altered mental status or a loss of airway reflexes.

TABLE 6-4. Management of Acute Poisonings and Ingestions

TREATMENT	INDICATIONS	MECHANISM OF ACTION	DOSING AND ADMINISTRATION	CONTRAINDICATIONS	NOT TO BE USED WITH
Activated charcoal	Emergency decontamination of any substance that can be bound by charcoal.	Adsorbs toxins, thereby preventing systemic absorption.	1 g/kg PO or NG **or** 10 g charcoal per gram of drug ingested. **Note:** Repeat dose if emesis occurs within one hour of the first dose. Can be repeated q 2–4 h.	Any risk of aspiration. Any anatomical or physical obstruction of the GI tract (e.g., ileus).	**CHEMICAL CAMP:** Cyanide Hydrocarbon Ethanol Metals Iron Caustics Airway Lithium CAMphor Potassium

TABLE 6-4. Management of Acute Poisonings and Ingestions *(continued)*

TREATMENT	INDICATIONS	MECHANISM OF ACTION	DOSING AND ADMINISTRATION	CONTRAINDICATIONS	NOT TO BE USED WITH
Gastric lavage	Emergency treatment of a recent ingestion (e.g., < 1 hour) and/or patients who are obtunded.	Removal of ingestus.	Lavage with NS via NG/orogastric tube until gastric contents are cleared.	Ingestion of foreign material with sharp edges. Any risk of aspiration (consider intubation to protect airway, especially if the patient is obtunded).	Hydrocarbons, caustics.
Ipecac	Home treatment of recent ingestion (< 30 min) in consultation with Poison Control.		**6–12 months:** 10 mL. **1–12 years:** 15 mL. **> 12 years:** 30 mL. **Note:** Can cause drowsiness.	Any history of hematemesis. Preexisting or potential for altered mental status. Risk or potential risk of airway compromise. Bleeding disorder.	**4 C's:** **C**omatose **C**onvulsing **C**orrosive Hydro**C**arbon
Whole bowel irrigation	In an emergency setting when charcoal is not effective (e.g., packets of illegal substances).		Polyethylene glycol (PEG) electrolyte lavage via an NG tube at a continuous rate for 4–6 hours or until rectal output is clear.	GI disorders, including bleeding and obstruction. Any risk of aspiration (the procedure should be done with the patient intubated).	
Urinary alkalinization	As an adjunct to GI decontamination.	Enhances the elimination of weak acids such as barbiturates, methotrexate, TCAs, and salicylates.	IV fluids with the addition of bicarbonate at 1.5–2.0 times maintenance to goal of urine pH of 7–8.	Preexisting electrolyte disturbances; renal failure.	
Hemodialysis	As an adjunct to GI decontamination.	Removes small substances such as lithium, alcohols, aspirin, theophylline, and phenobarbital.	Consult with a nephrologist.		

Specific Poisonings

Table 6-5 outlines treatment guidelines for specific poisonings.

TABLE 6-5. Management and Treatment of Specific Poisonings

POISONING	TOXIDROME	MANAGEMENT AND TREATMENT
Acetaminophen (the most common overdose in children < 6 years of age)	Evaluate any child receiving > 150 mg/kg/dose: ■ **0–24 hours:** Nausea, vomiting. ■ **24–36 hours:** Nausea and vomiting improve but clinical evidence of hepatic impairment begins, as indicated by an ↑ in INR and AST.	Charcoal decontamination (avoid use within one hour of *N*-acetylcysteine). Gastric lavage if ingestion is large. Serum level at four hours postingestion is the most accurate predictor of hepatic toxicity. *N*-acetylcysteine is the mainstay of treatment; guided by nomogram.
Aspirin	Presents with nausea, vomiting, low-grade fever, tinnitus, and seizures; can progress to lethargy, cerebral edema, pulmonary edema, and coma. Anion-gap metabolic acidosis, respiratory alkalosis.	Decontaminate with charcoal or gastric lavage. Monitor serum levels, especially the six-hour level (for prognosis and need for hemodialysis). Alkalinize urine. Hemodialysis in severe situations.
Anticholinergics (including TCAs and carbamazepine)	**"Mad as a hatter, red as a beet, blind as a bat, hot as a hare, dry as a bone."** Delirium, hallucinations, flushing, tachycardia, blurred vision, mydriasis, fever, thirst, dry mucous membranes, ileus, urinary retention. **TCAs = 3 C's and an A: C**ardiac (prolonged PR and QRS intervals, life-threatening dysrhythmias), **C**oma, **C**onvulsions, **A**cidosis (metabolic).	Activated charcoal early; consider gastric lavage. Benzodiazepines for agitation. Physostigmine with significant ingestions. Sodium bicarbonate for acidosis caused by TCA ingestion.
β-blockers	Respiratory depression, bronchospasm, hypotension, bradydysrhythmias, hypoglycemia, seizures, altered mental status, coma.	Activated charcoal or whole bowel irrigation (especially for sustained-release formulations); consider gastric lavage. Glucagon to reverse bradycardia, hypotension, and hypoglycemia. Sympathomimetics if bradycardia persists; may require pacing.
Calcium channel blockers	Hypotension, bradycardia, hyperglycemia, seizures, altered mental status, coma.	Activated charcoal or whole bowel irrigation (especially sustained-release formulations); consider gastric lavage. Give calcium if bradycardia and/or hypotension is present. Glucagon can be given if patients are unresponsive to supportive measures.

TABLE 6-5. **Management and Treatment of Specific Poisonings** *(continued)*

EMERGENCY AND
CRITICAL CARE MEDICINE

POISONING	TOXIDROME	MANAGEMENT AND TREATMENT
Caustics	Airway complaints: stridor, drooling, dyspnea, chest pain. Nausea, vomiting. Patients may be asymptomatic early in the course.	Airway management, CXR to evaluate for perforation, NPO. Consider steroids if airway is compromised.
Digoxin	Therapeutic serum levels 0.5–2.0 ng/mL. Rhythm disturbances (multiple types), nausea, vomiting, lethargy, seizures, visual changes, electrolyte abnormalities.	Decontaminate with activated charcoal. Monitor and treat electrolyte imbalances; calcium can potentiate rhythm disturbances and should be avoided. Digoxin-specific Fab in the presence of cardiovascular instability, rhythm disturbances, or hyperkalemia.
Hydrocarbons (aliphatic: gasoline, kerosene, mineral oil, lighter fluid; aromatic: benzene, turpentine; halogenated)	Airway complaints: dyspnea, tachypnea, cyanosis, grunting, cough, wheezing. Lethargy, seizures, coma, vomiting, hepatic toxicity, cardiac instability, fever. **A**liphatic = **A**spiration (greatest risk for pulmonary disease). **A**romatic = **A**re systemic (greatest risk for systemic disease).	**Avoid** charcoal, emesis, or lavage 2° to aspiration concerns. Protective intubation may be needed. Observe for a minimum of six hours. CXR lags 4–6 hours behind clinical symptoms. Can progress to a chemical pneumonitis, hypoxia, and ARDS. Prophylactic steroids may be given; antibiotics are not recommended.
Iron	Four stages: ■ **30 minutes – 6 hours:** GI toxicity. ■ **6–24 hours:** Latent; relative stability. ■ **6–48 hours:** Systemic toxicity (acidosis, hepatic compromise, hypoglycemia, bleeding, coma). ■ **4–8 weeks:** Late complications (GI stenosis, strictures).	Obtain CXR/KUB if ingested pills are radiopaque. Obtain level 2–4 hours postingestion. If the patient ingested < 20 mg/kg, treatment is supportive only. For unknown quantities or 20–60 mg/kg, consider ipecac. If the patient ingested > 60 mg/kg, consider gastric lavage or whole bowel irrigation. Deferoxamine if significant clinical symptoms and/or serum levels > 500 µg/dL.
Methanol, ethylene glycol	Both have an ↑ anion gap **and** an ↑ osmolar gap. Methanol ingestion may present with visual complaints. Ethylene glycol can cause hypocalcemia.	Rapidly absorbed, so charcoal is not effective. Use fomepizole if levels are > 20 mg/dL and/or there is a metabolic acidosis with a high anion gap. Ethanol should be considered with caution when fomepizole is unavailable. Can progress to renal failure requiring dialysis.

TABLE 6-5. Management and Treatment of Specific Poisonings *(continued)*

POISONING	TOXIDROME	MANAGEMENT AND TREATMENT
Methemoglobinemia	Clinical symptoms depend on the percent methemoglobin: ■ **< 10%:** No symptoms. ■ **10–20%:** Cyanosis. ■ **20–30%:** Tachycardia, headache, agitation. ■ **30–50%:** Lethargy, confusion, dyspnea. ■ **50–70%:** Stupor, seizures, acidosis, severe dyspnea. ■ **> 70%:** Death.	Normal Pao_2 and normal O_2 saturation, but abnormal oximetry O_2 saturation. If level > 30%, give methylene blue. Hyperbaric oxygen and exchange transfusion have been used in severe cases.
Opiates	**DOPE: D**ecreased respiratory drive, **O**btunded, **P**inpoint pupils, **E**uphoria. Also ↓ bowel sounds.	Naloxone has a short half-life, can be given via endotracheal tube, and can precipitate withdrawal in chronic opiate users.
Organophosphates	Cholinergic symptoms—**DUMBBELS: D**iarrhea, **U**rination, **M**iosis, **B**radycardia, **B**ronchospasm, **E**mesis, **L**acrimation, **S**alivation. Also hypotonia, hyporeflexia, hypertension, seizures, and bradycardia.	Decontaminate by removing clothing. Consider charcoal or lavage. Measure plasma or RBC pseudocholinesterase activity. Administer atropine and pralidoxime.
Phenothiazine	Altered mental status, miosis, hypotension, extrapyramidal symptoms, neuroleptic malignant syndrome, ECG changes.	Activated charcoal decontamination. Obtain an ECG. Extrapyramidal symptoms can be treated with diphenhydramine. Supportive measures for neuroleptic malignant syndrome; also consider dantrolene.
Theophylline	Emesis, GI bleeding, cardiovascular instability, dysrhythmias, acidosis, hypokalemia, hyperglycemia, altered mental status.	Activated charcoal decontamination. Obtain serial serum levels. Monitor electrolytes. Hemodialysis.

EMERGENCY AND CRITICAL CARE MEDICINE

Specific Antidotes

Table 6-6 lists antidotes for specific poisons.

Foreign Body Aspiration

Foreign body aspiration is one of the leading causes of death in children < 5 years of age and accounts for 10% of deaths in infants < 1 year of age.

SYMPTOMS/EXAM

■ Commonly aspirated objects include peanuts, hot dogs, vegetables, popcorn, seeds, toys, crayons, and coins.
■ Depending on object size and location, patients may exhibit drooling, stridor, wheezing, respiratory distress, or chest pain.

*The anion gap and the osmolar gap are useful adjuncts in the diagnosis of toxidromes. Anion gap = serum [**Na⁺**] − [(**Cl⁻**) + (**HCO₃⁻**)]. Osmolar gap = measured serum osmolality − calculated serum osmolality (2 × [Na⁺] + glucose/18 + BUN/2.8)*

TABLE 6-6. Antidotes for Specific Agents

ANTIDOTE	POISONING TREATED	MECHANISM
N-acetylcysteine	Acetaminophen	Restores hepatic stores of glutathione and/or inhibits toxic metabolites.
Fomepizole	Methanol and ethylene glycol	Inhibits alcohol dehydrogenase to ↓ the formation of toxic metabolites.
Ethanol	Methanol and ethylene glycol	Ethanol competitively inhibits the metabolism of methanol; consider using folate as well to ↑ formic acid elimination.
Physostigmine	Anticholinergics	Prolongs the effects of acetylcholine by blocking cholinesterase activity.
Atropine	Organophosphates	Blocks acetylcholine activity.
Pralidoxime	Organophosphates	Reactivates cholinesterases to ↓ acetylcholine activity.
Glucagon	β-blockers	Inotropic and chronotropic effects as well as prevention of hypoglycemia.
Digoxin-specific Fab	Digitalis	Binds unbound digitalis and promotes renal excretion of bound drug.
Flumazenil	Benzodiazepines	Antagonist at GABA/benzodiazepine-specific receptor
Deferoxamine	Iron	Complexes with trivalent ionic form to be renally excreted.
Methylene blue	Methemoglobinemia Cyanide	Speeds conversion of methemoglobin to hemoglobin. Forms a complex with cyanide that cannot interact with the cytochrome system.
Naloxone	Opiates	Receptor antagonist.
Calcium	Calcium channel blockers	Restores calcium levels.
Vitamin K	Warfarin	Restores vitamin K–dependent coagulation factors.

DIAGNOSIS

- Obtain a CXR and a lateral neck film. Radiopaque objects are visible on x-ray, while radiolucent object are not (but the effect on the local anatomy may be evident).
- Inspiratory and expiratory or lateral decubitus films can be helpful, as there will be air trapping on the involved side and shifting of the trachea to the opposite side.

TREATMENT

- Bronchoscopy should be performed if the patient is in significant distress. For the patient with acute and near- or complete obstruction, promptly perform the ABCs. If the patient is in distress, the Heimlich maneuver or back blows/abdominal thrusts (depending on patient age) should be performed.

- Esophageal foreign bodies frequently lodge at one of three sites: the thoracic inlet, the aortic arch (origin of the left mainstem bronchus), or the gastroesophageal junction. Lodged objects often require endoscopic retrieval. Objects in or distal to the stomach may be managed with observation.
- Ingestion of a battery can cause GI burns; batteries should thus be retrieved if lodged in the esophagus. If the battery is past the esophagus, the patient may be observed for passage of the battery.

INJURIES

Wound Care and Suturing

- Copious and high-pressure irrigation of a wound prior to suturing is mandatory. Injuries to the face, lip (especially if the vermillion border is involved), hands, genitals, or periorbital area may require consultation with a specialist.
- Bite wounds should be sutured only if they are in an area of cosmetic concern or on the hand or foot.
- Puncture wounds are of special concern given the high risk for infection (e.g., cellulitis or osteomyelitis) and retained foreign body.
  - In general, a radiograph should be obtained followed by cleaning, debridement, and removal of any foreign body.
  - *Pseudomonas aeruginosa* is the most common cause of osteomyelitis following a puncture wound to the foot.
  - Many advocate administration of prophylactic antibiotics, and close follow-up is advised.
- Sutures should be removed as soon as possible to prevent scarring or infection.
- Tetanus prophylaxis should be considered (see below).

Tetanus Immunoprophylaxis

The patient's tetanus status must be addressed with all wounds and injuries (see Table 6-7). For children < 7 years of age, DTaP is given; Td is given for all children ≥ 7 years of age.

TABLE 6-7. Guidelines for Tetanus Prophylaxis

PRIOR TETANUS DOSES	CLEAN, MINOR WOUND		ALL OTHER WOUNDS	
	VACCINE	TIG[a]	VACCINE	TIG
Unknown or < 3	Yes	No	Yes	Yes
3+, last < 5 years ago	No	No	No	No
3+, last 5–10 years ago	No	No	Yes	Yes
3+, last > 10 years ago	Yes	No	Yes	No

[a]TIG = tetanus immunoglobulin.

Burns

SYMPTOMS/EXAM

- Presentation varies according to the degree of burn.
  - **First-degree burns** involve only the epidermis and are painful and erythematous on examination.
  - **Second-degree** or **partial-thickness burns** extend into the dermis. Superficial second-degree burns are painful and blister, while deep second-degree burns are white and painless. Note that any blistering constitutes a second-degree burn.
  - **Third-degree** or **full-thickness burns** extend through the dermis into the subcutaneous tissues. These burns are pale, charred, and painless.
- Burns may result from a flame, scald, chemical, electrical, or cold exposure injury.
  - **Flame injuries:** Most common.
  - **Electrical injury:** Can lead to muscle damage and fatal cardiac arrhythmias; should be evaluated for exit-site injuries.
  - Suspect child abuse if the burn pattern is not consistent with the child's developmental age or with the history or mechanism of injury.
- **Inhalation injury** can cause carbon monoxide poisoning.
  - Blood carboxyhemoglobin levels and arterial oxygen tension should be assessed.
  - Pulse oximetry may read as normal, since carboxyhemoglobin, like methemoglobin, absorbs light at the same wavelength as oxyhemoglobin.
  - Cyanide poisoning is another potential problem if combustible industrial materials are inhaled.

TREATMENT

- For burns involving > 15% of total body surface area or smoke inhalation injury, IV fluids should be initiated promptly and fluid status closely monitored owing to high insensible water losses.
- If initiated promptly, cooling the patient provides analgesia and reduces the severity of the burn. Any chemical burn should be promptly treated with removal of affected clothing and lavage of the area.
- Criteria for hospitalization include partial-thickness burns > 10%, any full-thickness burns, areas of injury at high risk for poor cosmetic outcome and/or disability (e.g., facial, circumferential), evidence of smoke inhalation injury, significant pain, or suspected child abuse.
- Tetanus status should be reviewed and immunoprophylaxis given if indicated.
- The mainstays of outpatient management are cleansing, pain control, and topical antibiotics (e.g., silver sulfadiazine, bacitracin).

Drowning and Near-Drowning

- **Drowning** is a term used to describe death due to asphyxia that occurs within 24 hours of the submersion event. **Near-drowning** is characterized by survival for > 24 hours.
- Risk factors include age, male gender, substance abuse, warm weather, lack of adult supervision, lack of safety barriers enclosing a body of water, and predisposing medical conditions (e.g., mental retardation, epilepsy).
- Age distribution is bimodal, with peaks in children 1–4 years of age and in adolescents 15–19 years of age.

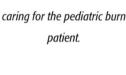

Approximately 20% of all pediatric burns are inflicted; hence, a high suspicion of child abuse is indicated in caring for the pediatric burn patient.

Any patient with a large burn or a burn acquired in an enclosed space should be assumed to have an inhalation injury while further examination and evaluation is performed.

EMERGENCY AND CRITICAL CARE MEDICINE

- The most important determinant of outcome is administration of basic life support at the scene of the submersion. Rescue breaths should be administered as soon as possible and should be given in the water if the rescuer is able to do so. Outcomes are better for cold-water submersions.
- The pathophysiology of near-drowning is due to the multiorgan effect of hypoxemia. A common complication of near-drowning is ARDS.

Environmental Injuries

HUMAN AND ANIMAL BITES

- The decision to close a bite wound depends on the type, age, location, and severity of the wound. Cat bites are usually **puncture wounds** and are best left to heal without suturing. Dog bites may be closed up to 12 hours after the injury. However, dog bites to the hand should be left unsutured. Human bites may also be closed provided that the hand is not involved.
- Cat bites are classically infected with *Pasteurella multocida*, whereas dog bite infection may result from a variety of organisms, including *Staphylococcus* and *Streptococcus* spp. Human bite wounds may also be infected with *Staphylococcus* or *Streptococcus*; *Eikenella corrodens* is another common bacterium.
- **Antibiotic prophylaxis is indicated for cat and human bites.** Dog or rodent bites should be treated with antibiotics only if there is evidence of infection. Antibiotic options include penicillin, amoxicillin +/– clavulanic acid, first-generation cephalosporin, or erythromycin in the penicillin-allergic patient. Tetanus prophylaxis should also be considered.
- Rabies prophylaxis depends on the type of animal and the regional rabies prevalence.
    - **No suspicion of rabies:** No treatment is necessary.
    - **Any suspicion of rabies:** Animal control should be contacted and the animal quarantined for observation.
    - **High suspicion of rabies** (because of local prevalence, the type of animal involved, or the results of testing on a quarantined animal): Give a dose of human rabies immunoglobulin plus five IM injections of human diploid cell vaccine over the course of two weeks.

COLD AND HEAT INJURIES

- **Heat injuries:**
    - Heat injuries appear on a spectrum from mild heat cramps to life-threatening heat stroke. In all instances, normalization of body temperature is the first step in therapy.
    - **Heat cramps:** Self-limited and self-resolving cramps that are most common in athletes. Treatment is supportive.
    - **Heat exhaustion:** Characterized by dizziness, nausea, weakness, and possibly syncope, but mentation remains normal. Body temperature is normal to slightly ↑, and perspiration is common. Electrolytes should be drawn and any imbalances corrected with appropriate fluids.
    - **Heat stroke:** A severe form of heat injury that has a high mortality rate. This form of heat-related injury has symptoms similar to those of heat exhaustion but also includes changes in mental status and/or seizures. Body temperature is almost always ↑. Complications include renal insufficiency, rhabdomyolysis, hepatic injury, coagulation abnormalities, CNS damage, and even shock. Treatment includes the ABCs of resus-

The most common complication associated with bite wounds is infection, the rates for which are as high as 30% for dog bites, 50% for cat bites, and up to 60% for human bites. Irrigation of wounds has been shown to significantly reduce infection rates.

Any wound that appears infected should be left open.

Babies and infants are especially susceptible to heat- and cold-related injuries owing to their poorly developed thermoregulatory systems and relatively high surface area compared to body mass.

citation and fluid replacement therapy. Multisystem monitoring is indicated, and admission to an ICU may be necessary.

- **Cold injuries:**
  - Hypothermia is defined as a core temperature of < 35°C (95°F).
  - For any seriously ill patient, attention to rewarming and ABCs is critical. Defibrillation and emergency medications may not be effective at or below 30°C, so CPR should continue while the patient is warmed.
  - Rewarming measures depend on the severity of the cold injury and on the patient's core temperature.
    - O_2 and IV fluids should be warmed before administration. In severe cases, additional measures may include rewarming of the stomach, bladder, and colon.
    - Peritoneal lavage with heated fluid is particularly useful.
    - Extracorporeal membrane oxygenation (ECMO) has been utilized in extreme cases.
    - Recent literature in adults, however, has demonstrated a neuroprotective effect of maintaining a low body temperature after cardiac arrest.
  - In the absence of an obvious exposure to a cold environment, other causes of hypothermia should be considered, particularly sepsis.
  - Frostbite is treated by rewarming the body part, usually in a circulating warm-water bath. Pain control will likely be needed. Debridement of nonviable tissue is usually done days to weeks after initial insult.

CHILD MALTREATMENT

Risk factors for maltreatment include child stressors such as a medical condition; social stressors such as poverty; and parental factors such as domestic violence, substance abuse, mental illness, or a history of abuse. Siblings of the victim are also at an ↑ risk of abuse.

Health care workers are required to report any suspicion of child abuse or neglect to the authorities. Of all reports made to authorities, roughly 25% originate from health care professionals.

> A 10-month-old girl is brought into the urgent care clinic with a chief complaint of "rash." The mother says that she noticed a new rash on her daughter's back and buttocks yesterday afternoon. She also states that the patient's 17-year-old cousin was baby-sitting the child yesterday afternoon but did not notice the rash. Exam reveals multiple linear, brownish-blue abrasions over the child's back and buttocks. What is in your differential diagnosis? What other studies would be indicated? A hematologic disorder is possible, but child abuse should be a leading concern. Given the age of the patient, a skeletal survey, head CT, and retinal exam should be performed.

A related caregiver is the abuser in 90% of child abuse cases.

Child Abuse

Head injuries due to abuse are the leading cause of morbidity and mortality in the pediatric population. Visceral injuries are the second leading cause of death from child abuse.

SYMPTOMS/EXAM

- A thorough history and physical examination is essential. Special care should be taken to corroborate the physical examination findings and his-

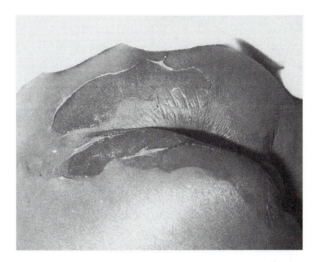

FIGURE 6-4. Burns on buttocks.

(Reproduced, with permission, from Weinberg S et al. *Color Atlas of Pediatric Dermatology*, 3rd ed. New York: McGraw-Hill, 1998:240.) (Also see Color Insert.)

tory with the caretaker, in conjunction with law enforcement and protective services agencies.

- Cutaneous findings may indicate underlying injuries (see Figures 6-4 and 6-5). Noninflicted bruises tend to occur over a bony prominence such as the shin or elbow. Skin findings may occur in a pattern that is suggestive of abuse, such as an area of erythema in the shape of a curling iron or cigarette burn. Human bites and burns may have characteristic patterns that differentiate the injury from another cause.
- **Shaken-baby syndrome,** or shaken-impact syndrome, is most frequently encountered in children < 2 years of age and may be associated with blunt trauma. ↑ ICP → lethargy and vomiting. Retinal hemorrhages and/or skeletal fractures may also be present, and identifying these injuries is an important part of the clinical and evidentiary evaluation. A head CT may reveal subdural hematoma or subarachnoid hemorrhage.

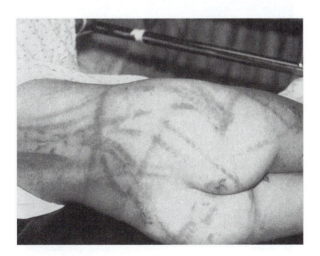

FIGURE 6-5. Loop marks from a hanger.

(Reproduced, with permission, from Weinberg S et al. *Color Atlas of Pediatric Dermatology*, 3rd ed. New York: McGraw-Hill, 1998:240.) (Also see Color Insert.)

DIFFERENTIAL

- Skin findings can mimic true disease, and these possibilities should also be addressed. Bruising may be a presentation of a bleeding diathesis, "mongolian spots," coining/cupping, or urticaria pigmentosa. Burns can be confused with impetigo, HSV, contact dermatitis, or toxic epidermal necrolysis.
- In the case of fractures, medical conditions such as osteogenesis imperfecta, rickets, and osteoid osteoma must also be excluded.

DIAGNOSIS

- Usually based on the history and physical findings. Individual family members should be interviewed independently. Repeated interviews may be helpful in that stories evolve or change.
- Workup should include a radiographic skeletal survey and a thorough retinal exam for hemorrhages.
- The following fractures should raise suspicion of abuse:
  - Fractures in patients < 2 years of age.
  - Fractures of the rib (see Figure 6-6), scapula, vertebral body, spinous process, or sternum.
  - Metaphyseal injuries, including a chip fracture or bucket-handle fracture that results from wrenching or pulling.
  - Spiral or transverse diaphyseal fractures may be due to twisting forces.
  - Multiple fractures of different ages.

TREATMENT

Refer to social workers and/or Child Protective Services for any suspicious cases.

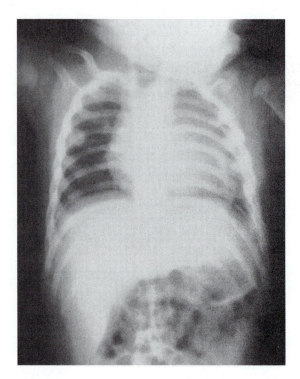

FIGURE 6-6. Rib fractures.

(Reproduced, with permission, from Skinner HB et al. *Current Diagnosis & Treatment in Orthopedics*, 4th ed. New York: McGraw-Hill, 2006:644)

Child Neglect

- Child neglect can be loosely categorized into five areas: medical, supervisory, physical, abandonment, and failure to thrive.
- The possibility of neglect must be considered in any workup involving an infant or child with failure to thrive. Hospitalization may be necessary, and weight gain in the hospital setting suggests that a degree of neglect is responsible for the patient's situation.

Neglect is the most common form of maltreatment and is also most frequently reported to authorities.

Sexual Abuse

- An estimated 10–20% of children (~ 80% female) have been sexually misused. The abuse is often repetitive and performed by a family member, and the perpetrators are almost always known by the child prior to the abuse.
- In half of all cases, sexual abuse has occurred despite the absence of clinical findings.
- On physical exam, careful inspection of the external structures, vaginal opening, hymen, and anorectal region is performed. Forensic evidence should be collected at this time, including samples for STD analysis.
- In the prepubescent child, a ⊕ STD screening is highly suspicious for sexual abuse. Note, however, that babies can acquire a congenital chlamydial infection that persists after birth.

PEDIATRIC CRITICAL CARE

A 10-year-old boy presents to the ER with one week of polydipsia, polyuria, and fatigue. On exam, he appears dehydrated, tired, and tachypneic. What is your diagnosis? What would you expect his ABG to be? What about the serum anion gap? ABGs reveal a pH of 7.10, a $Paco_2$ of 20, an HCO_3 of 9, and a Pao_2 of 84. His anion gap is 28. This patient has a 1° metabolic acidosis with respiratory compensation, and the acidosis has an ↑ anion gap 2° to DKA.

Blood Gases and Acid-Base Disorders

- The range of normal values for an ABG should be memorized:
  - pH 7.35–7.45
  - $Paco_2$ 35–45
  - HCO_3 22–26
  - Pao_2 80–100
- The steps for interpretation are as follows (see also Table 6-8):
  - Use pH to determine if the patient is acidotic (pH < 7.35), alkalotic (> 7.45), or normal/compensated.
  - Use $Paco_2$ to analyze the respiratory component. A low $Paco_2$ → an alkalosis that is either 1° if pH is high or an attempt to neutralize a low pH as a compensatory effect. A high $Paco_2$ suggests acidosis that is 1° if the pH is low or 2° if the pH is high.
  - Use HCO_3 to evaluate the metabolic component. As with $Paco_2$, HCO_3 can be abnormal for 1° or 2° (compensatory) reasons.
  - If $Paco_2$ is abnormal but pH is normal, there is metabolic compensation.
  - If HCO_3 is abnormal but pH is normal, there is respiratory compensation.

TABLE 6-8. ABG Interpretation

If the pH Is	And the $Paco_2$ Is	And the HCO_3 Is	It Is a 1°
> 7.45	High	High	Metabolic alkalosis
> 7.45	Low	Normal to low	Respiratory alkalosis
< 7.35	High	Normal to high	Respiratory acidosis
< 7.35	Low	Low	Metabolic acidosis

Differential diagnosis for anion-gap acidosis—MUDPLIERS

Methanol ingestion
Uremia
Diabetic ketoacidosis
Paraldehyde
Lactic acidosis
INH or **I**ron overdose
Ethylene glycol ingestion
Rhabdomyolysis
Salicylates

An eight-year-old boy with ALL is seen in clinic. He has a central venous catheter for administration of chemotherapy. You note on his intake sheet that he has a temperature of 38.9°C, a heart rate of 145 bpm, and a BP of 85/32. When you step into the room, he is lying in his mother's lap, and you note that he is pale and not answering any of your questions. What should you be worried about? What else might you find on this patient's exam? This patient likely has septic shock. The physical exam often shows warm skin and bounding pulses.

Shock

- Shock is broadly defined as inadequate delivery of substrates to tissues. It may be classified as compensated (normotensive with adequate essential organ blood flow although abnormal perfusion patterns exist), decompensated (hypotensive with poor or absent perfusion), or terminal (irreversible).
- There are three major categories of shock: hypovolemic, distributive, and cardiogenic (see Table 6-9). Hypovolemia is the most common explanation for shock in children.
- All types of shock (except possibly cardiogenic shock) should initially be treated with 20 mL/kg of lactated Ringer's or saline, with frequent assessment for additional boluses. If the immediate cause is not evident, broad-spectrum antibiotics are recommended.

Respiratory Disorders

RESPIRATORY FAILURE

The anatomy of pediatric patients differs from that of adults, involving smaller, more collapsible airways; a more compliant chest wall; a relatively large tongue; and accessory respiratory muscles that fatigue more easily—all of which make them more prone to respiratory failure. Because of limited alveolar space, the pediatric patient augments minute ventilation (tidal volume × respiratory rate) by ↑ respiratory rate. Therefore, a high respiratory rate may be the earliest and most sensitive sign of respiratory insufficiency. Causes of respiratory failure can be grouped as follows:

- Inadequate respiratory drive (drugs, ↑ ICP)
- Neuromuscular (myasthenia gravis, Guillain-Barré syndrome)

TABLE 6-9. Categories of Shock

	HYPOVOLEMIC	DISTRIBUTIVE	CARDIOGENIC
Examples	Dehydration, burns, hemorrhage.	Anaphylaxis, neurogenic, drugs, sepsis.	Congenital heart disease, ischemic heart disease, cardiomyopathy.
Heart rate	↑	↑	↑
Cardiac output	↓	↓	↓
Systemic vascular resistance (SVR)	↑	↓	↑
Mean arterial pressure (MAP)	Normal or ↓	Normal (early) or ↓ (late)	↓
Central venous pressure (CVP)	↓	Normal or ↓	↑
Physical exam	Prolonged capillary refill, cool extremities, mottled skin, lethargy.	Warm skin, bounding pulses, altered mental status.	Prolonged capillary refill, mottled skin, diaphoresis, +/– crackles.
Therapy	Volume replacement, pressors; treat the underlying process.	Volume replacement, pressors; treat the underlying process.	Cautious volume replacement, pressors; treat the underlying process.

EMERGENCY AND CRITICAL CARE MEDICINE

- Extrinsic factors (flail chest, scoliosis)
- Airway obstruction (foreign body, croup, asthma)
- Parenchymal (pneumonia, pneumothorax)
- Metabolic demands (sepsis, toxins such as aspirin)

SYMPTOMS/EXAM

Examination should include assessment of mental status, respiratory rate, use of accessory muscles (retractions, nasal flaring), any audible breath sounds (wheezing, stridor, grunting), and careful auscultation.

DIAGNOSIS

- CXR, ABGs, and pulse oximetry are useful adjuncts.
- Pulse oximetry may be undetectable if peripheral perfusion is poor.
- Methemoglobin or carboxyhemoglobin leads to overestimation of O_2 saturation.

TREATMENT

Direct treatment toward the underlying etiology; should include supplemental O_2 and assisted ventilation.

Respiratory failure is the leading cause of cardiorespiratory collapse in children.

EMERGENCY AND CRITICAL CARE MEDICINE

Causes of ARDS— CARDS? HOPE IT'S NOT ARDS!

CNS disorders,
  Contusion
  (pulmonary)
Aspiration
Radiation
Drugs
Smoke, toxin inhalation
Hypotension, shock
Other, **O**xygen toxicity
Pneumonia,
  Pancreatitis
Emboli (venous, fat)
Infection, sepsis
Transfusion reaction
Surgery
Near-drowning
Organ failure or trauma
Thermal injuries, burns
Altitude sickness
Renal failure
DIC
SLE

Management of severe asthma—BATHE SOME

Beta-agonist (albuterol)
Anticholinergic
  (ipratropium bromide)
Terbutaline
Heliox
Epinephrine
Steroids
Oxygen
Magnesium
Expect intubation

ACUTE RESPIRATORY DISTRESS SYNDROME (ARDS)

- A clinical syndrome characterized by acute lung injury that result in pulmonary inflammation and hypoxemic respiratory failure.
- **Dx:** Diagnostic criteria used include an acute onset of respiratory symptoms, bilateral pulmonary infiltrates on radiographs, and a PaO_2-to-FiO_2 ratio (PFR) of < 200. A subset of ARDS is acute lung injury, which is differentiated by a PFR of 200–300.
- **Tx:** Treatment consists of addressing the underlying etiology and strategies of mechanical ventilation that reduce barotrauma.

SEVERE ASTHMA

The management of severe asthma can be described in the mnemonic **BATHE SOME**. Additional information can be found in the chapter on respiratory disorders.

PNEUMOTHORAX

The causes of pneumothorax are described in the mnemonic **SIT ABC**. Additional information can be found in the discussion of respiratory disorders.

PULMONARY EMBOLISM (PE)

In the pediatric population, pulmonary emboli are more likely due to endovascular damage (e.g., trauma, indwelling catheters) than to peripheral vascular disease. Hematologic abnormalities are being recognized more often as a culprit.

SYMPTOMS/EXAM

The presentation of pediatric PE is similar to that of adults but often goes unrecognized in the younger patient. Chest pain, dyspnea, cough, and hemoptysis are frequent symptoms. Tachypnea and fever are variably present.

DIAGNOSIS

- Maintain a high index of suspicion and obtain a ventilation/perfusion (V/Q) scan or angiography.
- D-dimers and CRP are often ↑.
- ECG may show an S1Q3T3 pattern—prominent S in lead I; Q and inverted T in lead III.
- ABGs reveal hypoxia, and the CXR is abnormal in 50%.

TREATMENT

Anticoagulation with heparin or warfarin. Prophylactic measures in high-risk patients can reduce the risk of PE.

Heart Failure

Heart failure (or CHF) results when the heart is unable to provide adequate support for the body's metabolic demands. Etiologies include congenital disease (congenital heart disease), infectious disease (sepsis, myo- or pericarditis), hypertension, acute rheumatic fever, Kawasaki disease, toxins, collagen vascular disease, valvular disease, lung disease, and arrhythmias. It may also be idio-pathic (e.g., dilated cardiomyopathy).

SYMPTOMS

Failure to thrive, poor feeding, exercise intolerance, shortness of breath, or-thopnea, abdominal pain (from poor gut perfusion), agitation/lethargy.

EXAM

Tachypnea, tachycardia, hyperdynamic precordium, murmur/rub (depending on the cause), gallop, hepatomegaly, JVD, crackles, delayed capillary refill, cool extremities, weak pulses. Altered mental status.

DIAGNOSIS

- **CXR:** Reveals cardiomegaly, pulmonary vascular congestion, and effu-sions.
- ECG/echocardiography.
- **Labs:** Obtain cardiac enzymes, lactate, mixed venous oxygen saturation (low in CHF), LFTs, and BUN/creatinine to assess end-organ perfusion.

TREATMENT

- Follow the ABCs of resuscitation.
- Refer to the treatment for cardiogenic shock.
- Diuretics, supplemental O_2, and blood transfusions are useful adjuncts.
- In severe cases, mechanical ventilation and sedation +/− paralysis may be necessary to ↓ the work demands of the heart.

Neurologic Disorders

REYE SYNDROME

Primarily affects preteens and toddlers.

SYMPTOMS/EXAM

- **Acute onset of encephalopathy two weeks after a viral illness.** Risk is ↑ when the patient has been using aspirin, although the exact pathophysiol-ogy is unclear.
- Symptoms begin with vomiting and can progress to lethargy, altered men-tal status, seizures, or coma. ICP is ↑.

DIAGNOSIS

- Laboratory abnormalities include ↑ liver enzymes and ↑ serum ammonia.
- Hypoglycemia may be profound. However, jaundice is rare, and bilirubin is usually normal.

TREATMENT

Management of ↑ ICP, reversal of hypoglycemia, supportive therapy.

Causes of pneu-mothorax—SIT ABC

Spontaneous (think tall, thin male)
Iatrogenic
Trauma
Asthma
Badness (tumor)
Cystic fibrosis

EMERGENCY AND
CRITICAL CARE MEDICINE

ALTERED MENTAL STATUS (AMS) AND COMA

A disturbance in the level of consciousness that spans a spectrum ranging from confusion to delirium to coma. The etiologies of AMS and coma are numerous and are described in the mnemonic **MOVE, STUPID.**

SYMPTOMS/EXAM

- After attention to basic life support, a detailed physical examination should be performed. Attention to vital signs and the neurologic exam may reveal abnormalities suggestive of the underlying process causing the derangement.
- As part of a detailed history, the child's parents should be questioned about potential ingestions, trauma, medication/drug use, or infections. The GCS (see the section on trauma) should be performed and monitored.

DIAGNOSIS

- The workup should focus on the underlying disorder.
- A Dextrostix strip should be used during the initial evaluation. Other laboratory studies could include a CBC, electrolytes, LFTs, ammonia, lactate, and ABGs.
- A toxicology screen (blood and urine) may be useful. Cultures of urine, blood, and CSF may be indicated.
- An emergent head CT is often performed while awaiting the results of any laboratory testing.
- While not performed emergently, an EEG may be part of the workup if a neurologic disorder is suspected.

TREATMENT

Focus on supportive care and on finding the underlying cause. If ingestion is suspected, empiric therapy and gastric decontamination should be strongly considered. If a narcotic ingestion is suspected, for example, the patient should be given naloxone.

HEAD TRAUMA

- Common subtypes are as follows:
    - **Basilar skull fractures:** Usually occur in the temporal bone. Findings include hemotympanum, CSF otorrhea, periorbital ecchymoses ("raccoon eyes"), or postauricular bruising (Battle's sign). Diagnosis is made by CT scan.
    - **Epidural hematoma** (see Figure 6-7): Incidence in children is similar to that in adults. Some 75% of cases occur in combination with a skull fracture and subsequent middle meningeal artery bleeding.
    - **Subdural hematomas:** Result from bleeding of the bridging veins; more common in adults. When they do occur in children, **abuse** should be ruled out.
    - **Diffuse cerebral edema:** Much more common in children; usually the result of abuse.
- Tx: Treat with neurosurgical consultation, close observation with frequent neurologic checks, and ICP management (see below).

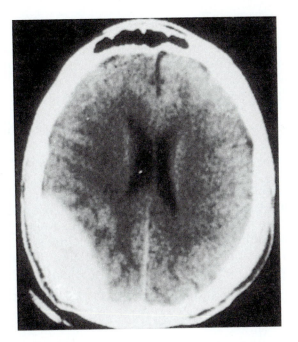

FIGURE 6-7. Epidural hematoma with classic biconvex lens shape.

(Reproduced, with permission, from Aminoff MJ et al. *Clinical Neurology*, 3rd ed. Stamford, CT: Appleton & Lange, 1996:296.)

ACUTE INTRACRANIAL HYPERTENSION

Etiologies include child abuse, Reye syndrome, intracranial hemorrhage, infection, hydrocephalus, metabolic abnormalities (e.g., DKA), and mass.

SYMPTOMS/EXAM

- Headache, nausea, vomiting, diplopia, cranial nerve findings, bulging fontanelle, gait abnormalities, progressive decline in mental status, papilledema (late finding).
- Central or transtentorial herniation can result when the damage is diffuse. This may lead to:
  - Decorticate (flexor) posturing or decerebrate (extensor) movements.
  - Cheyne-Stokes respirations (↑ and deeper respirations followed by periods of apnea).
  - With progression, the pupils become fixed and dilated and muscle tone is flaccid. Breathing slows and becomes irregular.
- In the early stages, uncal herniation is characterized by hyperventilation, a unilaterally dilated and sluggish pupil, and decorticate or decerebrate responses. In the late stages, it may be difficult to distinguish from transtentorial herniation.

DIAGNOSIS

- Head CT acutely.
- MRI can better define structural abnormalities, especially in the posterior fossa.

Cushing's triad is an ominous sign of ↑ ICP characterized by hypertension, bradycardia, and irregular respiratory rate.

TREATMENT

- Follow the ABCs and 2° survey (including assignment of a GCS score).
- If rapid-sequence intubation is performed, ketamine and succinylcholine should be avoided, as they will ↑ ICP.
- The head should be kept midline and the head of the bed elevated to 30 degrees.
- Hyperosmolar agents such as mannitol or hypertonic saline should be administered.
- Seizures should be anticipated and medications made available for treatment.
- Hyperventilation will ↓ ICP acutely but has not been demonstrated to improve outcomes and is not recommended for prolonged periods.
- Sedation should be provided and noxious stimuli avoided.
- BP should be sufficiently high to maintain cerebral perfusion pressure. Invasive ICP monitoring is often necessary. BP and ICP are related by the following equation:

$$\text{Cerebral perfusion pressure (CPP)} = \text{MAP} - \text{ICP}$$

BRAIN DEATH

Brain death criteria have evolved over time. Recent guidelines for the determination of brain death, derived from the President's Commission for the Study of Ethical Problems in Medicine and Biomedical Behavioral Research (*JAMA* 246:2184–2186, 1981) are as follows:

- Absence of hypothermia, shock, or drug intoxication.
- Cerebral unresponsiveness.
- Apnea and $Pa_{CO_2} > 60$.
- Absent brain stem reflexes (pupillary, corneal, oculovestibular, oculocephalic, oropharyngeal).
- Observe for six hours if corroborative testing is used (EEG, angiography, radionuclide flow study).
- Observe for 12 hours if no corroborative testing is used.

Miscellaneous Disorders

MALIGNANT HYPERTHERMIA

Defined as a hypermetabolic response by skeletal muscle to certain medications—e.g., inhaled anesthetics (especially halothane) or a neuromuscular blocking agent such as succinylcholine. Associated risk factors include muscular dystrophy, scoliosis, ↑ muscle mass, and a ⊕ family history.

SYMPTOMS/EXAM

- Sudden onset; often occurs in the PACU.
- Occasionally, masseter spasm is seen during induction in the OR.
- Hypertension, tachycardia, muscle contractions, and arrhythmias are also seen.
- Hyperthermia may be a late sign, so a normal temperature should not exclude the diagnosis.
- If untreated, symptoms progress to renal failure, shock, and even cardiac arrest.

DIAGNOSIS

Labs reveal hypercarbia, hypoxemia, acidosis, DIC, myoglobinuria, hyperkalemia, and renal failure.

TREATMENT

- Dantrolene, treatment of acidosis, cooling measures, and aggressive fluid management.
- Follow-up includes avoidance of halothane anesthetics and succinylcholine; first-degree family members should be screened.

NEUROLEPTIC MALIGNANT SYNDROME (NMS)

- Resembles malignant hyperthermia, but the time until onset of symptoms is usually more insidious, occurring over days to months. The pharmacologic trigger is also different, as neuroleptic agents such as haloperidol are implicated. Symptoms are similar to those of malignant hyperthermia. Therapy is similar and includes dantrolene or bromocriptine.
- Patients should be considered susceptible to malignant hyperthermia as well.

Critical Life Events

A three-month-old infant is found face down in a crib. When the EMS team arrives, the infant is apneic and pulseless with no movement or response to interventions, including intraosseous administration of medications and endotracheal intubation. The infant is transported to the ER and receives chest compressions and ventilatory support en route. What are likely causes of this child's arrest? What interventions lead to a reduction in the number of SIDS deaths? What are risk factors for SIDS? The most likely cause of arrest is SIDS, although abuse, infection, ingestion, metabolic disease, and cardiac causes should be considered. The "Back to Sleep" campaign has led to a dramatic reduction in SIDS deaths. Risk factors are social, environmental, and economic.

SUDDEN INFANT DEATH SYNDROME (SIDS)

- SIDS is the sudden death of an infant, generally between one month and one year of age, that is unexpected and unexplained by the history or by other causes after an autopsy. SIDS is the leading cause of death in infants < 6 months of age. The pathophysiology is unknown.
- Several risk factors have been identified, including prone sleeping position, low birth weight, apnea, a history of an apparent life-threatening event (ALTE), male gender, maternal tobacco or drug use, winter months, poverty, and sleeping on or near soft surfaces. Of these, the prone sleeping position is considered the strongest risk factor for SIDS.
- SIDS accounts for 5000 deaths per year in the United States. The peak incidence is at 2–4 months of age, and the vast majority of cases occur before six months of age.

- The differential diagnosis includes infection, environmental factors, trauma, metabolic disorders, congenital heart disease, adrenal insufficiency, and arrhythmia.
- The "Back to Sleep" campaign, which began in 1992, has led to a 50 percent ↓ in the number of SIDS deaths.

APPARENT LIFE-THREATENING EVENT (ALTE)

- An ALTE is an episode in which a patient has apnea, color changes such as cyanosis or pallor, and a change in muscle tone. The parents or witness genuinely believes that the event was life-threatening and may have attempted stimulation or CPR. There is a weak association between ALTEs and SIDS.
- In 50% percent of cases, an exact diagnosis is not found. The differential diagnosis is lengthy and includes neurologic, metabolic, cardiac, endocrine, and infectious disorders.
- Underlying disorders should be treated appropriately. When no cause is identified, it is appropriate to teach parents CPR. Home monitoring is controversial.

CHAPTER 7

Endocrinology

Ryan Miller, MD
Elizabeth Tan Rosolowsky, MD
reviewed by Louise Greenspan, MD, and Leslie Plotnick, MD

PREMATURE THELARCHE

Defined as isolated breast development before age seven in Caucasian girls and before age six in African-American girls. Often due to the development of a small ovarian cyst or to brief LH and FSH secretion. However, it is essential to rule out exposure to exogenous estrogens such as creams and OCPs.

SYMPTOMS/EXAM

Unilateral or bilateral breast development with no other signs of puberty.

DIAGNOSIS

- GnRH stimulation test is prepubertal.
- Bone age correlates with chronological age.
- Pelvic ultrasound may or may not show ovarian cysts.

TREATMENT

Management consists of reassurance and close follow-up after precocious puberty has been ruled out.

Isolated premature thelarche most often regresses within six months without treatment.

A seven-year-old boy presents with a six-month history of pubic hair and adult body odor. He has no significant family or medical history. Physical examination reveals a healthy-appearing boy with mild facial acne and a slight amount of pubic hair. Testes measure 2 cm bilaterally. How would you proceed? Bone-age x-ray equals eight years (within normal). DHEAS and 17-hydroxyprogesterone (17-OHP) are normal, and FSH, LH, and testosterone are all prepubertal. The diagnosis of premature adrenarche is made. Two years later the boy's exam is unchanged, and bone age is equal to chronological age. He undergoes normal puberty at age 11.

PREMATURE ADRENARCHE

Isolated development of pubic hair prior to age six in African-American girls, age seven in Caucasian girls, and age nine in boys.

SYMPTOMS/EXAM

- Growth velocity is normal or slightly ↑.
- Axillary hair, acne, body odor, and oily skin may be seen.
- Breast/genital development is prepubertal.
- No virilization or clitoromegaly is seen.

DIAGNOSIS

- Plasma DHEAS correlates with stage of pubic hair.
- Bone age is within 2 SDs of chronological age (not advanced).

TREATMENT

Management consists of reassessment of growth velocity and pubertal status at three- to six-month intervals.

In premature adrenarche, 17-OHP and DHEAS may be ↑ for age but normal for sexual maturity rating (SMR). An ACTH stimulation test can differentiate congenital adrenal hyperplasia (CAH) from premature adrenarche. In CAH, 17-OHP will hyperrespond, whereas in premature adrenarche it will not ↑ significantly.

More than 75% of healthy boys in stages 2 and 3 of puberty have unilateral or bilateral breast development that is benign and self-limited. The etiologies of pathologic gynecomastia are as follows:

Galactorrhea or other signs of feminization are indicators of pathologic gynecomastia.

- 1° hypogonadism (including Klinefelter syndrome)
- Familial aromatization excess
- Exogenous:
    - Estrogen exposure (including marijuana)
    - Anabolic steroids
    - Androgen antagonists (spironolactone, ketoconazole)
- Any tumor secreting hCG or estrogen (e.g., adrenal, testicular)
- Sertoli cell tumor
- Liver disease

DIAGNOSIS

If no abnormalities are found on exam, reassess in six months. If gynecomastia progresses, proceed with evaluation:

- ↑ **hCG or estradiol:** Obtain a testicular ultrasound to evaluate for tumor. If ⊖, consider further studies for a germ cell tumor (e.g., CXR, CT of the abdomen).
- ↑ **LH:** Consider 1° hypogonadism or Klinefelter syndrome.
- If prolactin is ↑, order a brain MRI to look for a prolactinoma.

TREATMENT

Surgery is indicated in the most severe and persistent cases. Antiestrogens and aromatase inhibitors are of questionable efficacy.

Sexual development prior to the age of **six in African-American girls, seven in Caucasian girls,** and **nine in boys** is considered precocious. The effects of ↑ sex steroids include a faster rate of growth than appropriate for age and rapid bone-age advancement. Puberty in Caucasian girls 7–8 years of age and in African-American girls 6–8 years of age is rarely pathologic when the pace of puberty is normal and there are no other suspicious findings (e.g., neurologic findings or signs of ↑ ICP).

SYMPTOMS/EXAM

- SMR 2 or greater breast/genital development.
- Pubic hair.
- Pink, estrogenized vaginal mucosa.
- Sebaceous activity (acne, oily skin).

Central Precocious Puberty (CPP)

CPP is gonadotropin dependent and indicates premature activation of the hypothalamic-pituitary-gonadal (HPG) axis. It is more common in girls (5:1). Although CPP is idiopathic in the majority of girls, up to 50% of boys with CPP have a demonstrable abnormality. Any CNS disease that interferes with normal inhibition of the HPG axis can → CPP. The condition may be idiopathic or caused by the following:

- **Congenital CNS anomalies:** Hypothalamic hamartoma (visualized by MRI or CT), hydrocephalus, arachnoid cyst.
- **Acquired CNS lesions:** Cranial irradiation, trauma, granuloma.
- **Tumors:** Astrocytoma, glioma, craniopharyngioma, ependymoma.
- Chronic exposure to sex steroids, as in CAH.

DIAGNOSIS

- **FSH, LH:** Secretion is pulsatile, and therefore random levels may be pre-pubertal or ↑. If levels are prepubertal and CPP is suspected, perform a GnRH stimulation test, which will show ↑ **FSH/LH.**
- Testosterone or estradiol levels correspond to pubertal stage.
- Obtain TFTs.
- Bone age is advanced in relation to chronologic age.
- MRI of the brain (hypothalamus/pituitary) may reveal a tumor or structural abnormality.

TREATMENT

- **GnRH analogs** (e.g., leuprolide acetate).
- Adequate treatment is indicated by suppressed LH on repeat GnRH testing; prepubertal levels of testosterone or estradiol; and slowing of bone-age advancement and growth velocity.
- Puberty will commence once treatment is discontinued.

Gonadotropin-Independent Precocious Puberty

Caused either by an endogenous, peripheral source of sex steroid or by ongoing exposure to exogenous hormone. Specific etiologies include the following:

- **Ovarian cysts:** Most resolve spontaneously.
- **Congenital adrenal hyperplasia** (see below): Causes virilization resulting from excess androgen secretion from the adrenals.
- **Genetic disorders:**
    - **Familial gonadotropin-independent sexual precocity:** An LH receptor–activating mutation that affects only males.
    - McCune-Albright syndrome.
- Germ cell tumors.
- **Exogenous sex steroids:** Always ask about this in the history!

DIAGNOSIS

FSH and LH are suppressed to undetectable levels, while sex steroid concentrations (estradiol, testosterone) can be extremely ↑.

Tumors in the region of the hypothalamus or pituitary can present with headache, visual disturbance, and DI.

CPP is most commonly idiopathic, with the next most frequent cause hypothalamic hamartoma.

Peripheral precocious puberty, café-au-lait spots with irregular borders, and bone lesions on x-ray point to McCune-Albright syndrome.

ENDOCRINOLOGY

> A 14-year-old girl new to your practice presents for routine care. Her height is well below the third percentile for age, and you note that there is no breast development and a slight amount of pubic hair. On further questioning, the parents report that the girl also underwent repair of an aortic coarctation at two weeks of age. Your workup reveals a delayed bone age at 11.5 years, estradiol < 20 pg/mL, FSH 150 mIU/mL, and LH 22.6 mIU/mL; karyotype is 45,XO. What is your diagnosis? Delayed puberty 2° to Turner's syndrome. She is started on growth hormone (GH) therapy with a plan to initiate estrogen replacement in 1–2 years.

A full evaluation of delayed puberty is warranted if:

- There are no physical changes of puberty by age 14 in boys.
- There are no physical changes of puberty by age 13 in girls.
- Menarche has not occurred by age 16 within five years of the first sign of puberty in girls.

A persistently low LH suggests a central hormonal defect; an ↑ LH over time suggests constitutional delay; and an extremely ↑ LH suggests 1° gonadal failure.

Table 7-1 outlines the etiologies of pubertal delay.

SYMPTOMS/EXAM

- No pubic hair; no breast or genital development.
- No acne or sebaceous activity; no facial hair.

DIAGNOSIS

- Obtain LH/FSH.
- Evaluate growth and bone age.
- Obtain TFTs.
- Karyotype if Klinefelter or Turner syndrome is suspected.
- See Figure 7-1 for an evaluation algorithm.

TREATMENT

- **Girls:** Start hormone replacement with low-dose ethinyl estradiol and gradually ↑ the dosage. Start cycling after one year if indicated.
- **Boys:** For patients who will require lifetime testosterone replacement, slowly work up to an adult replacement dose of 200 mg IM every two weeks.

Constitutional Delay of Growth and Puberty (CDGP)

By definition, CDGP is a nonpathologic condition. Patients are healthy but have short stature in comparison to familial height and have a significant delay in pubertal development. Often there is a family history of constitutional delay.

DIAGNOSIS

Skeletal maturation (as measured by bone age) is delayed. Height is typically shorter than average for age but is appropriate for bone age.

TREATMENT

In the majority of patients, the only treatment required is reassurance and close follow-up.

TABLE 7-1. Etiologies of Pubertal Delay

HYPOGONADOTROPIC HYPOGONADISM	HYPERGONADOTROPIC HYPOGONADISM
Chronic disease	Gonadal dysgenesis
Anorexia nervosa	1° ovarian failure (including Turner syndrome)
Exercise-induced amenorrhea	
Isolated gonadotropin deficiency	1° testicular failure
Hypopituitarism, septo-optic dysplasia	Klinefelter syndrome
Kallmann syndrome	
CNS tumors	
Chemotherapy, CNS irradiation	

ENDOCRINOLOGY

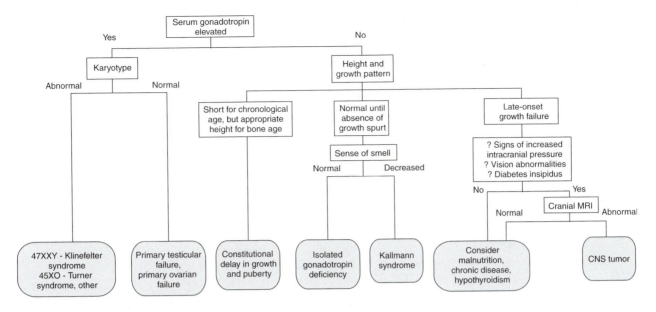

FIGURE 7-1. Evaluation of the absence of 2° sexual development.

(Adapted, with permission, from Rudolph CD et al. *Rudolph's Pediatrics*, 21st ed. New York: McGraw-Hill, 2002:2104.)

Kallmann Syndrome

Defined as hypogonadotropic hypogonadism associated with anosmia. Associated with X-linked transmission via the KAL1 gene, but there are also autosomal-dominant and autosomal-recessive forms (whose genes have not been identified).

SYMPTOMS/EXAM

- Delayed puberty, eunuchoid habitus, gynecomastia, reduced sense of smell.
- Cryptorchidism and micropenis are seen in affected male infants.
- Unilateral renal agenesis is seen in 40% of cases.

TREATMENT

Testosterone replacement in males; estrogen replacement in females.

ANTIDIURETIC HORMONE (ADH) DISORDERS

Vasopressin (ADH) is made in the posterior pituitary. It is essential for fluid balance, and its 1° action is on the kidney.

Syndrome of Inappropriate Antidiuretic Hormone Secretion (SIADH)

A condition in which ADH concentrations are ↑ in relation to plasma osmolality. Causes include the following:

- Head trauma, infections, CNS tumors, and surgery near the hypothalamus.
- Drugs (including lithium).

- Lung disease (tuberculosis).
- Severe hypothyroidism.

SYMPTOMS/EXAM

- ↓ urine output.
- Hypervolemia, weight gain, nausea, vomiting, headache, malaise.

DIAGNOSIS

Hyponatremia (Na < 135 mmol/L), low serum osmolality, high urine osmolality.

If patients with SIADH are water restricted, sodium and osmolality return to normal.

TREATMENT

- Correct hyponatremia slowly with fluid restriction.
- Initiate strict intake/output measurements.
- Daily weights; frequent serum sodium measurements.

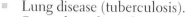 A 15-year-old girl presents with gradually worsening thirst over the past several months, accompanied by excessive urination that now requires several trips to the bathroom overnight. She denies weight loss, fatigue, medication use, or recent head trauma. Initial labs reveal glucose 85 mg/dL, sodium 138 mEq/L, serum osmolality 280 mOsm/L, and urine osmolality 204 mOsm/L. After three hours of water deprivation, urine osmolality is unchanged, serum osmolality is 315 mOsm/L, and serum sodium is 155 mEq/L. What would be the appropriate next step? Desmopressin acetate (DDAVP) administration. One hour after starting DDAVP, serum osmolality is 290 mOsm/L and urine osmolality 415 mOsm/L. MRI of the brain reveals a lesion involving the sella turcica that is consistent with craniopharyngioma.

Central Diabetes Insipidus (DI)

Vasopressin deficiency. Etiologies include the following:

- Midline brain abnormalities (e.g., septo-optic dysplasia).
- Surgical or accidental trauma involving the neurohypophysis.
- Tumors (germinomas often present with DI).
- Infiltrative disease (histiocytosis, lymphocytic hypophysitis).
- Gene mutations.

SYMPTOMS/EXAM

- **Infants:** Failure to thrive, vomiting, constipation, poor growth.
- **Older children:** Abrupt onset of excessive thirst, nocturia, 2° enuresis, polyuria, lethargy.
- Dehydration can occur if there is damage to the thirst mechanism or if fluid intake is not sufficient to keep up with urinary losses.

DIAGNOSIS

- DI is confirmed when hypotonic urine is accompanied by hypertonic serum in the setting of polyuria.

DI often follows resection of craniopharyngiomas.

- Screen first-morning urine and serum for osmolality and sodium levels.
- A formal water deprivation test can be performed in the hospital.
- When a diagnosis of central DI is made, an MRI of the brain should be performed to evaluate for tumors or infiltrative processes.

TREATMENT

- **DDAVP** can be administered orally, intranasally, or subcutaneously.
- Infants should be treated with ↑ free water rather than with DDAVP in light of the high risk of fluid overload and hyponatremia.

TYPE 1 DIABETES MELLITUS

Caused by immune-mediated destruction of pancreatic islet cells. The prevalence among U.S. school-aged children is approximately 2 in 1000. The risk of diabetes for a sibling is 3–6%. Associated with HLA-DR3 and -DR4.

SYMPTOMS/EXAM

Classic symptoms are polyuria, polydipsia, hyperphagia, and weight loss.

DIAGNOSIS

- Criteria for the diagnosis of DM are as follows:
  - Fasting plasma glucose > 126 mg/dL.
  - Random glucose > 200 mg/dL (or two hours after an oral glucose load).
- Other labs at diagnosis should include a complete UA (including ketones and glucose), a comprehensive metabolic panel, blood pH, and bicarbonate to check for acidosis.
- Glycosylated hemoglobin (HbA_{1c}).
- **Autoantibodies:** Islet cell antibodies, insulin antibodies, glutamic acid decarboxylase (GAD65).
- Obtain TFTs at diagnosis.
- Screen for celiac disease (endomysial antibodies or tissue transglutaminase) at diagnosis or shortly thereafter.

TREATMENT

- See the discussion below for the treatment of DKA.
- If the patient is adequately hydrated and has a normal blood pH, SQ insulin can be started. Most children require 0.5–1.0 unit/kg/day.
- **Insulin regimens:** A combination of short- and long-acting insulins is typically used that covers basal and meal-time insulin needs (see Figure 7-2).
- **Insulin pump:** Provides SQ infusion of rapid-acting insulin. Pumps are programmed to administer insulin at variable basal rates; the user enters bolus doses with meals.
- **Dietary measures:** Carbohydrate counting is recommended.
- Home glucose measurements should be made at least four times daily.

COMPLICATIONS

On **sick days,** the following adjustments should be made:

- Insulin doses may have to be ↑ by 20% or more even with mild illness.
- Urine ketones should be checked in the presence of vomiting or other illness or if blood glucose > 250 mg/dL. The presence of ketones indicates the need for additional insulin.
- Intake of clear fluids must be ↑ to maintain hydration status.

Following a positive water deprivation test, obtain plasma vasopressin level, administer vasopressin, and measure urine and serum osmolality to distinguish between central and nephrogenic DI.

Transient hyperglycemia can occur with illness. Blood glucose determinations must be repeated to confirm the diagnosis of diabetes.

ENDOCRINOLOGY

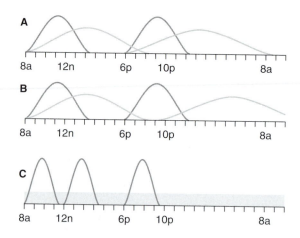

FIGURE 7-2. **Commonly used insulin regimens for patients with type 1 DM.**

(A) Standard twice-daily regimen with rapid-acting and intermediate-acting (NPH) insulins given before breakfast and dinner. (B) Three-shot regimen with the NPH moved to bedtime to prevent nocturnal hypoglycemia and to provide better coverage in the early morning. (C) Basal-bolus regimen with 24-hour insulin (e.g., glargine) and rapid-acting insulin (e.g., lispro) for meals and snacks provides a better approximation of endogenous insulin secretion. (Reproduced, with permission, from Rudolph CD et al. *Rudolph's Pediatrics*, 21st ed. New York: McGraw-Hill, 2002:2125.)

Health Supervision for Type 1 Diabetes

Even if glucose values are not ↑, patients must continue to take insulin on sick days to cover basal needs in order to avoid ketoacidosis.

- Schedule a diabetes-focused visit every three months.
- Review insulin doses and blood sugars on each visit.
- Monitor weight, body mass index (BMI), height, and BP on each visit.
- Monitor blood glucose control with HbA_{1c} on each visit.
- All patients ≥ 10 years of age should have a dilated eye exam annually.
- TFTs should be monitored yearly as indicated.
- A lipid panel should be ordered starting at age 12 and should be repeated every five years (or yearly if abnormal).
- Celiac screening should be conducted at diagnosis and then as indicated.
- Urine microalbumin should be monitored yearly.

Diabetic Ketoacidosis (DKA)

Up to 1% of DKA cases result in fatalities, primarily as a result of cerebral edema or electrolyte disarray.

Defined as insulin deficiency that → a catabolic state. An ↑ of counterregulatory hormones (epinephrine, cortisol, GH, glucagon) antagonizes insulin action and promotes glycogenolysis, gluconeogenesis, lipolysis, and ketogenesis.

- Glucosuria (renal threshold approximately 180 mg/dL) → osmotic diuresis, urinary loss of electrolytes, and dehydration.
- Exacerbated by urinary ketone excretion.
- A combination of dehydration and ↑ stress hormones → metabolic decompensation.

TREATMENT

- Restore fluid volume with NS, 10–20 cc/kg in the first hour. Replace the remaining fluid deficit plus maintenance over 48 hours. Do not exceed 40 cc/kg in the first four hours given the danger of cerebral edema.

- Regular insulin should be given IV at a rate of 0.1 units/kg/hr. Blood glucose levels should be measured hourly. If blood glucose falls faster than 150 mg/dL/hr or drops to < 250 mg/dL, add dextrose to IV fluids. The insulin infusion should not be discontinued until pH is > 7.30.
- **Replacement of body salts:** Sodium, potassium, and phosphorus are lost in the urine with ketones and are depleted.
    - **Sodium:** Rehydration fluid is usually adequate for replacement.
    - **Potassium:** Potassium levels may initially be ↑ because of acidosis even if total body potassium is low. Monitor hourly, and when the potassium level becomes low or returns to normal, begin replacement. It may be useful to replace some potassium as potassium phosphate.

COMPLICATIONS

Cerebral edema is a rare, unpredictable complication of DKA that is associated with high morbidity and mortality rates.

- Rapid rehydration and rapid correction of serum osmolality may contribute to the risk of cerebral edema. Low pH, low bicarbonate, sodium bicarbonate therapy, and hyponatremia have been identified as possible risk factors.
- Early neurologic signs include severe headache, lethargy, altered mental status, and dilated pupils.
- If cerebral edema is suspected, begin treatment immediately by raising the head of the bed followed by mannitol and hyperventilation. A head CT should then be performed.

A 16-year-old girl presents to the ED with nausea and vomiting accompanied by a three-week history of thirst and urination. She also reports fatigue and a 20-pound weight loss over the past several months. She appears ill but not toxic. Examination is notable for tachycardia, acanthosis nigricans, and obesity (BMI 97th percentile). Labs reveal a glucose level of 457 mg/dL and a CO_2 of 12 mEq/L with an anion gap of 22. She is given a bolus of NS and started on an insulin drip. After correction of the anion gap and hyperglycemia, she is started on a SQ insulin regimen and given diabetes education. Labs reveal that her HbA_{1c} is 9.7%, her C-peptide level is 1.8 ng/mL, and her GAD antibodies are weakly ⊕. What is the most likely diagnosis? You decide that she most likely has type 2 DM and start her on metformin. At her follow-up visit three months later, her BMI has ↓ to the 90th percentile; the patient reports that she was able to discontinue insulin, and her HbA_{1c} has improved to 7.8%.

TYPE 2 DIABETES MELLITUS

Due to a heterogeneous group of disorders of carbohydrate metabolism → insulin resistance and/or impaired insulin secretion.

SYMPTOMS/EXAM

Obesity and acanthosis nigricans are frequent physical findings in type 2 DM.

Type 2 DM now accounts for nearly half of all cases of newly diagnosed diabetes in adolescents.

TREATMENT

- Management of impaired glucose tolerance consists of lifestyle changes, including nutritional education, ↑ physical activity, and ↓ sedentary activity.
- Oral medication is indicated if HbA_{1c} is abnormal despite lifestyle changes.
    - **Metformin** is the only approved medication for pediatric patients. It is contraindicated in the presence of liver or renal impairment and should be discontinued during illnesses involving vomiting. It should also be discontinued 72 hours before surgery or the use of iodine-containing contrast.
    - Sulfonylureas and glitazones are also available but are not approved for use in children.
- Treat with insulin under the following conditions:
    - In the presence of DKA.
    - If type 1 DM is suspected.
    - If fasting glucose is > 250 mg/dL or postprandial glucoses are > 300 mg/dL.

HYPOGLYCEMIA

Defined as a blood glucose level < 45 mg/dL in neonates and < 50 mg/dL in older infants and children. Can be ketotic or nonketotic (see Table 7-2). See Table 7-3 for risk factors.

SYMPTOMS/EXAM

- **Infants:** High-pitched cry, diaphoresis, poor feeding, tremors, irritability/jitteriness, exaggerated Moro reflex, lethargy, hypotonia, seizures, cyanosis, pallor, tachypnea.
- **Older children:** Sweating, anxiety, tachypnea, weakness, headache, irritability, confusion, abnormal behavior, seizures.

DIAGNOSIS

- Obtain the critical sample at the time of hypoglycemia:
    - Serum insulin, cortisol, GH, electrolytes, glucose, C-peptide.
    - Urine ketones, organic acids.
    - Serum β-hydroxybutyrate, free fatty acids, amino acids, acylcarnitine profile, lactic acid, pyruvic acid.
- Glucagon stimulation test at the time of hypoglycemia:
    - Give glucagon 0.03 mg/kg (up to 1 mg) SQ.
    - Measure serum glucose at 15 and 30 minutes.

An ↑ in glucose of > 30 mg/dL in response to a glucagon stimulation test is indicative of hyperinsulinism.

TABLE 7-2. Ketotic vs. Nonketotic Hypoglycemia

KETOTIC	NONKETOTIC
Benign ketotic hypoglycemia	Infant of diabetic mother
Hormonal deficiencies	Hyperinsulinism
Glycogen storage disease	Fatty acid oxidation disorders
Abnormalities of gluconeogenesis	Hyperinsulinism-hyperammonemia

MATERNAL	NEONATAL
DM	Small for gestational age
Tocolytic therapy	Large for gestational age
Hypertension in pregnancy	Smaller of discordant twins
Substance abuse	Perinatal distress
Previous hypoglycemic infant	Anterior midline defects
	Microphallus
	Macroglossia or gigantism

Congenital Hyperinsulinism

Presents in the first several days of life or at a time when length between feedings is ↑.

DIAGNOSIS

- Insulin > 2 µIU/mL at the time of hypoglycemia and ⊕ response to a glucagon stimulation test.
- Focal or diffuse pancreatic involvement may also be seen.

TREATMENT

- **Medical: Diazoxide** and **octreotide** act by ↓ insulin secretion.
- **Surgical:**
  - If a focal lesion can be located intraoperatively, partial pancreatic resection can be curative.
  - For diffuse disease, near-total pancreatectomy may be effective, but DM may follow.

Benign Ketotic Hypoglycemia

Thought to be due to ↓ substrate for gluconeogenesis. Most often presents during an illness in which oral intake is ↓. Usually resolves by 5–6 years of age.

TREATMENT

- Avoid prolonged periods of fasting.
- Slowly digested carbohydrate (e.g., corn starch) can be provided at bedtime.

HYPOCALCEMIA

Etiologies of hypocalcemia include the following:

- **Neonates:**
  - Antenatal maternal illness (DM, pregnancy-induced hypertension, hyperparathyroidism, familial hypocalciuric hypercalcemia).
  - Perinatal asphyxia, respiratory distress, sepsis.
  - Transient neonatal hypoparathyroidism.
  - Excessive phosphate intake from formula.
  - Structural abnormality of the parathyroids or gene mutation.

ENDOCRINOLOGY

- **Children:** Vitamin D deficiency, inadequate calcium intake, hypoparathyroidism, pseudohypoparathyroidism.

SYMPTOMS/EXAM

- Neonates may be asymptomatic or present with irritability, tetany, apnea, or seizures.
- Children may be asymptomatic or present with muscle cramps, dry skin, abdominal pain, paresthesias, or tetany.
- Physical findings may also include ⊕ Chvostek's sign and ↑ ICP.

DIAGNOSIS

- Measure total and ionized serum calcium and urine calcium.
- Obtain serum PTH, phosphorus, magnesium, creatinine, and alkaline phosphatase.

Obtain a fluorescence in situ hybridization (FISH) study for DiGeorge syndrome if any other features are present.

HYPOPARATHYROIDISM

Inappropriately **low levels of PTH** → **hypocalcemia and hyperphosphatemia.** Etiologies include DiGeorge syndrome, congenital absence or autoimmune destruction of the parathyroid, mutations in the gene for PTH, and gain-of-function mutations in calcium-sensing receptor (CASR).

Pseudohypoparathyroidism is due to a signaling defect → resistance to PTH.

DIAGNOSIS

- **Labs:** Low calcium, PTH, and magnesium; ↑ phosphorus.
- **Imaging:** May reveal metastatic calcifications.

TREATMENT

- Calcitriol, ergocalciferol, calcium, magnesium replacement.
- Monitor the following:
  - Serum PTH, calcium, phosphorus, magnesium, alkaline phosphatase.
  - Urinary calcium, phosphate, creatinine.

HYPERCALCEMIA

Etiologies include hypervitaminosis D, familial hypocalciuric hypercalcemia (FHH), prolonged immobilization, 1° hyperparathyroidism, and Williams syndrome.

Williams syndrome is suggested by elfin facies and supravalvular aortic stenosis.

SYMPTOMS/EXAM

- Patients with mild hypercalcemia (< 12 mg/dL) usually have no symptoms but may present with renal calculi, pathologic fractures, or osteopenia.
- Signs and symptoms associated with severe hypercalcemia include the following:
  - Anorexia, nausea, vomiting, constipation, nocturia, thirst.
  - Dehydration, muscle weakness, diminished reflexes.
  - **Neurologic impairment:** Confusion, difficulty concentrating, irritability.

DIAGNOSIS

- History may reveal excessive intake of vitamin D, vitamin A, calcium, or thiazide diuretics along with a ⊕ family history of FHH or renal calculi.

- **Labs:**
    - ↑ serum calcium, PTH, urinary calcium.
    - ↓ serum phosphate; normal or low alkaline phosphatase.
- A parathyroid adenoma can be localized with ultrasound, CT, MRI, or radionuclide imaging with sestamibi.

TREATMENT

- **Acute therapy: IV isotonic saline and furosemide** stimulate calcium clearance.
- If serum calcium level does not respond to the above measures, calcitonin or bisphosphonates can be used. Calcitonin acts rapidly but transiently. Pamidronate has been found to be effective in children.
- Patients with parathyroid hyperplasia (including MEN) require total parathyroidectomy with implantation of a small amount of parathyroid tissue in the forearm.
- Hypervitaminosis D or hypercalcemia associated with granulomatous or chronic inflammatory disease can be managed with glucocorticoids.

An 18-month-old boy presents for routine well-child care. At this visit, his parents are concerned that he started walking late at 16 months, is unable to run, and falls over frequently. He has no significant medical history, and other developmental milestones have been met on time. His exam is notable for wobbly gait, tibial bowing, and widening at the wrists. X-rays reveal cupping of the tibial metaphyses, and the distal radial physes appear sclerotic. Further history reveals that the patient was breast-fed until 15 months of age and did not receive vitamin D supplementation. Labs reveal an alkaline phosphatase of 945 IU/L, calcium 9.5 mEq/L, phosphate 4.2 mg/dL, vitamin D (25-hydroxy) 13 ng/mL (normal 20–67), and vitamin D (1,25-dihydroxy) 36 pg/mL (normal 27–71). What is the appropriate initial treatment? As this is consistent with vitamin D–deficient rickets, he is started on supplementation with ergocalciferol. Several months later, the tibial bowing is much improved, gait is normal, and radiographic findings have resolved.

RICKETS

A disorder of growing bone characterized by deficient mineralization of the bone matrix due to inadequate calcium, phosphorus, or both. Risk factors include breast-feeding (especially without vitamin D supplementation), prematurity/low birth weight, lack of sun exposure, and anticonvulsant use.

SYMPTOMS/EXAM

- May present with failure to thrive and seizures.
- Examination may reveal gross motor delay, waddling gait, and fractures.
- Bony abnormalities include the following:
    - Widening of the extremities of the long bones (wrists and ankles).
    - Enlarged costochondral junctions ("rachitic rosary").
    - Tibial and femoral bowing.
    - Ulnar and radial bowing.
- **Dental abnormalities:** Delayed eruption, enamel hypoplasia, caries.

- Wrists and knees show cupping, fraying, and widening of the epiphyses on x-ray.
- Osteopenia and rachitic rosary of the costochondral junctions are also seen on x-ray.
- See Table 7-4 for lab abnormalities associated with rickets.

Vitamin D–Deficient Rickets

SYMPTOMS/EXAM

Key components of the history are as follows:

- **Breast-fed infant**
- Dark skin
- Mother/infant with poor sun exposure
- Lack of vitamin D supplementation
- Inadequate dairy intake in older children (including lactose intolerance)

TREATMENT

- Ergocalciferol and supplemental calcium until physical, radiologic, and biochemical evidence of rickets has reversed.
- Follow serum 25(OH) vitamin D, PTH, calcium, and alkaline phosphatase levels and urinary calcium.

X-Linked Hypophosphatemic Rickets

Due to a defect in the kidney → massive renal phosphate losses.

TREATMENT

- Treat with phosphate replacement and calcitriol.
- Monitor PTH, calcium, phosphorus, and alkaline phosphatase.

Vitamin D–Dependent Rickets

Due to a rare inborn error of vitamin D metabolism in which patients are unable to generate $1,25(OH)_2$ vitamin D in the kidney.

SYMPTOMS/EXAM

Clinically, signs and symptoms are the same as those of vitamin D deficiency, but patients do not respond to vitamin D therapy at the usual dose.

TREATMENT

- Treat with calcitriol, ergocalciferol, and calcium supplementation. It may be necessary to continue treatment into adulthood.
- Monitor 25(OH) vitamin D, PTH, calcium, and alkaline phosphatase levels at each visit.

ENDOCRINOLOGY

TABLE 7-4. Lab Differentiation of Rickets

TYPE	25(OH) VITAMIN D	1,25(OH)₂ VITAMIN D	PTH	CALCIUM
Vitamin D deficient	↓	Normal or ↑	↑	↓
X-linked hypophosphatemic	Normal	Normal or ↓	Normal or ↑	Normal
Vitamin D dependent	Normal	↓	Normal or ↑	Normal or ↓

DISEASES OF THE THYROID AND THYROID HORMONE

Thyroid Hormone Synthesis

The hypothalamus releases thyrotropin-releasing hormone (TRH), which stimulates the pituitary to release thyroid-stimulating hormone (TSH). TSH stimulates the thyroid to produce and release T_4 and a small amount of T_3. Thyroid hormone synthesis begins with the production of thyroglobulin by the follicular cells. Iodine trapping and organification involve thyroid peroxidase (TPO) and pendrin. Most T_3 is produced via peripheral conversion of T_4, and both T_3 and T_4 circulate primarily by binding to thyroid-binding globulins (TBG).

The most common cause of congenital hypothyroidism is thyroid dysgenesis (ectopic, hypoplastic, or absent gland).

Hypothyroidism

CONGENITAL HYPOTHYROIDISM (CH)

CH presenting in the newborn period is due to **lesions in the thyroid gland (1°)** or in the **pituitary (2°)** or **hypothalamus (3°)**. Transient CH can occur with fetal exposure to maternal antithyroid medications, maternal ingestion of excess iodine, and transplacental passage of maternal TSH receptor antibodies that antagonize the fetus's TSH receptors (TSH_R). Approximately 80% of CH cases are due to an absent, hypoplastic, or ectopically placed thyroid gland; about 15% are due to a defect in any of the steps of thyroid hormone synthesis; and the remaining 5% stem from other causes.

The most common cause of endemic hypothyroidism globally is iodine deficiency.

SYMPTOMS/EXAM

Most affected infants have a normal appearance; however, the **most sensitive findings** for hypothyroidism include a large (> 1 cm) posterior fontanelle, hypoplastic or absent epiphyseal centers of the distal femur and proximal tibia, and jaundice lasting > 1 week. Macroglossia, hoarse cry, an enlarged umbilical hernia, constipation, and dry skin are infrequent signs.

DIAGNOSIS

- Newborn screening with measurements of T_4 and/or TSH in blood spots. Given the physiologic surge of TSH, T_4, and T_3 following delivery, screening should take place within the first 24 hours following birth, usually between 24 and 48 hours of age. See Table 7-5 for lab findings in CH.
- A thyroid scan with ^{99}Tc will demonstrate the absence or presence of thyroid gland.

In some states, newborn screening measures only TSH, which can miss the diagnoses of 2° and 3° CH.

ENDOCRINOLOGY

TABLE 7-5. Laboratory Findings in Congenital Hypothyroidism

	T$_4$	Free T$_4$	TSH	TBG
1° CH	↓	↓	↑	Normal
2°/3° CH	↓	↓	Normal or ↓	Normal
TBG deficiency[a]	↓	Normal	Normal	↓
TBG excess[a]	↑	Normal	Normal	↑
Total thyroid hormone resistance	↑	↑	↑	Normal

[a] Patients with TBG deficiency and excess are clinically euthyroid.

*Congenital hypothyroidism is the most common cause of **preventable** mental retardation.*

TREATMENT

- Administer T$_4$ in form of L-thyroxine. Adjustments are based on TSH and FT$_4$ levels (the latter is maintained in the upper half of normal range).
- Organification defects are usually permanent, whereas hypothyroidism due to an ectopically placed gland may be transient. Therefore, a trial of L-thyroxine at three years of age may be attempted for those with ectopic thyroid glands.
- Thyroid hormone is involved in neuronal synaptogenesis. Thus, the goal of treatment is to prevent loss of cognitive function. Most neonates in whom treatment is instituted early have normal IQs and motor development as children.

Infants found to have 2° or 3° CH should be evaluated for panhypopituitarism.

ACQUIRED HYPOTHYROIDISM

Etiologies of acquired hypothyroidism include postviral illness, neck radiation, iodine excess, and iodine deficiency. Excess iodine leads to an acute block in the release of thyroid hormone, referred to as the **Wolff-Chaikoff effect.** Iatrogenic causes of excess iodine include amiodarone (contains 37% iodine) and povidone-iodine (Betadine) skin preps. Hypothalamic and pituitary dysfunction may also arise, leading to 2° and 3° acquired hypothyroidism.

SYMPTOMS/EXAM

↓ growth velocity, delayed bone age, myxedema, constipation, cold intolerance, ↓ energy, delayed or precocious puberty, goiter.

The magnitude of growth retardation is proportional to the duration of untreated hypothyroidism.

DIAGNOSIS

- 1° **hypothyroidism:** ↓ FT$_4$, ↑ TSH.
- 2°/3° **hypothyroidism:** ↓ FT$_4$, ↓ TSH.

TREATMENT

L-thyroxine.

ENDOCRINOLOGY

Hashimoto's Thyroiditis

Characterized by **antibodies against thyroid gland, TBG, or TPO,** with **lymphocytic infiltration** leading to **thyromegaly.** May be **associated with other autoimmune diseases,** such as type 1 DM, Addison's disease, vitiligo, hypoparathyroidism, celiac sprue, and juvenile rheumatoid arthritis. Seen primarily in adolescents; affects females more often than males.

SYMPTOMS/EXAM

- Most affected children present with a diffusely enlarged thyroid that is firm and nontender with a "pebbly" consistency. A sensation of neck fullness or dysphagia may also develop.
- Patients may be **euthyroid** or have symptoms of **hypothyroidism.** Some develop **hashitoxicosis,** which causes transient symptoms of hyperthyroidism from the sudden release of preformed thyroid hormone during immunologic destruction of the thyroid gland.

DIAGNOSIS

FT_4, TSH; thyroid antibodies.

TREATMENT

- If patients are hypothyroid, treatment is with L-thyroxine.
- Monitor euthyroid patients for the development of hypothyroidism.

Hyperthyroidism

Leading causes include Graves' disease and neonatal thyrotoxicosis.

> A 16-year-old who presented with tachycardia, palpitations, weight loss, and nervousness was diagnosed with Graves' disease. What intervention will give the fastest symptomatic relief? Propranolol.

GRAVES' DISEASE

Defined as hyperthyroidism caused by **IgG antibodies that stimulate the TSH receptor.**

SYMPTOMS/EXAM

- Poor concentration, weight loss, polyphagia, palpitations, exercise intolerance, ↑ stool frequency, oligomenorrhea, emotional instability, nervousness, warm skin, tachycardia, proptosis, symmetrically enlarged thyroid.
- Exophthalmos may be seen but is much less common in children than in adults.

DIAGNOSIS

- ↓ TSH; ↑ total T_3 and FT_4 (although in some cases only T_3 may be ↑ and T_4 may be normal).
- ↑ uptake of ^{99}Tc on thyroid scan.

TREATMENT

- **Antithyroid medications are first-line treatment for children.**

The most common cause of goiter and hypothyroidism in childhood and adolescence is Hashimoto's (autoimmune) thyroiditis.

Children with trisomy 21 have a 35-fold greater risk of hypothyroidism than the general population.

The most common cause of hyperthyroidism in childhood is Graves' disease.

ENDOCRINOLOGY

173

- Medications include **propylthiouracil (PTU) and methimazole,** which prevent organification and peripheral conversion of T_4 to T_3. Methimazole has a longer half-life than PTU, is more potent, and is less likely to cause severe hepatitis. Serious complications of these medications include **agranulocytosis,** which is often reversible, and **hepatitis,** which may not be reversible and may become fulminant.
- Both medications inhibit hormone formation but do not prevent release. Therefore, **β-blockers** may be employed to reduce symptoms produced by extant circulating hormone.
- **Radioiodine:** ^{131}I trapped in follicular cells → thyroid destruction. A more favorable response is obtained in smaller glands.
- **Surgery: Total or near-total thyroidectomy to prevent recurrences.** Complications of surgery include hypocalcemia (hypoparathyroidism) and vocal cord paralysis.

NEONATAL THYROTOXICOSIS

Defined as severe and life-threatening hyperthyroidism due to **transplacental transfer** of TSH receptor–stimulating antibodies from a mother with a history of Graves' disease.

SYMPTOMS/EXAM

Intrauterine growth retardation (IUGR), premature fusion of cranial sutures, mental retardation, tachycardia.

TREATMENT

Methimazole, β-blockers, and/or potassium iodide.

Thyroid Mass

Although the prevalence of thyroid nodules is greater in adults than in children, the **risk of malignancy is higher in children.** Radiation is a risk factor for neoplasm. However, most patients with thyroid nodules do **not** have a history of irradiation. Other risk factors include female gender, puberty, and a family or personal history of thyroid disease. Thyroid masses are subdivided into hot, warm, and cold nodules. Hot nodules have activating mutations in TSH_R.

DIAGNOSIS

- **Ultrasound:** Cystic lesions are less likely to be malignant than solid lesions.
- **Radionuclide scan:** Can distinguish hot from cold nodules, but cannot differentiate benign from malignant lesions.
- Fine-needle aspiration (FNA).

TREATMENT

Because of the higher risk of malignancy in children, some clinicians opt for removal of all nodules, while others try to suppress TSH (and thus nodule growth) with exogenous thyroid hormone if FNA demonstrates benign features.

The thyroid nodules that are most likely to be malignant in children are solitary nodules and lateral neck masses with prominent cervical adenopathy.

Target adult height or midparental height is computed as follows:

- **Target height for males** = (father's height + mother's height + 13 cm) ÷ 2.
- **Target height for females** = (father's height + mother's height − 13 cm) ÷ 2.

A 14-year-old girl presents for a routine physical and is noted to have a height at the third percentile and weight at the fifth percentile. Her mother is 4′11″ and her father is 5′4″. The patient's birth weight and length were at the 40th percentile at birth and slowly dropped to their current percentiles by 18 months of age. Her weight and length have continued along the third to fifth percentile. What is the most likely diagnosis? Familial short stature.

Short Stature

Short stature is defined as follows:

- Absolute height < 2 SDs mean for age (or < 3% for age).
- Height that decelerates greater than two growth channels over time or height velocity < 2 SDs for age.

Etiologies include the following;

- **Chromosomal:** Turner syndrome, trisomy 21.
- **Syndromic:** Silver-Russell syndrome
- **Osteochondroplasias:** Defects in bone, cartilage, or both. Include achondroplasia.
- **Chronic disease:** Examples include congenital heart disease, chronic lung disease, renal failure, DM, and malabsorption syndromes such as celiac disease.
- **Endocrinopathies:**
    - **Hypothyroidism:** Height is more significantly affected than weight. Delay in skeletal age may be significant (> 2 years); replacing thyroxine produces catch-up growth.
    - **Cushing syndrome:** Glucocorticoid excess delays skeletal growth at the level of the growth plate.
    - **Growth hormone (GH) deficiency.**
- **Variants of normal:**
    - **Constitutional delay:** The most common cause of short stature. Associated with a ⊕ family history of "late bloomers." Bone age lags chronological age. Characterized by delayed puberty with no endocrinopathy. Target height is usually attained (see Figure 7-3).
    - **Familial short stature:** Typically a small child who grows and maintains growth along his own growth channel. Puberty is normal; other family members are small. Patients are expected to reach target adult height; bone age is seldom > 1 year behind chronological age (see Figure 7-4).
    - **Idiopathic short stature:** Height < 3% and growth velocity < 25% for age. Patients may have delayed skeletal maturity and puberty without a ⊕ family history.

The most common cause of short stature is constitutional delay of growth.

Children with short stature due to an endocrinopathy tend to be overweight.

ENDOCRINOLOGY

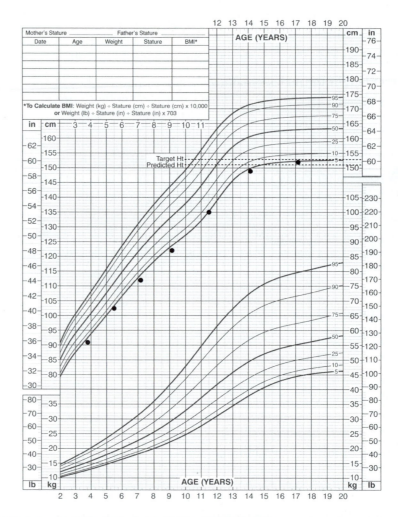

FIGURE 7-3. Growth chart of constitutional growth delay.

(Reproduced, with permission, from Hay WW et al. *Current Pediatric Diagnosis & Treatment*, 17th ed. New York: McGraw-Hill, 2005:966.)

DIAGNOSIS

See Table 7-6 for the diagnostic evaluation of short stature.

TREATMENT

- Gear treatment toward the underlying cause of short stature.
- GH therapy is approved by the FDA for the following conditions:
  - **Idiopathic short stature:** < −2.25 SDs below the mean and adult height prediction of < 5'3" for boys and < 4'11" for girls.
  - GH deficiency from hypothalamic-pituitary disease.
  - Chronic renal failure before transplantation.
  - Small for gestational age not demonstrating catch-up growth by two years of age.
  - Turner syndrome, Prader-Willi syndrome.
  - AIDS-related wasting.

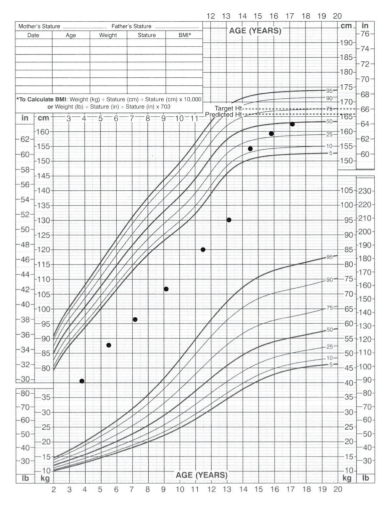

FIGURE 7-4. Growth chart of familial short stature.

(Reproduced, with permission, from Hay WW et al. *Current Pediatric Diagnosis & Treatment,* 17th ed. New York: McGraw-Hill, 2005:965.)

TABLE 7-6. Studies to Consider in the Evaluation of Short Stature

STUDY	SUSPECTED PATHOLOGY
Karyotype	Short stature in females should prompt workup for Turner's syndrome.
Bone age	Bone age that lags chronological age by > 2 years may be seen with an endocrinopathy or constitutional delay of growth.
TSH, FT$_4$	Hypothyroidism.
CBC, UA, BUN/creatinine, serum electrolytes, ESR	Anemia, inflammation, RTA, and renal failure may stunt growth.
IGF-1 and IGF-BP3 +/− provocative testing	GH deficiency.

Growth Hormone Deficiency and Insensitivity

May be due to central (hypothalamic-pituitary) disturbance or to a downstream problem with recognizing and responding to GH (see Table 7-7).

SYMPTOMS/EXAM

- Characterized by subnormal growth velocity.
- Truncal adiposity and/or hypoglycemia may be seen.
- Hypoglycemia, hypovolemia, microphallus, and midline defects may be seen if associated with panhypopituitarism.
- Bone age may be delayed by as much as half of chronological age.

DIAGNOSIS

- **Provocative GH testing:** Uses levodopa, clonidine, arginine, and insulin. Arbitrary cutoff of $< 7–10$ µg/L for GH deficiency.
- **Random serum GH level:** Difficult to interpret given that **GH secretion is pulsatile** and the normal physiologic nadir for GH is below the detection threshold of most standard assays. **Twenty-four-hour GH profiles** can plot and account for GH pulsatility but are rarely performed.
- **IGF-1 and IGF-BP3:** Unlike GH, these proteins are not secreted episodically, and their half-lives are longer than GH, obviating the need for provocative testing.
- **MRI of the hypothalamus and pituitary:** May reveal a congenital defect or tumor.

Children with precocious puberty will be tall for their age, but their final height will be shorter than predicted due to premature closure of growth plates.

Tall Stature

Defined as follows:

- Absolute height > 2 SDs from the mean for age (or $> 97\%$ for age).
- Height that accelerates > 2 growth channels over time or height velocity > 2 SDs from the mean for age.
- See Table 7-8 for various etiologies and their associated features.

TABLE 7-7. Central vs. Peripheral GH Deficiency

LOCATION OF LESION	TYPE OF LESION	DESCRIPTION
Hypothalamus/pituitary	Hereditary defects	Mutations in genes encoding for GH synthesis and release.
	Congenital malformations	**Septo-optic dysplasia:** Absence or hypoplasia of the septum pellucidum or corpus callosum and optic chiasm accompanied by hypothalamic insufficiency.
	Acquired defects	Tumors, trauma, sarcoidosis, fungal infections.
	GH deficiency not otherwise defined	**Prader-Willi syndrome:** Central GH deficiency in the absence of MRI findings.
Peripheral	Hereditary defects	GH receptor defects and defects in signal transduction.
	Acquired defects	Antibodies against GH or GH receptor.

TABLE 7-8. Etiologies of Tall Stature

SYNDROME	CLINICAL FEATURES	PATHOPHYSIOLOGY/ABNORMAL FINDINGS
Cerebral gigantism (Sotos syndrome)	Prominent forehead, macrocephaly, hypertelorism, large hands and feet with thickened subcutaneous tissue, mental retardation.	No known cause. GH and IGF are normal. Early puberty; final adult height usually within normal.
Familial (constitutional) tall stature	No syndromic features.	GH and IGF are usually upper normal. Family history of tall individuals.
Marfan syndrome	Arachnodactyly, hypermobile joints, subluxation of ocular lenses, pectus carinatum, aortic aneurysms.	An autosomal-dominant disorder of fibrillin gene. Sporadic cases have been described.
Klinefelter syndrome	Small testes, delayed puberty, gynecomastia, disproportionately long legs, delayed emotional development.	Karyotype 47,XXY; sporadic inheritance. Testosterone levels are ↓.

DISORDERS OF THE ADRENAL GLAND

Glucocorticoid Excess

Cushing syndrome refers to the constellation of physical and clinical findings of glucocorticoid excess. **Cushing disease** specifically refers to glucocorticoid excess due to an ACTH-secreting pituitary lesion. The majority of these lesions are microadenomas.

SYMPTOMS/EXAM

As shown in Table 7-9, multiple systems are affected by glucocorticoid excess.

DIAGNOSIS

- **Plasma cortical concentrations:** Will be ↑ with loss of diurnal variation.
- **Serum electrolytes:** ↓ chloride and potassium and ↑ sodium and bicarbonate may be seen.
- **Urinary free cortisol:** Will be ↑. This is the most useful initial diagnostic test.
- **Urinary 17-ketosteroid excretion:** Will be ↑ in adrenal tumors.
- **Dexamethasone suppression test:** Dexamethasone is normally a potent downregulator of ACTH and cortisol, so in the setting of autonomous glucocorticoid excess, suppression will not be seen.
- **Pituitary and/or adrenal imaging.**

TREATMENT

- Surgical resection of pituitary adenomas and adrenal tumors is the treatment of choice. Intraoperative and postoperative glucocorticoid treatment is necessary to prevent adrenal crisis until the hypothalamic-pituitary-adrenal (HPA) axis returns to its normal function. After pituitary resection, complete panhypopituitarism may occur.
- Radiation therapy.

The most common cause of glucocorticoid excess in children is exogenously delivered synthetic glucocorticoid.

TABLE 7-9. Systems Affected by Glucocorticoid Excess

SYSTEM	CLINICAL EFFECT	PROPOSED MECHANISM[a]
Constitutional	↑ weight but ↓ height, i.e., ↑ BMI; moon facies, buffalo hump.	⊗ GH and IGF-1.
Dermatologic	Striae, thin skin, acne, hirsutism.	⊗ collagen synthesis; ACTH may ↑ adrenal androgens.
Cardiovascular	Hypertension.	Cross-reacts with mineralocorticoid receptor.
Endocrine	Glucose intolerance; menstrual irregularities and/ or delayed puberty; hypothyroidism.	⊗ insulin; ⊗ HPG axis; ⊗ $T_4 \rightarrow T_3$ conversion.
Musculoskeletal	Osteoporosis, osteopenia, proximal myopathy.	⊗ intestinal absorption of Ca^{2+} and osteoblast activity.
Neuropsychiatric	Pseudotumor cerebri, depression, OCD.	

[a] ⊗ = "inhibition of."

> An 11-year-old girl with Addison's disease on hydrocortisone requires surgery to fix a supracondylar fracture. What should be done with her steroid dose in the perioperative period? Stress doses of IV hydrocortisone must be given one hour before and during surgery. Once the patient can tolerate oral medication, oral hydrocortisone must be given at 50 mg/m²/day for at least 24 hours after the acute stress has resolved.

Adrenal Insufficiency

1° insufficiency is due to defects of the **adrenals**, whereas 2° **insufficiency** is due to defects of the **hypothalamus and/or pituitary**. Both 1° and 2° insufficiency may be inherited or acquired.

- 1° inherited adrenal deficiencies:
  - **Congenital adrenal hyperplasia:** See the discussion below.
  - **Adrenoleukodystrophy:** Accumulation of very long chain fatty acids in the CNS and adrenal gland → demyelination and adrenal insufficiency. Presents from the neonatal period to early adulthood with neurologic decline and symptoms of adrenal insufficiency. Follows X-linked or recessive inheritance.
- 1° acquired adrenal deficiencies:
  - **Addison's disease:** Autoimmune destruction of the adrenal gland; has exceeded TB as the most common cause. May occur as part of an autoimmune polyendocrinopathy syndrome (APS).
    - **APS type I: hypoadrenocorticism, hypoparathyroidism,** and **candidiasis** (aka **APECED syndrome:** Autoimmune Polyendocrinopathy–Candidiasis–Ectodermal Dystrophy). Autosomal-recessive inheritance. Associated with hypogonadism, vitiligo, and alopecia.

- APS type II: Characterized by **hypoadrenocorticism, thyroid disease (Schmidt syndrome), and/or type 1 diabetes (Carpenter syndrome)**. Multigenetic inheritance.
  - **Waterhouse-Friderichsen syndrome:** An intra-adrenal hemorrhage that may occur during sepsis (especially meningococcemia) and ischemia.
- **2° adrenal insufficiencies:**
  - Mutations → CRH or ACTH deficiency.
  - Traumatic, neoplastic, or autoimmune destruction of the hypothalamus or pituitary.
  - Iatrogenic.

Exogenous glucocorticoids that are given for chronic disease and are then suddenly discontinued will → iatrogenic 2° adrenal insufficiency.

SYMPTOMS/EXAM

Table 7-10 lists symptoms and exam findings associated with adrenal insufficiency. The symptoms may be chronic. During times of stress such as that induced by illness or surgery, an adrenal crisis may occur → severe, life-threatening symptoms. Adrenal crisis is much more common in 1° adrenal insufficiency because mineralocorticoid activity usually remains intact in 2° adrenal insufficiency.

DIAGNOSIS

- **ACTH stimulation test:** In 1° adrenal insufficiency, an ↑ in cortisol and aldosterone will not be seen in response to ACTH.
- **Serum ACTH:** Will be ↑ in 1° adrenal insufficiency.
- **Urinary free cortisol:** Will be ↓.
- **Metyrapone test:** Can be used to diagnose 2° adrenal insufficiency. A test dose of metyrapone given at midnight suppresses cortisol production. If the HPA axis is intact, ACTH secretion should ↑ and will → an ↑ in 11-deoxycortisol measured in the morning. In hypopituitarism, urinary 11-deoxycortisol is ↓.
- **CRH test:** Can be used to diagnose 2° adrenal insufficiency. Serum ACTH and cortisol are measured after a dose of CRH is given.

Hyperpigmentation is seen only in 1° adrenal insufficiency because it results from excess ACTH stimulating the melanocyte-stimulating hormone receptors in the skin.

TABLE 7-10. Symptoms and Exam Findings in Adrenal Insufficiency

SYSTEM	SYMPTOMS/EXAM
Constitutional	Weakness, fatigue, weight loss.
GI	Vomiting, anorexia, abdominal pain.
GU	Polyuria, dehydration.
Dermatologic	Hyperpigmentation.
Musculoskeletal	Myalgia, bone pain.
Cardiovascular	Hypotension.
Neurologic	Coma, confusion.

TREATMENT

- The maintenance hydrocortisone dose is 8–15 mg/m²/day, while stress dosing, 50 mg/m²/day, should be used during times of illness and surgery.
- Fludrocortisone must be added for 1° adrenal insufficiency in order to replace mineralocorticoid activity.

> A newborn infant was found to have bilateral cryptorchidism and proximal hypospadias. What life-threatening diagnosis should be considered and ruled out first? Salt-wasting CAH, which leads to adrenal crisis.

The most common cause of CAH is 21-hydroxylase deficiency.

Congenital Adrenal Hyperplasia (CAH)

A group of **autosomal-recessive enzyme deficiencies** → disorders in adrenal hormone synthesis. Most forms of CAH → cortisol deficiency. Depending on the enzyme deficiency involved, mineralocorticoid deficiency or excess may occur as well as androgen deficiency or excess. See Figure 7-5 for the steps in adrenal hormone synthesis. Table 7-11 outlines the characteristics of various subtypes of CAH.

21-hydroxylase deficiency is the most common cause of ambiguous genitalia.

21-HYDROXYLASE DEFICIENCY

Characterized by ↑ 17-OHP, androstenedione, and sex hormones. Adrenal hyperplasia results from ACTH stimulation. CAH-related forms of 21-hydroxylase deficiency are as follows (see also Table 7-12):

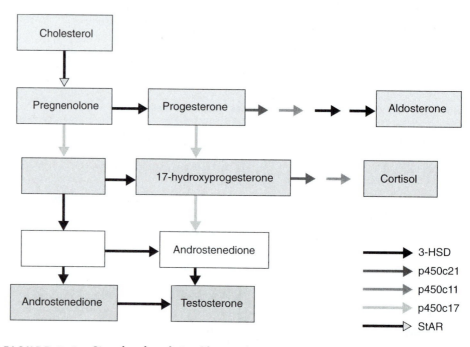

FIGURE 7-5. **Steps in adrenal steroidogenesis.**

Some steps have intentionally been left blank for simplification.

TABLE 7-11. Hormone Deficiencies and Clinical Findings in Additional Types of CAH

TYPE	HORMONE DEFICIENCY	CLINICAL FINDINGS
11β-hydroxylase deficiency	Aldosterone and glucocorticoid.	Hypertension, hypoglycemia, and signs of masculinization in XX infants. Precocious puberty in males. Not salt wasters.
17-hydroxylase deficiency	Glucocorticoid and sex hormones.	Hypertension, hypoglycemia, hypokalemia, XY infants with undermasculinized genitalia. 1° hypogonadism in females. Not salt wasters.
3β-hydroxysteroid dehydrogenase deficiency	Mineralocorticoid, glucocorticoid, sex hormones.	Hypotension, hypoglycemia, XY infants with undermasculinized genitalia. Most waste salt → adrenal crisis.
Lipoid adrenal hyperplasia[a]	Mineralocorticoid, glucocorticoid, sex hormones.	Hypotension, XY infants with undermasculinized genitalia, salt waste → adrenal crisis.

[a] Results from a mutation in the StAR protein, which carries cholesterol across the mitochondrial membrane to be converted into pregnenolone.

TABLE 7-12. CAH Subtypes Resulting from 21-Hydroxylase Deficiency

VARIABLE	CLASSIC SALT WASTING	CLASSIC NON–SALT WASTING OR SIMPLE VIRILIZING	NONCLASSIC
Time to medical attention	Early onset.	Early onset.	Late onset.
Symptoms/exam	**Males:** No obvious signs as newborn; may present with precocious puberty. **Females:** Virilization, ambiguous genitalia, menstrual irregularities, hirsutism, acne. **Both:** Poor feeding, failure to thrive, vomiting, fatigue, dehydration, hypotension.	**Males:** No obvious signs as newborn; may present with precocious puberty. **Females:** Virilization, ambiguous genitalia, menstrual irregularities, hirsutism, acne.	**Males:** Infertility, acne, precocious puberty. **Females:** Mild clitoromegaly, premature adrenarche, irregular menses, acne, PCOS. **Both:** May be asymptomatic.
Risk of adrenal crisis	↑↑	Not typical.	Not typical.
Laboratory findings	↑↑ serum 17-OHP.[a] Hyponatremia, hyperkalemia. ↑ renin.	↑↑ serum 17-OHP.	↑ serum 17-OHP.
Treatment	Glucocorticoids and mineralocorticoids.	Glucocorticoids only.	Glucocorticoid treatment is **not** essential (given if the patient is symptomatic).

[a] 17-OHP is highest in classic salt wasters, followed by simple virilizers, and is lowest in nonclassic forms.

- **Classic salt wasting (75%):** Blockage → a deficiency of aldosterone and cortisol.
- **Classic non–salt wasting or simple virilizing (20%):** Blockage → a deficiency of cortisol only.
- **Nonclassic (1–5%):** Blockage leads to excessive androgens only.

Diagnosis

- **ACTH stimulation test:** Measures 17-OHP levels at 0 and 60 minutes and plots these values against a nomogram.
- **Newborn screening:** Measures 17-OHP in blood spots obtained in the first 24–48 hours of life.
- **Prenatal diagnosis:** Measurement of amniotic fluid 17-OHP or chorionic villus sampling for restriction fragment–length polymorphisms.

Treatment

- **Replace glucocorticoid deficiency: Hydrocortisone** is the **drug of choice.** The goal is to provide enough to suppress ACTH, thereby suppressing adrenal androgen production, without providing too much and stunting growth.
- **Replace mineralocorticoid for those with the salt-wasting subtype: Fludrocortisone** and **salt supplementation.**
- **Management of acute crisis:** IV saline boluses; glucocorticoid and mineralocorticoid replacement given as hydrocortisone 50 mg/m² bolus (at this dose, hydrocortisone provides mineralocorticoid as well; no IV form of fludrocortisone is available).
- **Stress-dose/sick-day management:** Shock, surgery, febrile illness. Hydrocortisone 50 mg/m²/day; an IM form (**Solu-Cortef**) may be given if the patient is unable to tolerate PO medication.

NORMAL SEXUAL DETERMINATION AND DIFFERENTIATION

- Early embryos possess **bipotential gonads** and both **müllerian** and **wolffian** internal genital structures (see Table 7-13). Genetic makeup determines whether the bipotential gonad differentiates into testes or ovaries, and subsequently whether internal and external sexual organs appear male or female.
- The **default pathway is along the female pathway** with preservation of müllerian structures and loss of wolffian structures. Differentiation into testes requires the presence of the **testis-determining factor,** which is regulated by the **sex-determining region on the Y chromosome (SRY).**
- Sertoli cells of the testes produce müllerian inhibiting substance (MIS), which induces the regression of the müllerian structures. The Leydig cells of the testes produce testosterone, which stabilizes the wolffian structures and potentiates the effects of MIS.

Ambiguous Genitalia

A term used to describe sexual organs that appear neither completely male nor completely female. Subtypes include the following:

- **True hermaphroditism:** Both testicular and ovarian tissue are present; external genitalia may be ambiguous, completely male, or completely female.

TABLE 7-13. Structures Derived from Müllerian and Wolffian Ducts

Müllerian-Derived Structures	Wolffian-Derived Structures
Fallopian tubes	Epididymis
Uterus	Vas deferens
Cervix	Seminal vesicles
Upper two-thirds of vagina	

- **Pseudohermaphroditism:** Either ovarian or testicular tissue is present, but not both; phenotypic appearance is ambiguous.

Symptoms/Exam

Clitoromegaly, micropenis, cryptorchidism, hypospadias, rugated labia major, and/or bifid scrotum.

Differential

The following are causes of ambiguous genitalia that may present in the newborn period (see also Table 7-14):

- **Lesion or insult to the hypothalamic-pituitary stalk:** Any lesion of this kind may give rise to deficient testosterone. **Panhypopituitarism** may be

TABLE 7-14. Causes of Ambiguous Genitalia in the Newborn Period

	Chromosomal	Müllerian	Wolffian	External
Klinefelter syndrome	XXY	Absent	Absent	Micropenis
Panhypopituitarism	XY	Absent	Present	Micropenis
21-hydroxylase deficiency	XX	Present	Absent	Ambiguous, virilized
11β-hydroxylase deficiency	XX	Present	Absent	Ambiguous, virilized
17-hydroxylase deficiency	XY	Absent	Present	Ambiguous
StAR protein deficiency	XY	Absent	Absent	Female
Complete androgen insensitivity syndrome	XY	Absent	Absent	Female
Partial androgen insensitivity syndrome	XY	Absent	Variable	Ambiguous
5α-reductase deficiency	XY	Absent	Present	Ambiguous
Vanishing testes syndrome	XY	Absent	Absent	Anorchid, micropenis
Placental aromatase deficiency	XX	Present	Absent	Ambiguous, virilized

seen as micropenis in an XY infant who also has hypoglycemia, hypotension, and failure to thrive.
- **Congenital adrenal hyperplasia.**
- **Placental aromatase deficiency:** Aromatase normally converts fetal androgens into estrogen; therefore, a deficiency → the buildup of androgens and virilization of the female fetus.
- **Complete androgen insensitivity syndrome from failure of receptors to respond to testosterone:** Presents with unambiguously female external genitalia; **partial androgen insensitivity syndrome** presents with ambiguous genitalia.
- **5α-reductase type 2 deficiency:** In this deficiency, dihydrotestosterone (DHT) (testosterone → DHT) is not made in sufficient quantities at birth to complete external genital differentiation in an XY infant. However, masculinization may occur during puberty owing to activity of the type 1 isozyme found in skin on ↑ circulating testosterone.
- **Maternal ingestion of androgens or excess maternal endogenous production of androgens.**

DIAGNOSIS

- Determine karyotype.
- Evaluate for CAH (e.g., 17-OHP and electrolytes).
- Ultrasound to delineate internal genital structures and to determine the presence of ovaries or undescended testes.
- Measuring testosterone before and after hCG stimulation can demonstrate testosterone synthesis defects.

TREATMENT

- **A social emergency and potentially a medical emergency as well** (e.g., salt wasting with virilization, adrenal insufficiency in panhypopituitarism).
- Treatment should be administered with a **multidisciplinary team** consisting of a pediatrician, an endocrinologist, a urologist, and a social worker.
- Although sensitivity must be employed in addressing parents' concerns over determining the sex of their infant, a thorough and prudent attempt at clarifying the diagnosis and etiology should be made before subjecting the infant to a premature gender label and to potentially unnecessary or unwanted gender reversal surgery.

CHAPTER 8

Gastrointestinal System and Nutrition

Shervin Rabizadeh, MD, MBA
reviewed by Patricia DeRusso, MD

Abdominal Pain

Vomiting that precedes pain is usually associated with acute gastroenteritis, whereas pain most often precedes vomiting in GI obstruction.

The signs and symptoms of pediatric abdominal pain vary according to the disorder. Listed below are some common signs and symptoms of GI disorders affecting the pediatric population. Specific diagnoses are described in the section on GI disorders. Figure 8-1 shows an algorithmic approach to the evaluation of abdominal pain.

ACUTE APPENDICITIS

Inflammation of the appendix resulting from obstruction of the lumen. If left untreated, it can → appendiceal perforation and subsequent peritonitis. Occurs twice as frequently in males than in females; most common among adolescents.

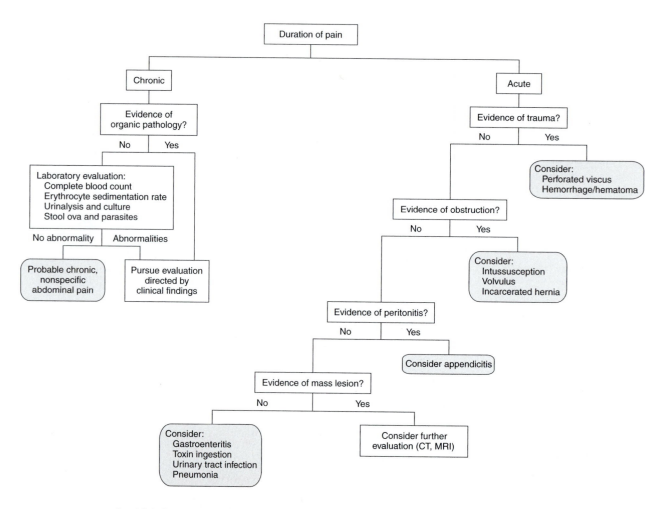

FIGURE 8-1. Algorithm for evaluation of abdominal pain in children.

(Reproduced, with permission, from Rudolph AM et al. *Rudolph's Fundamentals of Pediatrics,* 3rd ed. New York: McGraw-Hill, 2002:488.)

SYMPTOMS/EXAM

- Starts with crampy periumbilical pain, nausea, vomiting, and fever.
- Localizes to the RLQ at McBurney's point.
- Rectal exam may reveal tenderness.

DIAGNOSIS

- **Labs:** Neutrophilic leukocytosis is often found, but in some cases the CBC may be normal.
- **Imaging:**
  - AXR may show a calcified fecalith but is not a sensitive test; ultrasound may demonstrate dilation of the appendix.
  - Abdominal CT is a sensitive test and is being used more frequently; sensitivity ↑ with use of rectal contrast.

TREATMENT

Surgery is the definitive treatment.

ACUTE PANCREATITIS

Defined as acute inflammation of the pancreas. The mechanism is not well understood but is thought to be related to the autodigestion of tissue from pancreatic enzymes. The etiology may be idiopathic, infectious, pharmacologic, traumatic, metabolic, anatomic, or associated with cystic fibrosis (CF). Pancreatitis should always be considered in the differential diagnosis of acute abdominal pain.

Think of mumps and pancreatitis.

SYMPTOMS/EXAM

- Presents with mild to severe abdominal pain in the LUQ or epigastrium with radiation to the back.
- Low-grade fever may be present.

DIAGNOSIS

- **Labs:** Amylase and lipase levels are 3–4 times higher than normal (amylase is not as specific).
- **Imaging:** Ultrasound is the initial diagnostic study and can be used to rule out abscess, cysts, or stones; CT can also be used.
- ERCP may be necessary when repeated episodes of pancreatitis are unexplained and anatomical causes are being investigated.

TREATMENT

- Supportive measures; can feed via tube in the jejunum.
- Institute NG tube suctioning if the patient is vomiting.
- Narcotics should be administered as needed but with caution; hydromorphone hydrochloride (Dilaudid) may be better than morphine. The latter is speculated to induce sphincter of Oddi spasm/dysfunction.

COMPLICATIONS

Complicatons may result from infection, abscess formation, pseudocyst, or phlegmon. Can be life threatening.

CHOLECYSTITIS

- Acute inflammation of the gallbladder, most commonly caused by gallstones.
- Has ↑ in incidence.
- **Sx/Exam:** Presents with RUQ pain and a ⊕ Murphy's sign on exam. If pain is of > 3 months' duration, consider a diagnosis of chronic cholecystitis.
- **Dx:** Abdominal ultrasound.
- **Tx:** Surgery. Evaluate for an etiology of gallstones.

LACTOSE INTOLERANCE

- Defined as inability to digest lactose-containing substances; results from a shortage of the enzyme lactase.
- More commonly affects older children.
- **Sx/Exam:** In the absence of lactase, lactose is digested by bacteria, releasing hydrogen and CO_2. This → discomfort, bloating, gassiness, and eventual diarrhea.
- **Dx:** Diagnosed by the breath hydrogen test.
- **Tx:** Treat by eliminating offending substances from the diet or supplementation with lactase enzyme.

DYSPEPSIA

- **Sx/Exam:** May present as nausea, heartburn, regurgitation, belching, bloating, or hiccups.
- **Dx:** Rule out organic causes.
- **Tx:** Treat in accordance with the etiology.

IRRITABLE BOWEL SYNDROME (IBS)

- **Sx/Exam:**
  - Presents as episodic pain, typically crampy, that may be felt in any part of the abdomen.
  - Can be accompanied by constipation or diarrhea.
  - Episodes are often associated with stressful situations.
- **Tx:** Treat with reassurance, a high-fiber diet, and medication (not very effective).

RECURRENT ABDOMINAL PAIN

- Involves the interaction of physical and psychosocial stressors and the ANS-controlled motor activity of the intestines.
- **Dx:** A diagnosis of exclusion.
- **Tx:** Treat by addressing stressors, instituting therapy, and initiating a high-fiber diet. Medication is not very effective.

Vomiting

Vomiting may result from a variety of disorders affecting pediatric patients. A key is to use the history and physical to distinguish nonbilious from bilious causes (proximal vs. distal to the ampulla of Vater). Table 8-1 lists the various causes of vomiting.

TABLE 8-1. Causes of Vomiting and Regurgitation

GASTROINTESTINAL TRACT DISORDERS

Esophagus:
Achalasia
Gastroesophageal reflux (chalasia)
Hiatal hernia
Esophagitis
Atresia with or without fistula
Congenital vascular or mucosal rings, webs
Stenosis
Duplication and diverticulum
Foreign body
Periesophageal mass

Stomach:
Hypertrophic pyloric stenosis
Pylorospasm
Diaphragmatic hernia
Peptic disease and gastritis
Antral web

Duodenum:
Annular pancreas
Duodenitis and ulcer
Malrotation
Mesenteric bands
Superior mesenteric artery syndrome

Intestine and colon:
Atresia and stenosis
Meconium ileus
Malrotation, volvulus
Duplication
Intussusception
Foreign body
Polyposis
Soy or cow's milk protein intolerance
Gluten enteropathy
Food allergy
Hirschsprung's disease
Chronic intestinal pseudo-obstruction
Appendicitis
IBD
Gastroenteritis, infections

Other abdominal organs:
Hepatitis
Gallstones
Pancreatitis
Peritonitis

EXTRAGASTROINTESTINAL TRACT DISORDERS

Sepsis
Pneumonia
Otitis media
UTI
Meningitis
Subdural effusion
Hydrocephalus
Brain tumor
Reye syndrome
Rumination
Intoxications
Alcohol
Aspirin

Acetaminophen
Adrenal insufficiency
Renal tubular acidosis
Inborn errors
Urea cycle disorders
Phenylketonuria
Maple syrup urine disease
Organic acidemia
Galactosemia
Fructose intolerance
Tyrosinosis
Scleroderma
Epidermolysis bullosa

Reproduced, with permission, from Hay WW et al. *Current Pediatric Diagnosis & Treatment,* 17th ed. New York: McGraw-Hill, 2005:626.

GASTROESOPHAGEAL REFLUX

See the section on GI disorders.

ACHALASIA OF THE ESOPHAGUS

See the section on GI disorders.

CAUSTIC BURNS OF THE ESOPHAGUS

Ingestion of caustic solids or liquids → lesions that may range from superficial inflammation to coagulative necrosis and ulceration, perforation, and mediastinitis.

SYMPTOMS/EXAM

- Edema and exudates → obstruction that can occur as quickly as 24 hours after ingestion.
- Strictures of the esophagus can occur quickly or may develop gradually over months.

DIAGNOSIS

The severity of oral or laryngeal lesions does not correlate well with the degree of esophageal injury.

The child should have endoscopy within 24–48 hours to assess the degree of burn.

TREATMENT

- The role of corticosteroids in preventing stricture formation is controversial, and they should not be used to treat first-degree burns.
- Antibiotics are mandatory when perforation occurs.
- When esophageal stricturing occurs, long-term treatment may require repeated esophageal dilation, an esophageal stent, or surgical replacement of the esophagus with a segment of the colon.

HIATAL HERNIA

Hiatal hernia may arise in children who have had previous Nissen fundoplication.

- Protrusion of a portion of the stomach into the chest through an opening in the diaphragm. Subtypes are as follows:
  - **Paraesophageal:** The esophagus and the gastroesophageal junction are normally placed, but the gastric cardia is herniated beside the esophagus through the diaphragmatic hiatus (uncommon in children).
  - **Sliding:** The gastroesophageal junction and a portion of the proximal stomach are herniated through an esophageal hiatus (more common in children; associated with GERD).
- **Treatment:** Treat hernias surgically if medical management fails.

PYLORIC STENOSIS

See the section on GI disorders.

Constipation

Defined as a reduction in number of bowel movements with changes in consistency, volume, and passage. In the vast majority of cases, constipation is a functional disorder (i.e., one without a recognizable underlying organic disorder) characterized by ≥ 2 weeks of ≤ 2 bowel movements per week with hard, large, or pellet-like stools. Functional fecal retention → fecal soiling.

DIAGNOSIS

- Obtain a detailed history and exam, including a rectal exam.
- Chronic constipation → poor anal sphincter tone on digital exam and dilated rectal vault.
- Rule out organic causes.

TREATMENT

- The 1° goal is to empty the rectal ampulla, thereby producing painless bowel movements with a frequency of > 3 per week.
- Enemas, nonabsorbable osmotically active sugars, behavioral training, and fiber. (Avoid phosphate enemas, as they may → hypocalcemia.)

When diagnosing constipation, rule out organic disorders such as Hirschsprung disease, hypothyroidism, cow's milk protein intolerance, CF, celiac disease, and spina bifida (always inspect the spine).

Upper GI Bleeding

Defined as bleeding above the ligament of Treitz. Upper GI bleeding is less common in children than lower GI bleeding. Its etiologies vary with age:

- **Neonates:** Swallowed maternal blood, hemorrhagic disease of newborn, cracked/irritated nipple, stress gastritis/ulcer, cow's milk protein sensitivity, anatomic deformity.
- **Infants:** Stress gastritis/ulcer, dyspepsia, Mallory-Weiss tear, vascular anomalies, GI duplications, obstruction.
- **Children/adolescents:** Mallory-Weiss tear, dyspepsia, variceal bleeding, ingestions, vasculitis, Crohn's disease, vascular anomalies.

DIAGNOSIS

- Obtain a gastric and/or stool occult blood test to confirm the presence of blood.
- Gastric lavage can confirm upper GI bleed and help assess the activity of the bleed.
- Upper endoscopy is the preferred means of evaluating the upper GI tract but should be performed only if it is likely to change management.

TREATMENT

- Evaluate ABCs.
- Treat according to the cause.

The color of the stool or blood can be a clue to the location of the bleed. The brighter red the blood, the more likely it is from a distal source.

Lower GI Bleeding

Defined as bleeding distal to the ligament of Treitz. The etiology varies with the patient's age:

- **Neonates:** Necrotizing enterocolitis, malrotation with volvulus, allergic colitis, Hirschsprung's disease enterocolitis, hemorrhagic disease of the newborn.

Meckel's diverticulum and polyps commonly present with painless bleeding without diarrhea. Bleeding associated with Meckel's is usually a maroon color, reflective of its location in the distal small bowel, whereas polyps are usually bright red, which is representative of the more usual distal colonic location.

- **Infants:** Anal fissure (the most common cause), infectious colitis, intussusception, Meckel's diverticulum, lymphonodular hyperplasia, intestinal duplication, allergic colitis.
- **Preschoolers:** Polyps (the most common cause after two years of age), infectious colitis, anal fissure, Meckel's diverticulum, Henoch-Schönlein purpura (HSP), hemolytic-uremic syndrome (HUS), lymphonodular hyperplasia.
- **School-age children:** IBD, anal fissure, infectious colitis, polyps, HSP, HUS.
- **Rare causes:** Vascular abnormalities, traumatic rectal lesions, neoplasms.

DIAGNOSIS

- Always rule out an upper GI bleed (gastric lavage and gastroccult).
- Obtain a stool occult blood test to confirm the presence of blood.
- Conduct a thorough history and physical to narrow the differential and to guide testing (e.g., order a stool culture for patients with bloody diarrhea; order a Meckel's scan for patients with maroon blood that is not accompanied by pain; perform a colonoscopy for patients with painless bright red blood without diarrhea in whom polyps are suspected).

TREATMENT

- Evaluate ABCs.
- Treat according to the cause.

Diarrhea

An eight-month-old, former 28-week-premature male infant with a history of chronic lung disease is admitted for diarrhea and dehydration of five days duration. The patient had been doing well on regular formula prior to the onset of his symptoms. Stool studies are obtained, and the rotavirus antigen is found to be ⊕. Fluid resuscitation is initiated, and the patient improves slowly. The boy's parents want to know if there is any treatment for their child, whether any vaccine exists to prevent the recurrence of his symptoms, and whether they need to change his formula. What are the appropriate responses? The parents should be informed that treatment consists of supportive care. No antivirals are recommended for use with rotavirus. A rotavirus vaccine has been developed but was removed from the market in the United States 2° to the risk of intussusception. A new vaccine has been developed and will soon be on the market. The vaccine will not treat a current infection but will be used to prevent infections. Finally, there is no need for the child's parents to change his formula; lactose avoidance has not been shown to play a role in the treatment of rotavirus unless there is evidence of ongoing or worsening symptoms.

ACUTE DIARRHEA

Defined as fluid content greater than the norm of 10 mL/kg/day in children or 200 g/24 hours in adolescents and adults. More practical criteria involve a ↓ in consistency and an ↑ in frequency to ≥ 3 bowel movements per 24-hour period. Table 8-2 lists the most common etiologies of acute diarrhea that are unrelated to intestinal infection. However, infections are the most common cause.

- Rotavirus is the most pervasive cause of infectious diarrhea worldwide and peaks at 6–24 months.
- Bacterial infections are more common in the first months of life and in school-age children.

Tables 8-3 and 8-4 list the most common infectious causes of acute diarrhea in children and the pathogenic mechanisms and clinical features according to pathogen.

DIAGNOSIS

- The yield of stool cultures is low in acute diarrhea.
- Stool cultures are useful from an epidemiologic standpoint or when potentially treatable pathogens such as *Clostridium difficile* or *Shigella* are suspected.

C. difficile testing in infants < 6 months of age is unnecessary, as these patients will be colonized with the bacteria and are postulated to not have receptors for the toxins.

TABLE 8-2. Etiologies of Acute Diarrhea Unrelated to Intestinal Infection

Extraintestinal infections:
    UTIs
    URIs
    Otitis media
    Meningitis

Surgical conditions:
    Acute appendicitis
    Intussusception

Drug induced:
    Antibiotic associated
    Other drugs

Food allergies:
    Cow's milk protein allergy
    Soy protein allergy
    Multiple food allergies

Disorders of digestive/absorptive processes:
    Sucrase-isomaltase deficiency
    Late-onset (or "adult type") hypolactasia
    Malrotation
    Hirschsprung's disease (enterocolitis variant)
    Ileus
    Necrotizing enterocolitis
    Jejunal and ileal diverticula
    IBS

Reproduced, with permission, from Guandalini S. *Essential Pediatric Gastroenterology, Hepatology, and Nutrition.* New York: McGraw-Hill, 2005:16.

TABLE 8-3. Infectious Causes of Acute Diarrhea in Children

Bacteria:	Viruses:
Shigella	Rotavirus
Yersinia enterocolitica	Calicivirus
Clostridium difficile	Norwalk-like virus
Vibrio parahaemolyticus	Astrovirus
Aeromonas hydrophila	Enteric-type adenovirus
Plesiomonas shigelloides	
Campylobacter jejuni	**Parasites:**
Salmonella	*Cryptosporidium parvum*
Escherichia coli	*Giardia lamblia*
Enterotoxigenic (ETEC)	*Isospora belli*
Enteropathogenic (EPEC)	
Enteroaggregative (EAEC)	
Enteroinvasive (EIEC)	
Enterohemorrhagic (EHEC)	
Diffusely adherent (DAEC)	

Reproduced, with permission, from Guandalini S. *Essential Pediatric Gastroenterology, Hepatology, and Nutrition.* New York: McGraw-Hill, 2005:16.

Do not treat Salmonella *except in infants < 6 months of age or in children with sickle cell disease, malignant neoplasms, HIV, or immunosuppressive disease.*

TREATMENT

- Rehydration or maintenance of hydration is the cornerstone of treatment.
- Oral hydration solutions have been proven to be safe and effective, especially in cases of mild to moderate dehydration.
- Give IV hydration to patients with ≥ 10% dehydration, those in shock, those who are unconscious, and those in whom oral rehydration therapy has not been successful.
- Many controlled trials have demonstrated the benefit of early feeding.
- Do not withhold lactose unless the patient's diarrhea worsens after refeeding and shows evidence of reducing substances or low pH in the stool.
- The role of antibiotics is limited given that most cases of acute infectious diarrhea are self-limiting. However, antibiotics do play a role in shigellosis, suspected cholera, invasive *Entamoeba histolytica*, and proven *Giardia intestinalis* (see Infectious Disease chapter).
- Most antiemetics should be avoided because of their side effects; ondansetron has been proven efficacious but is costly.
- Antimotility substances should be avoided.
- There is a potential role for probiotics, especially in rotavirus.

> Divide the following into causes of secretory diarrhea, osmotic diarrhea, or mixed: VIPoma, IBD, cholestasis, graft-versus-host disease (GVHD), sucrase-isomaltase deficiency, lactose intolerance, cholera, toddler's diarrhea, laxative use, microvillus inclusion disease, tufting enteropathy.
> **Secretory:** VIPoma, cholestasis, GVHD, cholera, microvillus inclusion disease, tufting enteropathy.
> **Osmotic:** Sucrase-isomaltase deficiency, lactose intolerance, toddler's diarrhea, laxative use.
> **Mixed:** IBD.

TABLE 8-4. Mechanisms and Clinical Features of Intestinal Pathogens

PREDOMINANT PATHOGENESIS[a]	SITE OF INFECTION	AGENT	CLINICAL FEATURES
Direct cytopathic effect	Proximal small intestine	Rotavirus Enteric-type adenovirus Calicivirus Norwalk-like virus EPEC *Giardia*	Copious watery diarrhea, vomiting, mild to severe dehydration; frequent lactose malabsorption, no hematochezia. Course may be severe.
Enterotoxigenicity	Small intestine	*Vibrio cholerae* ETEC EAEC *Klebsiella pneumoniae* *Citrobacter freundii* *Cryptosporidium*	Watery diarrhea (can be copious in cholera or ETEC), but usually mild course. No hematochezia.
Invasiveness	Distal ileum and colon	*Salmonella* *Shigella* *Yersinia* *Campylobacter* EIEC *Amoeba*	Dysentery: very frequent stools, cramps, pain, fever, and often hematochezia with WBCs in stools. Variable dehydration. Course may be protracted.
Cytotoxicity	Colon	*Clostridium difficile* EHEC *Shigella*	Dysentery, abdominal cramps, fever, hematochezia. EHEC or *Shigella* may be followed by HUS.

[a] Elaboration of various types of enterotoxins affecting ion transport has been demonstrated as an additional virulence factor for almost all of the bacterial pathogens.

Reproduced, with permission, from Guandalini S. *Essential Pediatric Gastroenterology, Hepatology, and Nutrition*. New York: McGraw-Hill, 2005:17.

CHRONIC DIARRHEA

Defined as persistence of loose stools for at least two weeks; generally has a noninfectious etiology. May be secretory, osmotic, or both.

- **Secretory diarrhea** is an upregulation of the ion transport mechanisms involved in active secretion (e.g., the cystic fibrosis transmembrane regulator). This upregulation can be associated with enterotoxins. Clinically, secretory diarrhea is characterized by large volumes of watery stools, lack of dependence on oral food ingestion, and persistence during oral fasting.
- **Osmotic diarrhea** occurs in the presence of impaired intestinal digestion and/or absorption of nutrients (most often carbohydrates). It is usually associated with mucosal injury. Clinically, osmotic diarrhea improves following discontinuation of the offending nutrient.

In diagnosing chronic diarrhea, consider enterotoxins produced by Vibrio cholerae *and enterotoxigenic* E. coli.

Pay attention to blood tests in patients with chronic diarrhea (e.g., macrocytic anemia could point to vitamin B$_{12}$ deficiency in Crohn's patients).

- Secretory diarrhea can be distinguished from osmotic diarrhea through the measurement of stool sodium and potassium levels. If double the sum of stool sodium and potassium concentrations is within 50 mOsm/kg of plasma osmolality (which estimates osmolality of feces in the distal intestine), the disorder is likely a secretory process. If the difference is > 125, the picture is most consistent with an osmotic process. Anything in between signifies a mixed picture.
- Several tests can be done to further differentiate the causes of diarrhea:
    - Stool WBCs or a marker of WBCs, such as lactoferrin or calprotectin, point to an inflammatory process.
    - Stool α_1-antitrypsin is ↑ in protein-losing enteropathy.
    - Low stool pH (< 6) or the presence of reducing substances points to a carbohydrate malabsorption.
    - Fat globules are significant for steatorrhea.
    - Stool cultures, toxins, viral cultures, and O&P can be diagnostic.
    - Colonoscopy and endoscopy may be necessary to confirm the diagnosis, especially with noninfectious etiologies.

TREATMENT

- Treat the specific etiology.
- Intestinal transplantation is an option for severe chronic diarrheal diseases such as intractable diarrhea of infancy (see below).

INTRACTABLE DIARRHEA OF INFANCY

Table 8-5 shows the clinical and histologic features of intractable diarrhea of infancy.

Failure to Thrive (FTT)

Failure to thrive is defined as failure to achieve a normal rate of growth. It is a symptom or a descriptive term, not a disease or a diagnosis. Clinically, there are multiple definitions of FTT, such as falling below the third percentile for growth or crossing two or more percentile lines. Subtypes are as follows:

- A **wasted child** has a deficit in weight for height that is usually 2° to an acute etiology.
- A **stunted child** has a deficit in height and weight, but the weight for height is normal for age. This is usually 2° to a chronic process.

Tables 8-6 and 8-7 list the etiologies of FTT from both a metabolic and a system-based perspective.

DIAGNOSIS

- A proper dietary/feeding history is critical, as is a family and developmental history.
- On physical exam, it is essential to obtain proper markers of nutrition starting with anthropometrics (weight, height, head circumference, skin fold thickness). It is also important to look for signs of systemic illness and to observe feedings.
- Lab work should be based on the history and physical.

	ULTRASTRUCTURAL ENTEROCYTE DEFECTS		IMMUNE-MEDIATED ENTEROPATHY— AUTOIMMUNE	PHENOTYPIC DIARRHEA— SYNDROMATIC
	MICROVILLOUS INCLUSION DISEASE	TUFTING ENTEROPATHY		
Date of onset	Neonatal	Neonatal	3–12 months	1–3 months
Type of diarrhea	Watery (100 mL/kg per day)	Watery (100 mL/kg per day)	Watery (100–150 mL/kg per day)	Watery (50–100 mL/kg per day)
Family history	Frequent	Frequent	Rare	Rare-absent
Commonly associated symptoms	Mucus in the stools	Choanal atresia, keratitis		Low birth weight, facial dysmorphism (forehead, broad nose, hypertelorism), trichorrhexis nodosa, immunodeficiency
Villous atrophy	Moderate	Moderate	Moderate	Moderate
T-cell activation	Absent	Absent	↑↑↑	Absent
Intraepithelial lymphocytes	Normal	Normal or ↓	Normal or ↑	Normal
Epithelium	Abnormal PAS	Tufts	Normal to injured	Normal
Crypts	Normal	Hyperplastic, dilated branching	Hyperplastic, necrosis, abscess	Normal
Pathognomonic signs	Abnormal brush border, secretory granules, membrane inclusions lined by microvilli	Abnormal expression of $\alpha_2\beta_1$ integrin and desmoglein	Lamina propria T-cell activation; CD25+ T cells; ↑ HLA-DR	

Reproduced, with permission, from Guandalini S. *Essential Pediatric Gastroenterology, Hepatology, and Nutrition.* New York: McGraw-Hill, 2005:43.

- Consider CBC, ferritin, ESR, CRP, UA, TFTs, tissue transglutaminase and serum IgA (for celiac disease), and CXR as indicated by the history for first-line screening.

TREATMENT

- Treatment depends on the etiology, but general strategies should center on a multidisciplinary, collaborative approach.
- Increasing caloric intake is a strategy for "catch-up" growth.
- Particular attention should be paid to the replacement of micronutrients such as zinc, iron, and vitamin D when deficient.
- FTT can have an effect on cognition if it occurs early in life and is severe.

TABLE 8-6. Causes of FTT by Metabolic Process

INADEQUATE INTAKE	INADEQUATE ABSORPTION	EXCESSIVE LOSS	EXCESSIVE REQUIREMENT
Feeding mismanagement (e.g., errors in formula feed, bizarre/restricted diet, neglect, poverty)	Pancreatic insufficiency (e.g., CF, Schwachman-Diamond)	Vomiting (e.g., CNS abnormality, intestinal obstruction, metabolic abnormality, gastroesophageal reflux)	Chronic illness (e.g., CF, congenital heart disease, IBD)
Inability to feed optimally (e.g., developmental delay, cleft palate, bulbar palsy)	Small intestine disease (e.g., disaccharidase deficiency, cow's milk protein intolerance, celiac disease)	Protein-losing enteropathy	Thyrotoxicosis
Anorexia (e.g., chronic illness, "infantile anorexia nervosa")		Chronic diarrhea	Chronic infection (e.g., TB, HIV)
Diencephalic syndrome			Malignancy
			Burns

Reproduced, with permission, from Guandalini S. *Essential Pediatric Gastroenterology, Hepatology, and Nutrition.* New York: McGraw-Hill, 2005:57.

Intestinal Obstruction

Categorized as extrinsic or intrinsic compression:

- **Extrinsic compression:** Includes incarcerated hernia, malrotation, volvulus, superior mesenteric artery (SMA) syndrome, and perforated appendicitis.
- **Intrinsic compression:** Includes intussusception, intestinal stenosis and atresia, polyp, Hirschsprung's disease, and inspissation.

SYMPTOMS/EXAM

- Abdominal distention and emesis +/– passage of stool or gas are hallmarks of obstruction.
- Emesis can be nonbilious (proximal to the ampulla of Vater), bilious (distal to the ampulla), feculent (distal small bowel obstruction), or blood tinged (inflammatory).
- Periumbilical, crampy pain (colicky) is classic for obstruction.
- Peritoneal signs (rebound, rigidity, guarding) along with fever and tachycardia, as well as a lack of bowel gas, may indicate perforation.

DIAGNOSIS

Table 8-8 lists the age of presentation, clinical findings, and guidelines for the diagnosis of intestinal obstruction.

TREATMENT

- Initial management should include ABCs, fluid resuscitation, NG tube placement, NPO status, and broad-spectrum antibiotics.
- Indications for emergent exploratory laparotomy include malrotation with or without midgut volvulus, pneumoperitoneum, nonreducible intussusception, and peritonitis.

Diarrhea, especially if it is bloody, can be a finding of ischemia to the intestinal wall.

GASTROINTESTINAL SYSTEM AND NUTRITION

TABLE 8-7. Etiologies of FTT by System

Gastrointestinal	**Dysphagia:** Neuromuscular incoordination, cleft palate, micrognathia, postoperative esophageal atresia, tracheoesophageal fistula, esophagitis, achalasia. **Anorexia:** Gastritis, enteric infections, Crohn's disease, celiac disease, motility disorders. **Malabsorption:** CF, Schwachman, celiac, cow's milk–sensitive enteropathy, short gut, abetalipoproteinemia, lymphangiectasia, bacterial overgrowth, cholestatic liver disease. **Excessive losses:** Gastroesophageal reflux, pyloric stenosis, incomplete/recurrent obstruction.
Renal	Renal tubular acidosis, chronic renal disease, recurrent UTI.
Neurologic	Birth injury, asphyxia, chromosomal abnormalities, neurodegenerative diseases, hydrocephalus, intracranial lesions (e.g., diencephalic syndrome, myopathies).
Cardiovascular	Congenital and acquired congestive and cyanotic disease.
Endocrine	Hypo- and hyperthyroidism, hyperaldosteronism, hypopituitarism, growth hormone deficiency, exogenous hypercortisolism.
Respiratory	Chronic hypoxemia, bronchopulmonary dysplasia, CF.
Metabolic	Aminoacidopathies, inborn errors of metabolism, idiopathic hypercalcemia.
Immunologic	HIV, inflammatory joint disease.
Genetic	Fetal alcohol.
Chronic infection	TB, recurrent UTI.
Hematologic	Iron deficiency, malignancy.
Drugs and toxins	Lead.

Reproduced, with permission, from Guandalini S. *Essential Pediatric Gastroenterology, Hepatology, and Nutrition.* New York: McGraw-Hill, 2005:58.

Jaundice in the Infant

Neonatal jaundice is common, affecting approximately 50% of newborn infants and most often taking the form of unconjugated hyperbilirubinemia (see Neonatology chapter). Conjugated hyperbilirubinemia almost always indicates liver disease, and the etiologies are listed below.

INFECTIOUS CAUSES

Hypothyroidism is associated with conjugated hyperbilirubinemia.

- **TORCHeS infections** (toxoplasmosis, rubella, CMV, HSV/HIV, syphilis) are associated with the following liver pathology (see Infectious Disease chapter):
  - **Toxoplasmosis:** Congenital toxoplasmosis will → hepatomegaly, but jaundice is variable. Liver biopsy will demonstrate hepatitis and necrosis.
  - **CMV:** The most common congenital infection. Hepatosplenomegaly and cholestasis are common. Liver biopsy shows giant cell hepatitis and viral inclusions.

TABLE 8-8. **Intestinal Obstruction Findings and Diagnosis by Etiology**

ETIOLOGY	AGE	CLASSIC PRESENTATION	DIAGNOSIS
Malrotation with/ without midgut volvulus	Any age: 50–75% < 1 month; 90% < 1 year	Bilious emesis; minimal abdominal distention, with a late finding of blood in stool.	UGI: ligament of Treitz not located to left of midline; "bird's beak"/ "corkscrew" appearance.
Duodenal atresia or stenosis	First week of life	Bilious emesis. Epigastric distention only. Down syndrome.	UGI: blunt end termination of contrast.
Jejunoileal atresia or stenosis	First week of life	Bilious emesis and progressive abdominal distention. The more distal the obstruction, the later the onset of emesis and abdominal distention.	Contrast enema to distinguish small from large bowel obstruction. Presence of microcolon indicates unused colon due to proximal obstruction.
Meconium ileus	1–2 days	Absent or delayed passage of meconium. Bilious emesis; abdominal distention.	Barium enema for diagnostic and therapeutic purposes. Sweat test for CF.
Hirschsprung's disease	Any age	Delay or failure to pass meconium; sepsis, abdominal distention, bilious emesis.	Barium enema, rectal biopsy.
Pyloric stenosis	2–6 weeks	Projectile, nonbilious vomiting. Olive-shaped mass.	US. UGI.
Intussusception	5–9 months (range: 3 months to 3 years)	Colicky abdominal pain with periods of lethargy; bilious vomiting, "currant jelly" stool. Sausage-shaped mass.	US. Barium enema (or air inflation) for diagnosis and therapeutic reduction.
Incarcerated hernia	Any age	Inguinal mass.	Physical examination. Ultrasound.
Postoperative adhesions	Any age	Postoperative.	Barium enema or UGI.
Lap belt complex	Any age	Post-trauma.	Barium enema or UGI.
Perforated appendicitis	Any age	Anorexia, vomiting, abdominal pain.	US.
Meckel's diverticulum			Radionuclide scan.

UGI, upper GI barium study; US, abdominal ultrasound.

Reproduced, with permission, from Guandalini S. *Essential Pediatric Gastroenterology, Hepatology, and Nutrition.* New York: McGraw-Hill, 2005:98.

- **HSV:** Congenital herpes → severe liver disease with jaundice, hepatomegaly, and coagulopathy.
- **Syphilis:** Congenital syphilis may present at birth or over the first few weeks of life. Infants have hepatosplenomegaly and jaundice. Liver histology may demonstrate nonspecific hepatitis, but silver stain will show the spirochete.
- **Enteroviruses:** A rare cause of massive liver necrosis in the newborn. There have also been reports of liver disease with parvovirus B19 and HHV-6.
- **Systemic bacterial infections:** These can also → conjugated hyperbilirubinemia.

METABOLIC CAUSES

Following is a summary of liver pathology associated with metabolic disease (see also Human Genetics chapter).

- **Galactosemia:** Can present with cholestasis in the newborn period when infants are exposed to galactose. Conjugated hyperbilirubinemia and hepatomegaly develop over the first week of life.
- **Neonatal hemochromatosis (NH):**
  - A rare disorder that occurs 2° to iron overload in utero. Widely recognized to have a familial association.
  - **Sx/Exam:** Patients present with liver failure and are found to have splenomegaly and a small, firm liver.
  - **Dx:** Although lab studies will indicate liver failure (hypoglycemia, thrombocytopenia, coagulopathy, hypoalbuminemia), liver transaminases are usually normal. However, ferritin levels are significantly ↑. Diagnosis requires exclusion of other causes of neonatal liver failure. Coagulopathy usually precludes liver biopsy, which would demonstrate nodular cirrhosis with severe cholestasis and markedly elevated iron stores. Diagnosis is often made by iron deposition in salivary glands on lip biopsy or MRI demonstrating iron overload in several organs.
  - **Tx:** An antioxidant cocktail has been suggested as treatment with varying results. The patient should be listed immediately for liver transplantation, as the disease is usually fatal without transplantation. High-dose immunoglobulin is a promising therapy that has been given to mothers to prevent subsequent pregnancies resulting in an infant with NH.
- **Biliary atresia:**
  - Results from a destructive inflammatory process that affects intra- and extrahepatic bile ducts. Occurs in 1 in 10,000 live births; more common in females.
  - **Sx/Exam:** Patients are usually full-term babies of normal size who are jaundiced after two weeks of age and present with hepatomegaly, dark urine, and acholic stools.
  - **Dx:** Lab studies show conjugated hyperbilirubinemia, with total bilirubin most often in the range of 6–10 mg/dL and direct bilirubin in the range of 3–6 mg/dL, along with ↑ alkaline phosphatase, ↑ GGT, and mildly ↑ transaminases. Ultrasound is necessary to rule out other causes of cholestasis such as choledochal cyst, but in biliary atresia the gallbladder is usually not identified. Liver histology demonstrates bile duct proliferation, bile plugs, and portal tract edema; diagnosis can be confirmed with an intraoperative cholangiogram.

- **Tx:** Initial treatment is with a Kasai portoenterostomy, but in the long term patients most often require liver transplantation. Ursodeoxycholic acid (UDCA [Actigall]) may prevent hepatotoxicity from hydrophobic bile acids that can accumulate by assisting in the excretion of bile.
- **Neonatal hepatitis:** Also known as idiopathic hepatitis. Occurs in up to 25% of infants with cholestasis. Liver histology demonstrates giant cell transformation, generally with normal ducts. The prognosis is often good, with only 10% of patients developing progressive liver disease. Treatment is supportive.
- **Choledochal cyst:** Cystic dilation within the biliary tree. Shows a female predominance; diagnosis is made on ultrasound. Treated with surgical resection because of the risk of cholangiocarcinoma.
- **Alagille syndrome:**
  - Abnormal development of many organs (liver, heart, kidney, spine, eye) with liver disease manifested by cholestasis. There are characteristic facies (broad forehead, deep-set eyes, and small, pointed chin). Caused by a defect on chromosome 20 for the JAG1 protein.
  - **Sx/Exam:** Infants may present with jaundice, acholic stools, and poor growth. Clinical criteria have been established and include findings of jaundice (cholestasis), characteristic facies, cardiac anomalies, butterfly vertebrae, and posterior embryotoxin on eye exam. Additional findings may include FTT, renal disease, severe pruritus, and xanthomas.
  - **Dx:** Labs reveal high cholesterol levels, ↑ GGT and transaminases, conjugated hyperbilirubinemia, and ↑ alkaline phosphatase. Liver histology demonstrates paucity of bile ducts but may not be seen on liver biopsy when performed early in infancy (before six months of age). Intralobular bile ducts are lost over variable periods of time. Repeat biopsy may be necessary.
  - **Tx:** Treatment is supportive and includes medium-chain triglycerides for fat malabsorption, supplementation with fat-soluble vitamins, and UDCA to help improve bile flow and pruritus. Additional medications are used to help pruritus, but in severe cases, partial external biliary diversion is performed.
- **Progressive familial intrahepatic cholestasis (PFIC):**
  - Formerly known as Byler syndrome in Amish children.
  - Three forms have now been described: PFIC-1, PFIC-2, and PFIC-3. These have recently been renamed FIC1, BSEP, and MDR3, respectively. FIC1 and BSEP disease cause similar symptoms and together are called low-GGT PFIC because of their characteristic low GGT levels.
  - **Sx:** Cholestasis with average age at onset being three months, although symptoms may not occur until adolescence. Pruritus and growth failure are major features.
  - **Tx:** UDCA helps some mild forms. Special formulas with medium-chain triglycerides are given as well as fat-soluble vitamin supplementation. Surgical treatment with partial cutaneous biliary diversion has been shown to relieve pruritus and growth failure and arrest the progression of liver disease. Liver transplantation may be necessary in some patients.
- **α_1-Antitrypsin deficiency:**
  - An inherited disease in which patients have either two Z genes (called ZZ) or one S and one Z gene (called SZ) in the PI locus on chromosome 14.
  - Incidence is 1 in 1600; 15% will develop liver disease.

- **Sx/Exam:** Presents with prolonged jaundice in infants, mild elevation in aminotransferases in toddlers, and portal hypertension and severe liver dysfunction in children or adolescents.
- **Dx:** Blood test for α_1-antitrypsin phenotype. A distinctive histologic feature is periodic acid-Schiff-$\oplus$, diastase-resistant globules in the endoplasmic reticulum of the liver.
- **Tx:** Treatment is supportive. Avoid alcohol, tobacco smoke, and heavy air pollution. The prognosis is varied; half of patients with liver disease will do well.
- **Bile acid synthesis defects:**
  - A rare inherited disorder of bile acid metabolism.
  - Some patients have peroxisomal diseases, including Zellweger syndrome and neonatal adrenoleukodystrophy.
  - **Sx:/Exam:** Jaundice, poor growth, hepatosplenomegaly, bleeding, and/or rickets.
  - **Dx:** Abnormal bile acids through mass spectrometry of urine and serum.
  - **Tx:** Bile acid replacement therapy, medium-chain triglyceride–containing formulas and fat-soluble vitamins.

GI DISORDERS

Achalasia

A motor disorder of the esophagus characterized by partial or incomplete relaxation of the LES in response to swallowing, $\uparrow$ LES pressure, and abnormal peristalsis in the esophageal body.

- The etiology and underlying mechanism are not fully understood.
- The incidence of achalasia is 1 in 200,000, and its prevalence is 8 in 100,000.
- It is rarely seen in children < 5 years of age, and < 5% of patients are < 15 years of age.
- An $\uparrow$ incidence is seen with Down syndrome, Sjögren syndrome, and triple A syndrome (adrenal insufficiency, achalasia, alacrima); it can also result from Chagas' disease, which is caused by neuronal damage by the parasite *Trypanosoma cruzi*, as well as from malignancy or GERD surgery.

SYMPTOMS/EXAM

Presents with retrosternal pain, complaints of food sticking in the throat or upper chest, dysphagia relieved by forceful swallowing or vomiting, chronic cough, wheezing, and weight loss.

DIAGNOSIS

- Esophagography shows a dilated esophagus with a short, tapered beak at the distal end (see Figure 8-2).
- Esophageal manometry is abnormal with high resting pressure in the LES.

TREATMENT

- Nifedipine can be used to treat early disease.
- Patients generally require some form of invasive procedure, such as pneumatic dilation, botulinum toxin injected into the LES, or Heller myotomy

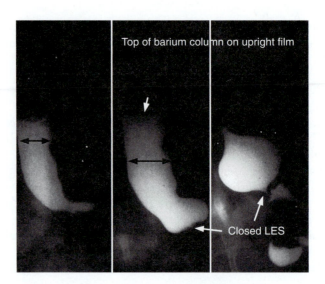

Top of barium column on upright film

Closed LES

FIGURE 8-2. **Barium esophagram in a patient with achalasia.**

Note the tapered beak formation at the closed LES. (Reproduced, with permission, from Guandalini S. *Essential Pediatric Gastroenterology, Hepatology, and Nutrition.* New York: McGraw-Hill, 2005:146.)

(surgical splitting of the LES). Heller myotomy usually requires partial fundoplication, since reflux is a major side effect of any procedure to relax the lower esophagus.
- Controversy exists regarding the role of annual endoscopy for the surveillance of long-standing achalasia.

COMPLICATIONS

Squamous cell carcinoma can occur in patients with long-standing achalasia.

Gastroesophageal Reflux (GER)

By definition, GER represents the retrograde passage of gastric contents into the esophagus. It can be asymptomatic or symptomatic. Gastroesophageal reflux disease (GERD) is defined as GER that occurs too frequently and damages the esophageal mucosa → clinical symptoms. GER is a physiologic event that can be seen in most neonates; > 50% of two-month-old infants regurgitate twice a day. The highest prevalence is at four months of age, when two-thirds of infants regurgitate. Prevalence starts to drop at six months of age. GERD affects a much smaller proportion of GER patients.

SYMPTOMS/EXAM

- The most common symptom is postprandial regurgitation or effortless spit-up.
- Although usually harmless, severe GERD may present with FTT, dysphagia, heartburn/chest pain or other signs of esophagitis, hematemesis, anemia, aspiration, chronic cough, and wheezing.
- GERD patients may also present with or develop apnea, colic, recurrent otitis media, chronic sinusitis, stridor, and dental erosion.

Sandifer syndrome, which is associated with GERD, is defined as stereotypical, repetitive stretching along with arching movements of the head and neck as the head tends to bend on the shoulder. These movements are often mistaken for seizure activity.

DIAGNOSIS

- Diagnosed clinically by a thorough history and physical.
- A pH probe is the best test for GERD short of invasive measures such as endoscopy, but it will miss cases of GERD with nonacidic fluid and will not be able to detect the amount of fluid refluxed or the distance the fluid travels in the esophagus, as in aspiration.
- Endoscopic evidence of esophagitis supports the diagnosis.
- Impedance studies measure fluid movements rather than luminal pH changes but have not been validated in children.

TREATMENT

- Some 85–90% of GER cases are self-limited, and the patient will outgrow the condition by one year of age.
- Small feedings, thickened feeds, H_2 receptor antagonists (e.g., ranitidine), and PPIs (e.g., omeprazole) may be effective. Metoclopramide (a promotility agent) may be used, but studies do not consistently support its efficacy. Erythromycin is another promotility agent that may assist in alleviating symptoms.
- Antireflux surgery (Nissen fundoplication) may work in selected cases but is associated with morbidity. Laparoscopic surgery has been associated with an ↑ rate of redo operations (vs. open surgery).

COMPLICATIONS

- Barrett's esophagus is metaplasia of the esophageal squamous epithelium that transforms to specialized columnar epithelium. This is a premalignant condition that is associated with a risk of dysplastic degeneration and adenocarcinoma.
- Peptic strictures can present in cases of severe but asymptomatic esophagitis.

Infantile Hypertrophic Pyloric Stenosis

A condition resulting from hypertrophy of the pylorus muscle in which the lumen becomes obstructed by mucosa. Affects 1.5–4.0 in 1000 live births; more common in males. Usually occurs in infants 3–5 weeks of age, but may affect infants anywhere between 2 and 8 weeks of age.

SYMPTOMS/EXAM

- Presents with nonbilious projectile vomiting.
- Coffee-ground emesis may be seen as a result of esophagitis or gastritis.
- Infants are generally not ill appearing unless undiagnosed for an extended period of time.
- On exam, the pylorus may be palpable as a small, hard mass or as an "olive."

DIAGNOSIS

- Labs demonstrate hypochloremic, hypokalemic metabolic alkalosis.
- Ultrasound is the gold standard and can reveal a thick pyloric muscle with a long pyloric channel and large pyloric diameter.
- A barium upper GI study will be ⊕ if there is a string sign through the pylorus (see Figure 8-3).

An upper GI series will rule out anatomic abnormalities; this will allow for the visualization of GER, although it is not a test for the condition. Sensitivity is approximately 30% and specificity 20%.

Very early postnatal exposure to erythromycin (between 3 and 13 days of life) has been associated with pyloric stenosis.

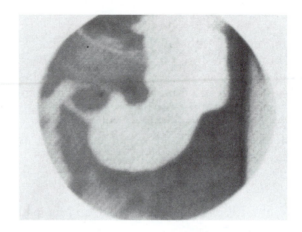

FIGURE 8-3. **UGI findings of pyloric stenosis.**

Note the string sign through the pylorus. (Reproduced, with permission, from Rudolph AM et al. *Rudolph's Pediatrics*, 18th ed. Norwalk, CT: Appleton & Lange, 1987.)

TREATMENT

- Ramstedt pyloromyotomy.
- Laparoscopic pylorotomy is gaining acceptance.

COMPLICATIONS

Mortality rates are low and are usually associated with perforation or infection.

Cow's Milk Allergy

Affects genetically predisposed patients when they are exposed to cow's milk protein. The most common type of food allergy in infancy, with an estimated prevalence of 2–3% in the first two years of life. The majority of patients have a ⊕ family history of atopy.

SYMPTOMS/EXAM

- Although the age of onset may range from a few days to several months after the introduction of cow's milk protein, it most often presents by the first month of life.
- Reactions can involve the GI tract as well as the respiratory system and the skin.
- Typical GI symptoms include GER, colitis, hematochezia, constipation, and colic.
- Pulmonary hemosiderosis, apnea, apparent life-threatening event (ALTE), and atopy may also be seen.

DIAGNOSIS

- The diagnostic gold standard, which is rarely done, is a double-blind, placebo-controlled food challenge that must be performed in the hospital.
- A history and physical can support the diagnosis.
- Lab studies have poor predictive value. Eosinophils may be seen on peripheral smear, but this is a nonspecific sign. Most available tests explore only IgE-mediated types of allergic reactions, but milk protein allergy of

infancy is often a non-IgE-mediated process. Hence, the skin prick test and radioallergosorbent test (RAST) are not sensitive in infancy when non-IgE-mediated reactions are suspected.

- Upper endoscopy and sigmoidoscopy can also aid in diagnosis. Eosinophils found in the upper GI tract, the small bowel, or the left side of the colon can be suggestive of the diagnosis.

TREATMENT

- If allergy is clinically suspected, the patient should be placed on a diet free of cow's milk protein. Within 2–3 weeks, there should be a clinical response. A rechallenge may be necessary to establish the diagnosis.
- Hydrolysate formulas are first-line therapy.
- Some 5% of patients will require elemental formulas.

Soy protein has ~50% cross-antigenicity with cow's milk protein and thus is not appropriate treatment for cow's milk protein allergy.

Eosinophilic Gastroenteritis

A disorder characterized by eosinophilic inflammatory infiltration of the tissues of the GI tract. It may occur in any age group. Food sensitivity plays a role in most cases; however, other causes should be considered (e.g., idiopathic, parasitic infection, connective tissue disease, IBD, vasculitis, malignancy).

SYMPTOMS/EXAM

Patients can present with any symptom of the GI tract, such as FTT, vomiting, or diarrhea.

DIAGNOSIS

- Diagnosis is based on a finding of eosinophils on biopsy of the GI tract.
- Eosinophils in the right colon can be a normal variant, but other locations—such as the esophagus, stomach, small bowel, or left colon—can also represent disease, and workup should be initiated for one of the possible causes, such as food allergies.

TREATMENT

- If food allergy is suspected, the patient should be tested for specific allergens and placed on an avoidance diet. The most common foods implicated are milk, soy, eggs, nuts, beef, wheat, fish, shellfish, and corn.
- If symptoms persist and are refractory to other measures, steroids may be tried. There is new evidence supporting the use of swallowed inhaled steroids for treatment-resistant disease.
- Some investigators advocate using an amino acid–based formula for a period of time and then reintroducing foods.
- Other treatments, such as leukotrienes and mast cell stabilizers, have not proven to be effective.

Peptic Disease

Peptic disease may occur at any age but is more commonly seen in children between 12 and 18 years of age; boys are affected more frequently than girls. Peptic disease can → ulcers, often 2° to illness, toxins, or drugs. Causes include the following:

- ↓ mucosal protection mechanisms (2° to aspirin use, NSAID use, or hypoxia).
- ↓ metabolic activity in mucosal cells, which allows for diffusion of hydrogen ions into the cells (→ hypoxia and hypotension).
- ↑ secretion of acid or pepsin.
- Reflux of bile from the duodenum to the stomach.
- ↓ neutralizing activity of duodenal secretions.

A close association exists between *H. pylori* infection of the gastric antrum and nodular antral gastritis, duodenal ulcer, and gastric ulcer, but there is no evidence that such infection → recurrent abdominal pain of childhood or dyspepsia without gastritis.

SYMPTOMS/EXAM

- Children < 6 years of age can present with vomiting and upper GI bleeding.
- Older children are more likely to present with abdominal pain.
- Peptic disease can be seen in association with other pathologic processes, such as Crohn's disease, hepatic cirrhosis, rheumatoid arthritis, burns, sepsis, and CNS disorders.

DIAGNOSIS

- Upper intestinal endoscopy is the most accurate diagnostic test.
- *H. pylori* can be diagnosed on antral biopsy. Stool antigen testing can also be used. Serum testing does not establish the existence of active infection.

TREATMENT

- Acid blockers such as H_2 receptor antagonists or PPIs.
- Caffeine should be avoided along with foods that → symptoms.
- Aspirin and NSAIDs should not be used.
- *H. pylori* can be treated with triple therapy, including antibiotics and PPIs.

A one-year-old child is brought to the pediatrician for a well-child visit. The physician notes that the patient's weight is below the fifth percentile for age but had been at the 25th percentile up to his four-month visit. The child's mother and father are of Irish descent. There is no family history of celiac disease. What are the appropriate steps in working up this patient for celiac disease? The patient should have a tissue transglutaminase (TTG) antibody and serum IgA level sent. The serum IgA level will help determine if the patient can have an appropriate TTG antibody response, as the most specific TTG is the IgA antibody. If the patient is IgA deficient, the TTG test will yield a high false-⊖ rate. Also, IgA deficiency is a risk factor for celiac disease. If the patient is IgA deficient or has a high TTG antibody in the face of a normal IgA level, he should have an endoscopy with multiple small bowel biopsies.

Celiac Disease

Enteropathy that occurs in genetically susceptible individuals and is triggered by the ingestion of gluten. Prevalence in the United States and in Western European countries is estimated to be 1 in 133.

SYMPTOMS/EXAM

- The classic form presents with symptoms between 6 and 24 months of age, usually soon after the introduction of foods containing gluten.
- Symptoms may include diarrhea, anorexia, abdominal distention, abdominal pain, poor weight gain, weight loss, and vomiting.
- Behavioral changes with irritability are common.
- Severe malnutrition is a sign of delayed diagnosis, and patients can present in crisis with explosive watery diarrhea, marked abdominal distention, dehydration, hypotension, and lethargy.
- Extraintestinal manifestations include short stature, delayed puberty, anemia, dental enamel hypoplasia, chronic hepatitis and hypertransaminasemia, arthritis, osteopenia, occipital calcifications, seizures, and infertility.
- Dermatitis herpetiformis is a blistering skin rash that involves the elbows, knees, and buttocks and is associated with dermal granular IgA deposits.
- Type 1 DM, Down syndrome, and IgA deficiency have all been associated with celiac disease.

Celiac disease has an association with HLA-DQ2 and -DQ8.

DIAGNOSIS

- TTG (IgA mediated) and antiendomysial antibodies (IgA mediated) are the most sensitive and specific screening tests. TTG is 99–100% sensitive.
- The gold standard involves small intestinal biopsies demonstrating villous atrophy with hyperplasia of crypts and intraepithelial lymphocytes while the patient is eating adequate amounts of gluten.

Oats should be avoided in celiac disease because of the risk of cross-contamination.

TREATMENT

Institution of a gluten-free diet (avoidance of wheat, barley, and rye) is the cornerstone of treatment.

Intestinal Obstruction

> A full-term baby presents with the following x-ray (see Figure 8-4). What would be the most common heart defect associated with the congenital disorder? The image demonstrates the "double bubble" sign, which is characteristic of duodenal obstruction. There is a high incidence of duodenal atresia in patients with Down syndrome. The heart defect most often associated with Down syndrome is endocardial cushion defect.

DUODENAL OBSTRUCTION

Extrinsic congenital obstruction is usually due to peritoneal bands associated with intestinal malrotation, annular pancreas, or duodenal duplication. Intrinsic congenital obstruction is a result of stenosis, mucosal diaphragm (wind sock deformity), or duodenal atresia. The obstruction may be proximal or distal to the ampulla of Vater.

DUODENAL ATRESIA

- A history of polyhydramnios is common.
- Duodenal atresia is commonly associated with congenital anomalies (30%). Prematurity is highly associated with the atresia.

211

GASTROINTESTINAL SYSTEM AND NUTRITION

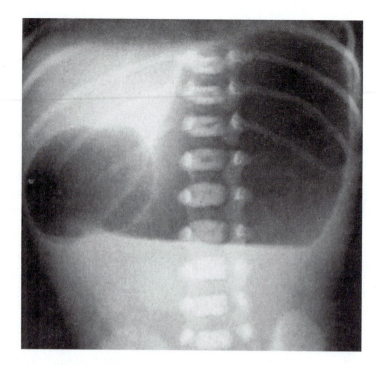

FIGURE 8-4. "Double bubble" sign of duodenal atresia.

(Reproduced, with permission, from Rudolph CD et al. *Rudolph's Pediatrics*, 21st ed. New York: McGraw-Hill, 2002:1403.)

- **Sx/Exam:** Vomiting can start a few hours after birth and may be accompanied by epigastric distention.
- **Dx:** AXRs show distention of the stomach and proximal duodenum with air ("double bubble" sign—see Figure 8-4). Paucity of gas in the distal intestine can be an indication of atresia.
- **Tx:** Surgery is performed to remove or bypass the obstruction. Thorough exploration is necessary to ensure that no additional anomalies are present.
- **Complications:** The mortality rate may be as high as 35–40%.

OTHER CONGENITAL INTESTINAL ATRESIAS AND STENOSES

Table 8-9 lists the localization and frequency of congenital atresias and stenoses. Polydyramnios during a pregnancy is often associated with congenital anomalies such as intestinal atresias and stenoses.

SYMPTOMS/EXAM

- Neonates present with abdominal distention, bilious vomiting, and obstipation or failure to pass meconium. Prematurity and other congenital anomalies may be present.
- Neonates usually have bile-stained emesis and abdominal distention.

DIAGNOSIS

- X-ray imaging shows dilated loops of small bowel and absence of colonic gas.

- Barium enema reveals a narrow-caliber microcolon if atresia is present in the distal small bowel.
- Some 10% of patients have absent mesentery and poor visualization of the SMA. The ileum coils around either the right colic or the ileocolic arteries, giving rise to a "Christmas tree" deformity. The tenuous blood supply often compromises surgical anastomoses.

TREATMENT

Surgery is mandatory.

COMPLICATIONS

Postoperative complications include short bowel syndrome and hypomotility.

MALROTATION

A condition in which the midgut (the duodenojejunal junction until the mid-transverse colon, which is supplied by the SMA) incompletely rotates during the 10th week of gestation. This → twisting of the bowel → a volvulus around the narrow mesenteric root that occludes the SMA. Malrotation accounts for 10% of neonatal intestinal obstructions; associated congenital anomalies occur in 25% of cases.

SYMPTOMS/EXAM

- Presents with recurrent bile-stained emesis or acute small bowel obstruction in the first three weeks of life.
- Later in life, the patient may present with intermittent intestinal obstruction, malabsorption, protein-losing enteropathy, or diarrhea.

TABLE 8-9. Localization and Frequency of Congenital GI Atresias and Stenoses

	AREA INVOLVED	TYPE OF LESION	RELATIVE FREQUENCY
Pylorus	—	Atresia; web or diaphragm.	1%
Duodenum	80% are distal to the ampulla of Vater.	Atresia, stenosis; web or diaphragm.	45%
Jejunoileum	Proximal jejunum and distal ileum.	Atresia (multiple in 6–29%); stenosis.	50%
Colon	Left colon and rectum.	Atresia (usually associated with atresias of the small bowel).	5–9%

Reproduced, with permission, from Hay WW et al. *Current Pediatric Diagnosis & Treatment,* 17th ed. New York: McGraw-Hill, 2005:630.

DIAGNOSIS

- An upper GI series shows the duodenojejunal junction inferior and on the right side of the spine.
- Barium enema may demonstrate a mobile cecum located in the midline, RUQ, or left abdomen.

TREATMENT

- Surgical treatment consists of a Ladd procedure in which the duodenum is mobilized and the short mesenteric root is extended.
- Midgut volvulus is a surgical emergency.

COMPLICATIONS

Bowel necrosis results from occlusion of the superior mesenteric artery.

SHORT BOWEL SYNDROME

- Defined as having < 50% of the small intestinal length remaining after resection. Patients are dependent on IV nutrition.
- The most common causes are necrotizing enterocolitis, intestinal atresias, gastroschisis, and volvulus.
- As the patient grows, the gut will grow and compensate resected sections.
- The presence of a colon dictates a more favorable prognosis.
- **Complications:** Liver failure is the most common cause of death and is usually 2° to parenteral nutrition and recurrent infections. Mortality is estimated at 10–15% of all patients.

MECKEL'S DIVERTICULUM

The most common of the omphalomesenteric duct remnants; usually found in the antimesenteric border of the mid- to distal ileum. It is present in 1.5–2.0% of the population but rarely causes symptoms. Diverticula may have gastric tissue that can → bleeding by irritating adjacent ileal mucosa. Complications occur three times more frequently in males than in females. Fifty to sixty percent of cases are diagnosed within the first two years of life.

SYMPTOMS/EXAM

- Patients normally present with painless passage of maroon blood per rectum.
- Intestinal obstruction occurs in 25% of symptomatic patients as a result of ileocolonic intussusception.

DIAGNOSIS

The Meckel scan uses ^{99m}Tc pertechnetate. This is taken up by the diverticulum, which is lined with heterotopic gastric mucosa. Cimetidine and pentagastrin can reduce the number of false-⊖ results.

TREATMENT

Surgical resection is curative, and the prognosis is good.

For Meckel's diverticulum, remember the rule of 2s: usually occurs in the first 2 years of life, affects ~ 2% of the population, usually 2 feet from the ileocolic junction, 2 cm in length, 2 types of abnormal tissue can occur (pancreatic and gastric).

A one-year-old boy presents with intermittent severe abdominal pain. His mother reports that the child has been vomiting but has been well in between the episodes of pain. She denies any changes in his stools and has not noted any bloody or black stools. The boy is not febrile, and his physical exam is normal. What is the best course of action?

Although this patient does not have bloody stools or ⊕ findings on his physical exam, his history is highly suspicious for intussusception. Diagnosis and treatment can be performed with a barium or air enema. In cases of small bowel intussusception (e.g., jejunojejunal), ultrasound can be considered. If enema reduction fails, the patient will require surgical intervention.

INTUSSUSCEPTION

One of the most common causes of intestinal obstruction in infants and young children. A portion of the intestine telescopes into another → invagination and obstruction of the small intestine, venous compression, and bowel wall edema. A lead point can be found in 2–10% of all cases but ↑ to as many as 22% of cases in children > 2 years of age. Intussusception resulting from lymphoid hyperplasia may be caused by a viral agent or may be idiopathic. The disorder has a male-to-female ratio of 3:2, with 70% of cases occurring in children < 1 year of age and 80% occurring in those < 2 years of age. Its incidence is 1–4 in 1000 live births.

Intussusception has a 5–7% recurrence rate (higher in older children and indicates a lead point).

SYMPTOMS/EXAM

- Associated with the classic triad of intermittent abdominal pain, vomiting, and "currant jelly" stool. However, this triad is seen in only 10–20% of patients.
- Pain is usually intermittent but is severe enough to make patients draw in their legs.
- In some cases, a sausage-shaped mass may be palpated in the upper abdomen.

DIAGNOSIS

- Ultrasound can reveal a target sign, which has good ⊕ predictive value.
- Air and barium contrast enemas are considered the gold standard for diagnosis and treatment.
- Intussusception can be seen on CT but may be an incidental finding.

Common lead points include Meckel's diverticulum, polyps, heterotopic pancreatic nodules, enterogenous cysts, adenomas, neurofibromas, hemangiomas, or enlarged hypertrophied ileal lymphoid patches.

TREATMENT

- Air and barium contrast enemas are first-line treatment.
- If enema reduction fails or if there is evidence of ischemia, the intussusception can be surgically reduced or resected.

- The postsurgical recurrence rate is approximately 3%.
- Delays in diagnosis → a high rate of complications (40%), including gangrene, ischemia, and perforation, eventually → death if the delay exceeds 2–5 days.
- The mortality rate is < 1%, with mortality occurring 2° to bowel ischemia and the presence of lead points.

HIRSCHSPRUNG'S DISEASE

A congenital aganglionic megacolon resulting from the absence of ganglion cells in the mucosal and muscular layers of the colon → failure of neural crest cells to migrate to the mesodermal layers. The rectum or the rectosigmoid is usually most often affected, but the disease affects the entire colon in 8% of cases. Hirschsprung disease → narrowing of the aganglionic segment with dilation of the proximal normal colon, as a result of which the patient can develop enterocolitis in that segment → diarrhea, protein loss, and bleeding. Hirschsprung disease is four times more common in boys than in girls, and a familial pattern has been described, particularly in total colonic aganglionosis. There is also a possible link to the *ret* proto-oncogene.

Some 10–15% of patients with Hirschsprung disease also have Down syndrome.

SYMPTOMS/EXAM

- Newborns present with failure to pass meconium followed by vomiting, abdominal distention, and reluctance to feed.
- Patients may also develop multiple episodes of enterocolitis, and older children can present with constipation.
- Encopresis occurs rarely.
- On digital exam, the anal canal and rectum are devoid of fecal material despite evidence of fecal impaction on x-ray, and there may be a gush of stool as the finger is withdrawn.

DIAGNOSIS

- Unprepped barium enema usually demonstrates the narrowed segment distally with a sharp transition to the proximal dilated colon.
- Rectal manometry will demonstrate failure of relaxation of the internal anal sphincter muscle following balloon distention of the rectum.
- Rectal biopsy can reveal an aganglionic bowel.

TREATMENT

Resection of the aganglionic bowel.

FOREIGN BODY

- Most foreign bodies can pass through the GI tract without difficulty. However, objects that are > 5 cm in length will have difficulty passing through the ligament of Treitz and will require endoscopic removal.
- Objects with diameters greater than that of a quarter (~ 2.5–3.0 cm) may have difficulty passing through the pylorus and may require endoscopic removal when they do not pass on their own or when there are signs of obstruction.

- Objects in the esophagus must be removed if there is evidence that the object has been lodged for > 24 hours or if the patient has symptoms such as drooling, pain, difficulty breathing, and/or shortness of breath.
- Disk-shaped batteries lodged in the esophagus should be removed immediately.

Polyposis

Polyps can be divided into two categories: hamartomas (juvenile polyps, Peutz-Jeghers polyps, and hyperplastic polyps) and adenomas. Adenomas are by definition dysplastic and are divided into tubular, tubulovillous, and villous, with the last category having the greatest risk of cancer. Hamartomas are nearly always stalked (those seen with Peutz-Jeghers syndrome may have a broad base) and are rarely associated with dysplasia. Multiple polyps usually suggest familial syndromes such as familial adenomatous polyposis or Peutz-Jeghers syndrome, which pose an ↑ risk of malignancy. Some 60–75% of all polyps are in the rectosigmoid colon. Polyposis is one of the most common noninfectious causes of rectal bleeding in toddlers and school-age children.

Solitary polyps in children are commonly juvenile hamartomas and are most often benign, posing no risk of malignant transformation.

SYMPTOMS/EXAM

- The most common symptom is painless rectal blood loss (usually bright red blood).
- Large polyps can be a lead point for intussusception (especially in Peutz-Jeghers syndrome).

DIAGNOSIS/TREATMENT

- For simple hamartomas, patients should undergo colonoscopy for both evaluation and removal.
- Multiple polyps may need to be removed. Consideration must be given to colectomy if there are dysplastic changes, > 100 polyps, or very large polyps that pose a risk of obstruction and cannot easily be removed by colonoscopy.

JUVENILE POLYPOSIS SYNDROME

- A rare autosomal-dominant disorder characterized by multiple (> 5) hamartomatous polyps in the colon.
- The mean onset of symptoms is nine years of age.
- **Dx/Tx:** Patients require regular screening colonoscopy with endoscopic polypectomy to reduce the risk of cancer, bleeding, and obstruction; colectomy may be required. Genetic testing is available, as two gene mutations have been identified.

PEUTZ-JEGHERS SYNDROME

- A rare autosomal-dominant disorder with an incidence of 1 in 120,000. Polyps may become cancerous.
- Associated with macular melanin pigmentation on the lips, buccal mucosa, hands, feet, and eyelids.
- **Sx/Exam:** Polyps arise in the small bowel and usually present with obstruction by intussusception.

Some 5–10% of girls with Peutz-Jeghers syndrome develop ovarian tumors → precocious puberty and irregular menstruation.

- **Dx/Tx:**
    - The diagnosis should be considered in family members of known Peutz-Jeghers patients.
    - Upper endoscopy, enteroscopy, and colonoscopy are used for evaluation and removal of polyps.
    - If a symptomatic polyp has a broad base and perforation is a risk, surgical resection is preferable.
- **Prevention:** Regular screening endoscopy for cancerous changes is recommended.

FAMILIAL ADENOMATOUS POLYPOSIS

Turcot syndrome is a combination of brain tumors and adenomatous polyposis.

- An autosomal-dominant syndrome occurring in 1 in 10,000 people. Caused by a defect in the APC gene.
- Hundreds or thousands of adenomatous polyps appear in the colon, having developed over time. Colon cancer occurs in all affected patients before 50 years of age. Patients are also at risk for hepatoblastoma.
- **Dx:**
    - α-fetoprotein and ultrasound are used to detect hepatoblastoma.
    - Endoscopic surveillance should be conducted every two years beginning at age 10–12 or earlier when symptoms are present.
    - Gene testing can be done if the familial gene defect is known.
- **Tx:** Patients should undergo colectomy when polyps are detected.

Inflammatory Bowel Disease (IBD)

Includes Crohn's disease, ulcerative colitis, and indeterminate colitis.

CROHN'S DISEASE

A chronic inflammatory disease that may involve any part of the GI tract from the oropharynx to the perianal area. In children, the ileocolonic area is the most common location of disease (40%). Crohn's disease occurs worldwide but is more common in the Northern Hemisphere, and its overall incidence is 1.6–5.4 in 100,000. Its peak incidence is in the second decade of life, but 25–50% of patients present in childhood. Younger children have a higher incidence of small bowel disease. Possible contributing etiologies are as follows:

- Immune-mediated bowel injury triggered by environmental factors in a genetically predisposed individual.
- The NOD2 (CARD15) gene mutation occurs in roughly 10% of Crohn's patients, with two variant alleles → a 20- to 40-fold ↑ in the risk for Crohn's.

SYMPTOMS/EXAM

- Depending on the location of the disease, patients can present with bloody diarrhea, nausea, emesis, epigastric pain, dysphagia, RLQ pain, and weight loss.
- On physical exam, patients can have diffuse abdominal tenderness along with clubbing of distal phalanges, rectal skin tags, deep anal fissures, and fistulas.

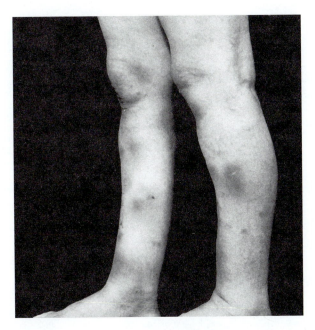

FIGURE 8-5. Erythema nodosum in a patient with Crohn's disease.

(Reproduced, with permission, from Freedberg IM et al. *Fitzpatrick's Dermatology in Medicine*, 6th ed. New York: McGraw-Hill, 2003:1056.) (Also see Color Insert.)

- Extraintestinal features may include fever, weight loss, growth failure, delay in sexual maturation, arthralgia, arthritis, oral aphthoid ulcers, erythema nodosum (see Figure 8-5), pyoderma gangrenosum (see Figure 8-6), autoimmune hepatitis, 1° sclerosing cholangitis, nephrolithiasis, and osteopenia.

DIAGNOSIS

- Diagnosis is based on clinical presentation, hematologic tests, radiologic imaging, and endoscopic evaluation.
- If the patient presents with bloody diarrhea, infectious etiologies must be ruled out.
- The hematologic workup should include a CBC for microcytic anemia, thrombocytosis, and leukocytosis; acute-phase reactants for ↑ ESR and C-reactive protein; serologic tests for ASCA (affects 50% of Crohn's patients) and p-ANCA titers; and chemistries for hypoalbuminemia and ↑ liver enzymes.
- Stool should be examined for the presence of fecal leukocytes and occult blood.
- Imaging studies include an upper GI series with small bowel follow-through, CT of the abdomen, and/or an MRI to rule out strictures.
- The gold standard involves biopsies during endoscopic evaluation (upper and lower) looking for signs of chronic inflammation in skip-lesion fashion (normal mucosa in between areas of abnormal mucosa) and granulomas, which differentiate Crohn's from ulcerative colitis.

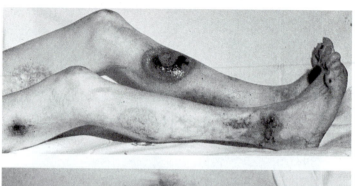

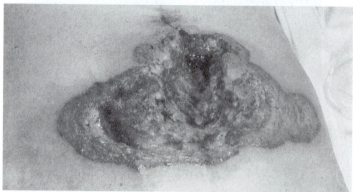

FIGURE 8-6. Pyoderma gangrenosum in inflammatory bowel disease.

(Reproduced, with permission, from Freedberg IM et al. *Fitzpatrick's Dermatology in Medicine*, 6th ed. New York: McGraw-Hill, 2003:971.) (Also see Color Insert.)

TREATMENT

- Corticosteroids can be effective in inducing remission, but long-term use → side effects.
- Sulfasalazine and mesalamine are local therapies that can help maintain remission, especially in mild to moderate cases.
- Antibiotics (metronidazole and ciprofloxacin) has been useful in perianal disease.
- Immunosuppressive therapy with 6-mercaptopurine (6-MP), methotrexate, or infliximab has been shown to be effective in maintaining remission.
- Other treatment modalities include nutritional programs.
- Surgery is reserved for medically intractable patients, those with a suspected perforation or abscess, and those with intestinal obstruction or hemorrhage.

COMPLICATIONS

Children with extensive disease have an ↑ risk of colon cancer.

ULCERATIVE COLITIS

A chronic inflammatory disease of the colon. Its incidence is 6.3–15.1 in 100,000. Ulcerative colitis shows a bimodal distribution, with the first peak occurring during the second and third decades of life and the second taking place in the sixth and seventh decades of life. Its etiology is unknown but is thought to result from immune-mediated bowel injury that may be triggered by environmental factors in a genetically susceptible host.

SYMPTOMS/EXAM

- Ulcerative colitis affects the rectum and extends proximally in a symmetric fashion in the colon.
- Patients can present with gross blood in the stool, tenesmus, and abdominal pain, especially LLQ pain.
- Fever, weight loss, anorexia, anemia, arthralgia, 1° sclerosing cholangitis, osteopenia, pyoderma gangrenosum (see Figure 8-6), and erythema nodosum (see Figure 8-5) may also be seen.
- Patients may develop toxic megacolon.

DIAGNOSIS

- Hematologic workup is similar to that for Crohn's but yields a high incidence of ⊕ p-ANCA.
- When patients present with bloody diarrhea, stool cultures must be obtained to rule out an infectious etiology before a diagnosis of ulcerative colitis can be made.
- Colonoscopy will reveal continuous lesions with acute and chronic inflammation of the mucosa.

TREATMENT

- Topical sulfasalazine and mesalamine may be adequate therapy for mild colitis.
- Steroids can be used to induce remission.
- Immunosuppressive therapy includes 6-MP, cyclosporine, and infliximab.
- About 5% of people with ulcerative colitis develop colon cancer. The risk of cancer ↑ with duration of disease and extent of disease in the colon.
- Colon cancer screening should occur approximately 8–10 years after initial diagnosis with regular screening every 1–2 years thereafter for those with severe disease.

Annular Pancreas

- Defined as incomplete rotation and fusion of the dorsal and ventral pancreas during embryology.
- The malformation results in pancreatic tissue surrounding a portion of the descending duodenum. Its etiology is not understood.
- **Sx/Exam:**
  - Patients present with symptoms of partial or complete duodenal obstruction.
  - Down syndrome and congenital anomalies of the GI tract occur frequently, and polyhydramnios is common.
  - Patients can present later in childhood.
- **Tx:** Treatment consists of duodenoduodenostomy or duodenojejunostomy without operative dissection or division of the pancreatic annulus.

Crohn's disease presents with skip lesions and may be seen throughout the GI tract; ulcerative colitis presents with continuous lesions and is confined to the colon.

> A previously healthy 16-year-old girl presents to the pediatrician because she has been feeling tired and is not doing as well in school. She appears pale, and there was no viral prodrome to her illness. A CBC reveals anemia with smear demonstrating extensive hemolysis without any other findings. What is the next step?
>
> The clinical presentation described can be typical of Wilson disease. A serum ceruloplasmin should be sent and a urine copper excretion test considered. If these are abnormal, a liver biopsy will help confirm the diagnosis, after which chelation treatment should be initiated. Family members should also be evaluated.

Wilson Disease

Also known as hepatolenticular degeneration, Wilson disease is characterized by ↓ hepatocellular excretion of copper into bile. It is caused by a mutation in the gene ATP7B, which is involved in copper transport, with accumulated hepatic copper → oxidant damage to the liver. Its incidence is 1 in 30,000. A family history is often present, as the disease is autosomal recessive, but sporadic cases may also be seen.

SYMPTOMS/EXAM

Individuals with Wilson disease can present with liver disease, progressive neurologic disease, or psychiatric illness. Patients present with variable degrees of liver disease ranging from asymptomatic elevation in liver enzymes to liver failure. There may be jaundice, hepatomegaly, cirrhosis, splenomegaly, Kayser-Fleischer rings (note that the absence of rings does not exclude the diagnosis), tremor, dysarthria, drooling, and deterioration in school performance.

DIAGNOSIS

- Lab studies may show a Coombs-⊖ hemolytic anemia with an ↑ in bilirubin and LFTs and low alkaline phosphatase (in acute presentation).
- Low serum ceruloplasmin and high urinary copper excretion are also seen.
- The gold standard is high tissue content of copper (> 250 μg/g dry weight) on liver biopsy.
- Biopsy can show variable findings such as mild steatosis, glycogenated nuclei, hepatocellular necrosis, and/or coarse nodular cirrhosis.

TREATMENT

- Copper chelation with D-penicillamine or trientine hydrochloride; dietary restriction of copper; zinc supplementation.
- Vitamin B_6 may be given to patients on penicillamine to prevent optic neuritis.
- Liver transplantation may be necessary for acute fulminant disease or progressive hepatic decompensation.
- If the disease is left untreated, the prognosis is poor.

Autoimmune Hepatitis (AIH)

Unresolving inflammation of the liver characterized by hepatitis, autoantibodies, hypergammaglobulinemia, and portal plasma cell infiltration on histologic examination. It is most common in adolescent girls, although it can occur in all age groups and in either sex. There is most likely a genetic susceptibility.

SYMPTOMS/EXAM

- Presents with fever, malaise, recurrent or persistent jaundice, skin rash, arthritis, amenorrhea, gynecomastia, acne, pleurisy, pericarditis, or ulcerative colitis.
- Can present as acute or chronic liver failure.
- Hepatosplenomegaly is often seen.

DIAGNOSIS

- Labs show a moderate ↑ in bilirubin, AST, ALT, and alkaline phosphatase. Serum albumin is low with ↑ or normal total protein 2° to hypergammaglobulinemia.
- Most patients have ⊕ ANA and/or anti–smooth muscle antibody associated with type 1 AIH or presence of anti–liver-kidney antibody, which is associated with type 2 AIH.
- Exclusion of genetic (α_1-antitrypsin deficiency, Wilson disease) and active viral hepatitis is essential.
- Liver biopsy shows piecemeal necrosis, bridging necrosis, and infiltration of plasma cells as signs of chronic inflammation.
- Portal fibrosis and bile duct and Kupffer cell proliferation may also be seen.
- Cirrhosis is found in 50% of patients.

TREATMENT

- Corticosteroids for induction.
- Azathioprine can be used for maintenance therapy.
- The goal of treatment is to induce remission. There is no prescribed minimum or maximum duration of therapy.
- Termination of medication after remission may be considered in only a small percentage of children because relapse is common.

COMPLICATIONS

- Relapses occur in approximately 60–80% of children, but remission can follow repeat treatment.
- Treatment failure is noted in 5–15% of children. Children who deteriorate despite therapy will require liver transplantation.
- A complication after transplantation is the development of AIH in the new liver.

NUTRITION

The nutrient requirements of children are substantially affected by growth rate and body composition.

Severe Malnutrition

- In chronic malnutrition, not only weight but also height and head circumference will ↓.
- Significant caloric deprivation will → severe wasting (marasmus).

- Significant protein deprivation in the face of adequate energy intake may → edematous malnutrition (kwashiorkor).

Energy

- Major determinants of energy expenditure include basal metabolism, metabolic response to food, physical activity, and growth.
- In the first several months of life, an infant's average energy requirement is 110 kcal/kg/day.
- As children get older, average energy requirements ↓ to 100 kcal/kg/day for children 1–3 years of age and to 90 kcal/kg/day for children 4–6 years of age.
- Protein requirements are 1–2 g/kg/day, with larger amounts necessary in infants and neonates.
- The American Academy of Pediatrics recommends that 30% of calories come from fats. In neonates, however, a higher percentage (40–50%) of energy requirements are provided by fats.
- Carbohydrates should contribute 40% of caloric intake in human milk while providing 55–60% after two years of age.
- Table 8-10 demonstrates the typical patterns of physical growth.

Breast-feeding

- **Advantages:** Immunologic factors (IgA, lysozyme, lactoferrin, macrophages) provide protection against GI and upper respiratory infections; allergic diseases are less common; promotes maternal-child bonding.
- **Contraindications:** TB in the mother; galactosemia in the infant; HIV; mothers receiving chemotherapy or radiation to the breast; drug-using mothers.

Pregestimil has a higher percentage of medium-chain fats than other hydrolyzed formulas, which is appropriate for patients with CF or liver disease.

Elemental formulas (Neocate and Elecare) are indicated in patients who are allergic to cow's milk protein but do not respond to hydrolyzed formulas (~ 5% of patients). These formulas are also useful for malabsorption syndromes.

Vitamin A deficiency is a leading cause of irreversible blindness in children worldwide.

TABLE 8-10. **Patterns of Physical Growth**

Weight	Birth weight is regained by the 10th to 14th day.
	Average weight gain/day: 0–6 mo = 20 g; 6–12 mo = 15 g.
	Birth weight doubles at ~ 4 mo, triples at ~ 12 mo, and quadruples at ~24 mo.
	During the second year, average weight gain/mo = ~ 0.25 kg.
	After age 2 years, average annual gain until adolescence = ~ 2.3 kg (5 lb).
Length/height	By the end of the first year, birth length increases by 50%.
	Birth length doubles by 4 years and triples by 13 years.
	Average height gain during the second year = ~ 12 cm (5 in).
	After age 2 years, average annual growth until adolescence ≥ 5 cm (2 in).
Head circumference	Average head growth/week: 0–2 mo = ~ 0.5 cm, 2–6 mo = ~ 0.25 cm.
	Average total head growth at 0–3 mo = ~ 5 cm, 3–6 mo = ~ 4 cm, 6–9 mo = ~ 2 cm, 9 mo–1 year = ~ 1 cm.

Reproduced, with permission, from Rudolph AM, Kamei RK, Overby KJ. *Rudolph's Fundamentals of Pediatrics*, 3rd ed. New York: McGraw-Hill, 2002:6.

Formulas

- Most common formulas are made with cow's milk protein and contain lactose.
- Soy-based formulas are recommended for galactosemia because the carbohydrate source is not lactose and therefore galactose is not present. However, soy-based formula is not appropriate for infants with cow's milk protein allergy given the 40–50% cross-antigenicity of soy and cow protein.
- Hydrolyzed formulas (Nutramigen, Alimentum, Pregestimil) have a hydrolyzed casein protein that is used in cow's milk protein allergy.

Vitamins and Micronutrients

Tables 8-11 and 8-12 outline the functions of various vitamins and micronutrients as well as the symptoms associated with their deficiencies. Vitamins A, D, E, and K are fat soluble.

Convulsions in infancy can be a manifestation of vitamin B_6 deficiency. INH can cause peripheral neuropathy that is responsive to vitamin B_6.

TABLE 8-11. Functions of Vitamins and Presentation of Deficiencies and Toxicities

VITAMIN	FUNCTION	SOURCE	DEFICIENCY	TOXICITY
Vitamin A	- Essential in vertebrates - Visual perception; functions in rods and cones of the retina - Cellular differentiation - Immune response - Used in the treatment of measles → a ↓ in morbidity and mortality	- Liver - Dairy - Fish - Yellow and green vegetables - β-carotene is the most efficient provitamin A	- Xerophthalmia—night blindness, conjunctival xerosis, Bitot's spots, corneal xerosis, ulceration, and scarring - Follicular hyperkeratosis	- Vomiting, nausea - ↑ ICP - Headache - Blurred vision - Emotional lability - Desquamating, dry skin - Myalgia and arthralgia - Cortical thickening of bones in the hands and feet - Liver abnormalities - Teratogenicity
Vitamin D	- Maintains serum calcium and phosphorus concentrations - Enhances small bowel absorption of calcium and phosphorus - Enhances bone release of calcium	- Fish liver oils - Flesh of fatty fish - Liver - Fat from aquatic mammals - Eggs - Sunlight - Supplementation is recommended for infants, especially if they are breast-fed	- Rickets - Osteomalacia - Bone demineralization	- Hypercalcemia - Deposition of calcium in soft tissues - Polyuria and polydipsia - Depression - Anorexia - Nausea, vomiting - Arteriosclerosis

VITAMIN	FUNCTION	SOURCE	DEFICIENCY	TOXICITY
Vitamin E	▪ Nonspecific antioxidant	▪ Vegetable oils (corn, soybean, safflower) ▪ Wheat germ ▪ Nuts	▪ Rare occurrence ▪ Hemolytic anemia ▪ Peripheral neuropathy ▪ Spinocerebellar ataxia ▪ Skeletal myopathy ▪ Pigmented retinopathy	▪ ↑ incidence of necrotizing enterocolitis in premature infants
Vitamin K	▪ Coenzyme during synthesis or coagulation proteins (2, 7, 9, 10, C, S)	▪ Leafy vegetables ▪ Soybean oil ▪ Fruits ▪ Seeds ▪ Cow's milk	▪ Bleeding ▪ Hemorrhagic disease of the newborn	▪ No adverse effects from consumption in food ▪ The synthetic form can cause hemolytic anemia, hyper-bilirubinemia, vomiting, and porphyrinuria
Vitamin B$_1$ (thiamine)	▪ Coenzyme in the metabolism of carbohydrates and amino acids	▪ Wheat germ ▪ Yeast extract ▪ Most animals ▪ Fortified flour ▪ Some green vegetables	▪ Cardiac failure, aphonia, pseudomeningitis in infants ▪ Dry beriberi—peripheral neuropathy, tingling, numbness, tenderness, weakness ▪ Wet beriberi—edema 2° to cardiac failure ▪ Wernicke-Korsakoff syndrome—encephalopathy and psychosis	▪ Very rare ▪ Anaphylaxis ▪ Respiratory depression
Vitamin B$_2$ (riboflavin)	▪ Catalyst for redox reactions	▪ Dairy products ▪ Meat ▪ Poultry ▪ Wheat germ ▪ Leafy vegetables	▪ Cheilosis ▪ Angular stomatitis (see Figure 8-7) ▪ Dermatitis ▪ Anemia ▪ Mental dysfunction	▪ None known

VITAMIN	FUNCTION	SOURCE	DEFICIENCY	TOXICITY
Vitamin B_3 (niacin)	▪ Precursor for NAD, which is critical for energy production ▪ Precursor for NADP, which is a major reducing agent used for biosynthesis (e.g., fatty acid synthesis)	▪ Meats ▪ Poultry ▪ Fish ▪ Legumes ▪ Wheat ▪ Yeast ▪ Milk ▪ Synthesized in the body from tryptophan	▪ The three D's—dermatitis, diarrhea, dementia ▪ Pellagra—dermatitis in sun-exposed skin (see Figure 8-8) ▪ Red tongue, diarrhea, vomiting, constipation ▪ Headache, fatigue, memory loss ▪ Common in populations with a maize-based diet	▪ Histamine release—cutaneous vasodilation ▪ Cardiac arrhythmias ▪ Cholestatic jaundice ▪ GI disturbance ▪ Hyperuricemia ▪ Glucose intolerance
Biotin	▪ Cofactor for 4-carboxylases	▪ Yeast ▪ Liver ▪ Kidney ▪ Legumes ▪ Nuts ▪ Egg yolks	▪ Patients who consume raw egg white for long periods of time ▪ Alopecia ▪ Hair thinning ▪ Loss of hair color ▪ Dermatitis—red, scaly skin rash ▪ Conjunctivitis ▪ Depression, lethargy, hallucinations, paresthesias ▪ Also a form of congenital deficiency	▪ None
Pantothenic acid	▪ Functions in the synthesis of coenzyme A, which is necessary for processes in fatty acid synthesis	▪ Ubiquitous	▪ Numbness and burning of feet and hands ▪ Headache ▪ Fatigue ▪ Insomnia ▪ Anorexia ▪ Impaired antibody production	▪ Diarrhea
Vitamin B_6 (pyridoxine)	▪ Coenzyme in metabolism of amino acids, glycogen, sphingoid bases	▪ All foods	▪ Seborrheic dermatitis ▪ Microcytic anemia ▪ Depression ▪ Confusion ▪ Peripheral neuritis	▪ Sensory neuropathy

VITAMIN	FUNCTION	SOURCE	DEFICIENCY	TOXICITY
Folic acid	■ Involved in DNA synthesis ■ ↓ in neural tube defects if pregnant women are supplemented	■ Leafy vegetables ■ Fruits ■ Whole grains ■ Wheat germ ■ Orange juice ■ Beans ■ Nuts	■ Megaloblastic anemia ■ ↓ WBCs and platelets ■ GI symptoms ■ Neural tube defects if pregnant women are deficient	■ Masking of B_{12}-deficient neuropathy ■ Hypersensitivity
Vitamin B_{12} (cobalamin)	■ Cofactor for two enzymes	■ Eggs ■ Diary products ■ Liver ■ Meats ■ None in plants	■ Megaloblastic anemia ■ Sensory disturbances of tingling and numbness in extremities ■ Vibratory and position sense disturbance ■ Motor disturbances ■ Cognitive changes of loss in concentration and memory loss ■ Disorientation ■ Frank dementia ■ Visual disturbances ■ Insomnia ■ Impotence ■ Impaired bowel and bladder control	■ None
Vitamin C	■ Refers to ascorbic acid and dehydroascorbic acid ■ Cofactor ■ Antioxidant ■ Participates in collagen hydroxylation, carnitine biosynthesis, and hormone and amino acid biosynthesis	■ Citrus fruits ■ Vegetables ■ Fortified products	■ Scurvy (see Figure 8-9) ■ Follicular hyperkeratosis ■ Petechiae ■ Ecchymoses ■ Coiled hairs ■ Inflamed and bleeding gums ■ Perifollicular hemorrhages ■ Joint effusions, arthralgia ■ Impaired wound healing ■ Weakness/fatigue ■ Sjögren syndrome	■ GI disturbances ■ Diarrhea ■ ↑ oxalate excretion ■ Kidney stones ■ ↓ vitamin B_{12} and copper status ■ ↑ O_2 demand ■ Erosion of dental enamel

TABLE 8-11. Functions of Vitamins and Presentation of Deficiencies and Toxicities *(continued)*

VITAMIN	FUNCTION	SOURCE	DEFICIENCY	TOXICITY
Carnitine	▪ Transfer of long-chain fatty acids from cytosol to mitochondria in β-oxidation	▪ Meats ▪ Diary products ▪ None in plants	▪ ↑ serum triglycerides and free fatty acids ▪ Fatty liver ▪ Hypoglycemia ▪ Muscle weakness ▪ Cardiomyopathy	▪ None

TABLE 8-12. Functions of Micronutrients and Clinical Presentation of Deficiencies

MICRONUTRIENT	FUNCTION	DEFICIENCY
Chromium	▪ Potentiates the action of insulin and beneficial effects on circulating glucose, insulin, and lipids ▪ Ubiquitous in environment	▪ Unexplained weight loss ▪ Peripheral neuropathy ▪ ↑ plasma free fatty acids ▪ Impaired glucose removal ▪ Low respiratory quotient
Copper	▪ An essential catalytic cofactor for selective oxidoreductases	▪ Rare ▪ Normocytic hypochromic anemia ▪ Leukopenia ▪ Neutropenia ▪ Osteoporosis
Iodine	▪ An essential component of thyroid hormone ▪ Deficiency occurs if a water source lacks iodine	▪ Mental retardation ▪ Hypothyroidism ▪ Goiter ▪ Cretinism ▪ Constipation ▪ Growth and developmental abnormalities ▪ Coexisting vitamin A, selenium, or iron deficiency exacerbates deficiency
Manganese	▪ Enzyme activator and metalloenzyme	▪ Not firmly established
Molybdenum	▪ Cofactor for oxidase reactions	▪ Possible mental disturbances and coma
Selenium	▪ Defends against oxidative stress; regulation of thyroid hormone action and regulation of redox status of vitamin C and other molecules	▪ Endemic cardiomyopathy (Keshan disease) ▪ Flaky skin ▪ Bilateral muscle pain

TABLE 8-12. Functions of Micronutrients and Clinical Presentation of Deficiencies *(continued)*

MICRONUTRIENT	FUNCTION	DEFICIENCY
Zinc	■ Functions in 100 specific zinc-dependent catalytic enzymes ■ Structural role in folding of certain proteins resulting in activation of the protein ■ Role in gene regulation ■ Essential in the function of many tissues, especially those with high turnover ■ Zinc supplementation prevents diarrhea and pneumonia in children and ↓ mortality in small-for-gestational-age infants	■ Acrodermatitis enteropathica (see Figure 8-10)—periorificial and acral dermatitis, alopecia, and diarrhea; symptoms usually occur a few months after birth ■ Bullous-pustular dermatitis ■ Alopecia ■ Retarded growth ■ Diarrhea ■ Recurrent infections ■ Male hypogonadism ■ Lethargy ■ Delayed wound healing ■ Impaired dark adaptation ■ Oligospermia ■ Immune function defects ■ Dwarfism ■ Iron deficiency

Menkes disease is an X-linked disorder that → an inability to transport copper across the gut epithelial cells and blood-brain barrier. It → neurologic, connective tissue, skeletal, and vascular abnormalities.

Low alkaline phosphatase may be due to zinc deficiency.

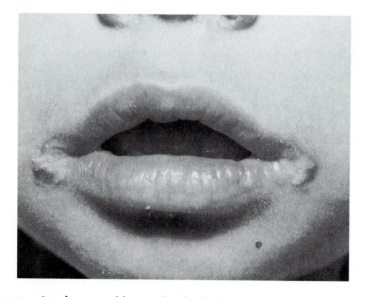

FIGURE 8-7. Angular stomatitis associated with riboflavin deficiency.

(Reproduced, with permission, from Freedberg IM et al. *Fitzpatrick's Dermatology in Medicine*, 6th ed. New York: McGraw-Hill, 2003:1407.) (Also see Color Insert.)

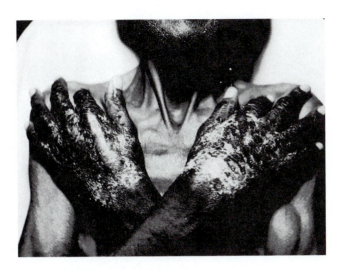

FIGURE 8-8. Pellegra with niacin deficiency.

(Reproduced, with permission, from Freedberg IM et al. *Fitzpatrick's Dermatology in Medicine,* 6th ed. New York: McGraw-Hill, 2003:1406.) (Also see Color Insert.)

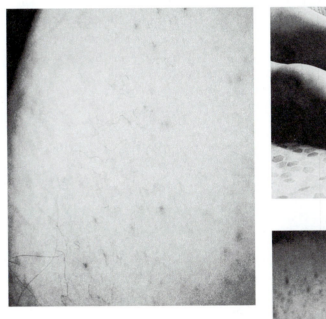

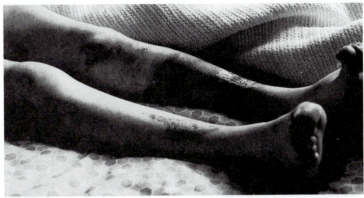

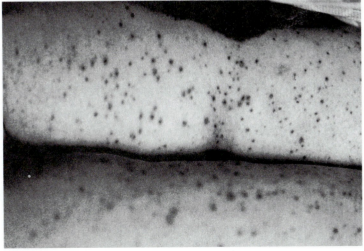

FIGURE 8-9. Evidence of scurvy in vitamin C deficiency.

(Reproduced, with permission, from Freedberg IM et al. *Fitzpatrick's Dermatology in Medicine,* 6th ed. New York: McGraw-Hill, 2003:1409.) (Also see Color Insert.)

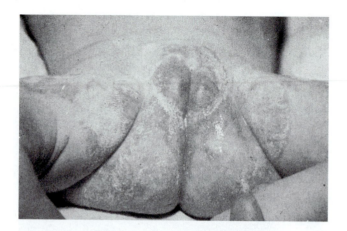

FIGURE 8-10. Acrodermatitis enteropathica in zinc deficiency.

(Reproduced, with permission, from Freedberg IM et al. *Fitzpatrick's Dermatology in Medicine*, 6th ed. New York: McGraw-Hill, 2003:1413.) (Also see Color Insert.)

CHAPTER 9

Growth, Development, and Behavior

Neal Rojas, MD
reviewed by Alison Schonwald, MD

Growth Indices

- Infant and child growth parameters include weight, length/height, head circumference, weight for height, and body mass index (BMI). Growth remains a 1° predictor of overall child health and well-being.
- Basic growth milestones and guidelines generally include the following:
  - Birth weight doubles by six months of age and triples by 12 months.
  - Poor growth or failure to thrive (see below) is a common pathway for many disorders and syndromes.

Growth velocities are at their highest during the first six months of life for all indices.

> A six-month-old boy born at term without complications presents with a weight at the 25th percentile (birth weight at the 75th percentile), a height at the 50th percentile (birth length at the 50th percentile), and a head circumference at the 50th percentile. The boy has no history of significant illness and has a caloric intake of 80 kcal/kg/day. His physical exam is normal. What would be the next appropriate step in management? Your recommendation is to ↑ his calorie count to > 100 kcal/kg/day and to reweigh him in one month. At seven months his growth percentiles are unchanged, and you start a workup that includes a CBC, an electrolyte panel, UA, ESR, and TFTs.

Poor Growth or Failure to Thrive (FTT)

DIAGNOSIS

- Measure growth percentiles and adjust for prematurity.
- Look for downward crossing of two percentile lines in ≥ 1 indices (usually weight falls off first, followed by height and then by head circumference; see Table 9-1).
- A thorough diagnostic workup begins with a general health, dietary, and social history. Additional workup may include calorie count, CBC, and an electrolyte panel, including measurement of acid-base status, UA, ESR, and TFTs.

TABLE 9-1. **Types and Features of FTT or Growth Deficiency**

TYPE	WEIGHT	HEIGHT	HEAD CIRCUMFERENCE	CAUSES
Caloric imbalance	Markedly ↓	Somewhat ↓	Normal (preserved)	Inadequate caloric intake (poverty, poor feeding); excessive loss of calories (malabsorption); excessive utilization of calories (↑ metabolic rate); inability to use calories (inborn errors of metabolism).
Physiologic limitation	Proportionally ↓	Proportionally ↓	Normal (but appears proportionally larger)	Genetically small; endocrinopathies; constitutional growth delay; skeletal dysplasia.
CNS limitation	↓	↓	↓	CNS abnormality; chromosomal defects; in utero or perinatal insults.

All cases of FTT represent a mismatch of caloric intake and caloric needs at some level of natural or physiologic growth (e.g., social, genetic, CNS, GI, skeletal, endocrine).

TREATMENT

- Requires early identification of the etiology as well as counseling.
- Closely monitor caloric intake (may require supplemental feeding with high-calorie formula, NG tube feeding, and hospitalization).
- Treat the underlying disease.

GENERAL DEVELOPMENTAL ISSUES

A five-year-old boy has recently started asking his parents to tell him "just one more story" every night at his bedtime of 7:00 PM. His mother and father are exasperated because the child becomes angry when they refuse to do so. The boy typically attempts to join his parents in their room at this time, and they occasionally allow him to fall asleep with them. When the child's grandparents come to visit, they let him stay up until 8:30 PM, at which point he "volunteers" to go to his own room for "only one bed story." When the boy asks for another story, what should his grandfather do? The grandfather tells him that he will get a prize in the morning (a sticker) if he goes to sleep in his own bed after only one story. The child's parents learn that a somewhat later bedtime, combined with limit setting and small incentives, will help this difficult but normal challenge pass more easily.

Sleep

- Definitions are as follows:
    - **Rapid eye movement (REM):** A sleep stage that generally represents lighter sleep in which dreams occur.
    - **Non-REM (NREM):** Stages I–IV of NREM sleep represent progressively deeper sleep.
    - **Sleep cycle:** Time between REM stages (usually ↑ with age).
- Infant and child sleep patterns follow a known developmental course (see Table 9-2).
- Disturbances of sleep patterns are often related to parental expectations, child illness, or familial disruption.
- Other sleep-related issues include the following:
    - **Night feeding:** Typically not needed past six months of age; may → night awakening thereafter.
    - **Cosleeping:**
        - The cultural norm in most of the world; rarely a health risk (smokers, drug and alcohol users, and "heavy adult sleepers" are known exceptions).
        - Can become habit forming if used to alleviate nighttime awakening problems or fears.
    - **Sleep associations:**
        - Defined as external stimuli that a child uses to sleep (e.g., pacifiers, feeding, rocking, music, visual or body contact with the parent).
        - The child can become dependent on such stimuli and can thus become less capable of putting himself to sleep.
    - **Nighttime awakening:**
        - Common in children up to 4–5 years of age; usually results from an inability to self-soothe back to sleep, often as a result of sleep associations.

- Can be treated with ↓ reinforcement and progressively longer intervals between brief comforting visits.
  - **Bedtime struggles:**
    - Defined as difficulty with sleep initiation 2° to sleep associations, fears, or ↑ wakefulness; often characterized by fussiness.
    - Common in children up to 4–5 years of age; usually results from lack of a routine and insufficient limit setting.
    - Can be treated with a somewhat later bedtime followed by a stricter routine and limit setting.
    - Can → difficulty getting back to sleep with normal nighttime awakening.

Colic

Defined as any recurrent, inconsolable crying in an otherwise healthy and well-fed infant that is considered a problem by the child's caretakers.

DIAGNOSIS

- Rule out other causes of crying with a thorough history and exam (classic causes are infections, GERD, anal fissures, hair tourniquets, corneal abrasions, and narcotic withdrawal).
- **Timing:** Most crying occurs during early evening hours (5:00–8:00 PM).
- **Quality of cry:** Can vary, but often characterized by a hyperirritable infant with ↑ tone.

> **Colic—the rule of 3s**
>
> Usually occurs for **3** hours or more at least **3** days a week.
> Usually occurs between the ages of **3** weeks and **3** months.

TREATMENT

- Family support involves demystifying the diagnosis, mitigating guilt, offering empathy, and providing close follow-up.
- Create a list of interventions that soothe the infant (generally, such interventions work in only 30% of infants), and use 1–2 items from this menu at any time to determine which is actually working (see Table 9-3).

TABLE 9-2. Sleep Development and Common Problems by Age

AGE	SLEEP STAGE DEVELOPMENT	AVERAGE SLEEP REQUIREMENTS (24-HOUR CYCLE)	COMMON PROBLEMS	COMMON SOLUTIONS
Infants	Up to 50% REM in 50-minute cycles.	15 hours.	Day-night reversal; nighttime awakening.	Daylight and stimulation; ↓ nighttime stimulation and sleep associations.
Toddlers	NREM > REM.	12 hours (including one nap).	Night terrors.	Scheduled awakenings.
School-age children	Longer cycles (> 1 hour).	10 hours (no longer napping).	Nightmares; night fears; limit setting.	Reassurance; routines and night lights.
Adolescents	Adult cycles (90 minutes); 20–25% REM.	8 hours.	Late nights; late weekend waking (delayed sleep phase).	Sleep hygiene; seven-day-a-week schedule.

TABLE 9-3. Commonly Used Methods to Soothe Colic

METHOD	COMMENTS
Formula switching	Works best as a last resort.
Changes in maternal breast-feeding diet	Stopping cow's milk and caffeine.
Changing feeding routine (bottle, nipple, burping)	Occasionally helps very gassy infants.
Supplemental carrying	May slightly ↓ cry time.
Stimulation (e.g., car ride, swing, rocking, vibrating)	Driver safety and the position of the child are paramount.
Swaddling	Good for hypersensitive infants.
White noise generator	May become habitual if used > 6 months.

■ Encourage caregivers to take necessary breaks, especially if they are overwhelmed or angry (excessive crying or colic can be a risk factor for child abuse).

Teething

Defined as a period of early tooth eruption (usually at 6–8 months) in which an infant has mild symptoms of gingival swelling and sensitivity, ↑ salivation, and irritability related to gum discomfort. There is no strong evidence for an association with diarrhea, rhinorrhea, rashes, or fever.

DIFFERENTIAL

Early gland development, which usually takes place 2–3 months before with ↑ secretions or mouth lesions associated with infections.

TREATMENT

Provision of a cool contact to gums with a chilled teething toy or a wet washcloth; judicious use of analgesics.

Discipline

■ Literally defined as to "teach or instruct," but often oversimplified and interpreted as punishment.
■ Tables 9-4 and 9-5 outline common methods of discipline as well as problem behaviors within various age groups.

*The American Academy of Pediatrics' three **essential elements** of discipline are as follows:*

■ *A ⊕ and supporting relationship with the child.*
■ *Use of ⊕ reinforcement to ↑ desired behaviors.*
■ *Removing reinforcement of undesired behaviors and using punishment to ↓ them.*

TABLE 9-4. Common Methods of Discipline

METHOD	DESCRIPTION
Time out	A quick intervention to remove the child physically from the undesired behavior and provide a ⊖ consequence for the action for one minute per year of age.
Time in	Immediate brief praise and physical contact for desired behaviors.
Natural consequences	The child learns via ⊖ reinforcement that directly results from his or her own behavior without parental intervention. Allows for learning when consequences are not particularly risky to the child's health or well-being.
Removal of privileges	Involves clear-cut consequences such as grounding the child or withdrawing TV.
Logical consequences	The child learns via ⊖ reinforcement that occurs in response to his or her misbehavior and prevents the opportunity for that behavior to recur.
Token economy	Use of a sticker-chart, point, or chip system to reward desired behaviors, with accumulated value and small prizes.

Temperament

- Defined as the style in which a child experiences and reacts to the environment. Determined largely by genetic factors. Approximately 65% of children fit into one of three **temperamental constellations:**
  - **The easy child** (40% of sample): A child who has a regular, ⊕ approach toward new stimuli, is highly adaptable to change, has mild to moderate intensity of reaction, and has a ⊕ mood.

TABLE 9-5. Problem Behaviors and Useful Discipline Techniques by Age

	TODDLERS (12–36 MONTHS)	PRESCHOOL AGE (3–5 YEARS)	EARLY SCHOOL AGE (6–8 YEARS)	OLDER SCHOOL AGE (9–12 YEARS)	ADOLESCENTS (13+ years)
Common problem behaviors	Dangerous behaviors, tantrums (hitting, limit testing).	Dangerous behaviors, tantrums, persistent defiance.	Lying, name calling, fighting.	Defiance, lying, rudeness.	Defiance, lying, rudeness, risk taking.
Useful disciplinary techniques	Time in.	Time out, time in, simple token economy.	Removal of privileges, time out, time in, advanced token economy, natural and logical consequences.	Natural and logical consequences, time in, removal of privileges.	Natural and logical consequences, time in, removal of privileges.

Seventy-five percent of children are toilet trained for both bowel and bladder by three years of age.

- **The difficult child** (10% of sample): A child who has an irregular, ⊖, or withdrawal response to new stimuli and who shows slow adaptability to new situations, intense ⊖ reactions, and a ⊖ mood.
- **The slow-to-warm-up child** (15% of sample): A child who has ⊖ (or withdrawal) but mild responses to new stimuli and slow adaptability to new situations even after repeated experiences.
- **Goodness of fit** refers to the match between a child's temperament and parental style/expectations; it is extremely important during stressful developmental periods such as toilet training (see below).

Toilet Training

A child's ability to maintain nighttime dryness usually follows his or her ability to maintain daytime dryness by 6–12 months.

- In most industrialized societies, toilet training is initiated in developmentally normal children at 2–3 years of age.
- **Methods of successful toilet training** are as follows (see also Table 9-6):
  - Use a **potty chair** beginning at 18 months of age, and allow for fun sitting time on a daily basis (using toys, books, and snack rewards as needed).
  - **Progress slowly** to remove clothes and eventually diapers, timing this activity to coincide with the usual bowel movement time.
  - Give ⊕ **feedback** at each stage for successful sitting periods of no longer than five minutes; then progress to longer periods, especially if the child is likely to produce spontaneous bowel movements in the diaper or toilet.

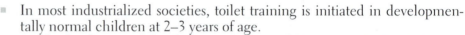

SPEECH AND LANGUAGE DEVELOPMENT

Key Milestones

Table 9-7 outlines language milestones by age and character.

Fractions for expressive-language milestones:

2 years = **2**/4ths (50%) intelligible speech

3 years = **3**/4ths (75%) intelligible speech

4 years = **4**/4ths (100%) intelligible speech

Reasons for Referral

- Any significant delay of speech or language milestone should be followed by a thorough history and physical as well as by a **hearing** evaluation.
- Although the differential diagnosis is broad, common red flags for serious language delay include the following:
  - **No babbling** or cooing by one year.
  - **No pointing or words** by 15 months.
  - No intelligible speech at two years.

TABLE 9-6. Prerequisites for Successful Toilet Training

BOWEL/BLADDER	MOTOR	COGNITIVE	MOTIVATION
Dry for several hours. No bowel movement during sleep.	Walks easily to bathroom. Bends down. Pulls down pants. Can sit still for 15 minutes.	Understands questions regarding "potty." Able to communicate the need to go.	Wants to give up diapers/pull-ups. Prefers to be clean and dry.

T A B L E 9 - 7. Key Language Milestones

AGE	EXPRESSIVE	RECEPTIVE
1 month	Makes small, throaty sounds.	Responds to sound of voice.
2 months	Coos spontaneously.	Coos more with vocal stimuli.
4–5 months	Squeals and laughs.	Turns to sound.
6–7 months	Pronounces single syllables (*ba, ga, da*).	Imitates sounds (cough, tongue click).
9–10 months	Polysyllabic babbling; nonspecific "mama/dada."	Inhibits to "no"; follows a one-step command with gesture.
12 months	Says first word; points.	Follows a one-step command without gesture (up to 14 months).
18 months	Says 4–6 words.	Points to > 1 body part.
24 months	Says sentences of 2–3 words; speech is 50% understandable.	Points to six body parts; follows two-step commands without gesture.
3 years	Says sentences of 3–4 words; speech is 75% understandable.	Repeats three digits forward; can carry on a simple conversation.
4 years	Names 3–4 colors; speech is 100% understandable.	Knows the names and uses of three objects.
5 years	Defines five familiar words.	Repeats four digits forward.

Reading Disorders (Dyslexia)

Defined as unexpected difficulty in reading despite adequate motivation, opportunity, and intellectual ability. The **most commonly diagnosed** learning disorder (up to 80% of all learning disorders), occurring in 5–10% of clinic- and school-selected samples. Shows a large **genetic** predisposition (one-fourth to two-thirds of patients have a parent who is also dyslexic), and may coexist with other learning disorders or behavioral problems (e.g., ADHD).

DIAGNOSIS

Diagnosed with testing that shows specific challenges in word decoding and phonemic awareness.

TREATMENT

Treated with diverse teaching methods that involve mastery of **phonological skills; academic accommodations** such as extra time for reading-based assignments; and augmentative learning aids (e.g., laptops, tape recorders, spell checkers).

Key Milestones

Table 9-8 outlines key motor milestones by age and character.

Reasons for Referral

- An unambiguously abnormal **exam finding** that is neurologically based (e.g., persistent primitive reflex, weakness, hypotonia).
- A history revealing significant **lack or loss of a motor milestone** with a correlating exam finding.
- Parental concerns regarding **poor fine-motor skills** such as cutting, drawing, and writing often reflect true developmental delays that may → ↓ preacademic skills.

- **Adaptive behaviors:** Behaviors that aid in the day-to-day self-care of an individual (e.g., eating, hygiene, dressing).
- **Social behaviors:** Behaviors that acknowledge interpersonal and intergroup relationships (e.g., eye contact, smiling, play, bonding).

TABLE 9-8. Key Motor Milestones

Age	Gross Motor	Fine Motor
1 month	Momentary head lift.	Fisted hands.
2 months	Lifts head 45 degrees while prone.	Regards hand.
4–5 months	Lifts head 90 degrees while prone; brings hands together.	Grasps objects with sustained regard; regards raisin.
6–7 months	Sits up for about one minute.	Palmar grasp of cube/rake a raisin.
9–10 months	Sits up from prone position; pulls up to stand; cruises with two hands.	Pincer grasp assisted by palm; bangs two cubes.
12 months	Stands alone for about 10 seconds.	Unassisted pincer grasp.
18 months	Walks up steps while holding onto rail.	Builds a tower of 3–4 cubes.
24 months	Jumps in place.	Builds a tower of 6–7 cubes.
3 years	Broad jump; throws ball.	Draws a circle.
4 years	Hops.	Draws a cross.
5 years	Walks stairs without railing.	Draws a triangle.

Key Milestones

Table 9-9 outlines key milestones pertinent to social and adaptive development.

Reasons for Referral

- ↓ eye contact with any combination of delayed social or adaptive milestones.
- ↓ communication (including gestures such as pointing) along with other delays.

Autism Spectrum Disorders

A group of biologically based developmental disorders of varying severity that include autistic disorder, Asperger disorder, pervasive developmental disorder not otherwise specified (PDD, NOS), Rett disorder, and childhood disintegrative disorder. Onset occurs by three years of age; estimated prevalence is at least 1 in 500, with a male-to-female ratio of 3–4:1. Characteristic features include impaired **social interaction, language,** and **behavior.** Distinguished as follows:

- **Autistic disorder:** Table 9-10 outlines the characteristics and features of autistic disorder.

TABLE 9-9. Key Social and Adaptive Developmental Milestones

AGE	SOCIAL	ADAPTIVE
1 month	Regards face.	Follows to midline.
2 months	Smiles responsively; vocalizes in response to social stimuli.	Regards hand briefly; follows to 90 degrees.
4–5 months	Smiles spontaneously; vocalizes at mirror.	Activates in response to toy/food; sustains regard for object in hand.
6–7 months	Reaches to pat mirror.	Feeds self cracker; looks after dropped object.
9–10 months	Gesture games (peekaboo); stranger anxiety.	Exploratory play by mouthing most objects.
12 months	**Initiates** gesture games; functional play (e.g., pushes car around, plays ball).	Object permanence (recovers object under cup or paper after visible displacements).
18 months	Imitative play (telephone, cleaning).	Drinks from cup, spilling less than half.
24 months	Symbolic play (pretends to feed or dress doll or animal).	Object permanence (recovers hidden object after invisible displacements).
3 years	Understands taking turns.	Puts on some clothing.
4 years	Plays cooperative games.	Dresses without help.
5 years	Follows rules.	Brushes teeth without help; prepares cereal.

TABLE 9-10. Characteristics of Autistic Disorder [a]

AREAS	SPECIFIC FEATURES
Qualitative impairments in social interaction	Marked impairment in use of nonverbal behaviors (eye gaze, facial expression).
	Failure to develop peer relationships appropriate to developmental level.
	Lack of spontaneous seeking to share enjoyment, interests, or achievements.
	Lack of social or emotional reciprocity.
Qualitative impairment in communication	Delay or lack of spoken language not accompanied by alternative attempts such as gesture or mime.
	Marked impairment in the ability to initiate or sustain conversation.
	Stereotyped and repetitive or idiosyncratic language.
	Lack of varied, spontaneous make-believe, imitative play appropriate to developmental level.
Restrictive, repetitive, stereotyped behaviors, interests, or activities	Encompassing preoccupation with stereotyped, restricted interests.
	Apparently inflexible adherence to specific, nonfunctional routines or rituals.
	Stereotyped and repetitive motor mannerisms.
	Persistent preoccupation with parts of objects.

[a] Based on *Diagnostic and Statistical Manual of Mental Disorders,* 4th ed. (DSM-IV) diagnostic criteria.

- **Asperger disorder:** Characterized by poor peer relationships with lack of empathy, overly focused interests, and no clinically significant delays in cognitive or language development.
- **PDD, NOS:**
  - Meets some but not all of the criteria for autistic disorder.
  - Not better explained by Rett's or childhood disintegrative disorder.
  - Sometimes used for very young children when the diagnosis is uncertain.
- **Rett disorder:**
  - A neurodegenerative disorder caused by a mutation on an X-linked gene.
  - Characterized by normal development up to five months of age followed by head growth deceleration, severe to profound mental retardation, hand wringing, impaired language and interaction, and loss of previously attained milestones.
  - Occurs primarily in females.
- **Childhood disintegrative disorder:**
  - Rare and somewhat controversial.
  - Characterized by normal development up to two years of age followed by marked regression in language, play, and motor skills.

DEVELOPMENTAL AND COGNITIVE ASSESSMENT TOOLS

Significance of Developmental Assessment

- Many studies have confirmed that **parental concern** for developmental delay is **highly sensitive** and specific. The pediatrician's role is to adequately screen, identify, and appropriately refer children with suspected delay.

- **Federal and state mandates for developmentally based services** are as follows:
  - Early intervention (children 0–3 years of age).
  - Early identification (children 3–5 years of age).
  - Schools must give disabled students equal access to services.

Developmental Screening

- Begins with a thorough history and physical examination.
- Specific high-risk factors for developmental delay include prematurity, genetic sensory or neuromuscular disease, lead exposure, chronic infections (including HIV), and a history of abuse or neglect. Also at risk are children whose parents are young or have a low educational level (< 10th grade).
- The most commonly used office-based screening instrument is the **Denver Developmental Screening Test II**. This test can, however, be highly insensitive to language delays; thus, other instruments are now gaining favor (see Table 9-11).
- The **PEDS** (Parents' Evaluation of Developmental Status) only takes < 5 minutes to score. Its **sensitivity is 74–79%** and its **specificity 70–80% across age levels.**

In general, developmental tests are not predictive of later cognitive functioning until after two years of age.

Referral

- Referral may be for further family assessment, auditory and visual testing, or global and specific diagnostic testing.
- The pediatrician may not be specifically skilled in the interpretation of developmental tests and may thus rely on the specialist (psychologist or developmentalist) to clearly state the rationale for specific testing, delineate results, and interpret findings for the family.

For children up to two years of age, most tests rely primarily on sensorimotor function; thereafter, the focus is on language.

School Readiness Screening

Defined as screening performed for the purpose of assessing the abilities that are required for academic achievement. These are as follows:

TABLE 9-11. Features of Commonly Used Developmental Tests

Test	Domains Assessed	Age Range	Administration
Battelle Developmental Inventory Screening Test	Global	0–8 years	By trained psychologist or developmentalist
Ages and Stages Questionnaire	Global	4–48 months	By parents
Bayley Scales of Infant Development II	Global	0–42 months	By trained psychologist
Parents' Evaluation of Developmental Status (PEDS)	Global	0–8 years	By trained pediatrician

- Visual-motor skills
- Number concepts
- Expressive language
- Verbal analogies
- Memory and sequencing
- Gross motor/body awareness
- Toilet training (now often mandatory)

Intelligence, Achievement, and Adaptive Testing

- **Psychological testing** is done for children with suspected mental retardation, early (preschool or kindergarten) social or behavioral difficulties, learning problems, or intellectual giftedness.
- **Cognitive or "intelligence" testing** is done for children with suspected mental retardation or specific academic difficulties.
  - Usually begins at four years of age but is more specific to true cognitive potential at school age.
  - **Mental retardation** is defined as an IQ < 70, impaired function, and age of initial insult < 18 years.
  - **Borderline intelligence** is defined as an IQ of 70–80.
- **Academic achievement tests** are usually administered by school specialists and assess specific areas, including reading, math, writing, and general-knowledge subject areas.
- **Adaptive behavior tests** provide functional assessments of daily living skills by means of standardized tools. A diagnosis of mental retardation requires low scores on **both cognitive ability and adaptive functioning.**

Learning Disabilities

- Defined as identified differences between intellectual ability and achievement, such as normal IQ and pronounced difficulty with math.
- Currently the DSM-IV and ICD-9 coding systems overlap somewhat for the following diagnoses:
  - Reading disability (dyslexia)
  - Writing disability (dysgraphia)
  - Mathematics disability (dyscalculia)
  - Learning disorder, not otherwise specified

SPECIAL DEVELOPMENTAL ISSUES

Enuresis

Defined as nocturnal bed-wetting after six years of age **or** daytime accidents after four years of age. Approximately 7% of eight-year-olds have occasional bed-wetting, but this rate drops by roughly 1% for each year thereafter. Only 10% of cases have an organic etiology. Clinically classified as follows:

- **1° enuresis:** The continuation of voiding accidents past appropriate ages for daytime and nighttime dryness.
- **2° enuresis:** Occurs after successful toilet training has been established for six months.
- **Complicated enuresis:** Involves frequent daytime accidents, abnormal physical findings, or recurrent UTIs.

DIFFERENTIAL

Table 9-12 outlines the differential diagnosis of enuresis.

DIAGNOSIS

- Conduct a complete history and physical that includes a voiding history, a developmental history, and GU and neurologic exams.
- Obtain a UA.
- Obtain a urine culture (for girls).

TREATMENT

- Education and destigmatization.
- Alarm system (up to 80% effective).
- Hypnotherapy.
- **Pharmacotherapy** (for short-term need or recalcitrant cases): TCAs (less favorable), vasopressin (DDAVP).

Radiologic or urodynamic studies are rarely needed to diagnose enuresis and should be guided by the history and exam.

> A toilet-trained, developmentally normal six-year-old boy is continent by day but has 5–7 bed-wetting episodes per week and 1–2 daytime stooling accidents per week. His exam reveals significant skin breakdown in his perineum as well as cloudy urine. After successful treatment of his skin rash and UTI, he returns with fewer episodes of bed-wetting but is still encopretic. What should his pediatrician do next? This time a KUB reveals large amounts of granular stool and dilatation of his rectum and distal colon. After further education of the family, a cleanout regimen is initiated with early follow-up in two weeks. At that point he begins a postprandial toilet-sitting program to prevent further constipation and encopresis. His enuresis improves thereafter.

Encopresis

Defined as repeated stooling in an inappropriate location after four years of age or after successful toilet training, and in the absence of any medical cause. Affects approximately 1–2% of school-age children (some studies cite a rate as high as 10%) and has a male-to-female ratio of 6:1.

TABLE 9-12. Differential Diagnosis of Enuresis

ANATOMIC/ MECHANICAL	DEVELOPMENTAL	MEDICAL	SOCIAL/OTHER
Ectopic ureter (vaginal)	Neurologic immaturity	Diabetes mellitus or insipidus	Psychosocial stressors
Chronic constipation		Sickle cell disease	Sexual abuse
Vaginal reflux		Frequent UTIs	Excessive nighttime drinking
Spastic bladder		Spina bifida	
		Seizure disorder	

Only 15% of families with encopretic children are aware of the problem.

DIFFERENTIAL

Constipation/obstipation, painful defecation (rectal fissures), physical or sexual abuse, neurologic abnormality (spina bifida), GI abnormalities (Hirschsprung disease or IBD), hypothyroidism, laxative abuse.

DIAGNOSIS

- Conduct a thorough history and physical with special attention to stooling history and rectal and neurologic exams.
- History often reveals late- or early-evening accidents, no perception of accidents or odor, abdominal pain if constipation is more recent, and overflow bowel movements in the toilet.
  - "Leakage" of loose stool around retained, compacted stool may be seen.
  - Some children withhold stool while at school → constipation.
- AXR often reveals right-to-left shift of granulated stool pattern and a markedly dilated rectum and colon.

TREATMENT

- Treatment follows a three-step plan consisting of the following:
  - Education and demystification (essential in breaking the pattern of blame and shame).
  - A colonic cleanout regimen (may include enemas, suppositories, stool softeners, or stimulants).
  - Early follow-up to ensure the success of the above measures; initiation of a morning and evening toilet-sitting routine.
- Prognosis is as follows:
  - Some 75–80% report improvement with the three-step plan above.
  - Risk factors for recalcitrant encopresis include bed stooling, lack of significant constipation, and other developmental and behavioral problems (e.g., ADHD).

Child Abuse

Child maltreatment involves acts of physical harm, sexual abuse, and general neglect.

- Data from 1995 suggest that 1 out of 25 children are reported for suspected abuse or neglect.
- Approximately 36% of these reports were substantiated.
- Approximately 2000 children die each year of abuse.

DIFFERENTIAL

- Misunderstanding, poor history.
- Cupping, coining, moxibustion (Asian traditional healing practices).
- Bleeding disorder (rare).

DIAGNOSIS

- Thorough history and physical with findings consistent with nonaccidental injury such as unexplained or implausible causes. May often present with delayed care.

- Laboratory workup includes a bone survey repeated in 7–10 days to reveal healing of more recent fractures, bleeding studies as needed for bruising, transaminases and pancreatic enzymes with imaging if abdominal trauma is suspected, and brain CT/MRI if an infant or as otherwise indicated.

TREATMENT

- Medical stabilization of the patient.
- Mandated reporting for suspected abuse.
- Security and safety measures.

Adoption/Foster Care

- Definitions are as follows:
  - **Adoption** is acquiring legal guardianship of an individual.
  - **Foster care** is a temporary placement of an individual who has been removed from an unsafe environment.
- Two percent of all children are adopted.
- Adopted children have a slightly higher prevalence of ADHD, fetal alcohol syndrome, mental retardation, and congenital malformations.
- The age at which children should be told they are adopted is somewhat controversial, but many agree that age 3–4, during the preschooler egocentric period, is recommended.
- It is important to convey understandable facts (if known) and to respect a child's eventual wish for privacy.
- Special-needs children are more difficult to place in adoption, as are paired siblings and children > 6 years old.

BEHAVIORAL AND PSYCHIATRIC DISORDERS

A seven-year-old boy is repeating the first grade because his teacher felt he was not "mature enough." Last year he was suspended for fighting and was found torturing a neighborhood dog on several occasions. This year his new teacher says he is quite fidgety in class and cannot sit still. His foster mother states that the boy has improved since he started taking medication for ADHD but is still having tantrums in which he hits and bites. His physical exam is normal, and he is growing well. What should his pediatrician do next? A new pediatrician realized that "all that is inattentive is not ADHD" and has decided to refer him to a psychiatrist for concerns regarding a mood disorder. His social history is explored there, and a new therapy and medication regimen is started by the psychiatrist.

Attention Deficit Hyperactivity Disorder (ADHD)

A chronic neurobehavioral disorder with difficulties in at least one of three main areas: focusing and sustaining attention, inhibiting impulsive behavior, and regulating activity level. The most commonly diagnosed behavioral disorder in childhood, it affects 4–12% of elementary school children; shows a male predominance (3:1 or higher); is present in 25% of first-degree relatives; and is associated with oppositional defiant disorder, conduct disorder, and mood disorders. Children often have poor self-esteem and can become socially isolated.

DIAGNOSIS

- There are three subtypes: predominantly inattentive, predominantly hyperactive/impulsive, and combined or mixed subtype (see Table 9-13).
- Symptoms causing impairment must be present before seven years of age.
- Symptoms must also be present in two or more settings for at least six months.
- Other disorders must be ruled out.

TREATMENT

- Treatment goals are as follows:
  - Demystify the condition for the child and caretakers.
  - Improve self-esteem, relationships, and academic performance.
  - ↓ disruptive behaviors and improve independence.
- **Mainstays of treatment** include the following:
  - A behavioral management plan in school and at home.
  - Classroom and academic accommodations as needed.
  - Pharmacologic therapy is most effective, with a 70–80% response rate (see Table 9-14).

TABLE 9-13. **Diagnostic Criteria for ADHD**

DIAGNOSTIC AREA	REQUIREMENT
Inattention	Must **often** have at least six of the following specific features:
	Lack of attention to detail/careless mistakes.
	Difficulty sustaining attention on tasks.
	Does not seem to listen.
	Does not follow through on instructions.
	Has difficulty organizing tasks.
	Avoids tasks that require sustained attention.
	Loses necessary items (homework, toys).
	Easily distracted by extraneous stimuli.
	Forgetful in daily activities.
Hyperactivity-impulsivity	Must **often** have at least six of the following specific features:
	Fidgets or squirms.
	Leaves seat in class or other situations.
	Runs about when inappropriate.
	Has difficulty playing quietly.
	Is on the go/"driven by a motor."
	Talks excessively.
	Blurts out answers.
	Has difficulty waiting in lines or for turn.
	Interrupts or intrudes on others.

TABLE 9-14. Common Pharmocotherapies for ADHD

DRUG CLASS	DURATION OF ACTION	TYPICAL SIDE EFFECTS
Methylphenidate	3–12 hours with different formulations.	Nervousness, insomnia, anorexia, tics.
Dextroamphetamine	3–12 hours with different formulations.	Palpitations, nervousness, insomnia, headache, worsened tics, anorexia.
Atomoxetine	24 hours.	Nausea, vomiting, headache, sleepiness.

Depression

Defined as pathologic sadness or despondency that cannot be explained as a normal response to stress and that → impairment in function. Affects at least 7% of the general pediatric population and 15–20% of adolescents. Males and females are affected equally until postpuberty, when the rate among girls is three- to fourfold higher than that in boys. Commonly recurrent and persists into adulthood; associated with a 15% annual risk of suicide attempts.

DIAGNOSIS

Requires at least two weeks of mostly depressed mood and at least four other depressive symptoms (see the mnemonic **SIG E CAPS**).

TREATMENT

- **Suicidal** or **homicidal** patients should always be **hospitalized.**
- Individual and family therapy as needed.
- **Cognitive behavioral therapy** (CBT) is the mainstay for older children (> 8 years of age).
- Despite recent concerns, **SSRIs** are still first-line pharmacotherapy.

Bipolar Disorder

Classified as two types: **type I,** which is characterized by depression plus mania; and **type II,** which is characterized by depression plus hypomania. Has a low prevalence in children (0.2–0.4%), but may be increasing.

DIAGNOSIS

- Symptoms include major somatic, thought, and behavioral changes.
- Symptoms often cycle fast but may also be slower.
- The mnemonic **DIG FAST** describes the classic symptoms of bipolar I disorder.

Schizophrenia

A chronic deterioration from a previous level of functioning for at least six months with psychotic features and without toxic causes (PCP, stimulants,

> **Depressive symptoms—SIG E CAPS**
>
> **S**leep problems
> **I**nterests (↓)
> **G**uilt
> **E**nergy (↓)
> **C**oncentration difficulties
> **A**ppetite changes
> **P**sychomotor retardation
> **S**uicidal ideations

> **Classic symptoms of bipolar I disorder— DIG FAST**
>
> **D**istractibility
> **I**nsomnia
> **G**randiosity
> **F**light of ideas
> ↑ in goal-directed
> **A**ctivities, psychomotor
> **A**gitation
> **S**peech (pressured)
> **T**houghtlessness

steroids) or organic etiologies (SLE, Wilson's disease, porphyria). Rare in childhood (< 5 in 10,000), but more common in adolescence. Boys have an ↑ incidence and a somewhat earlier onset than girls. Typical age at onset is late adolescence; earlier onset is associated with a worse overall prognosis. A parent with schizophrenia ↑ a child's risk from 1% to 10%.

DIAGNOSIS/TREATMENT

- Patients must see a child psychiatrist and have an adequate medical workup.
- Parent education and counseling are critical, as is close follow-up.
- Atypical antipsychotic medications are becoming popular but are associated with weight gain.

Generalized Anxiety Disorder

Estimated to affect 3–4% of children and adolescents; shows a female predominance, especially in adolescents.

DIAGNOSIS

Diagnosed in the presence of anxious mood for at least six months with at least four of the following:

- Worry about the future
- Concern about competence
- Concern about past behavior
- Somatic complaints
- Self-consciousness
- Continual need for reassurance
- Constant feelings of tension and/or inability to relax

TREATMENT

Can be treated with family therapy, CBT, and SSRIs if necessary.

CHRONIC ILLNESS IN CHILDHOOD

- Defined as any condition that limits the usual daily activities, requires special services, or limits the ability to do regular schoolwork (e.g., asthma, diabetes, epilepsy).
- **Developmental approach and regression:**
  - Hospitalization is associated with a normal period of regression in most children and with more prolonged regression in the chronically ill.
  - For toddlers, natural exploratory urges may be blunted by illness.
  - For adolescents, development of personal identity may be altered → rebellion or denial in terms of the illness itself.
- **Therapeutic and adaptive strategies:**
  - Family strength assessment and education about the illness.
  - Educational planning for the child (maximize participation).
  - Assisted technology (e.g., special wheelchairs, communication devices).
  - Coordinated care (a medical home that is involved with all services).

CHAPTER 10

Hematology

Wilbur Lam, MD
Debbie Sakaguchi, MD
reviewed by Robert E. Goldsby, MD

Defined as low hemoglobin, hematocrit, or RBC count for age and gender. Risk factors include a $\oplus$ family history (anemia, early gallbladder disease, splenectomy), a restricted diet (excessive cow's or goat's milk intake, vegan diet, pica), ethnicity (African-American, Mediterranean, or Southeast Asian descent), recent infection, chronic disease (renal or chronic inflammatory disease), prematurity, and a history of hyperbilirubinemia. Classified as follows:

- ↑ **RBC destruction:**
  - RBC membrane disorders (hereditary spherocytosis, elliptocytosis, pyropoikilocytosis).
  - Enzyme defects (G6PD deficiency, pyruvate kinase deficiency).
  - Hemoglobinopathies (sickle cell disease, α-thalassemia, β-thalassemia, hemoglobin E disease).
  - Autoimmune hemolytic anemia (AIHA).
  - Microangiopathic hemolytic anemia.
  - Blood loss.
- ↓ **RBC production:**
  - Nutritional anemias (iron, vitamin B_{12}, or folate deficiency; lead poisoning).
  - Anemia of inflammation (or chronic disease).
  - Defective marrow response (transient erythroblastopenia of childhood; Diamond-Blackfan anemia).

SYMPTOMS/EXAM

Fatigue, pallor, jaundice (hemolytic anemia), petechiae, ↑ heart rate, flow murmur, splenomegaly, dysmorphic features (facial changes, limb abnormalities).

DIAGNOSIS

- **Initial tests:** Hemoglobin/hematocrit, mean corpuscular volume (MCV), mean corpuscular hemoglobin concentration (MCHC), red cell distribution width (RDW), RBC count, peripheral smear, reticulocyte count.
- **Additional studies (depending on the above results):** Indirect bilirubin, LDH, haptoglobin, B_{12}, folate, ferritin, iron, total iron-binding capacity (TIBC), transferrin, lead, Coombs' test, hemoglobin electrophoresis., Heinz body preps.

RBC Membrane Disorders

Anemias related to RBC membrane disorders include the following:

- **Hereditary spherocytosis:** A primarily **autosomal-dominant spectrin deficiency** (RBC structural protein deficiency) that weakens the connection between the cell membrane and cytoskeleton. RBCs lose membrane surface area → poorly deformable spherocytes that are destroyed by the spleen. The clinical spectrum varies from mild to severe anemia; most patients have splenomegaly.
- **Hereditary elliptocytosis:** A primarily autosomal-dominant but heterogeneous group of disorders with a clinical spectrum ranging from chronic hemolysis to asymptomatic carrier states. Most patients are asymptomatic

with only incidental elliptocytes on smear. Defects in the RBC skeleton → ↓ mechanical stability.

- **Hereditary pyropoikilocytosis:** An uncommon disorder involving a spectrin deficiency or mutation that → ↑ **thermal sensitivity**. RBCs have a ↓ thermal threshold for fragmentation.

SYMPTOMS/EXAM

Mild to severe anemia (depending on the disease), intermittent jaundice, splenomegaly, and a ⊕ family history of anemia/jaundice/gallstones.

DIFFERENTIAL

AIHA; ABO/Rh incompatibility.

DIAGNOSIS

- **Hereditary spherocytosis:** Spherocytes, mild anemia (hemoglobin 9–12 g/dL), ↑ MCHC, ↑ RDW.
- **Hereditary elliptocytosis:** Elliptocytes; normal hemoglobin to severe anemia.
- **Hereditary pyropoikilocytosis:** Extreme poikilocytosis (budding RBCs, fragments, spherocytes, bizarre shapes), especially at high temperatures; extreme microcytosis; MCV < 50.
- **All types:** ↑ osmotic fragility; ↑ reticulocyte count, ↑ indirect bilirubin, ⊖ direct Coombs' test.

TREATMENT

Folate, transfusion, splenectomy (pneumococcal vaccination prior to and penicillin prophylaxis after surgery).

COMPLICATIONS

Neonatal hyperbilirubinemia; gallstones; splenomegaly → splenic rupture; aplastic crisis.

Spherocytes are seen not only in hereditary spherocytosis but also in immune-mediated hemolytic anemias, microangiopathic hemolytic anemias, and, occasionally, RBC enzyme deficiencies (with G6PD deficiency being the most common).

Enzyme Defects

G6PD DEFICIENCY

An X-linked recessive disorder; the most common RBC enzyme defect. Deficient RBCs are unable to generate adequate NADPH to prevent cellular damage from oxidative stress. Most common in those of Mediterranean, African, or Asian descent.

SYMPTOMS/EXAM

Neonatal hyperbilirubinemia; intermittent anemia; jaundice triggered by infections, drugs, and fava beans.

DIAGNOSIS

Bite cells, spherocytes, ↓ **RBC G6PD level,** ↑ reticulocyte count, ↑ bilirubin.

TREATMENT

Phototherapy; exchange transfusion for neonatal hyperbilirubinemia; transfusion; avoidance of oxidative drugs (sulfa drugs, antimalarials) and fava beans.

COMPLICATIONS

Neonatal hyperbilirubinemia, splenomegaly, gallstones.

PYRUVATE KINASE DEFICIENCY

An autosomal-recessive disorder in which a deficiency of pyruvate kinase → low adenosine triphosphate (ATP) levels. ATP depletion ↑ cellular potassium and water loss → inflexible, dehydrated, crenated RBCs that are destroyed in the spleen. Most common among those of Northern European descent.

SYMPTOMS/EXAM

Mild to severe anemia; jaundice, splenomegaly.

DIAGNOSIS

Occasional echinocytes (spiculated erythrocytes); ↑ RBC 2,3-DPG level; ↓ **RBC ATP level;** normal osmotic fragility test; ↑ reticulocyte count; ↑ bilirubin.

TREATMENT

- Phototherapy for newborns; exchange transfusion for neonatal hyperbilirubinemia; transfusion.
- Splenectomy (only for severe anemia; has no effect in mild anemia).

COMPLICATIONS

Neonatal hyperbilirubinemia, splenomegaly, gallstones.

Hemoglobinopathies

Caused by mutations in the α or β chains that cause structural changes in hemoglobin or alter oxygen-carrying capacity. Unbalanced production of α or β chains leads to the thalassemias.

A nine-month-old African-American infant develops painful swelling of the hands and feet. Hemoglobin electrophoresis confirms HbSS disease. What medications should this child receive on a chronic basis? Penicillin and folate.

SICKLE CELL DISEASE

Sickle cell anemia (HbSS disease) is an **autosomal-recessive** disorder (homozygous HbSS) that involves **polymerization of deoxygenated HbS** → distortion and ↓ deformability of RBCs, ↑ blood viscosity, and a predisposition to painful vaso-occlusive episodes. At highest risk are those of **African,** Mediterranean, Middle Eastern, and Indian descent. Associated with anemia, jaundice, recurrent pain episodes, splenomegaly in early childhood that disappears (→ functional asplenia), risk of sepsis, and gallstones. **Other sickle syndromes** include the following:

- **Sickle cell trait:** No ↑ morbidity or mortality; no anemia, abnormal RBC morphology, or ↓ RBC survival unless the patient is at high elevations. Involves HbS (40%) and HbA (60%).

A high rate of false-⊖ results occur when G6PD levels are measured during an acute hemolytic episode because older G6PD-deficient cells are destroyed, leaving only the young G6PD-⊕ cells in the circulation. This will falsely elevate G6PD levels to near normal. G6PD levels are most accurate when measured at steady state.

- **HbSC disease:** Mild chronic hemolytic anemia with variable vaso-occlusive complications. More common complications include eye disease, aseptic necrosis of the femoral heads, renal papillary necrosis, and splenomegaly with splenic sequestration. Associated with HbS (50%) and HbC (50%).
- **Sickle β^0-thalassemia:** Comparable to but distinguished from HbSS disease by microcytosis, splenomegaly, ↓ hemolysis, and lower reticulocyte count. Primarily involves HbS; also characterized by slightly ↑ HbA$_2$ and variable HbF.
- **Sickle β^+-thalassemia:** Comparable to HbSC disease; distinguished from HbSS disease by HbA, microcytosis, splenomegaly, and a benign clinical course. Distinguished from HbS trait by HbS > HbA, microcytosis, hemolytic anemia, and splenomegaly. Primarily involves HbS; also shows ↑ HbA$_2$ and variable HbF and HbA.

DIAGNOSIS

Newborn hemoglobin electrophoresis yields the following:

- **HbS and HbS-β^0-thalassemia:** HbS, HbF.
- **HbS-β^+-thalassemia:** HbS, HbF, HbA.
- **HbSC:** HbS, HbC.

TREATMENT

Acute complications of sickle cell anemia (HbSS disease) are as follows:

- **Vaso-occlusive crisis:** Painful episodes from intravascular sickling and tissue ischemia. Locations involved are the lumbosacral spine, knee, shoulder, elbow, and femur. Hand-foot syndrome (dactylitis) occurs in children < 5 years of age and presents with swollen, tender hands or feet as well as with leukocytosis, fever, and bony changes on x-ray (1–2 weeks later). Treat with hydration and analgesia.
- **Acute chest syndrome:** The **leading cause of morbidity and mortality.** Symptoms are cough, chest pain, tachypnea, fever, and new infiltrate on CXR. Etiologies include fat embolus (from bone marrow), atelectasis, dehydration/overhydration, pain crisis, and infection (viruses, *Chlamydia, Mycoplasma, Streptococcus pneumoniae, Haemophilus influenzae*). Treat with antibiotics, bronchodilators, incentive spirometry, hydration (but do not overhydrate), and analgesia.
- **Stroke:** The highest rate is in children 5–10 years of age. Presents with hemiparesis, speech problems, focal seizures, and gait abnormalities. Infarcts occur in areas supplied by narrowed internal carotid, middle cerebral, anterior cerebral, or watershed areas between the anterior and middle cerebral vessels. Diagnose with CT or MRI; treat with exchange transfusion followed by maintenance transfusions.
- **Priapism:** Prolonged, painful erection. Repeat episodes are associated with a high risk of irreversible fibrosis and impotence. Treat with analgesia, transfusion, corporal aspiration, and irrigation.
- **Splenic sequestration:** A major cause of death. Presents with a rapidly distending, painful abdomen and with vomiting, pallor, and shock. Diagnose by a low hemoglobin that is half of baseline, ↑ reticulocyte count, and a rapidly enlarging spleen. Treat with emergency transfusion and elective splenectomy to prevent recurrence.
- **Aplastic crisis:** Parvovirus B19 → temporary RBC aplasia, preventing the compensatory reticulocytosis needed to maintain baseline hemoglobin levels. Treat with observation and occasional transfusion.

Sickle cell trait is associated with a slightly ↑ risk of hyposthenuria; glaucoma and recurrent hyphema; bacteriuria in females; splenic infarction and sudden death at high altitudes or extreme hypoxemia; and renal medullary carcinoma (rare).

Poor prognostic indicators for vaso-occlusive events and stroke include ↑ WBC, hemoglobin < 7, and a history of dactylitis during infancy.

In HbSS disease, splenic sequestration ceases by the age of five owing to splenic autoinfarction. Sequestration may still occur in older children with milder forms of sickle cell disease.

- **Infections:** Sepsis related to splenic dysfunction is a major cause of mortality in children with sickle cell anemia. Evaluation of a febrile child should include CBC, blood culture, UA and urine culture, CXR, throat culture, and LP (if toxic). Treat with parenteral antibiotics pending cultures.

COMPLICATIONS

Chronic complications include the following:

- **Cardiovascular system:** Cardiomegaly with LVH from chronic anemia and ↑ cardiac output. Examination reveals systolic ejection murmur and split S1. Diagnose with echocardiography.
- **Renal system:** Hyposthenuria, hematuria, nephrotic syndrome, uremia. Hyposthenuria results from sickling, ↓ blood flow in the hypertonic medulla, and derangement of the concentrating mechanism. Hematuria results from papillary necrosis or (rarely) renal medullary carcinoma (more common in HbSS disease). Nephrotic syndrome is associated with more severe sickle cell disease. Uremia is rare and is associated with parvovirus and glomerulonephritis.
- **Hepatobiliary system:** Cholelithiasis, hepatic infarction, transfusion-related hepatitis.
- **Eyes:** Proliferative and nonproliferative retinopathy → blindness.
- **Skin:** Chronic leg ulcers in adolescents.
- **Skeleton:** Maxillary overgrowth; flattened "codfish vertebrae"; aseptic necrosis of the femoral head.
- **Pulmonary:** Obstructive and restrictive lung disease.
- **CNS:** Impairment of cognitive function and fine motor skills.
- **Growth and development:** Poor weight gain; delayed sexual development.

PREVENTION

Health care maintenance measures include the following:

- **Infection:** Pneumococcal, *H. influenzae*, HBV, and influenza vaccination; prophylactic penicillin until the age of five in addition to other routine immunizations.
- **Anemia:** Labs include initial red cell antigen typing and CBC every 1–2 years. Give folate daily to prevent deficiency. If needed, transfusions should be phenotypically matched RBCs that are screened for HbS.
- **Pulmonary:** Baseline CXR and PFTs every 3–5 years.
- **Ophthalmologic:** Eye examination every 3–5 years starting at five years of age; then yearly after ten years of age.
- **Liver function:** Screening labs yearly starting at five years of age.
- **Renal function:** Screening labs yearly starting at five years of age; UA yearly.
- **CNS:** Transcranial Doppler yearly to assess stroke risk starting at two years of age.

α-THALASSEMIA

Results from deletion of one or more α-globin genes (normally four genes are present). Divided into four categories: (1) silent carrier, which has one α-globin gene deletion; (2) α-thalassemia trait, which has two α-globin gene deletions (α-/α- or α α/--); (3) hemoglobin H disease, which has three α-globin gene deletions; and (4) homozygous α-thalassemia, which is characterized by deletion of all four α-globin genes.

SYMPTOMS/EXAM

The severity of the disease depends on the number of α-globin gene deletions (see Table 10-1).

DIFFERENTIAL

Iron deficiency anemia ($\downarrow$ iron and ferritin; $\uparrow$ free erythrocyte protoporphyrin); β-thalassemia trait (absence of Bart's hemoglobin; abnormal electrophoresis after 4–6 months of age).

TREATMENT

- **α-Thalassemia silent carrier: No treatment. Family counseling.**
- **α-Thalassemia trait:** No treatment. Family counseling.
- **Hemoglobin H disease:** Folate, transfusions, possible splenectomy. Family counseling.

COMPLICATIONS

Unnecessary iron administration from the incorrect diagnosis of iron deficiency anemia; splenomegaly that exacerbates anemia.

β-THALASSEMIA

Results from absent (β⁰-thalassemia) or $\downarrow$ (β⁺-thalassemia) β-globin production (normally two β-globin genes are present). This leads to excess α chains that precipitate and $\rightarrow$ RBC hemolysis.

SYMPTOMS/EXAM

Presentation varies by subtype (see Table 10-2).

TREATMENT/COMPLICATIONS

The treatment of β-thalassemia is outlined in Table 10-3.

TABLE 10-1. Presentation and Diagnosis of α-Thalassemia

SYNDROME	GENOTYPE	CLINICAL FEATURES	HEMOGLOBIN ELECTROPHORESIS
Silent carrier	α-/α α	No hematologic abnormalities.	**Neonatal:** 1–3% Bart's hemoglobin (four γ-globin chains).
α-Thalassemia trait	α-/α- or α α/–	Microcytosis; slightly low hemoglobin.	**Neonatal:** 5–10% Bart's hemoglobin.
Hemoglobin H disease	α-/–	Moderately severe hemolytic anemia; hepatosplenomegaly.	**Neonatal:** 15–25% Bart's hemoglobin. **Older:** 20–30% hemoglobin H (four β-globin chains).
Homozygous α-thalassemia	–/–	Fetal demise from hydrops fetalis.	Predominantly Bart's hemoglobin; no fetal or adult hemoglobin.

TABLE 10-2. Presentation and Diagnosis of β-Thalassemia

SYNDROME	GENOTYPE	CLINICAL FEATURES	DIAGNOSIS
Thalassemia minor (β-thalassemia trait)	Heterozygous.	Mild anemia; normal physical exam.	Mentzer index (MCV/RBC) < 11; normal iron studies. HbA_2 = 3.5–8.0%; HbF = 1–5%.
Thalassemia intermedia	Heterozygous or homozygous; variety of mutations.	Moderate microcytic anemia (not transfusion dependent), bony deformities, pathologic fractures, growth retardation.	HbA_2 > 3.5%; HbF = 5–15%.
Thalassemia major	Homozygous.	Severe anemia, jaundice, hepatosplenomegaly, bony deformities, fractures, growth retardation, iron overload.	HbF almost 100%; HbA_2 elevated; HbA little or none.

HEMOGLOBIN E DISEASE

A common hemoglobin variant that is frequently found in **Southeast Asia.**

SYMPTOMS/EXAM

Heterozygotes and homozygotes are both asymptomatic. Presents with mild anemia, microcytosis, and mildly ↑ reticulocyte count. Compound heterozygotes with HbE and β-thalassemia usually have a thalassemia major phenotype with severe hemolytic anemia.

DIAGNOSIS

Trait hemoglobin electrophoresis shows HbE comigration with HbA_2 of 19–34%. Homozygote electrophoresis shows ≥ 90% HbE and a varying amount of HbF.

TREATMENT

- **HbE (heterozygote and homozygote):** No treatment is necessary.
- **HbE/β-thalassemia:** Treatment is similar to that of β-thalassemia major.

TABLE 10-3. Treatment and Complications of β-Thalassemia

SYNDROME	TREATMENT	COMPLICATIONS
Thalassemia minor (β-thalassemia trait)	No treatment.	Unnecessary use of iron therapy.
Thalassemia intermedia	Intermittent transfusions.	Hemosiderosis (adult onset).
Thalassemia major	Chronic transfusion with iron chelation or bone marrow transplantation.	Hemosiderosis with cardiac, hepatic, and endocrine dysfunction; splenomegaly; viral infections.

Autoimmune Hemolytic Anemia (AIHA)

1° AIHA is defined as hemolytic anemia without systemic disease, such as warm-reactive AIHA ("warm AIHA"), paroxysmal cold hemoglobinuria, or cold agglutinin disease ("cold AIHA"). **2° AIHA** is defined as hemolytic anemia resulting from systemic disorders such as autoimmune disease (SLE), malignancy (lymphoma), infection (*Mycoplasma*, viruses), or drug-induced illness.

SYMPTOMS/EXAM

Fatigue, pallor, jaundice, dark urine, splenomegaly.

DIFFERENTIAL

Hereditary spherocytosis; microangiopathic hemolytic anemia.

DIAGNOSIS

Anemia ranging from mild to severe, ↑ reticulocyte count, ↑ bilirubin, ↑ LDH, ↑ AST, ⊕ Coombs' test, spherocytes on peripheral smear.

TREATMENT

See Table 10-4.

Microangiopathic Hemolytic Anemia

Defined as mechanical intravascular hemolysis within the small blood vessels. Occurs in disseminated intravascular coagulation (DIC), hemolytic-uremic syndrome (HUS), thrombotic thrombocytopenic purpura (TTP), tufted hem-

TABLE 10-4. Diagnosis and Treatment of AIHA

	WARM AIHA	COLD AIHA	PAROXYSMAL COLD HEMOGLOBINURIA
Immunoglobulin isotype	IgG	IgM	IgG
Temperature at maximum reactivity	37°C	4°C	4°C
Fixes complement	Variable	Yes	Yes
Pathophysiology	Extravascular hemolysis; destruction by the spleen.	Intravascular hemolysis.	Intravascular hemolysis.
Prognosis	Chronic; may be associated with systemic disease.	Acute, infection related.	Acute, infection related, self-limited.
Treatment	Transfusion (if needed), steroids, IVIG, splenectomy.	Transfusion (if needed); may benefit from plasmapheresis.	Transfusion (if needed); self-limited; symptomatic management.

angiomas or hemangioendotheliomas (Kasabach-Merritt syndrome), severe burns, heart valves, malignant hypertension, and connective tissue disease. May also be drug related (immunosuppressants).

Symptoms/Exam

Pallor, fatigue, dark urine; may have bruising.

Diagnosis

- Schistocytes, spherocytes, ↑ LDH, ↑ bilirubin, hemoglobinuria.
- Disease-specific findings are as follows:
  - HUS: ↑ BUN/creatinine.
  - DIC/TTP: ↓ platelets, ↑ PT/PTT, ↑ D-dimer.

Treatment

- Treat the underlying condition; initiate transfusion (use with caution).
- Exchange plasmapheresis removes RBC fragments and substances triggering intravascular coagulation and replaces coagulation factors with FFP infusion.

The pentad of TTP consists of fever, thrombocytopenia, microangiopathic hemolytic anemia, renal impairment, and neurologic dysfunction.

ANEMIA FROM ↓ RBC PRODUCTION

Nutritional Deficiencies

Iron Deficiency

Iron-rich foods include meats, beans, and leafy greens. Absorption in the duodenum ↑ with gastric acidity. Iron deficiency anemia is most common between 6 and 24 months of age 2° to ↑ iron demand during growth spurts → ↓ iron stores. Improved nutrition and iron-fortified formulas and cereals have ↓ the incidence of this type of anemia. Risk factors include ↑ cow's milk intake or early introduction of cow's milk; chronic blood loss; and prematurity. Risk factors in adolescence include growth spurts, menarche, and poor diet.

Symptoms/Exam

May be asymptomatic or may present with pallor/fatigue, irritability, and delayed motor development.

Differential

Thalassemia, lead poisoning, anemia of inflammation (see Table 10-5).

A low ferritin is very sensitive and specific for iron deficiency.

Diagnosis

Diagnosis is as follows:

- Microcytic hypochromic anemia, ↑ RDW, ↓ reticulocyte count.
- **↓ ferritin, ↓ transferrin saturation, ↑ free erythrocyte protoporphyrin (FEP).**

Treatment

Initiate a trial of iron therapy; repeat reticulocyte count in one week (↑ in 3–5 days). Anemia resolves in 4–6 weeks. Iron stores are replenished after three months of therapy.

HEMATOLOGY

TABLE 10-5. Laboratory Diagnosis of Microcytic Anemias

CAUSE OF ANEMIA	SERUM IRON	TIBC	FERRITIN	FEP	RETICULOCYTE COUNT
Iron deficiency	↓	↑	↓	↑	↓
Thalassemia trait	Normal	Normal	Normal	Normal	Normal or slightly ↑
Anemia of inflammation (chronic disease)	↓	↓	↑	Normal	↓
Lead poisoning	↓	↑	Normal or ↑	↑	↓

COMPLICATIONS

Cognitive delay; behavioral problems may occur if iron deficiency is prolonged or untreated.

VITAMIN B₁₂ DEFICIENCY

- Vitamin B_{12} is found in animal products and is produced by intestinal bacteria. Absorption requires intrinsic factor and occurs in the distal ileum. Risk factors for vitamin B_{12} deficiency include a vegan diet, pernicious anemia, and tapeworm. Deficiency occurs slowly.
- **Sx/Exam:** Pallor; mild jaundice; smooth, beefy-red tongue; paresthesias, weakness, and gait problems.
- **Ddx:** Folate deficiency, hypothyroidism, chronic liver disease, orotic aciduria.
- **Dx:**
  - Macrocytic anemia with large hypersegmented neutrophils.
  - ↓ serum B_{12}, ↑ serum methylmalonic acid, normal homocysteine, ↑ anti–intrinsic factor antibody (for pernicious anemia).
- **Tx:** Vitamin B_{12} injections.
- **Complications:** Irreversible neurologic damage (posterior and lateral spinal column demyelination).

FOLATE DEFICIENCY

- Folate is found in green vegetables and liver and is produced by intestinal bacteria. Absorption occurs in the duodenum. Risk factors for deficiency include ↑ cell turnover (sickle cell disease), poor diet (goat's milk intake), and drugs (trimethoprim, methotrexate, anticonvulsants). Deficiency can occur rapidly (limited folate stores).
- **Sx/Exam:** Pallor, mild jaundice.
- **Ddx:** Vitamin B_{12} deficiency, hypothyroidism, chronic liver disease, orotic aciduria.
- **Dx:** Macrocytic anemia with large hypersegmented neutrophils, ↑ homocysteine, and ↓ RBC folate.
- **Tx:** Folate supplementation; ↑ green leafy vegetables in diet.
- **Complications:** Folate treatment may mask vitamin B_{12} deficiency → permanent neurologic damage.

Infants who are primarily fed goat's milk have a high likelihood of developing folate deficiency.

Anemia of Inflammation (or Chronic Disease)

Associated with chronic infection, juvenile rheumatoid arthritis, and IBD. Results from cytokines → ↓ RBC survival, ↓ response to erythropoietin, ↓ erythropoietin production, and ↓ iron mobilization.

- **Sx/Exam:** Pallor, fatigue.
- **Dx:** Microcytic anemia, ↓ reticulocyte count, ↑ serum ferritin, ↓ serum iron.
- **Tx:** Treat the underlying disease. Iron and erythropoietin are ineffective.

Defective Marrow Response

TRANSIENT ERYTHROBLASTOPENIA OF CHILDHOOD

Acquired anemia 2° to ↓ RBC production usually occurring in healthy children 1–3 years of age prior to viral infection.

SYMPTOMS/EXAM

Pallor; no hepatosplenomegaly or lymphadenopathy; no dysmorphic features.

DIFFERENTIAL

Diamond-Blackfan anemia, anemia of inflammation, malignancy.

DIAGNOSIS

- Normocytic anemia without hemolysis; ↑ reticulocyte count; ⊖ Coombs' test.
- Normal RBC adenosine deaminase (ADA); normal fetal hemoglobin; normal "i" RBC antigen.
- Bone marrow reveals **initial RBC hypoplasia** with **subsequent RBC hyperplasia** on recovery.

TREATMENT

No treatment is necessary unless transfusion is needed; almost all cases spontaneously recover in 4–8 weeks.

 A six-month-old infant is noted to have triphalangeal thumbs, a hemoglobin of 5, and 1% reticulocytes. What is his most likely diagnosis? Diamond-Blackfan anemia.

DIAMOND-BLACKFAN ANEMIA

A rare congenital anemia affecting infants < 1 year of age. Associated with congenital anomalies.

SYMPTOMS/EXAM

Pallor, thumb anomalies (e.g., triphalangeal, bifid), short stature, congenital anomalies (wide-set eyes, thick upper lip, web neck, congenital heart defects, renal anomalies, hypogonadism), developmental delay.

DIFFERENTIAL

Transient erythroblastopenia of childhood.

DIAGNOSIS

Normocytic to macrocytic anemia, ↑ RBC ADA, ↑ fetal hemoglobin, ↑ "i" RBC antigen.

TREATMENT

Steroids; chronic transfusion and chelation; bone marrow transplant.

FANCONI'S ANEMIA

An autosomal-recessive, congenital pancytopenia 2° to ↑ chromosomal breakage. Affects children 2–15 years of age.

SYMPTOMS/EXAM

Pallor, petechiae, recurrent infections, café-au-lait spots, short stature, congenital anomalies (absent thumb and radius, renal anomalies).

DIAGNOSIS

Pancytopenia with macrocytosis, ↑ fetal hemoglobin, ↑ chromosomal breaks and rearrangements in lymphocytes, bone marrow aplasia.

TREATMENT

Supportive care with transfusions, antibiotics, androgen therapy, steroids, and bone marrow transplant.

COMPLICATIONS

Malignancy, death from bleeds, sepsis.

 A two-year-old boy is noted to have short stature, neutropenia, and fat malabsorption. What is his most likely diagnosis? Schwachman-Diamond syndrome.

NEUTROPENIA

Defined as an absolute neutrophil count (ANC) < 1500/mm³. Categorized as mild (1000–1500), moderate (500–1000), and severe (< 500). Only patients with severe neutropenia have ↑ susceptibility to life-threatening infections, especially if neutropenia is chronic. Etiologies are as follows:

- **Congenital:** Due to an intrinsic bone marrow defect (see Table 10-6). Include Kostmann syndrome (severe congenital neutropenia), Schwachman-Diamond syndrome, cyclic neutropenia, reticular dysgenesis, cartilage-hair hypoplasia, dyskeratosis congenita, hyper-IgM syndrome, Chédiak-Higashi syndrome, and Fanconi's anemia. Neutropenia in patients with congenital neutropenia is chronic, and patients have a much higher susceptibility to infections than do those with acquired neutropenia.

ANC = total WBC × (% segs + % bands).

*Neutrophil count is dependent on race; blacks may have lower neutrophil counts in the 1000–1400 range but **do not** have an ↑ risk for bacterial infections.*

Detection of antineutrophil antibody is not required for diagnosis of chronic benign neutropenia.

- **Acquired:** Due to extrinsic factors or a systemic disease (see Table 10-6). Include infection (usually viral—e.g., EBV), drug-induced neutropenia, chronic benign neutropenia (autoimmune neutropenia of childhood), alloimmune (neonatal) neutropenia, neutropenia associated with autoimmune disease (e.g., SLE), vitamin B_{12}/folate/copper deficiency, hypersplenism, and disorders infiltrating the bone marrow (e.g., malignancy, storage diseases).

DIAGNOSIS

See Table 10-6. Infections associated with neutropenia are characterized as follows:

- Usually occur only in those with severe or chronic neutropenia.
- Typically involve skin and mucous membranes → cellulitis, superficial and deep abscesses, furuncles, stomatitis, gingivitis, periodontitis, perirectal infection, otitis media, and pneumonia.
- Sudden onset of sepsis is rare (owing to intact monocytes and humoral and cellular immunity) but may occur if infection is untreated.
- The most commonly isolated organisms are S. *aureus* and gram-⊖ rods.

TREATMENT

- Aggressive initial management with broad-spectrum IV or IM antibiotics if signs of infection or fever are present.
- Treat the 1° cause in patients with acquired neutropenia.
- Good oral hygiene and antimicrobial mouthwashes to prevent oral infections in patients with chronic neutropenia.
- Consider TMP-SMX for prophylaxis in patients with chronic neutropenia and recurrent infections.
- G-CSF may be used to ↓ the severity of neutropenia in patients with congenital neutropenia who develop recurrent infections.
- The only curative option for patients with congenital neutropenia is bone marrow transplantation.

THROMBOCYTOPENIA

Immune-Mediated Thrombocytopenia

- The most common bleeding disorder; usually affects children 2–5 years of age, often prior to viral syndrome. Involves 2° splenic sequestration and removal of antibody-coated platelets.
- **Sx/Exam:** Acute-onset ecchymoses, petechiae, and epistaxis.
- **Ddx:** Leukemia, TTP, HUS, sepsis.
- **Dx:** ↓ platelets, normal WBC count, normal hemoglobin, ↑ mean platelet volume.
- **Tx:** Ranges from observation to treatment with IVIG, Rho immune globulin (hemolysis risk), steroids, or splenectomy (for chronic cases).
- **Complications:** Self-limited in almost all cases. Intracranial hemorrhage is rare.

TABLE 10-6. **Causes of Neutropenia**

	KOSTMANN SYNDROME (SEVERE CONGENITAL NEUTROPENIA)	CYCLIC NEUTROPENIA	SCHWACHMAN-DIAMOND SYNDROME	CHRONIC BENIGN NEUTROPENIA (AUTOIMMUNE NEUTROPENIA OF CHILDHOOD, IDIOPATHIC NEUTROPENIA)
Severity of neutropenia	ANC < 200 since birth.	Nadir < 200 for 3–5 days every three weeks; maximum ANC often remains < 1000.	Usually severe, but ANC may fluctuate.	ANC may be < 500 at diagnosis; spontaneous remission occurs in almost all patients within one year.
Risk of serious infection	High; patients often die of overwhelming infections.	Mild → high; 10% of patients die of infections, which occur during ANC nadir.	High.	Slightly higher frequency of infections, but despite low ANC, patients **do not** suffer serious infections and respond well to antibiotics.
Distinguishing clinical features		Cyclic fever, oral/mucosal ulcers, gingivitis, periodontitis, pharyngitis (occur during ANC nadir).	Exocrine pancreatic insufficiency → malabsorption and failure to thrive, metaphyseal dysplasia, and short stature.	Thought to result from autoimmune destruction of neutrophils due to transient antineutrophil antibody.
Diagnosis	Based on a history of severe infections and a persistent ANC < 200.	Obtain CBC 2–3 times per week for 6–8 weeks to document cycles and nadir.	Triad of chronic neutropenia, exocrine pancreas insufficiency, and metaphyseal dysplasia.	Patients are < 3 years of age and have not suffered a serious bacterial infection during the neutropenic period (usually several months); neutrophil morphology and other cell lines are normal.
Risk of leukemia	Yes.	No.	Yes.	No.

Amegakaryocytic Thrombocytopenia

An autosomal-recessive disorder involving ↓ platelets 2° to defective platelet production, together with ↓ megakaryocytes.

- **Sx/Exam:** Bleeding into skin, mucous membranes, and GI tract; no physical anomalies.
- **Dx:** ↓ platelets, normal WBC count, normal hemoglobin; bone marrow shows normal cellularity except for ↓ megakaryocytes.
- **Tx:** Steroids, androgens, bone marrow transplant.
- **Complications:** Aplastic anemia, bleeding, leukemia.

Thrombocytopenia with Absent Radii

A rare autosomal-recessive disorder involving ↓ platelets and skeletal anomalies.

- **Sx/Exam:** Bilateral absent radii; thumbs present; clinodactyly/syndactyly; bleeding in the newborn period (petechiae, GI bleeding).
- **Dx:** ↓ platelets, anemia, leukocytosis, normal fetal hemoglobin, no chromosomal breakage; bone marrow shows normal cellularity and no megakaryocytes.
- **Tx:** Transfusion, steroids, ε-aminocaproic acid, orthopedic procedures (after bleeding issues have improved).
- **Complications:** Malignancy (leukemia, neuroblastoma), bleeding; some patients may spontaneously improve or resolve.

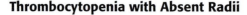

QUALITATIVE PLATELET DISORDERS

Glanzmann's Thrombasthenia

A rare, autosomal-recessive disorder involving an abnormal platelet receptor (GPIIb/IIIa receptor). Platelets cannot bind fibrinogen and von Willebrand's factor (vWF) → ↓ platelet aggregation. **Type I,** the more severe type, is associated with almost complete absence of platelet receptor; **type II** shows a relative deficiency of platelet receptor (10–20% of normal).

- **Sx/Exam:** Mucocutaneous bleeding (epistaxis, GI bleeds, menorrhagia); occasional joint bleeding.
- **Dx:** Platelet flow cytometry and immunoblot analysis to detect GPIIb/IIIa receptor.
- **Tx:** Platelet transfusion, factor VII (as supplement).
- **Complications:** Intracranial bleeding; joint bleeding.

Bernard-Soulier Syndrome

Another rare autosomal-recessive disorder involving an abnormal platelet receptor (GPIb-V-IX). Platelets cannot bind vWF → ↓ platelet aggregation.

- **Sx/Exam:** Mucocutaneous bleeding (epistaxis, GI bleeds, menorrhagia).
- **Dx:** ↓ platelet count; giant platelets; platelets fail to aggregate with ristocetin.
- **Tx:** Platelet transfusion, topical thrombin, desmopressin (DDAVP).

Wiskott-Aldrich Syndrome

An X-linked recessive disorder involving a defect in Wiskott-Aldrich protein (WASP), which is involved in signal transduction of the cytoskeleton. Associated with the triad of ↓ platelet count with small platelets, eczema, and immunodeficiency (cellular and humoral).

SYMPTOMS/EXAM

Bleeding (GI bleeding, bleeding after circumcision), eczema, recurrent infections, severe viral infections.

DIAGNOSIS

↓ platelet count, **small platelets,** ↓ IgM, ↑ IgA, ↑ IgE.

Supportive care (platelet transfusion, splenectomy, antibiotics, IVIG); bone marrow transplant.

COMPLICATIONS

Sepsis, severe bleeding, leukemia, and lymphoma (brain and GI) are associated with a poor prognosis.

Drug-Induced Platelet Dysfunction

Many drugs interfere with platelet function (see Table 10-7). The presentation of drug-induced platelet dysfunction ranges from asymptomatic (in normal individuals) to severe hemorrhage (in patients with underlying coagulopathy).

THROMBOCYTOSIS

Defined as a platelet count > 2 SDs above the mean. Results from ↑ platelet mass or ↑ platelet mobilization (since one-third are sequestered in the spleen). Causes are outlined in Table 10-8.

COAGULATION DISORDERS

Hemophilia A and B

X-linked recessive factor VIII (hemophilia A) and factor IX (hemophilia B) deficiencies.

TABLE 10-7. Common Medications That Interfere with Platelet Function

MEDICATION	MECHANISM
Anti-inflammatory medications (aspirin, NSAIDs)	Aspirin irreversibly inhibits cyclooxygenase (COX); NSAIDs reversibly inhibit COX.
Vasodilators (dipyridamole, methylxanthines)	Inhibit phosphodiesterase (PDE) → ↑ cAMP → ↓ platelet function.
Antibiotics (penicillin)	Mechanism is unclear.
Calcium channel blockers (nifedipine)	Interfere with thromboxane (TXA_2) receptor.
β-blockers (propranolol)	Alter the cell membrane.
Antidepressants (amitriptyline, imipramine, chlorpromazine)	Mechanism is unclear.
Anticonvulsants (valproic acid)	↓ platelet count.

TABLE 10-8. **Causes of Thrombocytosis**

TYPE	MECHANISM	DISORDER
1° thrombocytosis	Platelet production does not respond to the regulatory process.	**Myeloproliferative disorders:** Essential thrombocythemia, acute myelogenous leukemia (AML), chronic myelogenous leukemia (CML), polycythemia vera.
2° thrombocytosis	↑ megakaryocyte numbers.	**Inflammatory diseases:** Infection, rheumatoid arthritis, IBD, sarcoidosis, acute rheumatic fever, Kawasaki disease. **Hematologic disorders:** Iron deficiency, chronic hemolytic anemia, acute hemorrhage. **Drug related:** Steroids. **Malignancies:** Lymphoma, neuroblastoma. **Other:** Postsurgical, postexercise.
↓ splenic sequestration		Asplenia, drug related (epinephrine).

SYMPTOMS/EXAM

Frequent, spontaneous bleeding into skin, mucous membranes, joints, and muscles; ↑ bleeding with trauma or surgery. Categorized as follows:

- **Mild:** Bleeding with surgery or severe trauma.
- **Moderate:** Bleeding after mild to moderate injuries.
- **Severe:** Bleeding with minimal or unknown trauma.

DIAGNOSIS

- ↓ factor VIII or IX activity (mild = 5–40%; moderate = 1–5%; severe = < 1%).
- ↑ PTT, normal PT.

TREATMENT

DDAVP for mild hemophilia A; factor VIII or IX concentrate.

COMPLICATIONS

Intracranial bleeding, hemarthroses with joint destruction, inhibitor formation (acquired antibodies against factors), risk of blood-borne infections (HIV, HAV, HBV, HCV, parvovirus) if human-derived products are used (recombinant VIII and IX are now more commonly used).

DDAVP is contraindicated in vWD type 2B, as it can lead to ↑ thrombocytopenia and ↑ risk of bleeding.

von Willebrand's Disease (vWD)

The most common inherited bleeding disorder. Most cases are autosomal dominant. Involves a quantitative or qualitative abnormality in vWF, which is a cofactor for platelet adhesion and a carrier for factor VIII. Subtypes are as follows:

- **Type 1:** A partial quantitative deficiency (most common type).
- **Type 2:** A qualitative abnormality.
  - **Type 2A:** ↓ platelet-dependent function; reduction in intermediate/high-molecular-weight multimers. Most common form of type 2.

- **Type 2B:** ↑ affinity for platelet binding → thrombocytopenia.
- **Type 2M:** ↓ platelet-dependent function; normal multimers.
- **Type 2N:** ↓ binding to factor VIII.
- **Type 3:** Almost complete deficiency; most severe (autosomal recessive).

SYMPTOMS/EXAM

Bruising, epistaxis, bleeding after surgery, menorrhagia.

DIFFERENTIAL

Table 10-9 distinguishes vWD from hemophilia A.

DIAGNOSIS

- ↑ or normal PTT, normal PT, ↑ bleeding time, normal platelet count, ↓ vWF activity (ristocetin cofactor).
- **Types 1 and 3:** ↓ factor VIII; ↓ vWF level.
- **Type 2:** Normal factor VIII; normal vWF level.

TREATMENT

DDAVP for types 1 and 2; vWF-enriched concentrate; aminocaproic acid to stabilize clots.

 A 15-year-old girl develops a DVT after being immobilized after surgery. What is the most common cause of an inherited hypercoagulable state in children? Factor V Leiden mutation.

TABLE 10-9. von Willebrand's Disease vs. Hemophilia A

	vWD	HEMOPHILIA A
Symptoms	Mucosal bleeding, bruising	Muscle/joint bleeding
Inheritance	Autosomal dominant (most)	X-linked recessive
Bleeding time	↑	Normal
PTT	Normal or ↑	↑
Factor VIII activity	Borderline or ↓	↓
vWF antigen	↓	Normal
vWF ristocetin cofactor	↓	Normal
vWF multimers	Variable	Normal

THROMBOSIS

Uncommon in children. Associated with deep venous access, malignancy, infection, trauma, surgery, renal disease, sickle cell anemia, cardiac disease, and immobilization. Table 10-10 outlines the presentation, diagnosis, and treatment of common hypercoagulable states.

METHEMOGLOBINEMIA

Produced by the oxidation of O_2-carrying ferrous (Fe^{2+}) heme. The Fe^{3+} heme is unable to carry $O_2 \rightarrow$ functional anemia and cyanosis. Causes include congenital methemoglobinemia (hemoglobin M, NADH reductase deficiency), medications (benzocaine, antimalarials, nitrates, nitrites), and infections. Neonates are a high-risk group owing to immature NADH reduction.

SYMPTOMS/EXAM

Cyanosis (does not improve with O_2), headache, tachypnea, confusion, lethargy, seizure. Suspect when cyanosis is present without a history of cardiac or respiratory disease.

DIAGNOSIS

↑ methemoglobin, chocolate-brown blood, normal PaO_2.

TREATMENT

Removal of oxidant drugs; methylene blue (contraindicated in G6PD deficiency); ascorbic acid; exchange transfusion.

COMPLICATIONS

Coma, seizures, dysrhythmias, death.

TABLE 10-10. Causes of Hypercoagulable State

DISORDER	PATHOPHYSIOLOGY	SYMPTOMS/EXAM	DIAGNOSIS	TREATMENT
Protein C deficiency	Protein C is a vitamin K–dependent protein that is normally activated by thrombin. It inactivates factors V and VIII and stimulates fibrinolysis.	Venous thromboembolism (in autosomal-dominant form); neonatal purpura fulminans; CNS and retinal thrombosis; DIC (in homozygous recessive form).	↓ protein C.	FFP, heparin, warfarin.
Protein S deficiency	Protein S is a cofactor for protein C.	Similar to those of protein C deficiency.	↓ protein S.	Warfarin for recurrent events.
Antithrombin deficiency	Antithrombin is the most important thrombin inhibitor. Inhibits factors IX, X, XI, and XII.	Venous thromboembolism.	↓ antithrombin.	Heparin, warfarin, antithrombin concentrate if symptomatic. If asymptomatic, anticoagulate only if the risk of clotting is ↑.
Factor V Leiden mutation	A factor V mutation that → resistance to protein C inactivation.	Mild risk of venous thromboembolism in heterozygotes; higher risk in homozygotes.	Factor V mutation (molecular analysis).	Anticoagulate only if other risk factors are present.
Methylene tetrahydrofolate reductase (MTHFR) mutation	A mutation that → a mild ↑ in homocysteine.	Only homozygotes have a mild risk for venous thrombosis.	MTHFR mutation (molecular analysis).	Anticoagulate only if other risk factors are present.
Prothrombin 20210 mutation	A prothrombin mutation that → ↑ prothrombin levels.	Mild risk of venous thromboembolism in heterozygotes; higher risk in homozygotes.	Prothrombin 20210 mutation (molecular analysis).	Anticoagulate only if other risk factors are present.
Antiphospholipid syndrome/lupus anticoagulant	Antibodies are directed against phospholipid-binding proteins such as prothrombin, protein C, and protein S.	Venous thrombus; rarely, antiphospholipid syndrome → disseminated clotting, which → multisystem organ failure.	↑ PTT (no correction on 1:1 mix); ⊕ anticardiolipin; ⊕ RPR.	Warfarin for recurrent events.

HEMATOLOGY

HEMATOLOGY

CHAPTER 11

Human Genetics and Development

Ronald D. Cohn, MD
reviewed by Ada Hamosh, MD, MPH

Terminology

Forms of abnormal somatic development include the following:

- **Malformation:** Failure of proper or normal development. A 1° structural defect that results from a localized error in morphogenesis. Example: **cleft lip.**
- **Deformation:** Development is normal, but mechanical/extrinsic forces affect the fetus in utero. Example: ↓ amniotic fluid → **fetal akinesia** with **joint contractures.**
- **Disruption:** The developmental process is normal but is interrupted, and tissue is damaged. Example: **amniotic bands.**
- **Dysplasia:** Lack of normal organization of cells into tissue; abnormal tissue development. Example: **ectodermal dysplasia,** a condition in which tissues of ectodermal origin do not organize or form properly.
- **Association:** A grouping of congenital anomalies found together more often than expected, with no known common etiology. Two examples are given in the acronyms **VACTERL** and **CHARGE.**
- **Sequence:** A series of congenital anomalies derived from a single defect. Example: the Robin sequence, in which mandibular hypoplasia → posterior tongue displacement → cleft palate.
- **Syndrome:** A recognizable pattern of anomalies that are pathogenetically related. Example: trisomy 21.

Molecular Diagnosis and Genetic Testing

- The human genome consists of approximately 20,000 genes. Each gene is a unique sequence of a DNA macromolecule that is arranged in a double-stranded chain. Double-stranded DNA must **replicate** in order to produce new copies of genetic material for daughter cells.
- **Transcription** is the process of initiating protein synthesis by reading DNA and copying the future amino acid sequence encoded in the DNA onto a single strand of messenger RNA (mRNA). Mature mRNA from the nucleus then affixes to cytoplasmic ribosomes, where the genetic message is **translated** into a polypeptide chain of amino acids.
- Common terms used in genetic testing include the following:
  - **Fluorescence in situ hybridization (FISH):** Mapping of a gene by molecular hybridization of a cloned DNA sequence, labeled by fluorescence, to a chromosome spread or cell nucleus slide.
  - **Polymerase chain reaction (PCR):** A technique by which small amounts of genomic DNA or RNA sequences are amplified enormously. Simplifies subsequent analysis of DNA or RNA.
  - **Restriction fragment–length polymorphism (RFLP):** A polymorphic difference in DNA sequence between individuals that can be recognized by restriction endonucleases.
  - **Linkage analysis:** A statistical method in which the genotypes and phenotypes of parents and offspring in families are studied to determine whether two or more loci (positions of a gene on a chromosome) are separating independently or show **linkage** during meiosis.
  - **Southern blot:** Hybridization of single-stranded DNA to DNA following restriction enzyme digestion and gel electrophoresis; allows for the identification of specific (mutated) DNA molecules by labeled probes.

Nonrandom associ-ation of birth de-fects—VACTERL

Vertebral anomalies
Anus
   imperforate/**A**tresia
Cardiac anomalies
Tracheo**E**sophageal
   fistula
Renal and/or **R**adial
   anomalies
Limb anomalies

CHARGE associa-tion/syndrome:

Coloboma
Heart defect
Atresia choanae
Retarded
   growth/abnormal CNS
   development
Genital anomalies/
   hypogonadism
Ear anomalies/deafness

Mutations in the chromodomain-helicase-DNA–binding protein 7 gene have been identified as the cause of CHARGE syndrome.

HUMAN GENETICS AND DEVELOPMENT

- **Northern blot:** A technique analogous to the Southern blot, but involves the detection of RNA molecules by hybridization to a complementary DNA probe.
- **Western blot:** A technique used for the detection of proteins, usually by immunologic (antibody detection) methods.

Prenatal Diagnosis

- Prenatal diagnosis is a process for evaluating the health status of a fetus as early in gestation as possible.
- Within the last few years, **first-trimester screening (11–14 weeks)** has become available. This screening includes ultrasonographic measurement of **fetal nuchal translucency** as well as serum measurement of β-hCG and pregnancy-associated plasma protein A, which helps identify the risk for trisomies.
- Prenatal diagnosis may also include **chorionic villus sampling** (10th–12th week of pregnancy), **amniocentesis** (15th–16th week), and ultrasound. Maternal serum screening **(triple screen)** measures three blood markers and is made available to pregnant woman at **15–20 weeks' gestation** in order to identify those at risk for Down syndrome, trisomy 18, and neural tube defects. The three serum components measured are α-fetoprotein (AFP), unconjugated estriol (uE3), and hCG (see Table 11-1). (For a complete discussion of fetal assessment, see Neonatology chapter.)

A full-term infant presents after delivery with significant hypotonia, weakness, respiratory insufficiency, and feeding issues. The mother is noted to have mild mental retardation but no significant weakness. The clinical suspicion was myotonic dystrophy. What is the inheritance pattern? Myotonic dystrophy is an autosomal dominant disorder with evidence of genetic anticipation.

Autosomal Dominant Inheritance

- If one parent displays a dominant condition and is heterozygous for the gene, then each child has a **50% chance** of receiving the mutant gene allele and of manifesting the condition. **Not all patients** with the affected gene may be symptomatic (see Figure 11-1 and Table 11-2).

TABLE 11-1. Prenatal Diagnostic Measurements

	AFP	uE3	hCG
↑ risk for Down syndrome	↓	↓	↑
Trisomy 18	↓	↓	↓
Neural tube defects	↑	–	–
Twins	↑	–	–

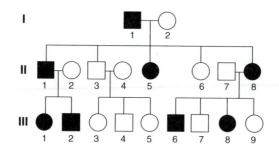

FIGURE 11-1. Example of an autosomal dominant pedigree.

- **Penetrance:** Reflects the percentage of patients with the gene who manifest symptoms or signs.
- **Expressivity:** The spectrum of severity among patients having clinical manifestations.
- **Anticipation:** Evident if the severity of the disease ↑ with each subsequent generation. An example of anticipation is **myotonic dystrophy**, an autoso-

TABLE 11-2. Common Autosomal Dominant Disorders

DISORDER	CHARACTERISTICS
Huntington disease	Chromosome 4p, 1 in 2500.
Adult polycystic kidney disease	Chromosome 16p, 1 in 1200.
Neurofibromatosis (NF)	Chromosome 17, 50% new mutations.
Vestibular schwannoma (NF2)	Chromosome 22q, 1 in 1×10^6.
Protein C deficiency	Chromosome 2p, spontaneous thrombosis.
Myotonic dystrophy	Chromosome 19q, 1 in 25,000.
Familial retinoblastoma	Chromosome 13q, 1 in 20,000.
von Willebrand disease	Chromosome 12, 1 in 100.
Tuberous sclerosis	Chromosome 9 and 16, tuberin and hamartin genes.
Marfan syndrome	Chromosome 15q, variable penetrance.
Achondroplasia	Chromosome 4p, 90% new mutations.
Hereditary spherocytosis	Spectrin deficiency, 1 in 5000.
Hereditary hemorrhagic telangiectasia (Osler-Weber-Rendu disease)	1–2 in 100,000, angiodysplasia.
Peutz-Jeghers syndrome	GI hamartomas, mucocutaneous pigment.

mal dominant disorder that is unusual in that a severe congenital form occurs by transmission from the **mother only** and not from the father. The expansion of the **CTG trinucleotide repeat** in a 3′ untranslated region of the myotonic protein kinase gene develops with each meiosis (mainly maternal), thereby explaining the genetic anticipation and ↑ severity in the next generation.

> A one-year-old infant presents with a disease that is classically an autosomal recessive trait (e.g., sickle cell disease). The father is tested and with 99% confidence is ⊖ for the carrier state. What is the explanation to be considered? Inheritance of two copies of the same affected chromosome from the mother is one possible explanation. Another would be nonpaternity, which should be considered as part of any genetic counseling process.

Autosomal Recessive Inheritance

- The phenotype is expressed when **two mutant alleles** are present. Consanguinity ↑ the risk of expressing an autosomal recessive disorder (see Figure 11-2 and Table 11-3).
- The risk of two carriers having a child with an autosomal recessive disorder is 1 in 4 (25%).

X-Linked Recessive Inheritance

- The incidence of the trait is much **higher in males** than in females.
- Heterozygous females are usually unaffected, but some may express the condition with variable severity, as determined by the pattern of X-inactivation (**Lyon hypothesis**).
- The gene responsible for the condition is transmitted from an affected male to **all** his daughters. Any of the daughters will then have a **50% chance** of transmitting it further.
- Ordinarily the gene is **never** transmitted directly from father to son.
- The gene may be transmitted through a series of carrier females; if so, the affected males in a kindred are related through females.
- A significant proportion of isolated cases (about 90%) are due to new mutations.
- Figure 11-3 gives an example of an X-linked recessive pedigree; Table 11-4 outlines common disorders associated with this mode of inheritance.

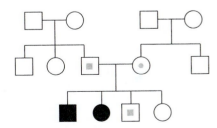

FIGURE 11-2. **Example of an autosomal recessive pedigree.**

TABLE 11-3. Common Autosomal Recessive Diseases

DISORDER	CHARACTERISTICS
Phenylketonuria (PKU)	Chromosome 12q, 1 in 14,000.
Sickle cell anemia	Chromosome 11, 1 in 625 African-Americans.
Congenital adrenal hyperplasia	Chromosome 6p, 1 in 5000–15,000.
Cystic fibrosis (CF)	Chromosome 7q, 1 in 2500.
Gaucher disease	Chromosome 1q, 1 in 2500 Ashkenazi Jews.
Tay-Sachs disease	Chromosome 15q, 1 in 3000 Ashkenazi Jews.
Galactosemia	Chromosome 9p, 1 in 60,000.
Wilson disease	Chromosome 1q, 1 in 200,000.
Fanconi anemia	Chromosomal breakage, absent thumbs.

Heteroplasmy is defined as the presence of > 1 type of mitochondrial DNA in the mitochondria of a single individual. Heteroplasmy is responsible for significant variation of the phenotype.

X-Linked Dominant Inheritance

- Daughters of affected males with normal mates are **all affected** but **sons are not.**
- **Both male and female** offspring of female carriers have a 50% chance of inheriting the phenotype. The pedigree pattern is the same as that seen with autosomal dominant inheritance (see Figure 11-4), except for the absence of male-to-male transmission.
- Example: **hypophosphatemic** (vitamin D–resistant) rickets.

Mitochondrial Inheritance

- Mitochondrial proteins and enzymes are encoded by nuclear genes, and 37 are encoded by **mitochondrial (mt) circular DNA.**
- Mitochondria are derived **exclusively from the mother;** defects in mtDNA therefore demonstrate **maternal inheritance** (see Figure 11-5).
- All children of a **female** with a mutation in mtDNA will inherit the muta-

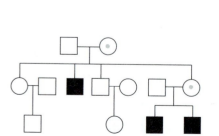

FIGURE 11-3. Example of an X-linked recessive pedigree.

TABLE 11-4. Common X-Linked Recessive Diseases

DISORDER	CHARACTERISTICS
Duchenne muscular dystrophy	Dystrophin gene, 1 in 5000.
Lesch-Nyhan syndrome	Hypoxanthine-phosphoribosyl transferase, 1 in 100,000.
Ornithine transcarbamoylase (OTC) deficiency	Hyperammonemia, urea cycle defect, females often affected.
Hemophilia A and B	Factor replacement necessary, 1 in 10,000.
Fragile X syndrome	Moderate to severe mental retardation, males often with macrocephaly and macro-orchidism; demonstrates anticipation.
Chronic granulomatous disease	Recurrent infections.
Bruton's agammaglobulinemia	Recurrent infections.
G6PD deficiency	Oxidant-induced hemolysis; affects 10% of African-Americans.
Color blindness	1 in 76.

tion, whereas none of the offspring of a **male** carrying the same mutation will inherit defective DNA.

- **Mitochondrial syndromes** include the following:
  - **Leber's hereditary optic neuropathy:** Characterized by rapid optic nerve death and blindness; usually **homoplasmic** (cells contain only abnormal mtDNA).
  - **NARP (Leigh disease):** Neuropathy, Ataxia, Retinitis Pigmentosa, developmental delay, mental retardation, lactic acidosis; heteroplasmic.
  - **MELAS:** Mitochondrial Encephalomyopathy, Lactic Acidosis, and Strokelike episodes; may manifest only as diabetes mellitus; heteroplasmic.

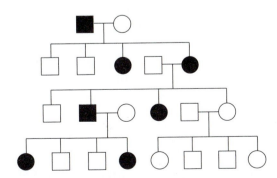

FIGURE 11-4. Example of an X-linked dominant pedigree.

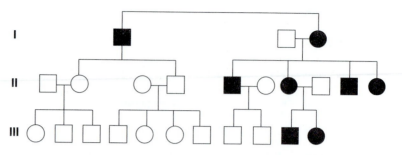

FIGURE 11-5. Example of a maternal inheritance pedigree.

- **MERRF**: **M**yoclonic **E**pilepsy, **R**agged **R**ed **F**ibers in skeletal muscle, ataxia, sensorineural deafness; heteroplasmic.
- **Kearns-Sayre syndrome**: Progressive external ophthalmoplegia, heart block, retinal pigmentation; heteroplasmic with sporadic mutations.

Inheritance of Complex Multifactorial Diseases

- **Not single-gene** disorders; recurrence risk is not based on mendelian genetic laws.
- Demonstrate **familial aggregation** because relatives of an affected individual are more likely than are unrelated individuals to have disease-predisposing alleles in common with the affected person.
- Pairs of relatives who share disease-predisposing genotypes at relevant loci may still show lack of penetrance because of the crucial role of **nongenetic factors** in disease causation.
- Example: **coronary heart disease.**
  - **Environmental factors**: Smoking, lack of exercise, obesity.
  - **Genetic factors**: LDL receptor mutations in familial hypercholesterolemia.

Terms Used in Cytogenetics

Cytogenetics is the study of chromosome **number** and **morphology**, which are generally analyzed in WBCs arrested in **metaphase**. Key terms used include the following:

The most common type of clinically significant chromosome abnormality is aneuploidy, which is due to an extra chromosome (most often trisomy) or a missing chromosome (monosomy).

- **Diploid (2n)**: Characteristic number of somatic cells.
- **Aneuploid**: Chromosomes with any chromosome number other than 46.
- **Reciprocal translocations**: An exchange of segments between nonhomologous chromosomes that generally lack any phenotypic abnormalities.
- **Unbalanced rearrangements**: Reflect additional or missing genetic information on a chromosome that usually has an impact on the clinical phenotype.
- **Robertsonian translocation**: The most common translocation; involves two of five acrocentric chromosomes—13, 14, 15, 21, and 22. Detected in 1 in 1300 persons; the carrier of the translocation is normal. Associated with a **risk of unbalanced offspring with genetic defects.**
- **Deletions**: Loss of a chromosome segment → chromosome imbalance.

- **Inversions:** Occur when a single chromosome undergoes two breaks and is then reconstituted with the segments inverted. Carriers of pericentric inversions (inversions involving the centromere) have a 5–10% risk of producing a child with an unbalanced karyotype.
- **Duplications:** Originate by unequal crossing over or segregation in meiosis. May disrupt genes and therefore → phenotypic abnormalities.

Terms Used in Dysmorphology

Table 11-5 lists common terms used in dysmorphology.

Chromosomal Abnormalities

All of the diseases listed below can occur via familial inheritance. However, they most often occur sporadically.

TABLE 11-5. Common Terms in Dysmorphology

TERM	DEFINITION
Plagiocephaly	Asymmetric head shape in the sagittal or coronal planes. Can result from suture closure or asymmetry of brain growth or abnormal positioning.
Brachycephaly	Shortened head shape from front to back; the skull is rounder.
Canthus	Lateral or medial angle of the eye formed by the junction of the upper and lower lids.
Telecanthus	Wide space between the medial canthi.
Glabella	Bony midline prominence of the eyebrows.
Ocular hypertelorism	↑ distance between the pupils of the eyes.
Palpebral fissure	Shape of the eyes based on the outline of the eyelids.
Philtrum	Vertical groove in the midline of the face between the nose and upper lip.
Synophrys	Eyebrows that meet in the midline.
Brachydactyly	Short digits.
Camptodactyly	A digit that is bent or fixed in the direction of flexion ("trigger finger").
Clinodactyly	A crooked digit that curves toward or away from adjacent digits.
Polydactyly	Six or more digits on an extremity.
Syndactyly	Two or more digits are at least partially fused; 2/3 syndactyly of the toes can be seen in Smith-Lemli-Opitz syndrome.

A newborn is noted to have dysmorphic features. The pregnancy was complicated by breech presentation, ↓ fetal movements, and polyhydramnios. The child demonstrates hypotonia, a flat face, plagiocephaly, epicanthal folds, and abdominal distention. What is the most likely cause of this condition? Trisomy 21.

DOWN SYNDROME (TRISOMY 21)

- The most common autosomal chromosomal abnormality in humans. A chromosomal nondisjunction during maternal meiosis is responsible for 80–90% of cases.
- Some **5% carry a translocation** in which an extra chromosome 21 is attached to another chromosome, yielding a chromosome count of **46.** Parents need to be tested for carrier status of **robertsonian translocation.**
- Has a prevalence of 1 in 700 live births, with incidence ↑ with maternal age (1 in 2000 at 20 years and **2–5% at > 40 years** of age).
- Patients with a mosaic karyotype may have a milder phenotype.
- Sx/Exam:
  - Short stature; central hypotonia.
  - Congenital heart disease; AV canal defect.
  - Mental retardation.
  - Structural abnormalities of the bowel (e.g., tracheoesophageal atresia, duodenal atresia, annular pancreas, duodenal web, Hirschsprung disease).
  - Brachycephaly; delayed closure of fontanelles.
  - Small midface, hypoplastic frontal sinuses, myopia, small ears.
  - Downslanting palpebral fissures; Brushfield spots (speckled iris).
  - Lax joints; laxity of atlantoaxial articulation, predisposing to C1–C2 dislocation.
  - Short, broad hands, feet, and digits; single palmar crease; clinodactyly.
  - Sandal toe (exaggerated space between the first and second toes).
  - Cutis marmorata; dry skin in adolescence.
  - ↑ risk for leukemia, Alzheimer's disease, and hypothyroidism.

AV canal defect is the most common heart defect associated with Down syndrome.

TRISOMY 18

- Sx/Exam:
  - Small for gestational age.
  - Narrow nose and hypoplastic nasal alae; **narrow bifrontal diameter.**
  - Congenital heart disease.
  - **Short sternum;** clinodactyly and **overlapping fingers** (index over third; fifth over fourth); **rocker-bottom feet.**
  - Hypoplastic nails.
- Only 5% of patients survive beyond the first year.

TRISOMY 13

- Sx/Exam:
  - Postnatal growth retardation.
  - Scalp defects, microphthalmia, microcephaly, holoprosencephaly.

- Sloping forehead; **cleft lip and palate (60–80%).**
- **Congenital heart disease (80%).**
- Thin and/or missing ribs, clinodactyly of the fingers and toes, polydactyly.
- Renal abnormalities.
- Only 5% of patients live > 6 months.

TURNER SYNDROME (MONOSOMY 45,X)

- Functional monosomy of the p arm of the X chromosome.
- Many affected females are mosaics 45,X/46,XX (most common).
- Risk **does not** ↑ with maternal age; in utero mortality is due primarily to generalized edema and cystic hygroma.
- Sx/Exam:
  - Short stature (height < 150 cm, adult height); growth hormone treatment is suggested.
  - Sexual infantilism.
  - Gonads are present at birth but **often regress** and become absent at puberty.
  - **Bicuspid aortic valve; coarctation of the aorta.**
  - **Lymphedema in infancy.**
  - Low hairline; webbed neck; widely spaced, hypoplastic nipples.
  - Horseshoe kidney.
  - Cubitus valgus of the elbow.
  - High frequency of hypertension.

As a consequence of the loss of the X chromosome, females with Turner syndrome are at risk for X-linked recessive disorders such as hemophilia A and B.

KLINEFELTER SYNDROME (47,XXY)

- Affects 1 in 1000 live male infants; has many chromosomal variants (e.g., 48,XXXY; 49,XXXXY; 48,XXYY).
- Infants and prepubertal boys have **no clinical signs;** postpubertal males show **infertility** resulting from hypogonadism with hypospermia/aspermia.
- Gonadotropin is ↑; testosterone is normal.
- Patients may have mild mental retardation, **gynecomastia,** small penis, and **long limbs.**

DiGEORGE SYNDROME (VELOCARDIOFACIAL SYNDROME, 22q112 SYNDROME)

- An autosomal dominant, contiguous-gene syndrome with variable expressivity that is caused by a deletion on chromosome 22q11.
- Deletions span about 3000 kb.
- Plays a role in as many as **5%** of congenital heart defects.
  - Some 40% with tetralogy of Fallot have a deletion of chromosome 22.
  - Some 60% with tetralogy of Fallot and absent pulmonary valve have chromosome deletion.
- Sx/Exam:
  - Postnatal short stature, microcephaly, hypertelorism.
  - **Long, tubular nose;** short philtrum.
  - Cleft palate; bifid uvula.
  - **Congenital heart defects:** Tetralogy of Fallot, truncus arteriosus, right aortic arch, interrupted aortic arch, VSD, PDA.
  - Mild mental retardation.
  - **Parathyroid absence; thymic hypoplasia.**

Diagnosis of DiGeorge syndrome—CATCH-22

Cardiac abnormalities
Abnormal facies
Thymic aplasia
Cleft palate
Hypocalcemia
22q11 deletion

- Immunodeficiency; T-cell defects.
- Neonatal hypocalcemia.
- Psychiatric disease, including bipolar disorder and schizophrenia.

CRI-DU-CHAT SYNDROME

- A contiguous-gene syndrome characterized by a deletion of chromosome 5p.
- Sx/Exam: Microcephaly, **cat cry in the newborn period**, epicanthal folds, cardiac defects, severe psychomotor retardation.

WILLIAMS-BEUREN SYNDROME

Williams-Beuren syndrome is also called "cocktail party syndrome" because patients generally have excellent social skills.

- A rare autosomal dominant, contiguous-gene syndrome characterized by a deletion of chromosome 7q.
- Sx/Exam:
    - Short stature; **periorbital fullness (puffy eyes).**
    - **Hypercalcemia.**
    - Stellate pattern of the iris, anteverted nares, thick lips, microdontia.
    - **Cardiac defects: Supravalvular aortic stenosis,** bicuspid aortic valve, mitral valve prolapse, peripheral pulmonary artery stenosis.
    - Pectus excavatum.
    - Nephrocalcinosis.
    - Mental retardation; poor visual-motor integration.

SMITH-MAGENIS SYNDROME

- A rare contiguous-gene syndrome characterized by interstitial deletion of chromosome 17p.
- Sx/Exam:
    - Brachycephaly; broad face.
    - Hearing loss.
    - Cardiac defects; renal abnormalities.
    - Mental retardation.
    - **Behavioral abnormalities** include self-destructive behavior (pulling out nails, wrist biting, head banging, insertion of foreign bodies into orifices).
    - **Sleep disturbances.**
    - ↓ pain sensitivity.

ALAGILLE SYNDROME

- An autosomal dominant disorder caused by mutations in the jagged-1 gene and characterized by a deletion of chromosome 20p12.
- Sx/Exam:
    - Triangular face.
    - Anterior chamber anomalies, posterior embryotoxon, chorioretinal atrophy on eye exam.
    - **Peripheral pulmonic stenosis (PPS), ASD, VSD.**
    - **Cholestasis with intrahepatic duct deficiency;** renal dysplasia.
    - **Vertebral anomalies.**
    - Mild mental retardation.
    - Hypercholesterolemia, hypertriglyceridemia, abnormal LFTs.

- Different expressions of alleles can cause different diseases depending on the parent of origin. Examples: Prader-Willi syndrome and Angelman syndrome on chromosome 15q11–q13.
- Prader-Willi syndrome:
  - Some 70% of cases are caused by a deletion of chromosome 15q11–q13 that is inherited by the patient's **father (missing paternal part)**.
  - Can also be caused by **uniparental disomy** (no deletion, but **two copies of chromosome 15 inherited from the mother**).
  - Sx/Exam:
    - Hypotonia and failure to thrive during infancy; subsequent hyperphagia.
    - Small hands and feet.
    - Mental retardation.
    - Hypogonadism.
- Angelman syndrome:
  - Some 70% of cases are caused by a deletion of chromosome 15q11–q13 that is inherited by the patient's **mother (missing maternal part)**.
  - Can also be caused by **uniparental disomy** (no deletion, but **two copies of chromosome 15 inherited from the father**).
  - Single gene mutations have also been described
  - Sx/Exam: Absent speech, distinctive facial appearance, seizures, mental retardation, laughter outbursts, ataxia.

COMMON GENETIC SYNDROMES

Achondroplasia

- An autosomal dominant disorder caused by mutations in the fibroblast growth factor receptor–3 gene (FGFR-3) and characterized by 80% new mutations.
- Sx/Exam:
  - Frontal bossing; megalencephaly and risk of foramen magnum stenosis.
  - Recurrent otitis media and conductive hearing loss.
  - Obstructive sleep apnea; hydrocephalus.
  - Rhizomelia.

Achondroplasia is the most frequent form of short-limb dwarfism.

Osteogenesis Imperfecta

- An example of **dominant** ⊖ disease, defined as a disease-causing allele, or the effect of such an allele, that disrupts the function of a wild-type allele in the same cell. Protein: type I collagen.
- Subtypes are as follows:
  - **Type I: Blue sclerae, brittle bones,** no bone deformities, presenile deafness.
  - **Type II:** Lethal in perinatal period.
  - **Type III:** Progressive structural bone deformities.
  - **Type IV:** Normal sclerae, brittle bones, tooth abnormalities.

Craniosynostosis Syndromes

Various FGFR-related craniosynostosis syndromes exist that are characterized by bicoronal craniosynostosis (cloverleaf skull), distinctive facial features, and variable hand and foot findings (see Table 11-6).

Beckwith-Wiedemann Syndrome

- Caused by a duplication or deletion at 11p15.5.
- Exhibits **uniparental disomy** for chromosome 11 (excess of paternal or loss of maternal contribution of genes).
- Sx/Exam:
    - **Exophthalmos, macroglossia, hypoglycemia,** and **macrosomia** in neonates.
    - Hemihypertrophy, cardiomegaly, hepatomegaly.
    - Pancreatic hyperplasia; renal abnormalities.
    - Gonadoblastoma.

Beckwith-Wiedemann syndrome is associated with an ↑ risk of Wilms tumor and hepatoblastoma.

Noonan Syndrome

- An autosomal dominant disorder caused by mutations in the protein-tyrosine phosphatase, nonreceptor-type 11 gene (PTPN11 in 60% of cases).
- Sx/Exam:
    - Short stature (postnatal onset); triangular face.
    - Down-slanting palpebral fissures; **hypertelorism.**
    - Dental malocclusion.
    - **Webbed neck;** low posterior hairline.
    - Congenital heart defects; **pulmonic stenosis.**
    - Shield chest; widely spaced nipples.
    - Cryptorchidism; vertebral abnormalities.
    - Wooly consistency of hair; **lymphedema.**
    - Mild mental retardation (25%).
    - Bleeding tendency.

TABLE 11-6. FGFR-Related Craniosynostosis Syndromes

	SYNDROME				
	MUENKE	**CROUZON**	**JACKSON-WEISS**	**APERT**	**PFEIFFER**
Thumbs	Normal	Normal	Normal	Occasionally fused to fingers	Broad, medially deviated
Hands	Carpal fusion	Normal	Variable	Bone syndactyly	Variable brachydactyly
Great toes	Broad	Normal	Broad, medially deviated	Fused to toes	Broad, medially deviated
Feet	Tarsal fusion	Normal	Abnormal tarsals	Bone syndactyly	Variable brachydactyly

Smith-Lemli-Opitz Syndrome

- An autosomal recessive disorder.
- Sx/Exam:
  - Short stature; birth weight < 2500 g.
  - Microcephaly; micrognathia.
  - **Hypotelorism,** ptosis, cataracts.
  - Anteverted nares; cleft palate.
  - **VSD, ASD,** coarctation of the aorta.
  - Poor suck; malrotation.
  - Hypospadias, ambiguous genitalia, **micropenis.**
  - Renal abnormalities.
  - **Syndactyly of the second and third toes.**
  - Mental retardation, seizures, hypotonia, self-injurious behavior.
  - **Low cholesterol;** ↑ 7-dehydrocholesterol.
- **Tx:** Behavioral problems may benefit from cholesterol supplementation.

Cornelia de Lange Syndrome

- An autosomal dominant disorder caused by a mutation in the Nipped B–like gene.
- Sx/Exam:
  - Microcephaly; long philtrum.
  - Hearing loss.
  - **Synophrys; long, curly eyelashes.**
  - Wide-spaced teeth.
  - GERD.
  - Finger abnormalities.
  - Cutis marmorata; **hirsutism.**

Russell-Silver Syndrome

- Isolated cases.
- Maternal uniparental disomy 7 (UPD 7) has been reported in some cases.
- Sx/Exam:
  - **Small-for-gestational-age infant** with **lateral asymmetry** and normal head circumference.
  - Cardiac defects.
  - Fifth-finger clinodactyly.
  - **Café-au-lait spots.**
  - Mental retardation.
  - Risk of neoplasm (Wilms tumor, craniopharyngioma, hepatocellular carcinoma).

Rubinstein-Taybi Syndrome

- An autosomal dominant disorder caused by mutations in the CREB-binding protein gene.
- Sx/Exam:
  - Postnatal growth retardation.
  - Microcephaly; large anterior fontanelle.
  - Eye abnormalities; **beaked nose.**
  - Cardiac abnormalities.
  - **Broad thumbs with radial angulation;** broad great toes.

- Mental retardation (average IQ 51).
- ↑ risk of tumor formation, especially of the head.

Klippel-Trenaunay-Weber Syndrome

- Large cutaneous hemangiomata, both capillary and cavernous.
- Lymphangioma.
- Asymmetric limb hypertrophy; macrodactyly.
- Mental retardation.
- Kasabach-Merritt syndrome.

Neurocutaneous Syndromes

NEUROFIBROMATOSIS

- An autosomal dominant disorder.
- Sx/Exam:
    - Lisch nodules (iris hamartomas); optic glioma.
    - Hypertension; renal artery stenosis.
    - Local bony overgrowth.
    - **Café-au-lait spots (> 5 mm)**, axillary freckling, plexiform neurofibromas.
    - Mental retardation (30%).
    - ↑ risk of neoplasms.

TUBEROUS SCLEROSIS

- An autosomal dominant disorder caused by mutations in the hamartin gene (TSC1) or the tuberin gene (TSC2).
- Sx/Exam:
    - Achromatic retinal patches.
    - Cardiac rhabdomyoma (regress during infancy); facial angiofibroma.
    - Hypopigmented ash leaf–shaped macules, shagreen patch, subcutaneous nodules, subungual fibromata.
    - Seizures (sometimes infantile spasms); mental retardation.
    - ↑ risk of giant cell astrocytoma and renal carcinoma.
- **Dx:** Intracranial calcification on x-ray or CT; subependymal nodules on MRI.

Sturge-Weber Syndrome

- Isolated cases.
- Sx/Exam:
    - Hemangiomata in at least the first (ophthalmic) branch of the trigeminal nerve distribution; generally unilateral but occasionally bilateral.
    - Choroidal hemangiomata; buphthalmos.
    - Arachnoid hemangiomata; mental retardation, seizures.

Ataxia-Telangiectasia (Louis-Bar Syndrome)

- An autosomal recessive disorder caused by mutations in the ataxia-telangiectasia mutated (ATM) gene.
- Sx/Exam:
    - Short stature, conjunctival telangiectasia.

- Hypogonadism.
- **Cutaneous telangiectasia**; progeroid skin changes.
- Cerebellar cortical degeneration; **cerebellar ataxia** (end of the first year).
- ↓ or absent DTRs.
- Thymus hypoplasia; ↓ numbers of T cells.
- Non-Hodgkin's lymphoma, leukemia, Hodgkin's lymphoma.
- ↑ levels of **AFP**; ↑ CEA.
- **Hypersensitivity to ionizing radiation.**

Ataxia-telangiectasia is associated with ↓ IgA, IgE, and IgG$_2$ levels → sinopulmonary infections.

von Hippel–Lindau (VHL) Syndrome

- An **autosomal dominant**, inherited familial **cancer syndrome** that is caused by mutations in the VHL gene and that predisposes to a variety of **malignant and benign tumors,** especially retinal, cerebellar, and spinal hemangioblastoma; renal cell carcinoma; pheochromocytoma; and pancreatic tumors.
- Subtypes are VHL type 1 (without pheochromocytoma) and type 2 (with pheochromocytoma):
    - **Type 1:** Renal carcinoma and hemangioblastoma.
    - **Type 2A:** Hemangioblastoma and pheochromocytoma.
    - **Type 2B:** Renal carcinoma and pheochromocytoma.
    - **Type 2C:** Pheochromocytoma only.

INBORN ERRORS OF METABOLISM

An 18-month-old male infant presents to the ER for emesis and diarrhea → dehydration and lethargy. His laboratory findings are significant for a serum glucose of 35, a bicarbonate of 10 with an anion gap of 32, hypocalcemia, and neutropenia. Which tests should his initial metabolic workup include? Plasma ammonium, urine organic acids, plasma amino acids, serum lactate, acylcarnitine profile.

Newborn Metabolic Screening

- All states screen for PKU and hypothyroidism; tandem mass spectrometry is currently available that ↑ the number of diseases detected (e.g., fatty acid oxidation disorders, organic acidurias, urea cycle defects).
- Additional conditions for which screening can be conducted include the following:
    - Galactosemia
    - Hemoglobinopathy
    - Tyrosinemia
    - Biotinidase deficiency
    - Congenital adrenal hyperplasia
    - Maple syrup urine disease
    - Homocystinuria
    - CF

Laboratory Tests

- Initial testing:
    - CBC with differential; serum electrolytes (**calculate anion gap**).
    - Blood glucose.
    - Liver enzymes, ALT, AST; total and direct bilirubin.
    - Blood gas.
    - Plasma ammonium; plasma lactate.
    - Acylcarnitine profile.
    - **Urine dipstick:** pH, ketones, glucose.
    - **Urine odor:**
        - **Acute disease:**
            - **Maple syrup urine disease:** Maple syrup; burned sugar.
            - **Isovaleric acidemia:** Cheesy; sweaty feet.
            - **Multiple carboxylase deficiency:** Cat urine.
        - **Nonacute disease:**
            - **PKU:** Musty.
            - **Hypermethioninemia:** Rancid butter; rotten cabbage.
            - **Trimethylaminuria:** Fishy.
    - Urine-reducing substances ($\oplus$ in galactosemia, hereditary fructose intolerance, diabetes mellitus, tyrosinemia)
- **Further testing:** Plasma amino acids; urine organic acids. If lactate is $\uparrow$, pyruvate levels should be obtained.
- Additional tools for the differential diagnosis of metabolic disease are listed in Table 11-7 and Figure 11-6.

TABLE 11-7. Differential Diagnosis of Suspected Metabolic Disease

	MAPLE SYRUP URINE DISEASE	TYPE 1 GLYCOGEN STORAGE DISEASE	MEDIUM-CHAIN ACYL-CoA DEHYDROGENASE DEFICIENCY	PROPIONIC ACIDEMIA	OTC DEFICIENCY
Mechanism	Amino acid metabolism	Carbohydrate metabolism	Fatty acid oxidation	Organic acid metabolism	Urea cycle defect
Test					
Blood pH	Acidosis	Acidosis	Variable	Acidosis	**Alkalosis**
Anion gap	$\uparrow$	$\uparrow$	$\uparrow$/Normal	$\uparrow$	Normal
Ketones	$\uparrow$	$\uparrow$	**Low**	$\uparrow\uparrow$	Negative
Lactate	Normal	$\uparrow$	Slightly $\uparrow$	Normal or $\uparrow$	Normal
Glucose	Variable	$\downarrow$	$\downarrow$	Normal, $\uparrow$, or $\downarrow$	Normal
NH$_4^+$	Slightly $\uparrow$	Normal	Moderately $\uparrow$	Normal or $\uparrow$	$\uparrow\uparrow\uparrow$
Neurologic findings	Lethargy, coma, developmental delay	Hypoglycemic seizures, **normal development**	Lethargy, coma, **normal development**	Lethargy, coma, developmental delay	Irritability, combative, coma, developmental delay

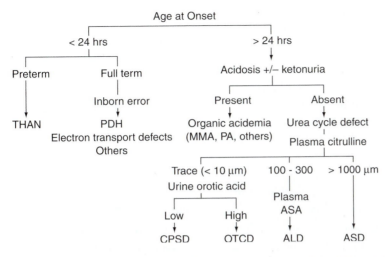

FIGURE 11-6. **Differential diagnosis of a hyperammonemic newborn (NH$_4$ > 50 µm).**

THAN, transient hyperammonemia of the newborn; PDH, pyruvate dehydrogenase deficiency; MMA, methylmalonic acidemia; PA, propionic acidemia; CPSD, carbamoyl phosphate synthetase deficiency; OTCD, ornithine transcarbamoylase deficiency; ALD, argininosuccinic acid lyase deficiency; ASD, argininosuccinic acid synthetase deficiency.

Overview of Metabolic Diseases

PHENYLKETONURIA (PKU)

- An autosomal recessive disorder caused by deficiency of phenylalanine hydroxylase in the liver. Its incidence is 1 in 10,000–15,000.
- Sx/Exam:
  - Affected infants are normal at birth but develop severe mental retardation if not treated.
  - Untreated children may have blond hair, blue eyes, eczema, and a mousy urine odor.
- Tx: A phenylalanine-restricted diet can prevent mental retardation.

HOMOCYSTINURIA

- An autosomal recessive disease caused by a deficiency of the enzyme cystathionine β-synthase → accumulation of homocysteine in the serum and urine → enhanced reconversion to **methionine** (newborn screening).
- Incidence is 1 in 200,000 live births.
- Sx/Exam:
  - **Marfanoid habitus:** Dislocated lenses, arachnodactyly, scoliosis, pectus deformities.
  - **Mental retardation** (one in three).
  - **Arterial and venous thrombosis.**
- Tx: Fifty percent of patients are vitamin B$_6$ responsive.

Pregnant women with PKU require rigorous management prior to conception and throughout pregnancy to prevent fetal brain damage and microcephaly.

Galactosemia is associated with an ↑ risk of E. coli sepsis and ⊕ urine-reducing substances.

GALACTOSEMIA

- An autosomal recessive disorder caused by a deficiency of galactose-1-phosphate uridyltransferase.
- Incidence is 1 in 60,000 live births.
- **Sx/Exam:** Clinical manifestations arise in neonates **after** they are milk fed and include **liver dysfunction with hyperbilirubinemia,** hypoglycemia, coagulation problems, renal tubular dysfunction, and cataracts.
- **Tx:** Elimination of dietary galactose.

> A previously healthy six-month-old infant presents with hepatomegaly, lethargy, ↑ jaundice, and severe emesis. The child appears dehydrated; the urine has a ⊕ reaction for reducing substances. The child's diet was solely breast milk until five months of age, when fruit juices and baby food were added to the diet. What is the most likely diagnosis? Hereditary fructose intolerance.

HEREDITARY FRUCTOSE INTOLERANCE

- A deficiency of fructose-1-phosphate aldolase characterized by accumulation of fructose-1-phosphate.
- **Sx/Exam:** Emesis, hypoglycemia, liver and kidney disease. Symptoms generally arise after the introduction of regular food and fruit.
- **Tx:** Dietary elimination of fructose **and** sucrose.

MAPLE SYRUP URINE DISEASE

- An autosomal recessive, branched-chain ketoaciduria caused by a deficiency of decarboxylase that initiates the degradation of leucine, isoleucine, and valine.
- Incidence is 1 in 250,000.
- **Sx/Exam:** Clinical manifestations usually occur within the first 5–14 days of life and include lethargy, irritability, seizures, opisthotonos, and coma.
- **Dx:** Definitive diagnosis is made through the measurement of plasma leucine concentration.
- **Tx:** Dietary restriction of leucine, isoleucine, and valine.

Dietary restrictions in MMA and PPA—
VOMIT

Valine
Odd-chain fatty acids
Methionine
Isoleucine
Threonine

ORGANIC ACIDURIAS

- Include methylmalonic acidemia (MMA), propionic acidemia (PPA), and isovaleric acidemia (IVA).
- **Sx/Exam:**
  - May have early or late onset.
  - Presentation usually involves anion-gap metabolic acidosis, hypo- or hyperglycemia, large ketones in urine, and mild hyperammonemia.
- **Dx:** Suspected diagnosis should be confirmed through analysis of plasma amino acids **and** urine organic acids.
- **Tx:**
  - Certain amino acids must be restricted in MMA and PPA.
  - Treatment during acute decompensation is intended to **stop catabolism.**

- Give high caloric glucose at 1.5 or 2× maintenance plus Na/K as needed.
    - Do not give any protein.
    - Provide IV carnitine (a detoxifying agent).
    - Replace HCO_3^- if necessary (pH < 7.1).
  - Long-term treatment consists of dietary restriction of relevant amino acids and carnitine supplementation.
- **Complications:** Patients are at risk of basal ganglia infarction during acute metabolic decompensation.

During acute episodes of decompensation, patients with an organic aciduria can present with pancytopenia and hypocalcemia.

UREA CYCLE DEFECTS

- The most common form is OTC deficiency. An **X-linked recessive** disorder with many clinically affected females.
- The liver is a mosaic of affected versus unaffected cells → variable severity of the phenotype.
- Sx/Exam:
    - Clinical manifestations range from neonatal onset (some lethal) to late onset in adulthood.
    - Features encompass emesis, irritability, lethargy, and psychiatric problems.
- **Dx:** Made by hyperammonemia and excretion of **orotic acid in urine** detected by urine organic acid chromatography.
- **Tx:** Generalized protein restriction during acute episodes to halt catabolism. Sodium benzoate, sodium phenylacetate can reduce plasma ammonium levels; hemodialysis should be used if above meds are ineffective.

NONKETOTIC HYPERGLYCINEMIA

- An autosomal recessive disorder caused by a defect in glycine cleavage.
- **Sx/Exam:** Characterized by clinically profound deterioration of the CNS in the neonatal period, as evidenced by seizures → respiratory depression, lethargy, and coma within the first few weeks of life.
- **Dx:** Made by **simultaneous** determination of glycine in both plasma and CSF.
- **Tx:**
    - No effective treatment is currently available.
    - Symptomatic treatment consists of administration of agents that ↓ glycine concentration (e.g., sodium benzoate) and dextromethorphan as an anticonvulsant.

BIOTINIDASE DEFICIENCY

- An autosomal recessive disorder.
- **Sx/Exam:** Clinical presentation may include seizures, hypotonia, alopecia, skin rashes, metabolic acidosis, and immunodeficiency.
- **Tx:** If provided early, oral supplementation of biotin ensures completely normal development and life.

TYROSINEMIA

- Takes various forms, including transient tyrosinemia of the newborn and tyrosinemia type I, II, and III.
- Associated with an ↑ risk of hepatocellular carcinoma (↑ AFP levels).

HUMAN GENETICS AND DEVELOPMENT

Hepatorenal tyrosinemia, or tyrosinemia I, exhibits a cabbage-like urine odor along with renal tubular dysfunction (Fanconi syndrome).

- **Sx/Exam:**
  - Fulminant liver failure.
  - ↑ succinylacetone causes inhibition of δ-aminolevulinate synthase and may → hematologic alterations and porphyria-like symptoms.
- **Dx:** Confirmed by ↑ succinylacetone in plasma and urine.
- **Tx:**
  - Administration of 2-(2-nitro-4-trifluoromethylbenzoyl)-1,3-cyclohexane-dione (NTBC) and dietary phenylalanine and tyrosine restriction.
  - May need liver transplantation.

FATTY OXIDATION DISORDERS

Several different disease groups are caused by enzyme deficiencies involved in the oxidative removal of acetyl groups (SCAD, MCAD, LCAD).

HEPATIC ENCEPHALOPATHY (COMPLICATION OF FATTY ACID OXIDATION DISORDERS)

Hypoketotic hypoglycemia is a common manifestation of fatty oxidation disorders.

- Fatty degeneration of viscera with severe liver dysfunction → hyperammonemia.
- **Similar to Reye syndrome** (caused by aspirin ingestion or viral infections such as influenza and varicella).
- Few SIDS cases are attributable to fatty acid oxidation disorders.
- **Dx:** Confirmed by acylcarnitine profile.

GLUTARIC ACIDURIA

- **Glutaric aciduria type I:**
  - **Sx/Exam:** Macrocephaly (at birth), dystonia, recurrent episodes of liver dysfunction with metabolic acidosis, hypoglycemia, and hyperammonemia.
  - **Dx:** Requires plasma amino acids and urine organic acids.
  - **Tx:** Consists of a low-lysine and -tryptophan diet, riboflavin, and agents that ↑ γ-aminobutyric acid in the brain, such as valproic acid and baclofen.
- **Glutaric aciduria type II:**
  - A defect in the transfer of electrons from flavine-adenine nucleotides to the electron transport chain.
  - Associated with an ↑ risk of cardiomyopathy.
  - **Sx/Exam:**
    - Congenital anomalies include renal cysts, facial dysmorphism, rocker-bottom feet, and hypospadias.
    - Infants may show **hypoglycemia without ketosis,** an odor of sweaty feet, and metabolic acidosis.
  - **Tx:** No effective treatment.

PEROXISOMAL DISEASES

- **Zellweger syndrome:**
  - An autosomal recessive disorder with an incidence of 1 in 100,000.
  - Also known as cerebrohepatorenal syndrome.
  - **Sx/Exam:**
    - Dysmorphic features include high forehead, flat orbital ridges, and widely open fontanelles.
    - Also associated with hepatomegaly, hypotonia and seizures, and migration disorders of the brain.

- Dx: ↑ very long chain fatty acids in plasma.
- Tx: No treatment is available.
- **Other peroxisomal diseases:** Adrenoleukodystrophy, Refsum disease, rhizomelic chondrodysplasia punctata.

GLYCOGEN STORAGE DISEASES

Table 11-8 outlines the presentation of common glycogen storage diseases.

TABLE 11-8. Overview of Glycogen Storage Disease

DISEASE	ENZYME DEFECT	ORGANS INVOLVED	PHENOTYPE	MANAGEMENT
Type I—von Gierke disease	Glucose-6-phosphatase	Liver, kidney, platelets, bones.	Hypoglycemia, lactic acidosis, doll-like face, hepatomegaly with risk of hepatic adenomas, hypotonia, ↑ uric acid, ↑ triglycerides, xanthomas.	Prevention of hypoglycemia with cornstarch and frequent meals.
Type II—Pompe disease	α-glucosidase **(lysosomal)**	Liver, skeletal muscle, cardiac muscle, peripheral nerves.	Profound hypotonia, enlarged tongue, cardiomegaly with short PR interval. The late-onset form is rare.	Enzyme replacement therapy is available; if no therapy is given, death occurs within the first year of life.
Type III—Forbes disease, Cori disease	Debranching enzyme	**IIIa:** Liver, skeletal muscle. **IIIb:** Only liver.	Hypoglycemia, ketosis, **no lactic acidosis, normal uric acid,** muscle weakness, risk of hepatic fibrosis and cardiomyopathy.	Liver symptoms improve with age; muscle weakness may persist.
Type IV—Andersen disease	Branching enzyme	Liver, skeletal and cardiac muscle, CNS.	Failure to thrive, liver cirrhosis, cardiomyopathy, muscle weakness, hypotonia, absent DTRs.	Symptomatic management of liver failure and cardiomyopathy.
Type V—McArdle disease	Muscle phosphorylase	Skeletal muscle.	Exercise-induced rhabdomyolysis; muscle weakness beginning in adolescence.	Sucrose supplementation may be beneficial.
Type VI—Hers disease	Liver phosphorylase	Liver.	Mild hypoglycemia and ketosis; hepatomegaly.	Good prognosis.
Type VII—Tarui disease	Muscle phosphofructokinase	Skeletal muscle.	Exercise-induced rhabdomyolysis; muscle weakness beginning in adolescence.	Avoid strenuous exercise.
Type VIII	Phosphorylase kinase	Liver.	Hypoglycemia, ketosis, **no lactic acidosis, normal uric acid.**	Good prognosis.

- **MPS I (Hurler syndrome):**
  - A deficiency of α-L-iduronidase.
  - **Sx/Exam:** Patients are normal at birth but subsequently present with **coarse facies, corneal clouding,** neurodegeneration, hernias, **dysostosis multiplex,** and hepatosplenomegaly.
  - **Dx:** Made by the detection of abnormal glycosaminoglycans in urine and confirmation of enzyme defect.
  - **Tx:** Bone marrow transplantation is recommended for severe infantile form. Enzyme replacement provides therapeutic benefit.
- **MPS II (Hunter syndrome):**
  - An **X-linked recessive** disease caused by iduronate-2-sulfatase deficiency.
  - **Sx/Exam:** Mild dwarfism, coarse facial features, macrocephaly, **no corneal opacities,** hepatosplenomegaly, dysostosis multiplex, claw hands, neurodegeneration → profound mental retardation.
  - **Dx:** Diagnosed by dermatan and heparan sulfate excretion in urine.
  - **Tx:** Enzyme replacement therapy
- **MPS III (Sanfilippo syndrome):**
  - A heparan N-sulfatase deficiency; various types exist.
  - **Sx/Exam:**
    - The presenting symptoms may include marked overactivity, destructive tendencies, and other behavioral aberrations such as sleep disturbances in a child 4–6 years of age.
    - Also presents with visceromegaly, mild corneal clouding, and claw hands.
  - **Dx:** Heparan sulfate excretion in urine.
- **MPS IV (Morquio syndrome):**
  - An N-acetylgalactosamine-6-sulfatase deficiency.
  - **Sx/Exam:** Short-trunked dwarfism characterized by mild coarse features, corneal clouding, restrictive lung disease, **no dysostosis multiplex,** and **normal intelligence.**
  - **Dx:** Chondroitin 6-sulfate excretion in urine.
- **MPS VI (Maroteaux-Lamy disease):**
  - An arylsulfatase B deficiency.
  - **Sx/Exam:** A short-trunked dwarfism that presents with corneal clouding, infantile cardiomyopathy, hepatosplenomegaly, dysostosis multiplex, and claw-hand deformities and normal intelligence.
  - **Dx:** Dermatan sulfate excretion in urine.
  - **Tx:** Bone marrow transplantation, enzyme replacement therapy.
- **MPS VII (Sly disease):**
  - A β-glucuronidase deficiency.
  - **Sx/Exam:** Short stature, mental retardation, coarse facial features, variable degree of corneal clouding, visceromegaly, anterior beaking of vertebrae.
  - **Dx:**
    - Dermatan and heparan sulfate, chondroitin 4-,6-sulfate excretion in urine.
    - Coarse metachromatic granules in WBCs.

MPS I is associated with an ↑ risk of upper airway obstruction.

Patients with MPS IV and VI have normal intelligence.

HUMAN GENETICS AND DEVELOPMENT

A 10-year-old girl is noted on routine physical examination to have splenomegaly. Laboratory findings reveal thrombocytopenia and moderate anemia. She also complains about bony lesions. Bone marrow shows ⊕ storage cells. What is an optional therapeutic approach for this disease? The case describes a patient with Gaucher disease. Enzyme replacement is available for this disorder and should be initiated after the diagnosis has been confirmed in symptomatic patients.

A seven-month-old boy has been healthy and developing normally since birth. His mother now reports that he has ↓ eye contact and startles very easily. Which diagnostic test is most likely to reveal a diagnosis in this case? The case described above is a child with Tay-Sachs disease. The diagnosis is confirmed by hexosaminidase A activity measurement in leukocytes.

LYSOSOMAL STORAGE DISEASES—LIPIDOSES

- Type I Gaucher disease:
  - A glucocerebrosidase deficiency.
  - Sx/Exam: Accumulation of Gaucher cells at the corneoscleral limbus; hepatosplenomegaly, osteolytic lesions, anemia and thrombocytopenia, ↑ risk of pathologic fractures.
  - Dx: Gaucher cells in the bone marrow.
  - Tx: Enzyme replacement therapy is available.
- Type A Niemann-Pick disease:
  - A sphingomyelinase deficiency that is more common among Ashkenazi Jews.
  - Sx/Exam: Hypotonia, hyperreflexia, cherry-red spots, hepatosplenomegaly, failure to thrive, profound loss of CNS function over time.
  - Dx: Multiple organs show foam cells, including the brain, lung, and bone marrow.
- Type B Niemann-Pick disease:
  - A sphingomyelinase deficiency that is also most commonly found among Ashkenazi Jews.
  - Sx/Exam:
    - Visceral form has no neurologic manifestations.
    - Hepatosplenomegaly and cherry-red spots are less common; frequent respiratory infections.
  - Dx:
    - Large vacuolated foam cells ("NP cells") on bone marrow biopsy.
    - Laboratory findings include ↑ LDL, ↑ triglycerides, and ↓ HDL.
- Type C Niemann-Pick disease:
  - Intracellular accumulation of cholesterol.
  - Highly variable phenotype with NPC-1 mutations.
  - Sx/Exam: Vertical supranuclear gaze palsy, hepatosplenomegaly, hypotonia, developmental delay, cerebellar ataxia, mental retardation, poor school performance, and behavioral abnormalities.
  - Dx: Foam cells on bone marrow biopsy.

- **Tay-Sachs disease (GM2 gangliosidosis):**
  - A hexosaminidase A deficiency that is more common among Ashkenazi Jews and French Canadians.
  - The infantile form is fatal by age five.
  - **Sx/Exam: Cherry-red spots and blindness,** ↑ startle response, hypotonia and poor head control, later spasticity.
  - **Dx:** GM2-ganglioside accumulation.
- **Metachromatic leukodystrophy:**
  - An arylsulfatase A deficiency.
  - Age of onset may vary; adult onset may present as psychiatric illness.
  - **Sx/Exam: Optic atrophy; biliary tract abnormalities;** severe CNS disease that includes hypotonia, seizures, loss of function, and progressive polyneuropathy.
  - **Dx:** ↑ protein in CSF; ↓ arylsulfatase A activity in urine, leukocytes, and fibroblasts; ↑ urinary sulfatide excretion.
- **Fabry disease:**
  - An X-linked recessive α-galactosidase deficiency.
  - **Sx/Exam:**
    - Delayed puberty.
    - Whorl-like corneal dystrophy in heterozygous females and hemizygous males.
    - Heart abnormalities, including CAD and cardiomyopathy.
    - Renal failure.
    - Autonomic dysfunction, **acroparesthesia,** ↑ risk for strokes.
  - **Dx:** Lipid-laden macrophages in bone marrow; glycosphingolipid deposition in all areas of the body.
  - **Tx: Enzyme replacement** therapy is available.
- **Krabbe disease:**
  - A β-galactosidase deficiency that takes four clinical forms: infantile, late infantile, juvenile, and adult.
  - **Sx/Exam:**
    - Failure to thrive.
    - **Optic atrophy; blindness.**
    - **Hyperirritability,** hypersensitivity to stimuli, mental deterioration, neurodegeneration, hypertonicity in early stage, seizures, decerebrate.
  - **Dx:** Diffuse cerebral atrophy on CT and MRI, ↓ nerve conduction velocity, ↑ **protein in CSF;** galactocerebroside β-galactosidase deficiency in serum, leukocytes, and fibroblasts.

CHAPTER 12

Infectious Disease

Allison George Agwu, MD
Sanjay Jain, MD

There has recently been widespread concern over the potential use of biological agents as weapons of terrorism. The clinical implications of two such agents are discussed in detail in Table 12-1.

ANTIMICROBIALS

Tables 12-2 through 12-4 outline common antibacterial, antiviral, and antifungal drugs and their mechanisms of action.

BITES AND INJURIES

Human and Animal Bites

Table 12-5 outlines the management of a variety of bites, both human and animal. Common categories of bites and their associated pathogens include the following:

- **Dogs and cats:** *Pasteurella* spp.
- **Humans:** *Eikenella*, anaerobes, *Streptococcus* spp., *S. aureus*.
- **Reptiles:** Enteric gram-⊖ organisms (*Salmonella* spp.).
- **Raccoons, bats, foxes:** Rabies (exposure to saliva alone is sufficient).

TABLE 12-1. Presentation, Diagnosis, and Treatment of Two Potential Bioagents

AGENT	INCUBATION/CLINICAL PRESENTATION	ISOLATION	DIAGNOSIS	PROPHYLAXIS/TREATMENT
Bacillus anthracis (anthrax)	**Incubation period:** 1–5 days. **Inhalation anthrax:** Presents with flulike symptoms with progression to mediastinitis and/or pneumonia, sepsis, shock, and meningitis. **Cutaneous anthrax:** Infection proceeds from papule to vesicle to ulcer, progressing to a depressed black eschar with edema.	Standard.	CXR shows a widened mediastinum, pleural effusion, and infiltrate. Obtain Gram stain and culture of vesicular fluid or blood; enzyme immunoassay (EIA) and immunohistochemistry are also available.	**Prophylaxis:** Give preexposure prophylaxis with vaccine to high-risk individuals; postexposure prophylaxis consists of ciprofloxacin or doxycycline. **Treatment:** Treat with ciprofloxacin or doxycycline.
Variola virus (smallpox)	**Incubation period:** 7–17 days. Presents with flulike symptoms with a **synchronous** vesiculopustular rash appearing predominantly on the face and extremities.	Airborne.	Obtain EIA, PCR, and viral culture of scab material and/or pharyngeal swab.	**Prophylaxis:** Give preexposure prophylaxis with live attenuated vaccine to high-risk individuals; postexposure prophylaxis consists of immunoglobulins. **Treatment:** Treatment consists of supportive care and possibly cidofovir.

TABLE 12-2. Mechanisms of Action of Common Antibacterial Drugs

CLASS	MECHANISM OF ACTION	COMMON AGENTS/ SPECTRUM OF ACTIVITY	COMMON RESISTANCE MECHANISMS	COMMENTS
β-lactams	Cell wall synthesis inhibition.	**Penicillin group:** Penicillin, ampicillin, oxacillin (anti-staphylococcal); ticarcillin/piperacillin (antipseudomonal). **Cephalosporins:** Cefazolin (gram-⊕ coverage); cefuroxime, cefotaxime/ceftriaxone (gram-⊖ coverage); ceftazidime (antipseudomonal); cefepime (broad spectrum; includes *Pseudomonas*). **Carbapenems:** Imipenem (↓ seizure threshold), meropenem.	β-lactamase or alteration of penicillin-binding proteins (PBPs). *Streptococcus pneumoniae* resistance results from alteration of PBP and can generally be overcome with ↑ concentrations of antibiotics.	The addition of a β-lactamase inhibitor (clavulanate, sulbactam, tazobactam) adds coverage for β-lactamase-producing organisms and gives additional anaerobic coverage. There is 10–15% cross-reactivity of cephalosporins with penicillins. In penicillin-allergic patients, there is up to 50% cross-reactivity of carbapenems with penicillins. Avoid ceftriaxone in neonates.
Glycopeptides	Cell wall synthesis inhibition.	Vancomycin.	Alteration of binding site.	"Red man syndrome" is not an allergic reaction and can be overcome by slowing infusion or through pretreatment with antihistamines.
Macrolides	Protein synthesis inhibition.	Erythromycin, clarithromycin, azithromycin (covers *Mycoplasma, Chlamydia,* and *Bordetella pertussis*).	Efflux pump and alteration of binding site.	Erythromycin has been associated with pyloric stenosis in infants and may alter the metabolism of other drugs. Use with caution in liver disease.
Aminoglycosides	Protein synthesis inhibition.	Gentamicin; tobramycin and amikacin.	Alteration of binding site.	Nephrotoxic and ototoxic; drug levels and kidney function must be monitored.
Tetracyclines	Protein synthesis inhibition.	Tetracycline, doxycycline, minocycline, and tigecycline.	Efflux pump.	Not to be used in children < 8 years of age or in pregnant mothers.
Chloramphenicol	Protein synthesis inhibition.	Broad-spectrum drug.	Alteration of binding site.	Can cause bone marrow suppression and gray baby syndrome; drug concentrations must be monitored.
Clindamycin	Protein synthesis inhibition.	Gram-⊕ and anaerobic pathogen; active against community-acquired methicillin-resistant *S. aureus* (MRSA), although susceptibility may vary with geographic location.	Alteration of binding site.	Good tissue penetration; classically associated with *Clostridium difficile* colitis.

CLASS	MECHANISM OF ACTION	COMMON AGENTS/ SPECTRUM OF ACTIVITY	COMMON RESISTANCE MECHANISMS	COMMENTS
Antifolate	Inhibition of dihydro-folate reductase.	Sulfonamides, tri-methoprim (TMP), cotrimoxazole (TMP-SMX).	Altered enzyme production or binding of drug with the enzyme.	Avoid in neonates and those with G6PD deficiency; may cause blood dyscrasias and Stevens-Johnson syndrome.
Fluoroquinolones	Inhibition of DNA unfolding.	Ciprofloxacin, levofloxacin, gatifloxacin.	Alteration of binding site.	Avoid in children < 18 years of age owing to concerns over the effect of fluoroquinolones on cartilage growth.
Metronidazole	Possible inhibition of the electron transport chain.	Excellent anaerobic coverage.	Alteration of binding site.	Antabuse effect with alcohol; good CSF penetration.

TABLE 12-3. **Mechanisms of Action of Common Antiviral Drugs**

CLASS	MECHANISM OF ACTION	COMMON AGENTS/ SPECTRUM OF ACTIVITY	COMMON RESISTANCE MECHANISMS	COMMENTS
Anti-HSV drugs				
Nucleoside analogs	Inhibition of DNA synthesis.	Acyclovir, ganciclovir (generally used against herpes group of viruses).	Alteration of viral thymidine kinase or DNA polymerase.	Acyclovir may crystallize in renal tubules if patients are not adequately hydrated; ganciclovir causes bone marrow suppression.
Pyrophosphate analogs	Inhibition of DNA synthesis.	Foscarnet (used for resistant herpes infections).	Alteration of viral DNA polymerase.	Nephrotoxic; cause electrolyte disturbances.
Anti-influenza drugs				
M2 inhibitors	Inhibition of viral uncoating and entry into cells.	Amantadine, rimantadine.	Alteration of binding site.	**Active only against influenza A.** Both have CNS effects, including seizures (more often with amantadine than with rimantadine).
Neuraminidase inhibitors	Inhibition of neuraminidase activity.	Oseltamivir, zanamivir.	Alteration of neuraminidase.	**Active against both influenza A and B.**

INFECTIOUS DISEASE

TABLE 12-4. Mechanisms of Action of Common Antifungal Drugs

CLASS	MECHANISM OF ACTION	COMMON AGENTS/ SPECTRUM OF ACTIVITY	COMMON RESISTANCE MECHANISMS	COMMENTS
Azoles	Inhibition of sterol synthesis.	Ketoconazole, fluconazole, itraconazole. Voriconazole (broad spectrum; good activity against *Aspergillus*).	↑ drug efflux.	Alter metabolism of other drugs. Ketoconazole is associated with gynecomastia. Use with caution in patients with liver disease.
Polyene	Alteration of cell permeability through interaction with ergosterol.	Amphotericin B (a broad-spectrum antifungal).	Alteration of binding site.	Causes infusional toxicity, nephrotoxicity, and hypokalemia.
Flucytosine	Inhibition of DNA and RNA synthesis.	Used only in combination with other antifungals because of the rapid development of resistance.	↓ penetration into cell; enzyme alteration.	Causes bone marrow suppression; drug levels must be monitored.
Griseofulvin	Mechanism is unclear, but thought to act through the disruption of spindle formation.	Used for tinea capitis and tinea unguium.		Contraindicated in porphyria and in liver disease; alters the metabolism of other drugs (e.g., OCPs). May have cross-reactivity in penicillin-allergic patients. A long course of treatment is usually required.
Echino-candins	Inhibition of glucan synthesis → cell wall damage.	Caspofungin, micofungin; broad spectrum for *Candida, Aspergillus,* no activity against *Rhizopus*.	Enzyme mutation.	Limited dosing data in pediatric patients.

TABLE 12-5. Management of Human and Animal Bites

MEASURE	PROCEDURES
Cleansing	Remove all visible dirt; irrigate with sterile saline. Puncture wounds should not be irrigated.
Culture	Culture if signs of visible infection and if wounds 8–24 hours old
Debridement	Debride devitalized tissue or bites on the head as well as injuries with metacarpal joint involvement.
Closure	Closure is appropriate for all bites, with the exception of puncture wounds and injuries of ≥ 8 hours' duration.
Tetanus	Assess risk (see p. 307 for postexposure management).
HBV	For human bites, assess risk and consider hepatitis B immunoglobulin (HBIG) and vaccine (see HBV, p. 319)
HIV	For human bites, assess risk. Postexposure prophylaxis is controversial.
Antibiotics	Give antibiotics for all moderate to severe (i.e., bite/crush injuries) wounds, puncture wounds, face/hand/genital bites, immunocompromised patients, or if the wound appears infected.
Rabies vaccine	Vaccine and immunoglobulin may be indicated (bite by wild animal or animal that cannot be observed, or animal with signs and symptoms of rabies; see p. 329).

Needlestick Injuries

The risk of disease transmission from needlestick injuries is greatest for HBV, followed by HCV and then by HIV. Local wound care and cleansing are required in all cases, and risk assessment should be done for HBV, HCV, and HIV.

- **HBV:** Assess the patient's immunization status (see p. 319).
- **HCV:** No postexposure prophylaxis is available.
- **HIV:** Postexposure prophylaxis for HIV is controversial.

> A three-year-old boy comes home from day care and reports that he was bitten by the day care provider's kitten during his lunch hour. It is now 8 PM. The child's mother sees a puncture wound in his left forearm. The boy is brought to the local ER, where examination reveals a 1-cm-diameter puncture wound with clean margins. What is the appropriate treatment? Following wound cleansing (not irrigation), the need for postexposure prophylaxis for tetanus and rabies should be assessed. Antibiotics should be administered.

Tetanus Prophylaxis for Wounds

Tetanus toxin → an inability to release activating neurotransmitters at synapses. This → overstimulation that manifests as local muscle spasms → generalized seizures and, if no intervention is initiated, → death. The need for postexposure tetanus immunization depends on prior vaccination history, the type of wound sustained, and the nature of the host (see Table 12-6). Tetanus immunization is available in various forms; the capitalized letters below indicate the emphasized component.

- Children ≤ 7 years of age should receive diphtheria and tetanus toxoids and acellular pertussis (DTaP), while those in whom acellular pertussis ad-

TABLE 12-6. Recommendations for Postexposure Tetanus Immunization

| VACCINE HISTORY | CLEAN WOUNDS | | DIRTY WOUNDS[a] | | COMMENTS |
	Tdap	TIG	Tdap	TIG	
< 3 doses or unknown history	Yes	No	Yes	Yes	Aggressive cleaning and debridement of necrosed/crushed tissue are necessary.
≥ 3 doses	No[b]	No	No[c]	No	If the child has received only three doses, a fourth dose should be administered.

[a] A dirty wound is defined as one containing dirt, saliva, or feces; the category also includes puncture wounds, crush injuries, burns, and frostbite.

[b] Yes, if > 10 years since last dose.

[c] Yes, if > 5 years since last dose.

ministration is contraindicated should receive diphtheria and tetanus toxoids (DT).

- Children > 7 years of age should receive tetanus-diphtheria toxoid and acellular pertussis (Tdap).
- Table 12-6 lists guidelines for the administration of tetanus immunoglobulin (TIG).

An 18-month-old boy presents with a two-day history of limp. The infant's mother states that her child has had a fever of up to 39.4°C for the past 2–3 days. The mother adds that the infant does not want to put weight on his right leg. A review of systems is otherwise unremarkable. On examination, you find that there is limited range of motion at the right hip along with pain, tenderness, and swelling. You order radiologic imaging and consult orthopedics. Which antibiotic combination would be appropriate for use after completion of the orthopedic procedure? Oxacillin plus ceftriaxone.

Acute Osteomyelitis

- **Dx:** The diagnosis of acute osteomyelitis is based on clinical evidence and supporting radiologic findings. Although radionuclide scans and MRI studies are more sensitive than plain radiographs, they are not always required for diagnosis. CRP is a useful marker for following the disease.
- **Tx:** Guidelines for antibiotic management according to pathogen and age group are listed in Table 12-7.

Septic Arthritis

- **Dx:** In septic arthritis, synovial fluid generally has > 50,000 WBCs/mm^3 with > 90% neutrophils.
- **Tx:** Antibiotic management for specific pathogens associated with each age group is outlined in Table 12-8.

TABLE 12-7. **Common Pathogens Associated with Acute Osteomyelitis**

Patient Age	Pathogens	Common Treatment Options
Neonates	*S. aureus*, group B streptococci, enteric gram-$\ominus$ organisms.	Oxacillin + gentamicin or oxacillin + cefotaxime
< 3 years of age	*S. aureus*, *Haemophilus influenzae* (unlikely in immunized children).	Oxacillin + ceftriaxone
> 3 years of age	*S. aureus*.	Oxacillin

Consider *Salmonella* spp. in patients with sickle cell disease.

TABLE 12-8. **Common Pathogens Associated with Septic Arthritis**

PATIENT AGE	PATHOGENS	TREATMENT OPTIONS
Neonates	*S. aureus*, group B streptococci, enteric gram-⊖ organisms.	Oxacillin + gentamicin or Oxacillin + cefotaxime
≤ 5 years of age	*S. aureus*, *H. influenzae* (unlikely in an immunized child), *Kingella kingae*, group A streptococci, *S. pneumoniae*.	Oxacillin + ceftriaxone
> 5 years of age	*S. aureus*, group A streptococci.	Oxacillin
Adolescents	Also consider *Neisseria gonorrhoeae*.	Ceftriaxone

Toxic Synovitis

■ **Sx/Exam:** Toxic synovitis is thought to be due to a viral or postinfectious process and typically affects the hip, often occurring after a respiratory infection.
■ **Dx:** ESR and peripheral WBC count are usually normal.
■ **Tx:** Management is symptomatic.

BOTULISM

■ Botulism is caused by *Clostridium botulinum* and results from the production of a neurotoxin that blocks the release of acetylcholine into the synapses. The pathogenesis of the disease varies according to type.
  ■ **Wound botulism:** This subtype is due to the spread of the causative organism from an infected wound (not discussed below).
  ■ **Food-borne botulism:** Food-borne botulism affects both children and adults, involving the ingestion of preformed toxin that is usually found in poorly canned foods.
  ■ **Infantile botulism:** This subtype is due to the ingestion of spores that germinate in the intestines and → toxin production.
■ **Sx/Exam:** Clinically, infantile botulism begins with constipation and develops into poor feeding, a weak suck, a weak cry, poor oral intake, hypotonia ("floppy baby"), ↓ movement, and ptosis. Older children and adults present with a self-limited illness that manifests as diplopia, blurry vision, dry mouth, dysphagia, dysphonia, and dysarthria.
■ **Dx/Tx:** Diagnosis is based on clinical suspicion, and treatment is supportive. For infant botulism, specific antitoxins should be sought and administered promptly.

Classically, ingestion of honey has been associated with infantile botulism, although other agents, such as corn syrup, may be associated with it as well.

CARDIAC DISEASES

Infective Endocarditis

The pathogenesis of infective endocarditis involves the trapping of pathogens in fibrin and platelet vegetation—factors that make it difficult to eradicate the infection. In general, pathogens involved in this disease adhere well to surfaces. Examples include oral streptococci and *S. aureus*, which can bind to endothelial cells as well as to collagen/fibronectin. Intravascular devices are a major cause of infective endocarditis and are often seen in hospitalized patients, especially in the neonatal population. Other common subtypes are as follows:

- **Native valve endocarditis:** This subtype is caused by turbulent flow that erodes the endothelium and therefore predisposes to infections and fibrin deposition. Congenital cardiac defects such as tetralogy of Fallot and VSD are major causes. Rheumatic heart disease, which is less common in the United States, is an important risk factor. Common organisms include S. *aureus* and oral streptococci, especially the viridans and HACEK (*Haemophilus aphrophilus/Haemophilus paraphrophilus, Actinobacillus actinomycetemcomitans, Cardiobacterium hominis, Eikenella corrodens,* and *Kingella kingae*) groups.
- **Postoperative endocarditis:** This subtype occurs in patients undergoing cardiac procedures. Skin flora plays an important role in postoperative endocarditis as well as in that related to intravascular devices; common causative agents include S. *aureus*, coagulase-⊖ staphylococci, *Candida* spp., and gram-⊖ bacilli.

SYMPTOMS/EXAM

- Patients typically have a history of fever, malaise, anorexia, heart failure, arthralgias, and skin lesions (petechiae).
- Patients should be asked about prior surgeries, including dental/oral procedures and injuries, as well as underlying cardiac defects and the use of indwelling lines.
- Physical examination may reveal fever, **heart murmur, splenomegaly,** Osler's nodes (small, tender nodules on the finger and toe pads), splinter hemorrhages (subungual petechiae), Janeway lesions (small, painless, peripheral hemorrhages), and Roth's spots (retinal hemorrhages).

DIAGNOSIS

A negative echocardiogram does not rule out infective endocarditis.

- CBC reveals leukocytosis with left shift and an ↑ ESR and CRP.
- Most patients have mild anemia, and 50% have microscopic hematuria as a result of embolic lesions of the kidney.
- Diagnosis is guided by the Duke criteria, which consist of two major **or** one major plus three minor or five minor criteria.
  - **Major criteria** include the following:
    1. ⊕ **blood cultures:** At least two sets separated in time with microorganisms consistent with infective endocarditis.
    2. **Echocardiogram findings:** These include vegetations, abscess, new valvular regurgitation, or new partial dehiscence of a prosthetic valve.
  - **Minor criteria** include the following:
    1. A predisposing heart condition or IV drug use.
    2. Fever.
    3. Vascular phenomenon (arterial emboli, pulmonary infarcts, mycotic aneurysms, conjunctival hemorrhages, Janeway lesions).
    4. Immunologic phenomena (Osler's nodes, Roth's spots, ⊕ RF).
    5. A ⊕ blood culture that does not meet the full criteria (separation in time) but shows serologic evidence of active infection with an organism consistent with infective endocarditis.
    6. Echocardiographic findings that do not meet the full criteria but are consistent with infective endocarditis.

Empiric IV antibiotic treatment is as follows:

- **Native valve endocarditis (community-acquired):** Oxacillin/nafcillin plus gentamicin.
- **Native valve endocarditis (nosocomial), intravascular device–related disease, early postoperative endocarditis:** Vancomycin plus gentamicin.
- Modify therapy once the organism is identified.

Myocarditis

Myocarditis can have infectious or noninfectious causes (e.g., autoimmune diseases, drug reactions, idiopathic factors). Etiologies are as follows:

- **Viral:**
    - The most important infectious cause is coxsackievirus B. Addition viral etiologies include other enteroviruses, CMV, influenza virus, parainfluenza virus, mumps, adenovirus, HIV, and parvovirus.
    - The pathogenesis of viral myocarditis may be acute infection or a postviral inflammatory process.
- **Bacterial:**
    - Bacteria may cause myocarditis by a variety of means. *S. aureus* and *Neisseria meningitidis* can form microabscesses in the myocardium, whereas diphtheria and tetanus can produce dysfunction by means of their toxins.
    - Toxic shock syndrome (*S. aureus*, *Streptococcus pyogenes*) may cause myocardial dysfunction. *Borrelia burgdorferi* and *Rickettsia* spp. may also cause myocarditis.
    - *Trypanosoma cruzi* is a major cause of myocarditis in South and Central America.
    - In immunocompromised patients, *Toxoplasma gondii* and CMV should also be considered.

SYMPTOMS/EXAM

- Clinically, myocarditis may present as an isolated finding but is often present as part of a systemic illness. Children may present with signs of heart failure and poor perfusion or with an acute, life-threatening event. Signs may be nonspecific in infants and neonates.
- Tachycardia is an important sign. Older children may have an audible S3 and/or S4.

DIAGNOSIS

- Lab tests include CK-MB isoform, which may be ↑.
- CXR may reveal cardiomegaly, while ECG and echocardiography may be more specific. A cardiac biopsy should be considered.

TREATMENT

- Management includes supportive care.
- Specific antimicrobial agents may be used in select situations.
- Use of immunosuppressive drugs or immunomodulators is controversial; some believe that high-dose pooled IVIG is useful, but this hypothesis has yet to be rigorously tested.

Pericarditis

- Pericarditis can be infectious or noninfectious. Infectious pericarditis can be benign (generally due to enteroviruses), purulent (i.e., of bacterial origin, in most cases *S. aureus*), or granulomatous (*Mycobacterium tuberculosis* and fungi).
- **Sx/Exam:** Clinical manifestations include chest pain (that may improve when sitting up and leaning forward) and exercise intolerance. Examination may also reveal a pericardial rub or distant heart sounds. Other manifestations include tachycardia and pulsus paradoxus.
- **Dx:** CXR may show an enlarged heart. ECG and echocardiographic studies are more useful. Tapping the pleural fluid may be diagnostic.
- **Tx:** Management depends on the etiology. Large quantities of pericardial fluid as well as purulent pericardial fluid require drainage. Specific antimicrobial agents may be used in select situations.

CATHETER-RELATED INFECTIONS

- Common pathogens associated with IV-related infections are skin commensals and include coagulase-⊖ staphylococci (CONS), *S. aureus*, *Candida* spp., and gram-⊖ organisms.
- Infection rates are higher for central venous catheters (especially those placed in the groin or jugular areas) than for peripheral or arterial catheters. Replacing catheters over a guide wire does not ↓ the risk of infection.
- Parenteral nutrition ↑ the risk for *Candida* infection. Lipid emulsions have classically been associated with *Malassezia* infections, although they also ↑ the risk for CONS.
- **Tx:** Management consists of removal of the infected catheter. Infections of tunneled catheters may require additional systemic therapy.

CNS INFECTIONS

A two-year-old African-American boy is brought to the ER by emergency medical technicians following a generalized tonic-clonic seizure. The child's grandmother states that he has had fever and a "cold" for the past 5–7 days. The grandmother adds that for the last two days the boy has "not been himself," has been sleepy, and has not eaten much. On examination, you find that the patient is obtunded and has neck stiffness. What is the appropriate treatment? Obtain LP, cell count and cultures, and then start the patient on vancomycin plus cefotaxime. Do not delay administration of antibiotics for obtaining CSF if the patient is very ill.

Encephalitis

- Defined as inflammation of the brain parenchyma. Noninfectious causes and toxic encephalopathies (e.g., pertussis, *Shigella* spp.) should always be ruled out.
- HSV is the most common cause of sporadic fatal encephalitis. HSV encephalitis in the neonate usually has an onset between 14 and 21 days.
- HSV-1 is the cause of HSV encephalitis occurring beyond the neonatal period and is a different disease that is usually due to reactivation of latent

virus. CSF findings in HSV encephalitis include ↑ RBC and WBC counts (usually in the hundreds) with lymphocytic predominance. Diagnostic workup includes HSV culture and PCR of CSF and skin lesions (if present).

- Other causes of encephalitis include enteroviruses, arthropod-borne viruses such as West Nile virus, and EBV. Many other viruses can cause postinfectious encephalitis, as can *Mycoplasma pneumoniae*. Opportunistic pathogens should also be considered in immunocompromised hosts.
- **Tx:** Management is symptomatic and also involves treatment of the specific pathogen.

"Alice in Wonderland syndrome" (the perception of objects as appearing substantially smaller than in reality) has been seen with EBV encephalitis.

Meningitis

Defined as inflammation of the leptomeninges (pia and arachnoid). Subtypes are as follows (see also Table 12-9):

- **Aseptic meningitis:** In this subtype, a pathogen is not isolated by routine bacterial cultures, and the etiologic agent is commonly found to be a virus (e.g., enteroviruses, herpesviruses, lymphocytic choriomeningitis virus, arboviruses). Other organisms that must be considered include *Borrelia burgdorferi* (Lyme disease), fungi, and TB. Noninfectious etiologies include drugs (e.g., NSAIDs, sulfa agents) and malignancy.
- **Bacterial meningitis:**
    - **Bacterial meningitis during the neonatal period:** Generally presents as part of a sepsis syndrome. Common causes include group B streptococci, enteric gram-⊖ organisms (especially *E. coli*), and *Listeria*. Antibiotic coverage should include meningitic doses of ampicillin plus cefotaxime ± gentamicin. In patients who have had prolonged hospitalization, *S. aureus*, *Enterococcus* spp., and resistant enteric gram-⊖ organisms should be considered.
    - **Bacterial meningitis beyond the neonatal period:** Commonly caused by *S. pneumoniae*, *N. meningitidis*, and *H. influenzae* type b (uncommon in the United States and in immunized children). Empiric antibiotics include meningitic doses of ceftriaxone/cefotaxime plus vancomycin. The role of steroids in bacterial meningitis is controversial. Steroids have been shown to be beneficial in children for *H. influenzae* meningitis only when given with the first dose of antibiotic (or 15–20 minutes prior). Prophylaxis of close contacts is needed for *N. meningitidis* (see the discussion of sepsis and shock) and *H. influenzae* (rifampin) meningitis.

TABLE 12-9. **Empiric Treatment of Bacterial Meningitis**

AGE	CAUSATIVE ORGANISM	TREATMENT
< 1 month	Group B streptococci, *E. coli*/gram-⊖ rods, *Listeria*.	Ampicillin + cefotaxime ± gentamicin.
1–3 months	Pneumococci, meningococci, *H. influenzae*.	Vancomycin IV + ceftriaxone or cefotaxime.
3 months – adulthood	Pneumococci, meningococci.	Vancomycin IV + ceftriaxone or cefotaxime.

Reproduced, with permission, from Le T et al. *First Aid for the USMLE Step 2 CK*, 5th ed. New York: McGraw-Hill, 2006:176.

INFECTIOUS DISEASE

Table 12-10 outlines the presentation, diagnosis, and treatment of common congenital infections, described by the mnemonic **TORCHeS:** *Toxoplasma gondii*, **O**ther (varicella, parvovirus, *Listeria*, TB, malaria, fungi), **R**ubella, **C**ytomegalovirus, **H**erpes simplex, and **S**yphilis.

TABLE 12-10. Diagnosis and Treatment of Common Congenital Infections

	TOXOPLASMA GONDII	RUBELLA VIRUS	CMV	HSV-1 AND -2	SYPHILIS (TREPONEMA PALLIDUM)
1° transmission	Transplacental.	The risk of transplacental transmission is highest in the first trimester.	Transplacental.	Intrapartum transmission generally occurs in the presence of active lesions; however, women can have asymptomatic shedding.	Transplacental.
Prevention	Pregnant women should avoid changing cat litterboxes and should avoid contact with raw or undercooked meat.	Vaccinate **prior to pregnancy.**	Ideally, avoid exposure.	Perform a C-section in the presence of active lesions.	Treat during pregnancy.
Eye findings	Chorioretinitis.	Cataracts.	Retinitis.	Keratoconjunctivitis.	Interstitial keratitis.[a]
Skin findings	None.	Blueberry muffin rash.[b]	Blueberry muffin–like rash.	Vesicular skin rash; mucocutaneous lesions.	Maculopapular skin rash.
CNS lesions and manifestations	Intracranial calcifications, ring-enhancing lesions, cognitive and motor dysfunction, microcephaly.	Mental retardation.	Periventricular calcifications, microcephaly, neurodevelopmental problems.	Mental retardation, seizures, microcephaly.	Mental, motor, and sensory deficits.
Hearing manifestations	Hearing loss.	Hearing loss.	Sensorineural hearing loss.	None.	Hearing loss.[a]

	TOXOPLASMA GONDII	**RUBELLA VIRUS**	**CMV**	**HSV-1 AND -2**	**SYPHILIS (TREPONEMA PALLIDUM)**
Skeletal manifestations	None.	None.	None.	None.	Osteitis, saddle nose, saber shins (bowing of shins). Hutchinson's teeth[a] (peg-shaped, notched central incisors).
Other manifestations	Anemia, jaundice, splenomegaly, lymphadenopathy, intrauterine growth retardation (IUGR).	PDA, stillbirth, spontaneous abortion, IUGR.	Hepatitis, hyperbilirubinemia, thrombocytopenia, IUGR.	Neonatal sepsis, hepatitis, pneumonia, IUGR.	"Snuffles" (mucopurulent rhinitis), lymphadenopathy, hepatomegaly, thrombocytopenia, hydrops fetalis, spontaneous abortion, IUGR.
Diagnostic tests	*Toxoplasma* serologies from mother and infant.	Rubella serologies.	Urine culture for CMV; CMV PCR; maternal and infant serologies.	Surface culture > 48 hours after birth; HSV PCR.	Darkfield microscopy of skin lesions; serologic testing on the mother and infant. Obtain the mother's prior serologies to assess adequate treatment response (fourfold ↓ RPR.
Treatment	Pyrimethamine, sulfadiazine.	None.	Ganciclovir (controversial).	Acyclovir.	Penicillin.[c]

[a] Hutchinson's triad.

[b] Extramedullary hematopoiesis.

[c] Treatment should be considered if 1) the mother was untreated; 2) mother was treated within the last month of pregnancy; 3) mother had inadequate treatment response; 4) mother/child have clinical signs or symptoms of disease; 5) mother was treated with erythromycin; 5) baby's RPR titers are fourfold > than its mother.

An infant was just born to a mother who developed varicella seven days prior to delivery, and you are the pediatrician on call covering labor and delivery. The infant appears well, but you are asked to make treatment recommendations for the infant. What should you recommend? How would your recommendations differ if the infant's mother developed varicella the day before delivery? In the first instance, recommend close monitoring with no intervention. In the second instance, recommend VZIG.

All congenital infections can be asymptomatic at birth.

Varicella

- The causative agent is varicella-zoster virus (VZV).
- The risk of transmission is highest in the presence of maternal infection five days before or two days after delivery; in such cases, there is no opportunity for transplacental transmission of IgG for protection.
- Remember that IgG transfer occurs after 28 weeks' gestation. This can → overwhelming and potentially fatal varicella infection (pneumonia, sepsis, transaminitis).
- 1° varicella infection describes infection that occurs prior to 20 weeks' gestation. Clinical manifestations can be severe and can include varicella embryopathy (limb atrophy, scarring of skin); CNS and eye manifestations may also be seen.
- **Dx:** Diagnosis can be made by isolating the virus from vesicular lesions through antigen detection or culture.
- **Tx:** Administer VZIG (IVIG should be used if VZIG is not available) in infants of women with disease. Acyclovir should be used only if the neonate develops varicella.

COMMUNITY-ACQUIRED PNEUMONIA

- Viruses are common causes of pneumonia in children and include RSV, influenza virus, and parainfluenza virus. Viral pneumonias may → superinfection with bacteria; common associations include influenza and *Streptococcus pneumoniae* or *S. aureus*.
- TB may cause pneumonias in any age group and should be considered in children with a high risk of exposure (see the discussion of tuberculin skin test interpretation) and in those for whom disease persists despite appropriate antibacterial therapy. Hospitalized patients or those with underlying disease (e.g., immunosuppression) are at risk for other pathogens.
- Antibiotic management and common pathogens associated with each age group are listed in Table 12-11.

TABLE 12-11. Pathogens Associated with Community-Acquired Pneumonia

PATIENT AGE	PATHOGENS	COMMENTS
Neonates (< 28 days)	Group B streptococci, enteric gram-⊖ organisms (especially *E. coli*), *Listeria*.	Consider viral pathogens causing disseminated viral infection—e.g., HSV, CMV.
1–3 months	*Chlamydia trachomatis, S. pneumoniae, S. aureus, Bordetella pertussis*.	
3 months – 5 years	*S. pneumoniae, H. influenzae* (nontypable), *M. pneumoniae*.	Think of *H. influenzae* type b in patients from outside the United States, where vaccination is less common.
5–15 years	*M. pneumoniae, Chlamydophila pneumoniae, S. pneumoniae*.	

Neonatal Conjunctivitis

Table 12-12 outlines the pathogenesis, diagnosis, and treatment of neonatal conjunctivitis.

Postneonatal Conjunctivitis

A high percentage of children with bacterial conjunctivitis have concurrent otitis media and often complain of early-morning crusting. The most common causative organisms are viruses such as adenovirus (hemorrhagic) and bacteria (nontypable *H. influenzae*, *S. pneumoniae*, other *Streptococcus* spp., *Moraxella catarrhalis*).

Non-typable H. influenzae *is the most common pathogen implicated in conjunctivitis-otitis syndrome.*

TABLE 12-12. Common Causes of Neonatal Conjunctivitis

	NEISSERIA GONORRHOEAE	CHLAMYDIA TRACHOMATIS	OTHER BACTERIA[a]	HSV	CHEMICAL
Age at onset	2–7 days	5–14 days (most common cause of infectious conjunctivitis)	6–14 days	Infants	24 hours (silver nitrate)
Keratoconjunctivitis	Yes	No	No	Yes	No
Discharge	Mucopurulent	Mucopurulent	Purulent	Serous	Serous
Corneal involvement	Yes (infiltrate and ulcerative)	No	No	Yes (dendrite, ulcer)	No
Diagnosis	Gram stain, culture	Giemsa staining of conjunctival scrapings, culture	Gram stain, culture	Culture of specimens; presence of multinucleated giant cells on microscopic exam	History
Treatment	Systemic third-generation cephalosporin	Oral and topical erythromycin	Topical ophthalmic ointments	Systemic acyclovir ± topical trifluridine	Supportive
Other manifestations	Rapidly progressive; can → blindness	Pneumonia (neonate)		Concurrent systemic illness	

[a] Other bacteria include *H. influenzae*, *S. pneumoniae* and other *Streptococcus* spp., and *Staphylococcus* spp.

A five-day-old Caucasian female presents to your clinic with a one-day history of fever (38.7°C axillary). The patient's mother says that she has not been feeding well. How would you manage this patient? Admit the child to the hospital; obtain blood, urine cultures, and LP and CSF cultures; and start parenteral antibiotics.

Subnormal temperatures and hypothermia should be considered signs of infection in neonates and are often referred to as temperature instability.

Fever is a manifestation of inflammation that may be due to an infectious or a noninfectious cause (e.g., rheumatologic, neoplastic). Several cytokines, including IL-1, IL-6, and TNF, are involved in the manifestation of fever. It should be noted that fever is a host-dependent process, and some groups of patients—such as neonates, neurologically impaired children, and those on immunosuppressive drugs—may not manifest fever in the same manner as other children.

Fever Without a Source

Fever is generally defined as a central temperature ≥ 38°C, although other definitions exist. Table 12-13 offers general guidelines for previously healthy children < 3 years of age who present with fever **without any localizing signs.**

Fever of Unknown Origin (FUO)

- There are several definitions of FUO, but a practical definition in children involves a daily fever of ≥ 38.3°C for ≥ 14 days without an apparent cause following repeated physical examinations and laboratory tests.

TABLE 12-13. Treatment of Fever Without a Known Source

PATIENT AGE	MANAGEMENT
< 28 days	Admit to hospital; obtain blood, urine cultures, and LP and CSF culture. Start parenteral antibiotics.
28–90 days	Obtain blood and urine culture, CBC, and UA. Patients who are **nontoxic in appearance with a WBC count < 15,000/mm³, < 10% bandemia, and a normal UA** can be managed on an outpatient basis with careful follow-up or may be admitted for observation. Patients treated on an outpatient basis generally receive a single dose of ceftriaxone (50 mg/kg) with follow-up in 24 hours. **Toxic-appearing patients** require admission with a full workup, including LP and CSF culture and parenteral antibiotics.
> 90 days	Patients who are **nontoxic in appearance with a fever < 39°C** require no workup. Such patients can be managed on an outpatient basis with careful follow-up. For patients who are **nontoxic in appearance with a fever ≥ 39°C,** obtain blood and urine cultures, CBC, and UA. Patients generally receive a single dose of ceftriaxone (50 mg/kg) if CBC is ≥ **15,000/mm³** with follow-up in 24 hours. **Toxic-appearing patients** require admission with a full workup, including blood and urine cultures, LP and CSF cultures, and parenteral antibiotics.

- Infections account for almost one-third of all cases of FUO; however, non-infectious causes should also be sought. Prominent among these are rheumatologic disorders, oncologic conditions, and periodic fever syndromes. Other causes may include physical stresses such as heat stroke, ingestion of poisons such as anticholinergics, drug fever, hyperthyroidism, and dysautonomia.
- **Sx/Exam:** Patients with FUO warrant a thorough evaluation. A detailed history with meticulous documentation is essential, as is a thorough physical examination.
- **Dx:** Testing should be based on clinical findings, but screening tests such as CBC, CRP, ESR, UA, and LFTs may be useful.
- **Tx:** Empiric antibiotic therapy should be avoided unless the patient is significantly compromised. Empiric therapy may be considered when a specific diagnosis such as TB is considered very likely.

GI INFECTIONS

Infectious Hepatitis

HEPATITIS A (HAV)

- Risk factors include exposure to day care centers with diapered children, restaurants with infected food handlers, and men who have sex with men (MSM). Transmission is by the fecal-oral route.
- **Sx/Exam:** Mostly subclinical but may present as an acute, self-limited illness with fever, anorexia, and jaundice (more common in adults and older children); fulminant hepatitis can occur but is less likely than with other forms.
- **Dx:** Diagnosed by the presence of HAV IgM (acute infection); IgG may develop shortly after IgM.
- **Prevention:** HAV is a preventable disease, and the HAV vaccine is recommended for travelers to endemic areas, high-risk populations (MSM), and workers in day care settings. Postexposure prophylaxis consists of HAV immune globulin, which can be administered within two weeks of exposure.
- **Complications:** There are no long-term manifestations.

HEPATITIS B (HBV)

- Transmitted via blood products, sex, or perinatal exposure.
- **Sx/Exam:** Presents with anorexia, nausea, malaise, and jaundice, but HBV may also be asymptomatic or present as fulminant, fatal hepatitis.
- **Dx:** Diagnosed by serology (see Table 12-14).
- **Prevention:** HBV is preventable, and therefore vaccine is recommended for all infants, children, adolescents, health care workers, and others who have had exposure to places in which HBV is endemic, as well as for IV drug users. Postexposure prophylaxis in the form of hepatitis B vaccine and HBIG should be given to infants exposed perinatally and to unvaccinated persons (or persons with inadequate antibody response to immunization) with high-risk contacts.
- **Complications:** Persistence of the infection over time can → the development of hepatocellular carcinoma.

TABLE 12-14. Serologic Diagnosis of HBV

	ACUTE INFECTION	PAST INFECTION	VACCINATED
HBsAg	+	+/− + in chronic infection; − in resolved past infection	−
Anti-HBsAg	+	+/− + in resolved infection; − in chronic infection	+
HBeAg	+ High risk of transmission	+/− Can be + in chronic infection with high risk of transmission	−
Anti-HBe	−	+ Low risk of transmission	
Anti-HBc IgG	+	+ Chronic or resolved	−
Anti-HBc IgM	+	−	−

HEPATITIS C (HCV)

- Transmitted via blood products, sex, or perinatal exposure (very unlikely).
- **Sx/Exam:** May present with anorexia, nausea, malaise, and jaundice, but most infections are asymptomatic.
- **Dx:** Diagnosed by ⊕ HCV IgG by enzyme immunoassay (EIA), recombinant immunoblot assay (RIBA), or HCV RNA.
- **Tx:** There are no approved therapies in children; however, interferon-α and ribavirin have been used with success in adults.
- **Prevention:** There is no vaccine, and no postexposure prophylaxis exists.
- **Complications:** Can → fibrosis and end-stage liver disease.

HEPATITIS D (HDV)

Transmitted only with HBV.

HEPATITIS E (HEV)

- Transmitted via the fecal-oral route.
- Fulminant hepatitis can occur in pregnant women.
- **Sx/Exam:** May present with abdominal discomfort, fever, jaundice, anorexia, nausea, and malaise. Infection can also be asymptomatic. It is rare in the United States but does occur among travelers to endemic regions.
- **Dx:** Diagnosed by ⊕ HEV IgM, IgG, or RNA.
- **Tx:** Supportive.
- **Prevention:** No vaccine or postexposure prophylaxis exists. Good hygiene is preventive.
- **Complications:** No chronic infection.

Gastroenteritis

Gastroenteritis can be parasitic, viral, or bacterial in origin.

- **Giardiasis,** caused by the parasite *Giardia lamblia*, is a common cause of gastroenteritis that may be exacerbated in the immunocompromised (see Figure 12-1).
- *Clostridium difficile:*
    - Causes diarrhea resulting from antibiotic use (antibiotic-associated diarrhea) → pseudomembranous colitis. It is classically associated with clindamycin; however, any antibiotic can cause the disease.
    - A significant number of patients (particularly infants < 1 year of age) have *C. difficile* in their flora with toxin that is not pathogenic. With use of antibiotics, however, other "normal flora" are eliminated, allowing for the overgrowth of this bacterium.
    - **Sx/Exam:** Clinical manifestations include watery diarrhea that may become bloody. A dreaded complication is toxic megacolon.
    - **Dx:** Diagnosed by the detection of *C. difficile* toxin.
    - **Tx:** Treat with metronidazole PO × 10 days. In the event of treatment failure, repeat the course; however, vancomycin PO × 10 days should be given for persistent treatment failure. **Note:** Testing for *C. difficile* should not be done following treatment, as the results could remain ⊕; the need for repeat treatment should be guided by the recurrence of symptoms.
- Tables 12-15 and 12-16 outline the treatment of gastroenteritis arising from a variety of bacterial and viral pathogens.

Peritonitis

- Defined as inflammation of visceral and parietal peritoneum, it may be caused by infectious or noninfectious etiologies.
- Two types of peritonitis exist.

Bacillus cereus *food poisoning has a presentation similar to that of* S. aureus *and is classically associated with fried rice.*

Management of hydration and electrolytes is the cornerstone of treatment of gastroenteritis.

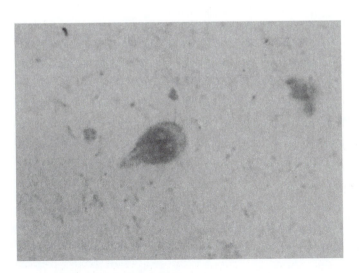

FIGURE 12-1. *Giardia* **trophozoite in stool.**

The trophozoite exhibits a classic pear shape with two nuclei imparting an owl's-eye appearance. (Reproduced, with permission, from Le T et al. *First Aid for the USMLE Step 2 CK*, 5th ed. New York: McGraw-Hill, 2006, Color Insert p. 14.) (Also see Color Insert.)

TABLE 12-15. **Diagnosis and Treatment of Bacterial Gastroenteritis**[a]

Organism	Mechanism	Source	Symptoms/Exam	Treatment
Campylobacter spp.	? toxin, invasion.	Food, poultry, animal contact (especially birds), untreated water, unpasteurized milk, person to person.	Fever, abdominal pain, bloody diarrhea.	Supportive +/– macrolides.
E. coli (EC)				
STEC (Shiga toxin–producing EC), previously known as EHEC (enterohemorrhagic)	Shiga-like toxin without invasion; O157:H7 is the most notorious.	Undercooked beef; unpasteurized milk and apple cider.	Bloody or nonbloody diarrhea, hemorrhagic colitis, hemolytic-uremic syndrome (HUS), thrombotic thrombocytopenic purpura (TTP).	Antibiotics should not be used, although definitive data are not available; supportive care.
ETEC (enterotoxigenic EC)	Cholera-like toxin without invasion.	Food, water.	A major cause of traveler's diarrhea; presents with watery diarrhea and abdominal cramps.	Supportive care, as the disease is self-limited; however, TMP-SMX or fluoroquinolones can be considered.
EPEC (enteropathogenic EC)	Attachment; enterocyte effacement without invasion.	Water, weaning foods (infants and toddlers transitioning from milk to other foods).	Watery diarrhea, dehydration; a major cause of infant morbidity and mortality in the developing world.	Supportive; TMP-SMX or fluoroquinolones.
EIEC (enteroinvasive EC)	Invasion, local spread.	Cheese, water, fecal-oral.	Fever, pain, bloody or nonbloody diarrhea, dysentery.	Supportive plus antibiotics: TMP-SMX, fluoroquinolones, macrolides for dysentery.
Salmonella	Invasion, translocation, dissemination.	Milk, beef, poultry, contact with reptiles.	Fever, bloody diarrhea, dysentery, extraintestinal spread.	Supportive. Antibiotics should generally be avoided, as they can perpetuate a carrier state; however, in high-risk populations (e.g., infants < 3 months of age, immunocompromised patients, or those with extraintestinal spread), antibiotics are indicated (amoxicillin, TMP-SMX in susceptible strains, third-generation cephalosporins).
Shigella	Invasion, local spread.	Person to person.	Bloody diarrhea, fever, dysentery, neurologic symptoms (seizures can occur).	Supportive, as the disease is usually self-limited. However, antibiotics should be administered to those with severe disease and should be based on local resistance patterns.

Organism	Mechanism	Source	Symptoms/Exam	Treatment [a]
S. aureus	Enterotoxin.	Food served by food handlers; inappropriate refrigeration or reheating.	Abrupt abdominal cramping and pain, nausea and vomiting +/– diarrhea shortly (30 minutes to 2 hours) after ingestion of contaminated food.	Supportive.
Vibrio spp., including V. cholerae	Invasion, enterotoxin without invasion.	Water, person to person, shellfish.	Watery diarrhea, cholera.	Supportive +/– antibiotics for moderately to severely ill patients, as antibiotics can limit both the extent and spread of disease (doxycycline is preferred; also treated with TMP-SMX and fluoroquinolones).
Yersinia spp.	Invasion, translocation.	Water, pig products (especially chitterlings).	Fever, abdominal pain, bloody diarrhea, extraintestinal spread.	Supportive + antibiotics (TMP-SMX, fluoroquinolones, third-generation cephalosporins).

[a] Fluoroquinolones should be avoided in children < 18 years.

TABLE 12-16. Diagnosis and Treatment of Viral Gastroenteritis

Virus	Symptoms/Exam	Transmission	Diagnosis/Treatment
Rotavirus	Nonbloody diarrhea, fever, emesis.	Fecal-oral, **day care centers.**	Diagnosed by rotavirus antigen detection; supportive treatment.
Norovirus (previously Norwalk-like virus)	Nonbloody diarrhea, vomiting, abdominal cramps, myalgias.	Person to person, foods contaminated by infected handlers; often associated with outbreaks in day care centers, cruise ships, and nursing homes.	Supportive treatment, hygiene. Highly infectious.
Astrovirus	Abdominal pain, nonbloody diarrhea, nausea, fever, malaise.	Fecal-oral, raw shellfish; peaks during winter.	Supportive treatment.
Enteric adenovirus	Abdominal pain, nonbloody diarrhea, nausea, fever, malaise; particularly affects young children < 4 years of age.	Fecal-oral.	Supportive treatment.

INFECTIOUS DISEASE

- **1°/spontaneous peritonitis:** Due to extension from a GU or bowel source, hematogenous/lymphatic spread, or direct inoculation from a foreign body in an **anatomically normal peritoneum.**
- **2° peritonitis:** Due to entry of organisms through rupture of the GI tract (ruptured appendicitis) or introduction of a pathogen through a foreign body (e.g., through a peritoneal or ventriculoperitoneal catheter).
- Common pathogens include the following:
  - **1° peritonitis:** *Streptococcus pneumoniae*, *S. aureus*, gram-⊖ bacteria.
  - **2° peritonitis:** Coagulase-⊖ staphylococci, *S. aureus* (most common), enteric pathogens.
- **Sx/Exam:** Clinical manifestations include abdominal pain and distention, fever, and irritability.
- **Dx:** Diagnosed by imaging to define abdominal pathology and sampling of peritoneal fluid (cell analysis and culture).
- **Tx:** Treatment is empiric and is aimed at covering the most likely pathogens (e.g., ceftriaxone for 1° peritonitis and vancomycin for catheter-associated peritonitis). Therapy should be modified on the basis of susceptibilities.

ANIMAL-, INSECT-, AND FOOD-BORNE PATHOGENS

Table 12-17 lists common food-, insect-, and animal-borne pathogens and their associated disease states.

IMMUNIZATIONS

A recommended vaccination schedule is shown in Figure 17-2 of the Preventive Medicine chapter (please refer to the latest immunization schedule from www.cdc.gov). Side effects and contraindications of common vaccines are outlined in Table 12-18. Local reactions are the most common side effects with many vaccines. For all vaccines, anaphylaxis to a prior dose or one of its components is a contraindication. Subtypes are as follows:

- **Active vs. passive: Active immunization** refers to a process in which the body develops antibodies or cell-mediated immunity following stimulation with a foreign antigen. **Passive immunization** (immunoglobulins) involves the direct administration of antibody to a specific pathogen. In general, active immunization is longer lasting than passive immunization.
- **Live vs. killed/inactivated vaccine:** In general, live vaccines provide more robust and longer-lasting immunologic response than killed vaccine owing to replication of the attenuated pathogen in vivo.
  - Live vaccines are generally contraindicated in immunocompromised hosts with 1° or 2° immunodeficiencies (e.g., HIV); in patients taking corticosteroids at doses ≥ 2 mg/kg/day of prednisone (or equivalent steroid) **or** a total of ≥ 20 mg/day (in children, > 10 kg × ≥ 14 days); and in patients taking immune-modulating agents (e.g., methotrexate, anti-TNF-α agents), pregnant patients, or the contacts of each.
  - Exceptions can be made on the basis of the specific immunodeficiency and degree of immunosuppression. Live vaccines are usually withheld for at least three months after immunosuppressive chemotherapy; however, the interval may vary with the degree of immunosuppression or the extent of underlying disease.

TABLE 12-17. Common Pathogens and Associated Diseases

CAUSATIVE AGENT	CLASSIC ASSOCIATIONS	CLINICAL SYNDROME	COMMENTS
Bacillus cereus	Fried rice, meats, stews, gravies, and vanilla sauce.	Gastroenteritis.	Enterotoxin-mediated illness.
Bartonella henselae (cat-scratch disease)	Kittens.	Lymphadenopathy; can cause Parinaud's oculoglandular syndrome.	Also a cause of bacillary angiomatosis in HIV patients.
Blastomyces dermatitidis (blastomycosis)	Soil.	Pulmonary and disseminated disease; may be asymptomatic.	Seen in the southeastern, central, and midwestern states bordering the Great Lakes.
Borrelia burgdorferi (Lyme disease)	Deer tick (*Ixodes scapularis*).	Erythema migrans (target lesion), arthritis, meningitis, carditis.	Seen in the northeastern United States (southern Maine to northern Virginia). The nymphal stage is the infective form.
Borrelia recurrentis (relapsing fever)	Human body louse.	Fever, chills.	*B. hermsii* is most common in the United States. Seen in western mountainous areas.
Brucella spp.	Contaminated dairy products or direct contact with tissue of infected farm animals.	Fever, malaise, lymphadenopathy, flulike syndrome.	Osteoarticular infection is the most frequent complication. Endocarditis is rare but accounts for most deaths.
Campylobacter jejuni[a]	Poultry, milk (unpasteurized).	Bloody gastroenteritis.	
Chlamydia psittaci (psittacosis)	Inhalation of dried bird feces (parakeets, parrots, pigeons, turkeys).	Acute febrile respiratory tract infection.	Infections are rare in children.
Clostridium botulinum	Canned food, honey.	Presents in infants with constipation and poor feeding; presents in older children and adults with descending paralysis.	Neurotoxin mediated; infants ingest spores that sporulate and produce toxin, while older children and adults ingest preformed toxin.
Coccidioides immitis (coccidioidomycosis)	Soil.	Usually asymptomatic; often the only lesions are calcified spots on CXR.	Found in the southwestern United States and Latin America.
Coxiella burnetii (Q fever)	Exposure to animals (cattle, sheep, goats) or tissue (urine, feces, amniotic tissue, placenta).	Fever, headache, flulike syndrome, hepatitis, pneumonia.	Consider in patients with both hepatitis and pneumonia.

INFECTIOUS DISEASE

TABLE 12-17. **Common Pathogens and Associated Diseases** *(continued)*

Causative Agent	Classic Associations	Clinical Syndrome	Comments
Cryptococcus neoformans (cryptococcosis)	Soil; associated with pigeon feces.	Pulmonary disease and meningitis, particularly in HIV patients.	India ink is used for diagnosis in CSF; cryptococcal antigen can be used for other sites (serum, CSF). Definitive diagnosis is by isolation from body fluid or tissue.
Ehrlichia chaffeensis, Anaplasma phagocytophilum (ehrlichioses)	Lone star tick and deer tick.	Fever, headache, myalgias, rash, sepsis (see p. 335).	Widespread in the United States; the treatment of choice is doxycycline.
Enterohemorrhagic *E. coli* (EHEC)	Apple cider (unpasteurized), hamburger.	Bloody diarrhea and HUS.	
Francisella tularensis (tularemia)	Bite by infected tick, direct tissue contact with infected animal (rabbit), inhalation.	Fever and lymphadenopathy, flulike syndrome; ulceroglandular syndrome, pneumonia.	
Giardia lamblia (giardiasis)	Camping, day care centers.	Diarrhea and flatulence.	*Giardia* stool antigen is the test of choice.
Hepatitis A	Shellfish.	Hepatitis.	Mostly asymptomatic in children.
Histoplasma capsulatum (histoplasmosis)	Birds, bats, construction sites.	Fewer than 5% of cases are symptomatic; often the only lesions are calcified spots on CXR.	Seen in the central and eastern United States (Ohio, Mississippi).
Leptospira interrogans (leptospirosis)	Rats (and other rodents), urine.	Self-limited systemic illness; conjunctival suffusion, fever, headache, nausea, vomiting.	
Listeria spp.	Milk (unpasteurized), soft cheeses, deli meats, hot dogs.	Sepsis and meningitis in neonates and immunocompromised hosts; gastroenteritis.	One of the rationales for using ampicillin in the empiric coverage for neonates; pregnant women are at ↑ risk.
Norovirus (previously Norwalk virus), calicivirus	Shellfish, salad bars, ice.	Gastroenteritis.	Recently reported aboard cruise ships.
Plasmodium spp. (malaria)	*Anopheles* mosquito; consider in returning travelers from endemic areas.	Fever and chills; multiorgan failure and shock are seen with *P. falciparum*.	Blood smear is the test of choice.
Rabies virus	Dogs, cats, foxes and raccoons, bats (spelunking).	Fatal encephalopathy.	Hydrophobia is a common manifestation; postexposure prophylaxis is vital.

TABLE 12-17. Common Pathogens and Associated Diseases *(continued)*

CAUSATIVE AGENT	CLASSIC ASSOCIATIONS	CLINICAL SYNDROME	COMMENTS
Rickettsia rickettsii (Rocky mountain spotted fever)	Dog tick (*Dermacentor variabilis*).	Fever, headache, myalgias, rash (palms and soles), sepsis (see p. 335).	Widespread in the United States, but most reported cases are from the south Atlantic, southeastern, and south central regions. The treatment of choice is doxycycline.
Salmonella (nontyphi)[a]	Poultry, reptiles.	Bloody gastroenteritis, sepsis/meningitis.	Sickle cell patients and children < 3 months of age are at especially high risk.
Shigella spp.	Egg salad; vegetables or scallions.	Bloody gastroenteritis.	Can cause seizures due to a toxin-mediated encephalopathy.
S. aureus	Picnics.	Gastroenteritis.	Preformed toxin; acute onset.
Toxoplasma gondii (toxoplasmosis)	Ingestion of undercooked meats; cat litter boxes.	Usually asymptomatic, but may present with lymphadenopathy and fever or with a flulike syndrome.	Causes congenital disease in infants born to mothers infected during pregnancy.
Vibrio parahaemolyticus	Contaminated seafood.	Gastroenteritis.	Reported on cruise ships in the Caribbean.
West Nile virus	Mosquitos.	Usually asymptomatic, but presents with febrile illness in some patients and with meningoencephalitis in a small proportion of cases.	Seasonal epidemics occur in the United States during summer and continue into fall. Not a common disease in children.
Yersinia enterocolitica [a]	Chitterlings.	Bloody gastroenteritis.	Think of it during the holiday season.
Yersinia pestis (plague)	Rat flea.	May occur in bubonic form (presents with a high fever and painful lymphadenopathy), septicemia form, or pneumonic form.	Rodents are the reservoirs for this disease; in the western United States (Colorado, New Mexico, California, Arizona) it is a rural disease associated with prairie dogs.

[a] Can be associated with immunoreactive syndromes such as Reiter or Guillain-Barré syndrome.

- MMR and varicella vaccines can be given to contacts of immunocompromised or pregnant patients as well as to HIV patients with only moderate immunodeficiency (CD4 > 25%). In addition, varicella vaccine should be considered in acute lymphoblastic leukemia (ALL) patients who are in remission and who lack any other evidence of active immunosuppression.

TABLE 12-18. Side Effects and Contraindications of Common Vaccines

Vaccine	Common Side Effects	Contraindications
DTaP	Local and febrile reactions.	Precautions should be exercised in patients with seizures; contraindicated in patients with progressive neurologic disorders or a history of encephalopathy within seven days of prior DTaP immunization.
Influenza (inactivated) vaccine	Fever; local reactions are rare in patients < 13 years of age.	Anaphylaxis to chicken or egg.
MMR vaccine	Fever; transient rash is reported in 5% of recipients.	Live vaccine precautions and contraindications.
Varicella vaccine	Fever; localized rash is reported in 3–5% of cases. An additional 3–5% have a generalized varicella-like rash.	Live vaccine precautions and contraindications.

There is no group B meningococcal vaccine.

- Because of concerns of diminished efficacy, patients who have received immunoglobulins should not receive live vaccines for several months. However, if exposure risk is very high, they should receive the vaccine and should then be reimmunized at the appropriate time.
- **Meningococcal vaccines:** Two vaccines against meningococcus groups A, C, Y, and W-135 are available. **Conjugate vaccine** has been recommended for children 11–12 years of age, teenagers entering high school, and college freshman living in dormitories. It is also recommended for high-risk groups, such as military recruits; those traveling to or residing in countries where *N. meningitidis* is epidemic; terminal complement deficient and asplenic patients; microbiologists; and those in outbreak situations. **Polysaccharide vaccine** is an acceptable alternative, although the conjugate vaccine is thought to be more immunogenic.
- Immunizations may also be used as postexposure prophylaxis for certain diseases (see Table 12-19).

IMMUNOCOMPROMISED STATES

A 15-year-old girl presents to the ER with a two-day history of fever, profound sore throat, and myalgias. On exam, she is found to have diffuse lymphadenopathy and significant pharyngitis without exudates. In your interview, you find that she is sexually active, with her last sexual activity having occurred approximately 3–4 weeks prior to her presentation. Which diagnostic measures would be appropriate? Appropriate tests may include a rapid streptococcal antigen test, bacterial throat culture, and Monospot test. An HIV RNA and antibody test should be considered.

TABLE 12-19. Postexposure Prophylaxis for Selected Diseases

IMMUNIZATION	ACTIVE	PASSIVE	COMMENTS
Measles	Live vaccine within 72 hours will provide protection in some cases.	IVIG for exposed patients < 1 year of age as well as for immunocompromised patients and pregnant women.	
Varicella	Live vaccine can be used in immunocompetent hosts within three days of appearance of rash in the index patient.	VZIG in immunocompromised patients within 96 hours.	
Rabies	Rabies vaccine.	Rabies immunoglobulin.	Administer active and passive immunization if the patient was bitten by a wild animal or by a domestic animal under observation that develops signs of rabies. High-risk animals include foxes, bats, raccoons, and skunks.
Tetanus			See the discussion of bites and injuries.
Hepatitis A			See the discussion of GI infections.
Hepatitis B			See the discussion of GI infections; consider other blood-borne pathogens.

Common Pathogens Seen in Immunodeficiencies

Table 12-20 outlines common conditions found in immunocompromised patients along with their associated pathogens.

Human Immunodeficiency Virus (HIV)

Infection in children occurs primarily by vertical transmission (mother to baby). The risk of transmission is ↑ in settings where the mother has a high HIV viral load, a low CD4 count, or premature and prolonged ROM; has had an emergent C-section (uncontrolled setting); or is breast-feeding. It should be noted that there is an increasing incidence of transmission in adolescent patients through behavioral exposures (sexual, drug use).

SYMPTOMS/EXAM

Children or infants may present with nonspecific symptoms such as weight loss, poor growth, fevers, night sweats, recurrent thrush, adenopathy, hepatosplenomegaly, and recurrent bacterial infections.

Avoiding breast-feeding is an effective means of preventing postnatal transmission from mother to fetus.

INFECTIOUS DISEASE

TABLE 12-20. Common Pathogens Seen in Immunodeficiencies

CONDITION	PATHOGEN
Asplenia (functional or anatomic)	Encapsulated organisms—e.g., *S. pneumoniae, H. influenzae, N. meningitidis.*
Chronic granulomatous disease	Catalase-⊕ organisms—e.g., *S. aureus, Aspergillus* spp., *Nocardia* spp., *Burkholderia cepacia.*
Cystic fibrosis	*Pseudomonas* spp., *S. aureus.*
Galactosemia	*E. coli* sepsis.
Myeloperoxidase deficiency	*Candida* spp.; deep infections.
Sickle cell disease and other hemoglobinopathies	See asplenia; *Salmonella* spp.
T-cell deficiencies (HIV/AIDS, SCID, DiGeorge syndrome)	*S. pneumoniae, Pneumocystis, Mycobacterium avium–intracellulare* (MAI), CMV (see the discussion of HIV for more details).
Terminal complement deficiency	Recurrent *Neisseria* spp.

Acute HIV infection can present as a flulike syndrome with fever, pharyngitis, myalgias, and diffuse lymphadenopathy and should particularly be considered in older children with risk factors. HIV antibody may be ⊖ with acute infection, and therefore HIV RNA should also be obtained.

For HIV-exposed neonate, viral diagnostic testing should be performed within 48 hours, 2 weeks (consider), 1–2 months, and 4–6 months of age. HIV infection can be reasonably excluded if an infant has had at least two negative virologic tests at ~ 1 month of age with at least one test performed at ~ 4 months of age.

DIAGNOSIS

- **Neonates:**
    - If an infant is shown to be HIV antibody ⊕ at birth, it confirms the mother's infection but does not necessarily indicate that the baby is infected.
    - Conversely, a ⊖ result could simply mean that the mother has not yet seroconverted and therefore does not refute infection in the baby.
    - HIV DNA PCR is preferred initially, as it may detect virus that may not yet have begun to replicate.
    - Screen by HIV RNA PCR and HIV antibody.
- **Beyond the peripartum period:**
    - **Dx:** HIV antibody by ELISA and confirmatory Western blot.
    - In children < 13 years of age, CD4 percentage is more reliable than CD4 count, with values < 15% categorized as severe suppression and values > 25% indicating no evidence of suppression. At 13 years of age, a CD4 percentage of < 15% corresponds to a CD4 count of < 200.

TREATMENT

HIV-exposed infants should receive the following:

- Zidovudine (AZT) starting at birth × 6 weeks.
- +/– nevirapine × 1–2 doses (controversial).

PREVENTION

In developed countries, perinatal transmission can be ↓ from approximately 35% to 5% or less with institution of the following measures:

- Highly active antiretroviral therapy (HAART) in the mother to suppress viral load.
- Peripartum AZT (initiated six weeks prior to delivery) and IV AZT given intrapartum.
- Elective C-section if viral activity in the mother is not suppressed at 38 weeks' gestation.
- **Note:** The use of nevirapine for the prevention of mother-to-child transmission of HIV is a controversial issue.

COMPLICATIONS

HIV-related opportunistic infections include the following:

- ***Pneumocystis carinii* pneumonia (PCP):** Recently renamed *P. jiroveci*, PCP is the most common initial manifestation of AIDS and is associated with an extremely high mortality rate, underscoring the importance of prophylaxis.
  - **Sx/Dx:** Infection presents with increasingly labored breathing and hypoxia with ground-glass infiltrates on CXR.
  - **Prevention:** TMP-SMX should be initiated at 4–6 weeks of age for the prevention of PCP. It should be noted, however, that severe anemia, GI symptoms, and hypersensitivity reactions can occur. TMP-SMX should also be avoided in patients with G6PD deficiency as well as in children < 2 months of age.
- Other opportunistic infections less commonly seen in infants include candidiasis, cryptococcosis, bacillary angiomatosis, toxoplasmosis, *Cryptosporidium*, MAI, CMV, and *Giardia*. There is also an ↑ risk of TB.

Neutropenic Fever

- Defined as a single oral temperature of 38.3°C or an oral temperature of 38.0°C for 1 hour in a patient who is neutropenic (neutrophil count < 500/mm^3). Chemotherapy-induced neutropenia is different from neutropenia resulting from other causes, since chemotherapy damages other mucosal surfaces (barriers), such as the GI tract. Chemotherapy also inhibits neutrophil function. The neutropenic nadir generally occurs 7–10 days after chemotherapy but depends on the regimen. Patients may also have indwelling catheters and skin breakdown. Therefore, the differential is very broad and includes gram-⊕ and gram-⊖ organisms as well as opportunistic fungi.
- **Sx/Exam:**
  - Neutropenic patients have minimal to absent signs of inflammation (e.g., pus, erythema).
  - Evaluation includes a thorough physical exam and history that should not include a rectal examination.
- **Tx:**
  - Empiric therapy includes use of a broad-spectrum antibiotic with antipseudomonal coverage (e.g., ceftazidime, cefepime, piperacillin/tazobactam). If the patient is toxic, an aminoglycoside may be added and vancomycin should be considered.
  - If the condition worsens in the next 72 hours, consider changing antimicrobials. If fever persists for five days or more, add an antifungal agent. Therapy should not be stopped until both fever and neutropenia have resolved.

- **Complications:** Patients with prolonged neutropenia who are on broad antibacterial coverage are especially prone to infections with filamentous fungi, including *Aspergillus*, *Mucor*, and *Rhizopus*. Voriconazole does not cover *Mucor* and *Rhizopus*.

LYME DISEASE

A zoonosis that is caused by *Borrelia burgdorferi*. Lyme disease is the most common tick-borne illness in the United States, where it is most often found in southern New England and the eastern mid-Atlantic states. Common vectors include the deer tick (*Ixodes scapularis*) in the Northeast and Midwest and the Western black-legged tick (*Ixodes pacificus*).

SYMPTOMS/EXAM

The disease is generally divided into three clinical stages with different presentations:

- **Early localized:** Presents with a single erythema migrans lesion ("bull's-eye" lesion; see Figure 12-2) as well as with regional lymphadenopathy and arthralgias.
- **Early disseminated:** Presents as single or multiple erythema migrans, radiculoneuritis (manifest as facial palsy), meningitis, and carditis.
- **Late:** Presents as arthritis that is usually mono- or pauciarticular and affects large joints.

DIAGNOSIS

- Testing for Lyme disease should be performed when specific symptoms and signs are present in consistent epidemiologic settings (e.g., location and time of the year).
- Testing includes an initial EIA for detection of antibodies followed by a confirmatory Western blot assay. This is necessary because EIA is fraught with false-⊕ results owing to cross-reactivity with other spirochetes (e.g., syphilis, leptospirosis, spirochetes of normal oral flora) and viral infections (e.g., varicella, autoimmune diseases such as SLE).

FIGURE 12-2. "Bull's-eye" lesion of Lyme disease.

(Reproduced, with permission, from Rudolph CD et al. *Rudolph's Pediatrics*, 21st ed. New York: McGraw-Hill, 2003, Color Plate 22.) (Also see Color Insert.)

- Antibody tests may be ⊖ in patients with early infection or in those treated with antibiotics early in the disease.
- There are several pitfalls inherent in serologic testing for Lyme disease, and therefore the results should be interpreted carefully even when the Western blot is ⊕.
- In addition, tests should be ordered only when there is sufficient cause to suspect Lyme disease on a clinical basis. Tests that are ⊕ in the setting of nonspecific symptoms such as fatigue, malaise, and headaches almost always yield false-⊕ results.
- Once the serologic tests become ⊕, they remain ⊕ for several months to years, making the diagnosis of a second episode very difficult.

TREATMENT

Treatment is dependent on the stage and form of the disease. In general, oral therapy with amoxicillin or doxycycline (for those ≥ 8 years of age) is sufficient.

- For early localized disease, oral treatment (14–21 days) is sufficient.
- Longer oral treatment (21–28 days) is required for multiple erythema migrans and isolated facial palsy (as part of early disseminated disease) as well as for arthritis (as part of late disease).
- Ceftriaxone is generally used for persistent or recurrent arthritis, carditis, and meningitis.

Consider bubonic plague in patients who have had contact with wild rodents and present with axillary and inguinal lymphadenopathy; also consider noninfectious causes (e.g., malignancy).

LYMPHADENITIS

Common causes and clinical presentations of lymphadenitis are outlined in Table 12-21.

PARASITIC INFECTIONS

 A three-year-old Caucasian male presents with perianal pruritus at night. Local examination reveals no lesions. What is the most likely diagnosis? The child most likely has pinworm.

Nematodes

PINWORM DISEASE (*ENTEROBIUS VERMICULARIS*)

- The most common helminthic infection in the United States; caused by ingestion of eggs.
- **Sx/Exam:** Patients present with perianal pruritus that is most prominent at night, when the adult female worm migrates to release eggs.
- **Dx:** Diagnosed through the detection of eggs on the skin (perianal area) with the "clear tape test."
- **Tx:** Treatment includes mebendazole or pyrantel pamoate.

ROUNDWORM DISEASE (*ASCARIS LUMBRICOIDES*)

- Caused by ingestion of eggs from soil contaminated by human feces. Seen in the southern United States.

TABLE 12-21. Causes and Clinical Presentation of Lymphadenitis

PATHOGENS	COMMENTS
Bartonella henselae (cat-scratch disease)	Enlargement of draining lymph nodes upstream from cat scratch; usually mildly painful. Suppuration can occur in up to one-third of cases; diagnosis is based on history, serology, and biopsy. Treatment is supportive, except in immunosuppressed patients or those with systemic illness (macrolides, doxycycline).
Cytomegalovirus (CMV)	Usually bilateral cervical adenopathy **(can be generalized)** in the setting of a viral syndrome, including pharyngitis and splenomegaly. Diagnosis is usually by serology—i.e., specific titers or Monospot test, which is usually $\ominus$ (see the discussion of viral syndromes).
Epstein-Barr virus (EBV)	Usually presents with bilateral cervical adenopathy **(can be generalized)** in the setting of a viral syndrome, including pharyngitis and splenomegaly. Diagnosis is usually by serology—i.e., Monospot or specific titers (see the discussion of viral syndromes for more details).
Gram-$\oplus$ organisms (*Streptococcus pyogenes*, group A streptococci, *S. aureus*)	Generally affect the cervical region, which is usually tender and highly inflamed; may be suppurative, especially with *S. aureus*. See the discussion of pharyngitis for more details about group A streptococci.
HIV	Presents with generalized painless lymphadenopathy as part of acute HIV (see the discussion of HIV for more details).
Mycobacterium spp.	Can be caused by *M. tuberculosis* or atypical mycobacteria such as MAI. The location is usually cervical with minimal inflammation, with the lymphadenitis typically described as "matted" nodes with overlying discoloration. A fistulous tract may be seen, as may superinfection with gram-$\oplus$ organisms. Diagnosis is made through consistent history, biopsy, and culture. Treatment depends on the organism isolated.
Toxoplasma gondii	Cervical or generalized; can be a part of a flulike syndrome. Diagnosis is based on a history of exposure and serology.

- **Sx/Exam:** Most infections are asymptomatic, but some may cause vague abdominal discomfort.
- **Dx:** Diagnosed through the detection of eggs in the stool.
- **Tx:** Treated with mebendazole or pyrantel pamoate.

HOOKWORM DISEASE (*ANCYLOSTOMA, NECATOR*)

- Caused by larval penetration of skin. *Necator* is endemic in the rural southern states.
- **Sx/Exam:** The disease leads to loss of blood in the intestines.
- **Dx:** Diagnosed through the detection of eggs in the stool.
- **Tx:** Treated with mebendazole or pyrantel pamoate.

Malaria

- Malaria is an important disease to consider in patients who present with fever and chills and have recently visited malaria-endemic areas (e.g., most parts of Africa, Southeast Asia, the Indian subcontinent, parts of the Middle East, South America, and the Caribbean).
- Transmitted by the bite of the female *Anopheles* mosquito; ultimately infects RBCs.
- **Sx/Exam:** Clinical manifestations may range from a spiking fever with chills to multiorgan system failure.
- **Dx:** Diagnosis is made by examining blood (thick and thin smears) for the parasite.
- **Tx:** Chloroquine-resistant malaria is becoming increasingly common in several parts of the world; antimalarial drugs are used in combination to treat such cases.
- **Prevention:** Chemoprophylaxis for travelers going to malaria-endemic areas is an important preventive measure.

RICKETTSIAL DISEASES

Rocky Mountain Spotted Fever (RMSF)

- RMSF is the most common fatal tick-borne disease in the United States. The causative organism is *Rickettsia rickettsii*, and transmission is mostly by the dog tick (*Dermacentor variabilis*).
- **Sx/Exam:** Clinical manifestations include **fever**, myalgia, and **rash** (a maculopapular rash involving the palms and soles that first appears on the extremities and then moves centrally) as well as CNS symptoms (lethargy, confusion), thrombocytopenia, leukopenia, hyponatremia, a sepsis-like syndrome, and multiorgan system dysfunction.
- **Dx:** Diagnosed by serology and immunofluorescence of the skin lesion (not very sensitive).
- **Tx:** Treated with doxycycline.

Ehrlichiosis

- Causative organisms are *Ehrlichia chaffeensis*, *Anaplasma phagocytophilum*, and *E. ewingii*; transmission is by the lone star (*Amblyomma* spp.) or deer tick (*Ixodes scapularis*).
- **Sx/Exam:** Presents as an acute febrile illness similar to RMSF, but with leukopenia, hyponatremia, hepatitis, thrombocytopenia, **fever,** and myalgia; less commonly, a variable **rash** may appear (approximately 60% of infected children present with a rash—as opposed to adults, in whom rash is less common). A sepsis-like syndrome and multiorgan system dysfunction may also be seen.
- **Dx:** Diagnosis is made by serology and by a peripheral blood smear showing a characteristic intraleukocytoplasmic cluster of bacteria called morulae.
- **Tx:** Treated with doxycycline.

If either ehrlichiosis or RMSF is suspected, they must be treated immediately, as both can be rapidly fatal, and waiting for a definitive diagnosis is not an option.

Chlamydia

- Chlamydia is caused by *Chlamydia trachomatis* and is one of the most common STIs in the United States, particularly among adolescents.
- Chlamydia can be transmitted perinatally and can persist until a child is roughly three years of age; therefore, a diagnosis of chlamydia in early childhood raises suspicion for, but does not automatically confirm, abuse.
- Sx/Exam:
  - Presents with a yellowish-greenish, mucopurulent discharge as well as with urethritis, cervicitis, endometritis, salpingitis, and epididymitis.
  - Chlamydial infection may be asymptomatic in women and is thus a leading cause of infertility and PID.
  - Other notable manifestations include the following:
    - **Lymphogranuloma venereum:** A suppurative, painful lymphatic infection of the femoral and/or inguinal nodes (usually unilateral) that follows the initial ulcerative genital lesion; more common in homosexual men.
    - **Reiter syndrome:** Characterized by the mnemonic "can't **pee** (urethritis), can't **see** (bilateral conjunctivitis), can't climb a **tree** (arthritis)."
  - Reinfection is very common, as the infection does not confer immunity.
- **Dx:** Diagnosed via antigen detection (EIA, DFA), DNA probe, PCR, or Giemsa staining of specimen.
- **Tx:**
  - A macrolide (e.g., azithromycin) and doxycycline are the treatments of choice.
  - When treating chlamydia, one should also treat for gonorrhea, as coinfection is common. Counseling and testing for other STIs and pregnancy should also be made available.

An 18-year-old girl presents to the adolescent clinic complaining of a vaginal discharge. She is sexually active and has recently been treated for gonorrhea with an oral drug whose name she cannot recall. She reports some relief followed by a recurrence of her symptoms. What factors could potentially explain her recurrence? The patient's symptom recurrence could be caused by medication noncompliance, an untreated sexual partner, reacquisition of her infection, or lack of treatment of concurrent chlamydia infection or fluoroquinolone-resistant gonorrhea.

Gonorrhea

- Sx/Exam:
  - **Females:** In postpubertal females, gonorrhea may present with vaginitis, cervicitis, erythema of the endocervix, dyspareunia, endometritis, salpingitis, urethritis, and proctitis. However, infection can often be **asymptomatic.** Extension of infection can → PID and perihepatitis (Fitz-Hugh–Curtis syndrome), which presents with RUQ abdominal discomfort.

- **Males:** Men are more commonly symptomatic, presenting with a yellowish-green mucopurulent discharge, urethritis, epididymitis, or proctitis.
    - Manifestations seen in both males and females include pharyngitis, arthritis (often sterile), and disseminated gonococcal infection → a maculopapular rash with necrosis, migratory arthritis, and tenosynovitis.
- **Dx:** Diagnosis is made by observation of gram-⊖ diplococci on a smear from an affected site as well as by nucleic amplification tests (PCR or ligase chain reaction assay).
- **Tx:**
    - An extended-spectrum cephalosporin (e.g., ceftriaxone) is the treatment of choice. Fluoroquinolones can be used in adults; however, resistance is emerging in certain parts of the country (e.g., Hawaii, the Pacific Islands, California).
    - Treatment for chlamydia should be instituted in both partners simultaneously; all sexual partners should be identified and treated.
- **Complications: Reinfection can occur.**

Unlike chlamydia, gonorrhea in a prepubertal child beyond the neonatal period is consistent with sexual abuse.

Pelvic Inflammatory Disease (PID)

- PID is usually a polymicrobial infection with causative organisms that include gonorrhea, chlamydia, and anaerobes.
- **Sx/Exam:** Signs and manifestations of PID include lower abdominal tenderness, cervical motion tenderness, adnexal tenderness, fever, and cervical/vaginal discharge.
- **Ddx:** The differential diagnosis of PID includes ectopic pregnancy, appendicitis, ovarian cyst (rupture, bleeding, torsion), dysmenorrhea, UTI, and endometriosis.
- **Dx:**
    - Diagnosis is based on a careful sexual history (often adolescents will not admit sexual activity or lack of protection); those with multiple partners or a history of IUD use are at ↑ risk.
    - Laboratory findings include ↑ WBC count, ↑ markers of inflammation, and culture/nucleic amplification testing that may be ⊕ for gonorrhea/chlamydia.
- **Tx:** Treatment varies according to the severity of disease.
    - **Outpatient:** Ceftriaxone IM plus doxycycline PO **or azithromycin.**
    - **Inpatient:** Ampicillin **plus** clindamycin **plus** gentamicin 2 **plus** doxycycline **or** azithromycin.
- **Prevention:** Pregnancy testing, testing for other STIs (e.g., syphilis, HIV), and counseling on safe-sex practices should be offered.
- **Complications:** Tubo-ovarian abscess, Fitz-Hugh–Curtis syndrome.

PID more commonly occurs after menses.

Human Papillomavirus (HPV)

- HPV has multiple serotypes, with serotypes 6 and 11 most often associated with genital warts and types 16, 18, and 31 associated with cervical cancer.
- **Sx/Exam:** Signs and manifestations include itching in the genital region and "genital warts" (pink or white cauliflower-like lesions; see Figure 12-3). HPV is associated with cervical and anal dysplasia and cancers. Lifelong infection can occur, with recurrences 2° to reactivation.

INFECTIOUS DISEASE

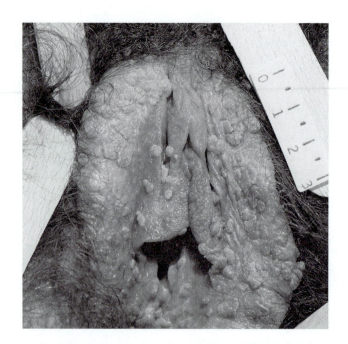

FIGURE 12-3. **Cauliflower-like lesions of HPV.**

(Reproduced, with permission, from Wolff K, Johnson RA, Suurmond D. *Fitzpatrick's Color Atlas & Synopsis of Clinical Dermatology*, 5th ed. New York: McGraw-Hill, 2005:889.) (Also see Color Insert.)

- **Dx:** Diagnosed by visualization of histopathologic changes characteristic of HPV and by DNA detection.
- **Tx:** Eliminate lesions (cryotherapy, podophyllin, salicylic acid). Spontaneous regression occurs in some cases, but monitoring and treatment are necessary for dysplasia.

Vaginitis

Vaginitis can be caused by a variety of pathogens, the most common of which are listed below and in Table 12-22.

TRICHOMONIASIS

- Caused by *Trichomonas vaginalis*, a flagellated protozoan.
- **Sx/Exam:** Presents with a gray-green, frothy vaginal discharge with vulvovaginal itching and a musty odor; a classic "strawberry cervix" is seen on exam along with erythema, friability, and petechiae. Most males are asymptomatic.
- **Dx:** A wet mount demonstrating motile flagella is diagnostic.
- **Tx:** Metronidazole should be given both to the patient and to sexual partners, as reinfection can occur.

BACTERIAL VAGINOSIS

- Most commonly caused by *Gardnerella vaginalis*.
- **Sx/Exam:** Presents with a white, thick, adherent vaginal discharge with a "fishy" odor; vaginitis and vulvitis may also be seen.

There is an ↑ risk of PID and preterm labor in patients with bacterial vaginosis.

TABLE 12-22. Causes of Vaginitis

	BACTERIAL VAGINOSIS	TRICHOMONAS	YEAST
Incidence	50% (most common).	25%.	25%.
Etiology	**Not an STI.** Caused by overgrowth of *Gardnerella* and other anaerobes.	Protozoal flagellates affect the vagina, Skene's duct, and lower urinary tract as well as the lower GU tract in men.	Not an STI. Usually *Candida.*
Risk factors	Pregnancy, IUD use, frequent douching.	Tobacco use, unprotected sex with multiple partners, IUD use.	**DM, antibiotic use, pregnancy, steroids,** HIV, OCP use, IUD use, young age at first intercourse, ↑ frequency of intercourse.
History	Odor.	Discharge.	Pruritus.
Exam	Mild vulvar irritation.	Strawberry petechiae in the upper vagina/cervix.	Erythematous, excoriated vulva/vagina.
Discharge	Homogenous, **grayish-white, fishy**/stale odor.	Profuse, malodorous, **yellow-green, frothy.**	Thick, white, **cottage-cheese texture.**
Vaginal pH	> 4.5 (5.0–6.0).	> 4.5 (5.0–7.0).	Normal.
Saline smear[a]	**"Clue cells"** (epithelial cells coated with bacteria).	**Motile trichomonads** (flagellated organisms that are slightly larger than WBCs).	Nothing.
KOH prep	⊕ whiff test (fishy smell).	Nothing.	Pseudohyphae.
Treatment	PO metronidazole or clindamycin × 7 days.	PO metronidazole. Treat partners and test for other STIs.	**Uncomplicated:** Topical azole × 1–3 days. **Complicated** (≥ 4 episodes in one year, noncandidal, HIV, DM, steroids, pregnancy): Two weeks of topical antifungals or fluconazole × 2 doses.
Complications	PID, endometritis, vaginal cuff cellulitis when invasive procedures are done (e.g., biopsy, C-section, IUD placement).		**No topical azole for pregnant women.**

[a] If there are many WBCs and no organism on saline smear, suspect *Chlamydia.*

Reproduced, with permission, from Le T et al. *First Aid for the USMLE Step 2 CK,* 5th ed. New York: McGraw-Hill, 2006:284.

- **Dx:** Diagnosed via wet mount showing clue cells with the addition of 10% KOH, a vaginal pH > 4.5, and a whiff test → a fishy odor with the addition of KOH.
- **Tx:** Treat with oral or intravaginal metronidazole.

Syphilis

- The causative organism is *Treponema pallidum*.
- **Sx/Exam:** Symptoms and manifestations are as follows:
    - **1°:** Presents with a **painless** ulcer (chancre) that is located at the site of inoculation and appears shortly (1–4 weeks) after infection (see Figure 12-4).
    - **2°:** Refers to the period 1–2 months after initial infection during which the patient can develop a maculopapular rash (including a rash on the palms and soles), generalized lymphadenopathy, fever, malaise, splenomegaly, constitutional symptoms, condylomata lata around the vulva or anus, and headache, which can be a sign of neurosyphilis.
    - **Latent period:** This is a period of varying length in which the patient remains asymptomatic.
    - **3°:** Characterized by gumma formation, cardiovascular syphilis (ascending aortic aneurysms), neurosyphilis (→ a generalized paresis with changes in affect, personality, and sensorium), and tabes dorsalis (demyelination of the posterior column and roots of the spinal cord).
- **Ddx:** RMSF also presents with a rash that involves the hands and the soles of the feet.
- **Dx:**
    - Diagnosed by visualization of spirochetes under darkfield microscopy and a ⊕ nontreponemal test (RPR, VDRL) followed by confirmatory treponemal testing (FTA-ABS).
    - Remember that the treponemal FTA-ABS will be ⊕ for life, while the nontreponemal test will ↓ with therapy (a fourfold ↓ in titer constitutes successful therapy) and can be used to monitor response to therapy as well as reinfection. The nontreponemal test can disappear over time and can ↑ with reexposure (patients can be reexposed and reinfected).

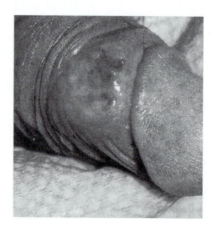

FIGURE 12-4. Primary syphilis.

(Reproduced, with permission, from Bondi EE. *Dermatology: Diagnosis & Therapy*. Stamford, CT: Appleton & Lange, 1991:394.) (Also see Color Insert.)

- Other factors that can cause $\oplus$ nontreponemal testing includes viruses (mononucleosis, hepatitis, varicella, measles), pregnancy, lymphoma, connective tissue disease, and $\oplus$ treponemal testing (Lyme disease and other spirochetal diseases).
- **Tx:** Treat with penicillin G parenterally; desensitization may be necessary in patients with penicillin allergy.

Herpes Simplex Virus (HSV)

- Genital herpes lesions are most commonly caused by HSV-2, but HSV-1 can → similar manifestations. Infection persists for life in the sensory (sacral) ganglia in the genital area.
- **Sx/Exam:**
  - Presents with vesicular/ulcerative lesions in the genital region.
  - Following the initial symptomatic infection, reactivation can occur asymptomatically, explaining why transmission can occur both sexually and perinatally in the absence of active lesions.
  - When recurrence occurs, it manifests as vesicular lesions on the genitalia and in the perineal region, often accompanied by pain or discomfort.
  - 1° genital infection with HSV-2 can be associated with self-limited meningitis with nonspecific clinical manifestations.
- **Dx:** HSV can be readily cultured in special viral culture media.
- **Tx:** Treated with acyclovir.

SHOCK AND SEPSIS

Toxic Shock Syndrome (TSS)

- TSS is an acute illness characterized by fever, rash, shock, and multiorgan system dysfunction. It is a toxin-mediated illness that is most commonly caused by S. aureus and Streptococcus pyogenes (group A streptococci). Its pathogenesis is thought to be related to a superantigen (toxin) → a cytokine storm that → capillary leakage and hypotension.
- **Sx/Exam:** Common clinical features include fever; a toxin-mediated, macular red rash that may subsequently desquamate; hypotension; and multiorgan system dysfunction that can manifest as renal and hepatic dysfunction, thrombocytopenia, myalgias (↑ CK), and mucosal inflammation (conjunctivitis, pharyngeal redness). Mucosal inflammation and myalgias are more common with S. aureus.
- **Dx:** Since this is a toxin-mediated illness, blood cultures may not definitively identify the causative agent, particularly with S. aureus.
- **Tx:** Treatment is supportive, and any source of infection should be debrided or removed. The choice of antibiotic therapy depends on the causative organism and includes use of vancomycin in areas with high MRSA prevalence. The use of adjunctive clindamycin should also be considered for the inhibition of toxin synthesis.

Think of S. aureus *TSS in females using tampons.*

Meningococcemia

- Meningococcemia is a fulminant illness with an acute onset followed by rapid progression. It is caused by *Neisseria meningitidis*.
- **Sx/Exam:** Characterized by fever, chills, malaise, and rash (maculopapular to petechial to purpuric; see Figure 12-5) rapidly progressing to shock,

341

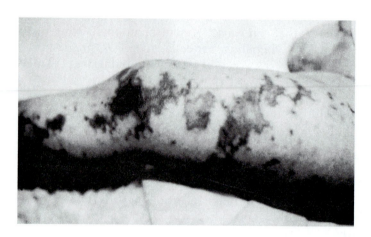

FIGURE 12-5. Characteristic rash of meningococcemia.

(Reproduced, with permission, from Freedberg IM et al. *Fitzpatrick's Dermatology in General Medicine*, 6th ed. New York: McGraw-Hill, 2003:1898.) (Also see Color Insert.)

DIC, coma, and death. Patients with terminal complement deficiencies and asplenia have a higher risk for this disease.

- **Dx:** Diagnosis is based on the clinical picture and on a culture of sterile sites, including skin lesions.
- **Tx:** Treatment includes supportive care and penicillin or third-generation cephalosporin.
- **Prevention:** Close contacts (including household members; day care/nursery school contacts; those who have had direct exposure to patient secretions via kissing, mouth-to-mouth resuscitation, and unprotected intubation; and those who frequently slept or ate in the same dwelling as the patient within seven days of the onset of illness) warrant chemoprophylaxis with rifampin, ceftriaxone, or ciprofloxacin (ciprofloxacin should be used only in nonpregnant adults).

Sepsis Syndromes and Empiric Therapy

Table 12-23 describes antimicrobial treatment regimens for sepsis syndromes.

In the differential diagnosis of sepsis, one should also consider overwhelming enteroviral sepsis in culture-⊖ neonatal infections that present with hepatitis, myocarditis, and/or encephalitis.

Most cases of enteric gram-⊖ bacteremia/sepsis require double coverage consisting of a cell wall–acting agent plus an aminoglycoside.

TABLE 12-23. Sepsis Syndromes and Empiric Therapy

GROUP	COMMON PATHOGENS	THERAPY
Community-acquired sepsis in a child	*S. pneumoniae, N. meningitidis, H. influenzae* type b (uncommon in the United States and in immunized children.	Ceftriaxone/cefotaxime +/– vancomycin.[a]
Sepsis in neonates	Group B streptococci, enteric gram-⊖ organisms (especially *E. coli*), *Listeria*.	Ampicillin + cefotaxime/aminoglycoside.

[a] Vancomycin should be considered in areas with high rates of pneumococcal resistance.

342

Scabies

- Caused by the adult form of the mite *Sarcoptes scabiei;* contracted through close personal contact.
- **Sx/Exam:** Clinical features include pruritic papules and burrows around the hand, especially the finger webs, wrists, axillae, and areolae (see Figure 12-6). Lesions are **intensely pruritic,** especially at night, and can also become superinfected.
- **Dx:** Diagnosis can be made clinically as well as by microscopic identification of the pathogen from skin scrapings.
- **Tx:** Topical application of 5% permethrin cream to all areas of the skin below the head is the treatment of choice. The medication is washed off 8–12 hours later and is then reapplied in 4–7 days. Successful treatment necessitates careful use and cleaning of all clothing, bedding, and the like. Family members and other close contacts must also be evaluated.

Lice

These insects attach themselves to the skin and release a salivary secretion that → pruritic dermatitis. Infection subtypes are as follows:

- **Pediculosis capitis:** Caused by *Pediculus humanus capitis;* commonly affects children. The treatment of choice is 1% permethrin cream that is applied to the hair and scalp and then washed off 10 minutes later. A second treatment is usually repeated 7–14 days later. Family members and close contacts should also be evaluated.

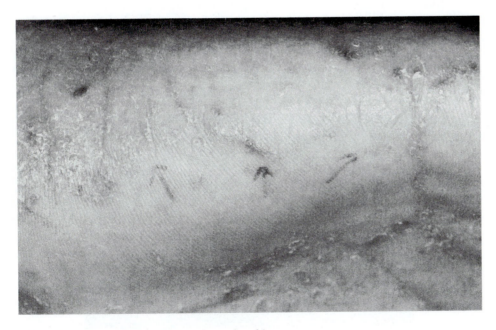

FIGURE 12-6. Characteristic lesions of scabies.

(Reproduced, with permission, from Wolff K, Johnson RA, Suurmond D. *Fitzpatrick's Color Atlas & Synopsis of Clinical Dermatology,* 5th ed. New York: McGraw-Hill, 2005:857.) (Also see Color Insert.)

INFECTIOUS DISEASE

- **Pediculosis corporis:** Caused by *Pediculus humanus corporis*; seen in people with very poor hygiene who do not change their clothes frequently.
- **Pediculosis pubis:** Caused by *Phthirus pubis*, which prefers to colonize areas of the body with shorter hair (e.g., pubic and axillary areas, eyelashes). It is spread primarily by sexual contact and fomites. Patients should thus be evaluated for other STIs. Treatment is similar to that for pediculosis capitis. Sexual partners should be treated simultaneously.

Tinea

- Tinea infections (e.g., ringworm, athlete's foot, jock itch) are superficial infections of the skin that are due to dermatophytic fungi.
- **Sx/Exam:**
  - Tinea lesions are characterized by pruritic papules and vesicles, broken hair, and thickened, broken nails (see Figure 12-7). Id lesions away from the 1° lesions are seen in some patients as a result of hypersensitivity to circulating antigen.
  - **Tinea versicolor** is caused by *Malassezia furfur* and presents as hypopigmented areas on the skin, usually occurring during the summer.
- **Dx:** Tinea infections are diagnosed clinically and by visualizing hyphae under the microscope from skin or nail scrapings treated with 10% KOH.
- **Tx:** Infections are treated topically with antifungal creams or systemically with griseofulvin (tinea capitis), generally for several weeks. Tinea versicolor is treated with topical antifungals.

*Several conditions ↓ response to the tuberculin skin test, and therefore **a nonreactive test does not exclude tuberculosis.***

TUBERCULIN SKIN TEST INTERPRETATION

- The tuberculin skin test determines whether an individual has latent TB (see Table 12-24). However, a ⊕ test **does not necessarily mean that the patient has active disease.**
- The standard PPD test uses five tuberculin units of PPD injected **intradermally** on the volar surface of the forearm, which raises a wheal 6–10 mm in size when administered appropriately. The diameter of **induration (not erythema)** is measured 48–72 hours after administration.

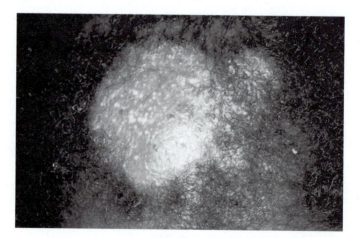

FIGURE 12-7. Characteristic lesions of tinea infection.

(Reproduced, with permission, from Freedberg IM et al. *Fitzpatrick's Dermatology in General Medicine*, 6th ed. New York: McGraw-Hill, 2003:1994.) (Also see Color Insert.)

TABLE 12-24. Tuberculin Skin Test

RISK CATEGORY	CUTOFF INDURATION (mm)
▪ Close contacts of known or suspected infectious cases of TB. ▪ Patient with suspected TB with: 　▪ Clinical evidence of TB disease. 　▪ Findings on CXR consistent with active or previously active TB. ▪ Immunosuppressed patients (e.g., those on immunosuppressive drugs, HIV patients).	≥ 5
▪ Patients with ↑ risk of dissemination: 　▪ Those < 4 years of age. 　▪ Those with concomitant medical conditions such as Hodgkin's disease, lymphoma, DM, malnutrition, and chronic renal failure. ▪ Patients with ↑ risk of exposure to TB: 　▪ Those born in a country with a high prevalence of TB. 　▪ Those who travel to a country with a high prevalence of TB. 　▪ Those with parents born in a country with a high prevalence of TB. 　▪ Those frequently exposed to adults with risk factors for TB, including the homeless, HIV-infected patients, illicit drug users, prisoners, and migrant farm workers.	≥ 10
▪ Children ≥ 4 years of age with no known risk factors.	≥ 15

UPPER RESPIRATORY TRACT INFECTIONS

Acute Pharyngitis

Table 12-25 distinguishes bacterial from viral pharyngitis.

TABLE 12-25. Differential Diagnosis of Pharyngitis

	GROUP A STREPTOCOCCAL PHARYNGITIS	VIRAL PHARYNGITIS
Causative organisms	Group A streptococci.	EBV, adenovirus, respiratory viruses, enterovirus.
Age	Mostly > 5 years.	All ages.
Symptoms	Acute onset; fever, severe sore throat, nausea, abdominal discomfort.	Less acute; variable fever, sore throat (often mild), myalgias, abdominal discomfort with certain viruses.
Exam	Palatal petechiae, pharyngeal erythema and exudates, tender cervical adenopathy, tonsillar hypertrophy, scarlet fever rash (sandpaper rash); no other symptoms (no cough, rhinitis, or conjunctivitis).	Pharyngeal erythema without exudates or ulcerative lesions; minimal adenopathy; variable tonsillar hypertrophy; variable exanthems; often presents with cough, rhinitis, and conjunctivitis.
Diagnosis	Rapid strep, throat culture.	Depends on the virus.
Treatment	Penicillin.	Supportive.
Complications	Rheumatic fever, poststreptococcal glomerulonephritis, reactive arthritis.	Depends on the virus; usually none.

INFECTIOUS DISEASE

Peritonsillar Abscess

Table 12-26 distinguishes peritonsillar from retropharyngeal and lateral pharyngeal abscess.

Otitis Externa

- Also called swimmer's ear; results from chronic irritation and maceration of the ear canal from excessive moisture. Most commonly caused by *Pseudomonas aeruginosa.* Other causative organisms include *S. aureus,* enteric gram-⊖ organisms, diphtheroids, and fungi such as *Candida* and *Aspergillus.*
- Sx/Exam:
  - Eczema can predispose to otitis externa, which presents as ear pain that is ↑ by application of pressure on the tragus. The pain may be greater than the observed inflammation because the skin is closely adherent to the underlying perichondrium.
  - There may also be conductive hearing loss due to edema and mechanical obstruction.
  - Rarely, facial nerve and other cranial nerve involvement may be seen; this is a medical emergency requiring IV antibiotics and possible surgical intervention.
- Tx: Treatment for otitis externa includes topical preparations consisting of neomycin and corticosteroids. If canal edema is marked, a wick can be inserted into the outer third of the canal and topical medication administered. Equally effective treatments are 2% acetic acid and half-strength Burow's solution.
- **Prevention:** Otitis externa can be prevented by instilling 2% acetic acid in the ear immediately after swimming or bathing.

TABLE 12-26. Differential Diagnosis of Tonsillar and Pharyngeal Abscess

	PERITONSILLAR ABSCESS	RETROPHARYNGEAL ABSCESS	LATERAL PHARYNGEAL ABSCESS
Age affected	Adolescents, adults.	< 14 years of age; usually < 4 years.	Older children (5–12 years of age), adolescents, adults.
Presentation	Tonsillar fullness, uvular deviation, muffled voice, odynophagia, trismus (difficulty opening the mouth).	Neck hyperextension, saliva pooling.	Swelling of the parotid area, trismus, prolapse of the tonsil and tonsillar fossa, septicemia.
Organisms	*Streptococcus* spp., *S. aureus,* anaerobes.	Same.	Same.
Treatment	Aspiration and drainage; antibiotics with coverage of typical pathogens (clindamycin, amoxicillin/clavulanic acid, nafcillin).	Same.	Same.

Acute Otitis Media

- Defined as inflammation of the middle ear. Bacterial causes include *S. pneumoniae* (25–50%), nontypable *H. influenzae* (15–30%), and *Moraxella catarrhalis* (3–20%).
- **Sx/Exam:** Patients present with fever, ear pain, and hearing loss.
- **Ddx:** Distinguish from serous otitis media, which involves the presence of fluid in the middle ear.
- **Dx:** Diagnosis requires a history of acute onset of signs and symptoms, the presence of middle ear effusion (bulging or limited motility of the tympanic membrane [TM]), an air-fluid level behind the TM, and signs of TM inflammation (e.g., erythema on exam or otalgia that → interference with normal activity or sleep).
- **Tx:**
  - Treatment includes use of analgesics when pain is present. Not all patients with acute otitis media require antimicrobials, and their use should be guided by the protocol listed in Table 12-27.
  - High-dose amoxicillin (80–90 mg/kg/day) is the initial antimicrobial choice. For severe illness, amoxicillin-clavulanate may be used instead.
  - The duration of therapy is 10 days for children < 5 years of age or for those with severe illness but 5–7 days for all others. If the patient cannot take oral medication, ceftriaxone IM can be used for three consecutive days.
  - Failure to respond in 48–72 hours can be managed as follows:
    - If no therapy was instituted initially, start antimicrobial therapy as indicated above.
    - If amoxicillin was used as initial therapy, switch to amoxicillin-clavulanate.
    - If amoxicillin-clavulanate was used as initial therapy, switch to ceftriaxone; alternatively, consider tympanocentesis.

Pertussis

- The causative organism is *Bordetella pertussis*, which is classically described as a gram-⊖ pleomorphic bacillus. It is transmitted by aerosolized droplets.
- An emerging issue is the problem of waning immunity among adolescents and young adults, who are most likely serving as the reservoir for the dis-

TABLE 12-27. Protocol for the Treatment of Acute Otitis Media

AGE	CONCLUSIVE DIAGNOSIS	INCONCLUSIVE DIAGNOSIS
< 6 months	Treat.	Treat.
6 months – 2 years	Treat.	May not treat; observe if not severe.[b]
> 2 years	May not treat; observe in the absence of severe illness.[a]	Observe.

[a] "Severe illness" is defined as moderate to severe otalgia or a fever ≥ 39°C.

[b] "Observe" means symptomatic relief only with deferral of antimicrobials and reevaluation at 48–72 hours.

ease and as transmitters for new infections to a younger, as-yet-unimmunized group. Recently, the Advisory Committee on Immunization Practices (ACIP) has recommended booster doses for adolescents.

- **Sx/Exam:**
  - Presents initially with mild upper respiratory symptoms but progresses to a cough that is classically described as paroxysms with a "whoop" at the end.
  - In infants, the disease can be associated with apnea, pneumonia, seizures, and encephalopathy (less commonly). Older children, particularly adolescents, can have atypical symptoms, most often prolonged cough without classic paroxysms.
- **Dx:** Diagnosed through DFA and PCR of nasopharyngeal secretions.
- **Tx:** Treated with macrolides, classically erythromycin, although azithromycin is associated with a similar level of efficacy. **Note:** Treatment that is initiated once the paroxysmal stage has begun does not shorten the duration of symptoms but ↓ bacterial shedding.
- **Prevention:**
  - Droplet precautions can prevent transmission.
  - Immunization is a significant preventive measure.
  - All household and close contacts should receive chemoprophylaxis (macrolides) to prevent transmission. Immunization should be administered to those who have not been fully immunized, and those who have not been vaccinated in the last three years should receive a booster.

Peripheral lymphocytosis is a classic finding in pertussis.

Sinusitis

- Acute sinusitis is defined as inflammation of the mucosa lining the sinuses.
- Some 5–10% of rhinitis cases in young children → acute sinusitis. Predisposing factors include cystic fibrosis, immotile cilia, mechanical defects in the nasopharynx, and immune disorders.
- Common causes include *S. pneumoniae*, nontypable *H. influenzae*, and *M. catarrhalis*. Less common causes include *S. aureus* and anaerobic bacteria, which generally cause long-standing sinusitis. *Pseudomonas* or other resistant organisms may be seen after multiple courses of antibiotics or with immunodeficiency.
- **Symptoms/Exam:**
  - Clinical manifestations of sinusitis include persistent nasal discharge and/or a cough that does not improve and is present for > 10 days. Severe symptoms include fever ≥ 39°C and purulent nasal discharge for > 3 days in addition to the above symptoms. Sinus headache or facial pressure may be present.
  - Examination reveals copious mucopurulent discharge accompanied by acute or serous otitis media and possibly tenderness over the paranasal sinuses.
- **Dx:** Diagnosis is usually clinical. A plain radiograph may be useful in patients > 6 years of age or in those with severe symptoms and may show mucosal thickening, complete opacification of the sinuses, or air-fluid level.
- **Tx:** Antimicrobial treatment includes high-dose amoxicillin, high-dose amoxicillin-clavulanate, or cefuroxime axetil. The last two should be considered in patients who do not improve with amoxicillin; those with *H. influenzae* and *M. catarrhalis* characterized by high β-lactamase production; and those with frontal/sphenoidal sinusitis or severe sinusitis.

- **Complications:** Common complications include subperiosteal abscess of the orbit and intracranial abscess.

- UTIs are a significant cause of FUO in young children and are more common among females. Common causes include enteric gram-⊖ organisms (e.g., *E. coli*, *Proteus* spp.). In postpubertal females, *Staphylococcus saprophyticus* should also be considered.
- **Sx/Exam:** Symptoms of UTI include fever, irritability, vomiting, and changes in urine color or odor. In older patients, urgency, ↑ frequency, abdominal pain, and dysuria are commonly seen.
- **Ddx:** Clinically, cystitis is differentiated from pyelonephritis by the absence of fever.
- **Dx:**
  - Diagnosis is made clinically as well as by urine analysis (↑ WBC count, presence of leukocyte esterase and nitrites) and culture (see Table 12-28).
  - Diagnostic imaging is required for young children with UTIs because of the potential for congenital or acquired abnormalities such as reflux and posterior urethral valves (in males). Imaging studies (renal ultrasound, voiding cystourethrography) are indicated with the first documented UTI in males and females < 5 years of age, and if anatomic or functional anomalies are found, their functional status should be further evaluated (via DMSA or an equivalent scan).
- **Tx:**
  - Management depends on the pathogen and on patient age. Generally, young children should receive parenteral therapy, whereas empiric outpatient antibiotics (e.g., TMP-SMX) may be appropriate for older children.
  - Patients with documented anomalies or frequent recurrences should be placed on prophylactic antibiotics (e.g., amoxicillin, TMP-SMX, nitrofurantoin).

TABLE 12-28. Diagnostic Criteria for the Evaluation of UTI

SPECIMEN	COLONY COUNT	PROBABILITY OF UTI (%)
Clean catch	Male: > 10,000	Infection likely
	Female: > 100,000	Infection likely
	10,000–100,000	Repeat culture
	< 10,000	Infection unlikely
Suprapubic	Gram-⊖ bacilli: any number	> 99%
	Gram-⊕ cocci: more than a few thousand	
Transurethral catheterization	> 100,000	95%
	10,000–100,000	Infection likely
	1000–10,000	Repeat culture
	< 1000	Infection unlikely

INFECTIOUS DISEASE

The common pediatric viral syndromes described below are diagnosed clinically and generally do not require any additional laboratory testing.

Coxsackievirus A16

- Also known as hand-foot-mouth disease. Transmitted by the fecal-oral route; peak incidence is in the summer and early fall.
- Sx/Exam:
  - Characterized by a brief prodrome with low-grade fever, malaise, sore throat, and anorexia followed 24–48 hours later by oral and skin lesions (erythematous, macular lesions on the palmar and plantar surfaces → gray vesicular lesions on an erythematous base appearing on the extremities and oral mucosa; see Figure 12-8).
  - May also present with herpangina (isolated oral lesions).
- **Tx:** Treatment is supportive.

Cytomegalovirus (CMV)

- Transmitted by saliva and blood; also transmitted perinatally. Seronegative pregnant women should avoid exposure to infected patients given the risk of congenital infection.
- Sx/Exam:
  - Most infections are asymptomatic; however, mononucleosis-like syndromes are characterized by fever, cervical or generalized lymphadenopathy, sore throat, fatigue, malaise, and hepatosplenomegaly.
  - In immunocompromised hosts, the disease can be severe and can include pneumonia, retinitis, thrombocytopenia, and colitis (see the discussion of congenital infections in neonates).
- **Dx:** Diagnosed by serology, culture, and a ⊖ Monospot; consider PCR in immunocompromised patients.
- **Tx:** Treatment is supportive unless patients are immunocompromised (e.g., transplant and HIV-⊕ patients), in which case ganciclovir is indicated.

Epstein-Barr Virus (EBV)

- Causes infectious mononucleosis, which is classically called the "kissing disease" because it often transmitted by intimate oral contact (e.g., sharing saliva through kissing, using the same eating utensils).
- Other EBV-associated conditions include post-transplant lymphoproliferative disease, Burkitt's lymphoma, nasopharyngeal carcinoma, and X-linked lymphoproliferative disease.
- Sx/Exam: Characterized by fever, exudative pharyngitis, cervical or generalized lymphadenopathy (can be significant tonsillar hypertrophy that can → airway obstruction), fatigue, malaise, splenomegaly, transaminitis, and exanthema (a diffuse, erythematous, maculopapular rash). Classic manifestations of infectious mononucleosis are most often seen in older children and adolescents, whereas in young children the disease often goes unrecognized.
- **Dx:** Diagnosed by serology and a ⊕ Monospot (see Table 12-29).

A child who is suspected of having streptococcal pharyngitis, and who develops a diffuse maculopapular rash after being administered antibiotics, is likely to have EBV.

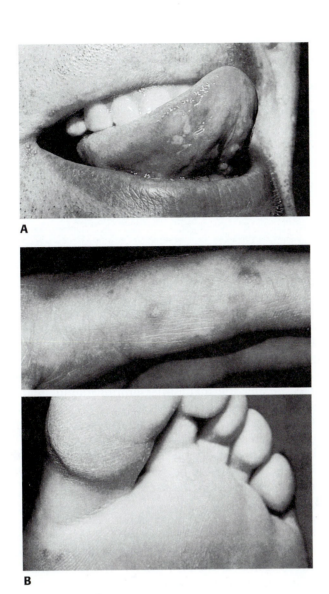

A

B

FIGURE 12-8. Characteristic lesions of coxsackievirus.

(A) Shallow ulcerations on the tongue. (B) Vesicular and popular lesions on the fingers and feet. (Reproduced, with permission, from Freedberg IM et al. *Fitzpatrick's Dermatology in General Medicine,* 6th ed. New York: McGraw-Hill, 2003:2050.) (Also see Color Insert.)

- **Tx:** Treatment is supportive. Initiate airway management in the presence of significant tonsillar hypertrophy; steroids may be needed. Patients should avoid contact sports if splenomegaly is present.

Human Herpesvirus 6 (HHV-6)

- Causes roseola infantum and exanthema subitum. Transmission occurs more commonly in late fall and early spring. Frequently affects children six months to three years of age.
- **Sx/Exam:** Classically characterized by rapid temperature elevation (≥ 39°C) followed by a erythematous maculopapular rash, with defervescence occurring within 72 hours. Patients do not appear toxic.
- **Tx:** Treatment is supportive.

HHV-6 is a common and important cause of febrile seizures.

TABLE 12-29. Laboratory Diagnosis of EBV

INFECTION	VIRAL CAPSID ANTIGEN (VCA) IgG	VCA IgM	EARLY ANTIGEN	EBV NUCLEAR ANTIGEN
No previous infection	–	–	–	–
Acute infection	+	+	+/–	–
Recent infection	+	+/–	+/–	+/–
Past infection	+	–	–	+

Influenza Virus

- Transmitted by respiratory droplet and contact with fomites. Peak incidence is in the winter months. The incubation period is 1–3 days, and patients are most infectious 24 hours prior to the onset of symptoms, with shedding continuing until seven days after symptom onset.
- Patients are predisposed to bacterial pneumonia with *Streptococcus pneumoniae* and *S. aureus*; the highest-risk groups include young and old patients as well as the immunocompromised.
- **Sx/Exam:** Characterized by sudden onset of fever, chills, diffuse myalgias, upper respiratory symptoms, headache, and malaise. Less common manifestations include Reye syndrome (encephalopathy and noninflammatory hepatic dysfunction; thought to be associated with the administration of aspirin in patients with influenza), encephalitis, myocarditis, myositis, and Guillain-Barré syndrome.
- **Dx:** Diagnosed via rapid antigen detection and culture.
- **Tx:**
  - The illness is usually self-limited, but its duration can be shortened by the administration of antivirals within 48 hours of symptom onset.
  - Amantadine and rimantadine are effective only against influenza A, while oseltamivir and zanamivir are effective against both influenza A and influenza B. Zanamivir is not approved for patients < 7 years of age; oseltamivir is not approved for patients < 1 year.
  - Therapy should be considered in healthy children with severe disease or in patients at risk for developing severe disease (e.g., immunocompromised patients, those with cardiopulmonary disease). Chemoprophylaxis is indicated in susceptible patients who are at high risk for developing severe disease or for those who are exposed during an outbreak.

Once the fever of rubeola peaks, it usually resolves rapidly. Therefore, the persistence of fever is an indicator of 2° bacterial infection.

Measles Virus (Rubeola)

- Transmitted by respiratory droplet. Patients are contagious from 1–2 days prior to the development of symptoms (3–5 days prior to the development of rash) until four days after the development of rash.
- **Sx/Exam:**
  - Characterized by fever, cough, coryza, conjunctivitis, an erythematous maculopapular rash (see Figure 12-9), and Koplik's spots (white, macular 1-mm lesions on the buccal mucosa).
  - After an incubation period of 8–12 days, fever, respiratory symptoms, and nonpurulent conjunctivitis develop, followed in 2–3 days by Kop-

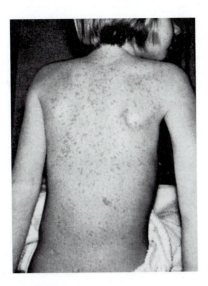

FIGURE 12-9. Generalized maculopapular rash of measles.

(Reproduced, with permission, from Freedberg IM et al. *Fitzpatrick's Dermatology in General Medicine*, 6th ed. New York: McGraw-Hill, 2003:2046.) (Also see Color Insert.)

lik's spots and subsequently (2–3 days later) by a generalized exanthem (forehead → trunk and extremities) that disappears in the same order 2–3 days later.

- **Tx:** Treatment is supportive; treat superinfection. Give vitamin A for severe measles. Postexposure prophylaxis is indicated for susceptible contacts (see the discussion of immunization).

Parvovirus B19

- Causes erythema infectiosum (fifth disease), which is transmitted by respiratory secretions and most often seen in preschool or school-age children.
- **Sx/Exam:**
  - Presents with arthropathy as well as with an exanthem that classically begins with a "slapped-cheek" appearance and develops into a lacy, erythematous rash on the extremities and extensor surfaces. Generally not associated with fever or constitutional symptoms.
  - Other manifestations include aplastic anemia, particularly in patients with ↓ RBC life spans, such as those with sickle cell anemia and other hemoglobinopathies, arthralgias, and nonimmune hydrops fetalis.
- **Dx:** Diagnosed by serology.
- **Tx:** Treatment is supportive.

Respiratory Syncytial Virus (RSV)

- Transmitted by respiratory droplets and fomites.
- **Symptoms/Exam:** An acute respiratory tract illness characterized by coryza, fever, and cough. In infants and young children, RSV is an important cause of bronchiolitis and pneumonia. It is also implicated as a cause of apnea.
- **Diagnosis:** Diagnosed by rapid antigen detection and culture.

Measles has a significant incidence in the developing world, where vaccination is not standard.

■ **Tx:** Treatment is supportive; palivizumab (a monoclonal RSV antibody) is indicated for patients at high risk of developing severe disease (e.g., those with cardiopulmonary disease and premature infants). Palivizumab is administered IM on a monthly basis during the RSV season (which may vary geographically) to high-risk patients.

Rubella (German Measles)

■ Transmitted by respiratory droplet. Rubella is an important cause of congenital infection.
■ **Sx/Exam:**
  ■ Characterized in older children by a prodrome of low-grade fever, occipital lymphadenopathy, sore throat, and coryza followed by a fine, erythematous maculopapular rash. The rash spreads to the face and then to the trunk and extremities, becoming generalized by 24 hours and resolving within 72 hours. A prodrome is not commonly seen in young children.
  ■ Other manifestations include arthritis and arthralgias, which are common in young female patients.
  ■ Some 25% of patients are asymptomatic but can transmit the disease.
■ **Tx:** Treatment is supportive.

Varicella-Zoster Virus (VZV)

■ Also known as chickenpox; transmitted by respiratory droplet and direct contact. The incubation period is 10–21 days; patients are infectious 1–2 days prior to the development of lesions until all lesions crust over.
■ **Symptoms/Exam:**
  ■ Presents with fever, coryza, and a progressive rash that is classically described as "dewdrops on a rose petal" (vesicles on an erythematous base).
  ■ The rash progresses from the trunk and scalp to the extremities (see Figure 12-10) and is characterized by crops of vesicles in different

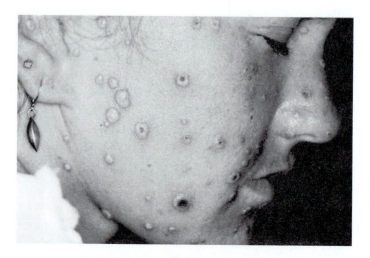

FIGURE 12-10. **Characteristic rash of varicella-zoster virus.**

(Reproduced, with permission, from Freedberg IM et al. *Fitzpatrick's Dermatology in General Medicine*, 6th ed. New York: McGraw-Hill, 2003:2074.) (Also see Color Insert.)

stages of healing, which effectively differentiates it from that of small-pox (in which the rash is in a uniform stage of healing). The rash of chickenpox is profoundly pruritic.

- Other manifestations include Reye syndrome (encephalopathy and noninflammatory hepatic dysfunction; thought to be associated with the administration of aspirin in patients with varicella), hepatitis, encephalitis, Guillain-Barré syndrome, and zoster (reactivation of varicella in a dermatomal distribution, often presenting with pain).
- **Tx:** Treatment is supportive; acyclovir may be given to immunocompromised patients and neonates.
- **Prevention:** Postexposure prophylaxis is indicated for susceptible contacts.
- **Complications:** Varicella rash tends to be worse in patients with prior skin conditions such as eczema. In patients with deficient cellular immunity, varicella is a severe and often fatal disease. Varicella can be complicated by superinfection with group A streptococci.

CHAPTER 13

The Musculoskeletal System and Sports Medicine

Maria Karapelou Brown, MD
reviewed by Teri M. McCambridge, MD

Developmental Dysplasia of the Hip (DDH)

A relatively common (1 in 1000 live births) spectrum of abnormalities that cause varying degrees of displacement of the proximal femur from the acetabulum. The hip may be unstable, partially dislocated (subluxation), or completely dislocated (luxation). DDH is not just congenital but can evolve over time and may arise at any point from infancy to childhood. Risk factors include female gender, Caucasian descent, first-born status, breech, and a ⊕ family history. It is more common in the left hip.

SYMPTOMS/EXAM

- Presents with an asymmetric number of skin folds in the thighs.
- **Allis' or Galeazzi sign:** Discrepant height of flexed thighs. The affected limb is shortened (see Figure 13-1).
- **Abduction/adduction:** Hips have < 75 degrees of abduction and < 30 degrees of adduction.
- **Provocative tests:** Most helpful before three months of age. With the infant supine on a firm surface, place fingers on the greater trochanters and thumbs on the knees.
- **Barlow's sign:** A ⊕ sign is **hip dislocation** and **clunk** with adduction of the legs and pushing down on the knees.
- **Ortolani's sign:** A ⊕ sign is **hip relocation** and **clunk** with abduction of the legs and lifting up on the trochanters.

DIAGNOSIS

Ultrasound is the screening modality of choice for infants < 4–6 months of age. Plain films can be used in infants > 6 months of age.

TREATMENT

The goal is to relocate and stabilize the femoral head in the acetabulum. In infants < 6 months, a Pavlik harness is used. After 6–12 months of age, a body cast is necessary. For infants > 1 year of age, surgery is likely required.

High-pitched clicks are commonly elicited in exam for DDH but are inconsequential.

Consider obtaining an ultrasound to screen girls born breech for DDH.

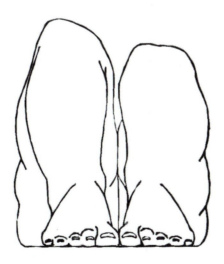

FIGURE 13-1. The Galeazzi test.

(Reproduced, with permission, from Rudolph AM et al. *Rudolph's Pediatrics*, 20th ed. Stamford, CT: Appleton & Lange, 1996:2136.)

THE MUSCULOSKELETAL SYSTEM
AND SPORTS MEDICINE

If left untreated, DDH can cause early degenerative hip arthritis.

> The parents of a two-week-old child seek evaluation of a previously healthy male infant who has a "lump" on his neck and apparent stiffness. They are concerned that the infant may have an infection or a tumor. What evaluation is necessary? For an afebrile well child with a normal neurologic exam, obtain cervical spine films. If these are normal, the child most likely has congenital torticollis.

Congenital Torticollis (Wry Neck)

Torticollis is the finding of a tilted and rotated neck. The most common cause of congenital torticollis is congenital muscular torticollis. The etiology is unknown, but its incidence is higher in children with breech presentation and forceps delivery.

SYMPTOMS/EXAM

Contracture of the sternocleidomastoid (SCM) muscle causes the head to *tilt* toward the affected side and *rotate* toward the unaffected side (the SCM flexes and contralaterally rotates neck). At 1–4 weeks of age, a well-circumscribed, firm lump or swelling ("tumor of SCM") may be felt in the muscle, which usually disappears within a few weeks.

DIFFERENTIAL

- **Benign paroxysmal torticollis:** Seizure-like episodes where intermittent torticollis is accompanied by vomiting, pallor, irritability, ataxia, or drowsiness.
- Congenital anomalies of the base of the skull.
- **Klippel-Feil syndrome:** Congenital fusion of cervical vertebrae.
- **Ocular disorders:** Children with disorders of ocular motility or alignment may tilt their heads to avoid diplopia.
- Brachial plexus palsy.

DIAGNOSIS

- Obtain AP and lateral radiographs of the cervical spine to rule out C1–C2 subluxation and underlying bony abnormalities.
- Associated disorders include DDH, metatarsus adductus, talipes equinovarus, C1–C2 subluxation, and plagiocephaly.

TREATMENT

After ruling out alternative diagnoses with C-spine radiographs, treat with frequent stretching exercises that tilt and rotate the head. If the condition persists after 12–18 months, surgical release may be required.

Foot Abnormalities

CLUBFOOT (TALIPES EQUINOVARUS)

Has four components: plantar flexion (equinus) of the ankle; adduction of hindfoot and forefoot (varu); plantar flexion of ankle (equinus); and arched midfoot (cavus) (see Figure 13-2 for an image of clubfeet). The tarsal bones are misshapen, irregular, and smaller in the affected foot. There is also ↓ musculature in the posterior compartment of the leg. The male-to-female ratio is 2:1, and there is an ↑ risk in those with a ⊕ family history. Most cases are idiopathic, but clubfoot can also be part of a syndrome or a neuromuscular disorder.

DIAGNOSIS

Consider radiographs.

TREATMENT

- Manipulation and casting are done immediately after diagnosis for 2–4 months.
- The success rate is 25%, with the remaining cases requiring surgery that lengthens or releases contracted tendons and ligaments.

OTHER ABNORMALITIES

- **Cavus foot:** A high-arched foot that is usually an inherited variation of normal; requires no treatment. Cases that are new onset, unilateral, or painful may point to other neurologic problems.
- **Calcaneovalgus foot:** Usually a packaging defect that resolves with time and spontaneously corrects.
- **Pes planus:** Commonly known as "flatfoot." Not a serious condition; shoe inserts may be used for patients with foot or knee pain.

There is an association between clubfoot and DDH, so carefully screen all children with clubfoot for DDH.

It is important to explain to parents of children with clubfoot that the affected foot and calf will always be smaller and less flexible than those of the unaffected side.

Clubfoot is NOT a packaging defect.

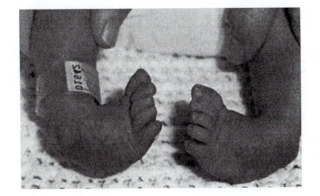

FIGURE 13-2. Bilateral clubfeet.

(Reproduced, with permission, from Rudolph CD et al. *Rudolph's Pediatrics*, 21st ed. New York: McGraw-Hill, 2002:2425.)

THE MUSCULOSKELETAL SYSTEM AND SPORTS MEDICINE

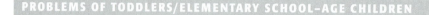

An asymmetric unilateral, painful or progressive angular deformity may be pathologic.

Tibial torsion is the most common cause of intoeing in children < 3 years. Medial femoral torsion is the most common cause of intoeing in children > 3 years.

Rotational Deformities

INTOEING

- Commonly referred to as "pigeon-toed"; the foot is turned in (see Table 13-1).
- More common than outtoeing.

SYMPTOMS/EXAM

- **Assess the foot progression angle:** This is the direction in which the child's feet point when he walks. Most adults have more than a 10-degree angle. Intoeing has a "negative" direction; outtoeing has a "positive" direction.
- **Assess for metatarsal adduction:** The heel bisector should be between the second and third rays of the foot.
- **Measure internal and external hip rotation:** Children > 2 years have a 50-degree internal rotation and 40-degree external rotation.

DIFFERENTIAL

Clubfoot.

DIAGNOSIS/TREATMENT

Table 13-1 outlines the presentation, diagnosis, and treatment of intoeing.

A two-year-old presents for a routine physical examination. You find that the child's left leg is bowed. The parents are not concerned because they are bowlegged as well. Should you reassure them that the child is normal? No, because the finding is unilateral. Radiographs should be obtained.

OUTTOEING

Results from an in utero packaging defect. Much less common than intoeing; usually improves within the first year of walking.

Angular Deformities

Two principal subtypes are genu varum (bowlegs) and genu valgum (knock-knees), both of which are usually variations of normal. Babies are born bowlegged, but by 2–3 years of age, most children are maximally knock-kneed and correct to a minimally knock-kneed adult position by seven years of age.

DIFFERENTIAL

Blount disease (tibia vara, an idiopathic deficiency in the medial tibial growth plate); tumor, infection, rickets, renal disease, dysplasias.

DIAGNOSIS

Radiographs are not necessary unless pathology is suspected.

Consider the possibility that an angular deformity is pathologic if it is asymmetric, unilateral, or painful or if it has an unexpected progression.

TABLE 13-1. Common Causes of Intoeing

	POINT OF ORIGIN	ETIOLOGY	SIGNS/EXAM	TREATMENT
Metatarsus adductus	Foot	Packaging defect; female > male, left > right.	Convexity along the lateral border.	**Actively correctable:** Baby straightens foot in response to tickling along the lateral border. Spontaneouly corrects. **Passively correctable:** Corrects with gentle pressure. Treatment is stretching exercises. **Uncorrectable:** Fails to correct after eight months of stretching. Requires casting.
Tibial torsion	Between the knee and ankle	Packaging defect; male = female.	Noticed by parents when the child begins to stand or walk.	Improves gradually within the first year of ambulation but may take up to eight years to completely correct.
Medial femoral torsion (femoral anteversion)	Between the knee and hip	Possibly acquired.	Sitting in the "W" position, increased internal rotation > 90 degrees.	Corrects spontaneously but slowly until age 8–10 years.

TREATMENT

Surgical correction of pathologic anomalies only.

Nursemaid's Elbow (Subluxation of the Radial Head)

The most common elbow injury in children < 5 years of age; associated with ↑ ligamentous laxity. The mechanism of injury is caused by a pull on the extended, pronated forearm. The annular ligament slips between the radius and ulna.

SYMPTOMS/EXAM

- The child will cry immediately after injury and not use the injured arm.
- Afterward, the child will be reluctant to use the arm but will not otherwise be in distress.
- On exam, the arm is held by the side with the elbow slightly flexed and the arm pronated. Tenderness over the radial head and resistance on attempted supination of the forearm are the only consistent findings. The child cannot supinate or fully flex the elbow.

DIAGNOSIS

Radiographs are not necessary but are normal if obtained.

In nursemaid's elbow, there is no tenderness or swelling of the elbow. If these symptoms are present, reduction should not be done and radiographs should be obtained.

- **Reduction:** Place the thumb over the radial head and supinate the forearm. If this fails, flex the elbow. Resistance may be perceived just before reaching full flexion; as the elbow is pushed through resistance, flex and supinate forearm. A palpable click is felt with reduction.
- If reduction is successful, the child will begin to use the affected extremity normally within a few minutes.

Legg-Calvé-Perthes Disease

Avascular necrosis of the femoral head. Occurs in children 2–12 years of age, typically in boys ages 4–8 years. Rare in African-Americans.

SYMPTOMS

The typical presentation is that of a child with limp. There is minimal pain in the groin and proximal thigh.

EXAM

Restriction of hip motion, especially abduction.

DIFFERENTIAL

Septic arthritis, Gaucher's disease, hypothyroidism, sickle cell disease, transient synovitis, epiphyseal dysplasias. See Table 13-3 for differential diagnosis of limp.

DIAGNOSIS

AP and frog-lateral radiographs of the pelvis (see Figure 13-3).

TREATMENT

- The goal is to contain the femoral head within the acetabulum and to maintain range of motion (ROM).
- For children < 6 years of age who lack significant subluxation and who have at least 40–45 degrees of abduction, observation is acceptable.
- For children > 6 years of age, containment with a brace is recommended until reossification or surgery.

Children with Legg-Calvé-Perthes disease who have bilateral hip involvement should have screening radiographs of the hand and knee to rule out skeletal dysplasia or hemoglobinopathy.

Perthes is **P**ainless.

THE MUSCULOSKELETAL SYSTEM AND SPORTS MEDICINE

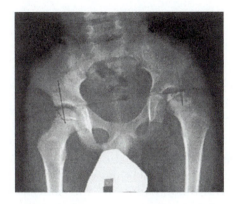

FIGURE 13-3. AP view of Legg-Calvé-Perthes disease with subluxation of the left hip.

(Reproduced, with permission, from Rudolph CD et al. *Rudolph's Pediatrics*, 21st ed. New York: McGraw-Hill, 2002:2438.)

Limp

Defined as uneven gait. Has a large differential diagnosis (see Table 13-2). The history should include the following:

- History of trauma or new activity.
- **Duration and course:**
  - Location/severity.
  - Effect on daily activities.
  - Use of new or poorly fitting shoes.
- **Associated symptoms:** Fever, anorexia, weight loss, back pain, arthralgia, incontinence.
- **Other factors:**
  - Recent viral or streptococcal infection.
  - New or ↑ sports activity.
  - Recent IM injection (can cause muscle inflammation or sterile abscess).

Hip pain is often referred from the knee.

TABLE 13-2. Presentation of Limp by Etiology

CONDITION	PRESENTATION
Juvenile rheumatoid arthritis (JRA), Legg-Calvé-Perthes disease, slipped capital femoral epiphysis (SCFE), Osgood-Schlatter disease, toxic synovitis	Pain is intermittent and mild to severe.
Fractures, dislocations, septic arthritis, osteomyelitis, sickle cell crisis	Pain is severe, constant, localized, and consistently reproducible.
Rheumatologic disorders	Symptoms are worse in morning and improve with activity.
Overuse injury	Pain/limp worsen with activity.
Neoplastic conditions	Nighttime symptoms that awaken the child.

CAUSES OF LIMP— STIFF SOLI

Sprain/**S**train

Tumor

Infected skin, soft tissue, bone, or joint

Fracture

Foreign body

SCFE and **S**ickle cell pain crisis

Overuse

Legg-Calvé-Perthes

Inflammation of bone or joints (JRA, SLE, toxic synovitis)

Initial x-rays may be normal in stress fractures, Salter-Harris type I fractures, early osteomyelitis, and septic arthritis.

- Endocrine dysfunction.
- A ⊕ family history of connective tissue disease, IBD, hemoglobinopathy, bleeding diatheses, or neuromuscular disorders.

SYMPTOMS

Symptoms vary with etiology (see Table 13-2).

EXAM

- Examination should include evaluation for rash, muscle strength, atrophy, joint tenderness, bony tenderness, bony deformity, joint effusion, active and passive ROM, inflammation of the joints/tendons/muscles, limb length discrepancy, and hip rotation.
- The soles of the feet should be examined for foreign bodies or calluses, and the shoes should be examined for wear pattern.
- Skin should be examined for rashes.

DIFFERENTIAL

See Table 13-3 for the differential diagnosis of a limp.

DIAGNOSIS

- Obtain AP and frog-lateral radiographs of pelvis.
- Consider ultrasound or MRI when plain x-rays are normal but suspicion of septic arthritis or transient synovitis is high.
- Laboratory evaluation is usually not indicated in an afebrile child with a normal physical exam, although CBC, ESR, and CRP may be helpful if history and physical are inconclusive.

TABLE 13-3. **Differential Diagnosis of Limp**

TYPE	EXAMPLES
Traumatic	Sprain/strain; contusion; fracture; foreign body, especially in the plantar surface of the foot; calluses/corns/ingrown toenails; poorly fitting shoes; stress fractures.
Infectious	Soft tissue or cutaneous infection, osteomyelitis, septic arthritis, appendicitis, Guillain-Barré syndrome, diskitis, myositis, gonococcal arthritis.
Inflammatory	Toxic synovitis of the hip, JRA, SLE, acute rheumatic fever.
Vascular	Legg-Calvé-Perthes disease, hemophilia, sickle cell vaso-occlusive crisis.
Overuse	Osgood-Schlatter disease, chondromalacia patellae, osteochondritis dissecans, shin splints, tendonitis.
Neoplastic	Leukemia, osteochondroma, osteogenic sarcoma.
Degenerative	SCFE.

- Obtain synovial fluid if septic joint is suspected because of a swollen or inflamed joint; effusion in a febrile child; or painful, limited ROM of the hip.
- CBC, ESR, and CRP may be helpful if the history and physical are inconclusive.

Slipped Capital Femoral Epiphysis (SCFE)

Displacement of the femoral head through the physis, typically posteriorly and medially. Most commonly seen in patients 10–16 years of age. Risk factors include obesity, male gender, African-American ethnicity, hypothyroidism, growth hormone deficiency, and renal osteodystrophy. Twenty-five percent of individuals develop SCFE in the other hip within two years.

SCFE is the most common nontraumatic hip disorder in adolescents. This diagnosis is frequently missed because of the vague symptoms and subtle initial radiographic findings.

SYMPTOMS/EXAM

- Pain exacerbated by activity is the most common presenting symptom.
- Child with limp who localizes pain to proximal thigh may have referred or localized knee pain.
- Loss of internal rotation is key.

DIFFERENTIAL

Endocrinopathy, Legg-Calvé-Perthes disease, neoplasm, myositis ossificans, muscle strain, avulsion fracture. See Table 13-3 for differential diagnosis of limp.

Pathognomonic sign of SCFE– the hip externally rotates with hip flexion.

DIAGNOSIS

AP and frog-lateral radiographs of the pelvis reveal Bloomberg's sign (widening or blurring of the epiphyseal plate) or an abnormal Klein's line, a line drawn along the superior border of the femoral neck (see Figure 13-4). In a normal hip, Klein's line should intersect the femoral head.

TREATMENT

- The goal is to prevent further epiphyseal displacement and to allow for physis closure.
- Most patients are treated with in situ stabilization with a single screw.

Osgood-Schlatter Disease

Osteochondrosis of a tibial tuberosity. Caused by overuse that → repetitive small avulsion injuries at the insertion point of the patellar tendon into the 2° aprophysis of the tibial tuberosity.

SYMPTOMS/EXAM

- Tenderness and swelling at the insertion of the patellar tendon of tibial tubercle.
- Pain with stair climbing and jumping.
- Pain with resisted knee extension.

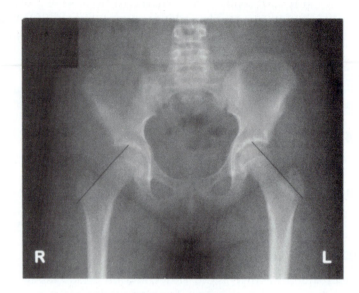

FIGURE 13-4. AP view of mild SCFE of the right hip.

Note that there is significantly less femoral head superior to the Klein's line on the right when compared to the normal left hip. (Reproduced, with permission, from Stead LG et al. *First Aid for the Pediatrics Clerkship*. New York: McGraw-Hill, 2004:336.)

DIFFERENTIAL

- See Table 13-3 for differential diagnosis of limp.
- Sinding-Larsen-Johansson syndrome (an overuse condition at the inferior pole of the patella that most commonly occurs in boys 9–11 years of age).

DIAGNOSIS

AP and lateral radiographs are typically normal but may show soft tissue swelling and heterotopic ossification anterior to tibial tuberosity (see Figure 13-5).

TREATMENT

Rest, ice after activity, NSAIDs; stretch hamstrings and strengthen quadriceps; brief immobilization in severe cases.

> A 14-year-old gymnast with a history of mild scoliosis presents for an annual exam. She informs you that she has frequent associated back pain but has not been concerned because she thought that this was to be expected with scoliosis. What should you tell her? The presence of pain in a patient with scoliosis suggests that the etiology is not idiopathic and requires further evaluation.

Scoliosis

Lateral curvature of the spine of > 10 degrees. Most cases are idiopathic and develop during adolescence. Other causes include congenital, neuromuscular, neoplastic, and infectious conditions; metabolic bone disease; and con-

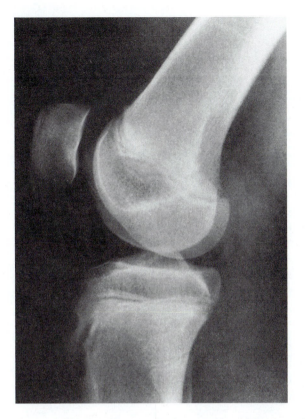

FIGURE 13-5. Osgood-Schlatter disease with heterotopic ossification of the tibial tuberosity.

(Reproduced, with permission, from Wilson FC, Lin PP. *General Orthopaedics.* New York: McGraw-Hill, 1997.)

nective tissue disorders. The incidence of mild curves of < 20 degrees is the same in both genders. Idiopathic scoliosis requiring treatment is 7–8 times more likely in girls.

SYMTPOMS/EXAM

- Typically asymptomatic.
- The forward bending test is the most sensitive clinical test. From behind, observe the patient's back as she bends forward with knees straight, feet together, and arms hanging free. ⊕ findings are elevation of the rib cage and prominence of the lumbar paravertebral muscle mass on one side.

DIAGNOSIS

- Obtain PA and lateral full-length radiographs with the patient standing and the knees straight.
- Determine the Cobb angle (see Figure 13-6).

TREATMENT

- No active treatment is necessary until the curve reaches 25 degrees.
- **Time for follow-up in months:** Computed as 25 − present curve magnitude (e.g., 15 months for a 10-degree curve).

The examination of patients with scoliosis should include evaluation for skin lesions, cavus feet, limb length discrepancy, abnormal joint laxity, and neuromuscular abnormalities.

Right-sided curves are more common. Left-sided curves require further evaluation.

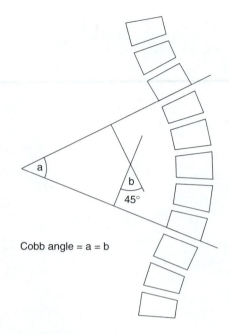

FIGURE 13-6. Determination of Cobb's angle.

(Reproduced, with permission, from Rudolph AM et al. *Rudolph's Fundamentals of Pediatrics,* 3rd ed. New York: McGraw-Hill, 2002:872.)

Girls who have been menstruating for two years have completed spinal growth.

↑ kyphosis does not lead to pulmonary function abnormalities.

The principal problem in advanced Scheuermann disease is pain with standing, which necessitates spinal fusion.

- Brace treatment 18–23 hours daily is recommended until growth is complete; associated with an 80% success rate.
- Curves of 40–50 degrees are likely to ↑ even after growth is complete.
- Surgery is recommended for curves of > 40 degrees.
- Clinical pulmonary restriction may become apparent with curves of > 75 degrees.

Kyphosis

Curvature of the thoracic spine beyond the normal range of 20–40 degrees. There are two main types of kyphosis in children and adolescents:

- **Postural:** More common in girls; more frequent in girls who are taller and have larger breasts than their peers. Postural kyphosis is flexible and can be corrected by hyperextension positioning.
- **Scheuermann disease:** A more fixed and less flexible right thoracic or thoracolumbar kyphosis. More common in boys. Lateral radiographs show irregular disk spaces and wedging of anterior vertebral bodies. In patients who are still growing, brace treatment is required.

Symptoms/Exam

- Patients present with poor posture that is sometimes associated with pain aggravated by activity.
- The Adams forward bend test is used to view the patient's spine from the side.

DIFFERENTIAL

Congenital anomalies, neurofibromatosis, neuromuscular conditions, pathologic fractures, Pott's disease.

DIAGNOSIS

Standing AP and lateral radiographs.

Congenital kyphosis may lead to stretching and dysfunction of the spinal cord.

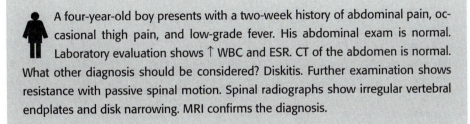

A four-year-old boy presents with a two-week history of abdominal pain, occasional thigh pain, and low-grade fever. His abdominal exam is normal. Laboratory evaluation shows ↑ WBC and ESR. CT of the abdomen is normal. What other diagnosis should be considered? Diskitis. Further examination shows resistance with passive spinal motion. Spinal radiographs show irregular vertebral endplates and disk narrowing. MRI confirms the diagnosis.

BACK PAIN

A child with back pain requires a detailed history and physical exam in order to determine the predisposing factors and diagnosis (see Tables 13-4 and 13-5).

EXAM

- Conduct a neurologic exam.
- Assess spinal flexibility and deformity, gait.
- Dermatologic abnormalities include spinal dimple, freckling, café-au-lait spots, and hairy patches.

Children < 10 years of age almost never have persistent muscular or ligamentous back pain. Further evaluation in these children is required.

TABLE 13-4. Differential of Back Pain

TYPE	EXAMPLES
Musculoskeletal	**Congenital:** Spinal anomalies, diastematomyelia (division of the spinal cord by a bony spur). **Developmental:** Scoliosis, kyphosis. **Traumatic:** Muscle strains, fractures, spondylolysis (separation in the vertebral pars interarticularis, i.e., L5), spondylolisthesis (slippage of the vertebral body), disk herniation.
Infectious	Diskitis, vertebral ostoemyelitis.
Neoplastic	**Benign:** Osteoid osteoma, osteoblastoma, histiocytosis. **Malignant:** Leukemia, spinal cord tumor, neuroblastoma, osteogenic sarcoma.
Rheumatologic	JRA, ankylosing spondylitis.
Neurologic	Syrinx.

TABLE 13-5. **Common Clinical Presentations of Back Pain**

CLINICAL SCENARIO	EVALUATION TIPS	DIAGNOSIS
Athletes who hyperextend: gymnasts, divers, dancers, football linemen, tennis players	Ipsilateral pain with one-legged hyperextension. Lumbosacral films.	Spondylolysis.
Gradual onset of pain; occasional fever accompanied by abdominal pain	Normal WBC but elevated ESR.	Diskitis.
Ten-year-old with nocturnal pain relieved by NSAIDs	Normal exam and labs. Bone scan with intense uptake.	Osteoid osteoma.

DIFFERENTIAL

See Table 13-4 for the differential diagnosis of back pain.

DIAGNOSIS

- Obtain AP and lateral radiographs of the spine. Obtain an oblique view if there is a concern for spondylolysis.
- Laboratory evaluation is usually reserved for cases in which an infectious or inflammatory process is suspected.
- See Table 13-5 for diagnostic tips for back pain.

PREPARTICIPATION PHYSICAL AND INJURY PREVENTION

A complete history and physical examination should be performed to identify conditions requiring limitation of sports participation (see Table 13-6).

HEAD AND NECK INJURY IN ATHLETES

Football, gymnastics, ice hockey, and wrestling are associated with the highest risk of head and spine injury. Other high-risk sports include rugby, horseback riding, baseball, boxing, pole vaulting, and soccer.

Neck Injury

SYMPTOMS

Neck pain, paresthesias, muscle weakness.

EXAM

- Check ABCs.
- Examine for neurologic deficits and cervical spine tenderness/ROM.
- Radiograph of cervical spine.

Children with Down syndrome are at risk for atlantoaxial instability. The Special Olympics Committee recommends preparticipation radiographic screening.

To prevent apophyseal avulsion fractures, preadolescents should not power lift.

TABLE 13-6. Medical Conditions and Sports Participation

CONDITION	PARTICIPATION	EXPLANATION
Bleeding disorder	Qualified yes	Requires full evaluation.
Carditis	No	
Hypertension	Qualified yes	If significant, avoid weight lifting.
Dysrhythmias	Qualified yes	Requires full evaluation.
Congenital heart disease	Qualified yes	Requires full evaluation.
Diabetes mellitus	Yes	
Diarrhea	No	↑ risk of dehydration.
One eye	Qualified yes	Use of an eye guard allows participation in most sports except wrestling.
Fever	No	
Hepatitis	Yes	Universal precautions.
HIV	Yes	Universal precautions.
Single kidney	Qualified yes	Most likely requires avoidance of contact sports; may consider participation based on individual patient.
Hepatomegaly	Qualified yes	Avoid contact sports.
Seizure disorder	Qualified yes	If poorly controlled, avoid archery, riflery, water sports, weight lifting, and adventure sports.
Single ovary	Yes	
Asthma	Qualified yes	Only the most severe cases require restriction.
Cystic fibrosis	Qualified yes	Patients may play if normal oxygenation is maintained during exercise test.
Splenomegaly	Qualified yes	Avoid contact sports.
Herpetic lesions	Qualified yes	No contact sports until lesions resolve.
Molluscum contagiosum	Qualified yes	Lesions must be covered.
Furuncles	Qualified yes	Avoid contact and water sports until lesions resolve.
Mononucleosis	No	No sports for 3–4 weeks from onset of illness.

TREATMENT

Any conscious athlete with neck pain, persistent numbness, or weakness requires spinal immobilization. Unconscious patients also require spinal immobilization.

Head Injury

Concussion is trauma-induced transient neurologic dysfunction. Loss of consciousness (LOC) is not necessary.

SYMPTOMS/EXAM

Headache, dizziness, nausea, vomiting, photosensitivity, blurred vision, amnesia, emotional lability, poor concentration. Perform complete neurologic and mental status exam.

DIAGNOSIS

A head CT should be considered in any athlete who has suffered LOC, has concern for a skull fracture, has focal deficit, has sustained multiple concussions in one season, or has an initial lucid interval followed by progressive decline.

TREATMENT

Table 13-7 outlines protocols for head injury.

Eye Injury

Protective eyewear should be worn by all athletes in eye-risk sports such as hockey, lacrosse, and racquetball. Athletes who are functionally one-eyed (i.e., those in whom vision in the affected eye is correctable to < 20/40) or who have a history of eye trauma or surgery require protective eyewear.

TABLE 13-7. Return-to-Competition Guidelines Following Concussion

GRADE OF CONCUSSION	SYMPTOMS	RETURN AFTER FIRST INJURY	RETURN AFTER SECOND INJURY
Grade 1	No LOC; confusion < 15 minutes.	Return to play in 15 minutes if exam is normal.	Return to play when asymptomatic for one week.
Grade 2	No LOC; confusion > 15 minutes.	Hospital evaluation if symptoms > 1 hour; head CT if symptoms > 2 weeks; return to play when asymptomatic for one week.	Return to play when asymptomatic for two weeks.
Grade 3	Any LOC.	Hospital evaluation; if few seconds of LOC, may return after asymptomatic for one week; if minutes of LOC, return when asymptomatic for two weeks.	Return to play when asymptomatic for one month; consider ending season.

Adapted, with permission, from Hay WW et al. *Current Pediatric Diagnosis & Treatment,* 17th ed. New York: McGraw-Hill, 2005:838.

TABLE 13-8. Diagnosis and Treatment of Common Eye Injuries

	SIGNS/SYMPTOMS	MANAGEMENT
Lid laceration	May be complicated by injury to the nasolacrimal system (medial lid and eye) or levator muscle (upper lid).	Repair by an ophthalmologist or plastic surgeon.
Corneal abrasions	Sensation of something in the eye or behind the eyelid; pain or blurred vision.	Fluorescein exam; antibiotic ophthalmic drops; patch for comfort in older children for 24–36 hours. Return to play is allowed for athletes with small abrasions, minimal discomfort, and no visual impairment.
Corneal foreign body	Same as above.	Gentle removal; antibiotic ointment and patching in older children.
Subconjunctival hemorrhage	No pain or vision impairment.	Treatment is symptomatic; no restriction from competition.
Hyphema	Hemorrhage in the anterior chamber. May cause blurred vision, pain, and photophobia.	Immediate referral to an ophthalmologist. The goal of treatment is to prevent rebleeding when hyphema resorbs. Return to play is determined by an ophthalmologist.
Ruptured globe	Eye pain, ↓ light perception, and ↓ visual acuity. May be characterized by a "teardrop-shaped" pupil.	Avoid any eye manipulation; patch without pressure and send for immediate ophthalmologic evaluation.
Orbital fracture	Periorbital hematoma and/or protruding/sunken eye; possible diploplia with upward gaze.	Unstable fractures require surgical repair and referral to an ophthalmologist.

DIAGNOSIS/TREATMENT

Table 13-8 lists guidelines for the diagnosis and treatment of common eye injuries.

SPRAINS AND STRAINS

Sprains

Defined as a ligamentous tear; categorized as first, second, and third degree (see Table 13-9). Treat with rest, ice, compression, and elevation (RICE). In general, return to play may occur when the athlete has no pain, full ROM, and strength equal to 85% of the uninjured extremity.

Strains

Defined as muscle tear; graded I–III. Treatment is similar to that of sprains.

> **Sprain treatment— RICE**
>
> **R**est
> **I**ce
> **C**ompression
> **E**levation

Sprains as isolated injuries are unusual in children until late adolescence. It is safer to assume Salter I fracture and splint injury.

THE MUSCULOSKELETAL SYSTEM AND SPORTS MEDICINE

TABLE 13-9. Categorization of Sprains

Sprain Type	Tearing	Pain/Swelling	Motion	Stability	Treatment in Addition to RICE
First degree	Minimal	None/little	Full	No laxity	Immobilization for comfort.
Second degree	Partial (5–99%)	Yes	Limited	Some instability	Immobilization for protection.
Third degree	Complete	Severe	Severely limited	Marked laxity	Immobilization for protection; possible surgical repair.

TABLE 13-10. Diagnosis and Treatment of Common Shoulder Injuries

	Mechanism	Signs/Symptoms	Radiographs	Management[a]
Acromioclavicular (AC) sprain	Fall or blow to the superior or lateral aspect of the shoulder or lateral deltoid.	Swelling and tenderness over the AC joint, pain with arm abduction, possible step-off at the AC joint, pain with crossover test.	May show elevation of the distal clavicle.	Immobilization; surgical correction for grades IV–VI.
Anterior shoulder dislocation	Blow or fall on the arm in external rotation, abduction, and extension; accounts for > 95% of shoulder dislocations.	Prominent acromion process with squared-off shoulder; the humeral head is palpable anterior, inferior, and medial to the glenoid fossa; the arm is held in abduction and external rotation; inability to touch the opposite shoulder.	AP, axillary; the humeral head is seen inferior to the coracoid process.	Reduction, shoulder immobilizer for four weeks, rehabilitation.
Posterior shoulder dislocation	Extreme internal rotation or trauma to shoulder with the outstretched arm.	The anterior shoulder is flat; the arm is held in adduction and internal rotation.	AP, axillary; the humeral head lies over the glenoid rim.	Reduction, shoulder immobilizer for four weeks, rehabilitation.
Rotator cuff injury	Muscles involved are the supraspinatus, infraspinatus, teres minor, and subscapularis (SITS); most from chronic impingement.	Recurrent shoulder pain, especially at night; limited active ROM, especially abduction and external rotation.	AP and lateral films are likely normal.	Rehabilitation, rest from offending activity.

	MECHANISM	SIGNS/SYMPTOMS	RADIOGRAPHS	MANAGEMENT*
Impingement syndrome (pitcher's/swimmer's/tennis shoulder)	Supraspinatus tendonitis from chronic anterior glenohumeral instability; subacromial bursitis.	Anterior shoulder pain is present only when the shoulder is abducted 90 degrees; tenderness over the greater tuberosity; pain with impingement tests.	AP and lateral films are likely normal.	Rest, rehabilitation.
Clavicle fracture	Fall or blow to the shoulder or outstretched arm.	Pain with arm and shoulder movement; point tenderness at the fracture site.	AP view of the clavicle; most common in the middle third of the clavicle.	Immobilization for 3–6 weeks in figure-of-eight splint or sling to maintain shoulder abduction.
Proximal humeral epiphyseal fracture	Blunt trauma to the arm or shoulder.	Pain with abduction; no obvious deformity.	Typically see Salter II fracture.	Shoulder immobilizer for minimal angulations; surgical correction for three-piece fractures.
Proximal humeral epiphysitis (Little League shoulder)	Overuse or stress fracture of the proximal humeral epiphysis due to overhead throwing during the growth spurt.	Pain in the proximal humerus while throwing. Exam may be ⊝ or relatively unremarkable; may have tenderness to palpation of the proximal humerus.	AP views with internal and external rotation may show widening of the proximal humeral physis.	Rest for 2–3 months; rehabilitation.

ª All injuries listed above also benefit from anti-inflammatory drugs.

SHOULDER INJURY

Table 13-10 outlines the diagnosis and treatment of common shoulder injuries.

ELBOW DISLOCATION

Typically occurs with a fall on a hyperextended arm. For children, most common joint dislocation.

SYMPTOMS/EXAM

- Deformity, swelling, and effusion of the elbow.
- Inability to bend the elbow.
- Assess for neurovascular compromise.

AC sprain is the most common acute shoulder injury.

DIAGNOSIS

Obtain AP, lateral, and oblique radiographs. A posterior fat pad or associated fracture may be seen.

TREATMENT

Orthopedic consultation, reduction under sedation, immobilization.

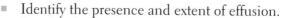

ACUTE KNEE INJURY

Table 13-11 outlines the diagnosis and treatment of common knee injuries.

EXAM

- Identify the presence and extent of effusion.
- In addition to routine musculoskeletal and neurovascular assessment of the lower extremity, the following should be performed:
  - **Lachman test:** Flex the knee 30 degrees. Pull the tibia forward with the medial hand and while stabilizing distal thigh. A ⊕ test points to ↑ anterior movement of the tibia with no endpoint.
  - **McMurray test:** Flex the knee to the maximum pain-free position. While extending knee, externally rotate foot to stress medial meniscus and internally rotate foot to stress lateral meniscus. Listen for click and assess pain.

TABLE 13-11. Diagnosis and Treatment of Common Knee Injuries

	MECHANISM	EXAM	TREATMENT
Anterior cruciate ligament (ACL) tear	Forced hyperextension or rapid deceleration.	**Large effusion:** Lachman test (most sensitive).	**Initial:** RICE, immobilization. **Definitive:** surgical repair.
Medial collateral ligament (MCL) tear	Valgus stress—blow to the lateral aspect of the knee.	**Trace to mild effusion:** Point tenderness.	RICE, immobilization; referral to an orthopedist.
Patellar fracture	Trauma to the anterior aspect of the knee.	Effusion.	RICE, immobilization; referral to an orthopedist.
Distal femur or tibial plateau fracture	Direct force/trauma; indirect valgus or varus stress.	Effusion; neurovascular compromise possible.	RICE, immobilization; immediate orthopedic consult.
Meniscal tears	Squatting or twisting injury.	Insidious onset of swelling and stiffness over 2–3 days; locking, catching, and popping of knee; tenderness over the medial or lateral joint; knee effusion; ⊕ McMurray test.	RICE, immobilization. Orthopedic referral for definitive surgical debridement or repair.
Patellar dislocation	Forced internal rotation of the leg or direct blow to the outer aspect of the knee.	Apprehension with patellar movement.	Reduction; RICE; rehabilitation.

DIAGNOSIS

- Obtain AP, lateral, tunnel, and patellar radiograph views.
- MRI is helpful to confirm ligamentous and meniscal injuries.

TREATMENT

RICE, immobilization. An orthopedic consult and surgical intervention are typically needed for ACL tears, meniscal injuries, and possibly fractures. Patellar dislocation requires reduction and rehabilitation.

ANKLE SPRAIN

Inversion (supination) is most common. Sprain injures the lateral ligaments.

SYMPTOMS/EXAM

- **Inversion injuries:** Look for tenderness anterior and inferior to the lateral malleolus where the anterior talofibular and calcaneofibular ligaments attach.
- **Eversion (pronation) injuries:** The deltoid ligament is injured. Patients may also sustain Maissonneuve fracture, which involves a fracture of the medial malleolus of the ankle with disruption of the tibiofibular syndesmosis and a fracture in the proximal third of the fibula.
- Anterior ankle drawer test for anterior talofibular ligament injuries.
- Talar tilt test for calcaneofibular ligament injuries.

DIAGNOSIS

- AP, lateral, and mortise radiographic views (while standing if possible) are generally indicated when there is tenderness over the distal fibula or ankle joint, syndesmosis, or other bony structure, or if there is significant swelling or inability to bear weight.
- Inspect for Salter-Harris and Maissonneuve fractures.

TREATMENT

- RICE for all sprains.
- For first-degree sprains, patients should avoid weight bearing for 3–4 days. Second-degree sprains require a splint for 3–4 weeks. Third-degree sprains often require surgical repair.

HEAT ILLNESS

Refers to a spectrum of conditions ranging from heat cramps to heatstroke (see Table 13-12). Several factors make children more susceptible than adults to heat injury:

- More metabolic heat per mass unit.
- Slower rate of acclimatization.
- Core temperature rises faster during dehydration.
- Insufficient fluid intake.
- Release most heat by convection.
- Lower sweat rate, and sweating starts at higher temperature.

To prevent heat illness, children should train in a similar environment prior to competition (10–14 days for acclimatization); practice in cool temperatures with low humidity; and take water breaks every 20–30 minutes.

Heat exhaustion is the most common heat disorder seen in children.

TABLE 13-12. Characteristics of Heat Illness

HEAT EXHAUSTION	HEATSTROKE
Core temperature between 38° and 40.5°C.	Core temperature > 40.5°C.
Profuse sweating.	Hot and dry skin.
Headache, dizziness, weakness.	Mental status changes ranging from confusion to coma. May cause rhabdomyolysis, renal impairment, hyperkalemia, and liver damage.

TREATMENT

- Obtain all vital signs, including core temperature.
- Move the patient to a cool area and remove clothing and protective equipment.
- Apply cold packs to the axillae, groin, and neck. Mist with water.
- Encourage drinking by mouth. If the patient is unable to drink, begin IV fluid resuscitation.
- The goal is to lower temperature to 38.9°C, at which point cooling measures can be stopped to avoid hypothermia.
- Heatstroke requires admission to the ICU for further evaluation and management.

NUTRITIONAL REQUIREMENTS IN ATHLETES

Fluid Restriction and Rehydration

Children have less tolerance for temperature extremes than do adults. The fluid needs of children must therefore be frequently assessed and fluid replaced to prevent dehydration. Children should drink at least 4–6 ounces and adolescents 8–12 ounces for every 20–30 minutes of exercise.

Weight Loss

Many athletes (e.g., wrestlers) participate in sports with weight categories. To lose weight, athletes combine exercise, fluid restriction, and methods of dehydration, including taking saunas and exercising in excess clothing or hot rooms. Some may use cathartics, laxatives, or diuretics. Weight reduction may lead to ↓ muscle strength and aerobic power capacity, ↓ endurance, impaired thermoregulation, and depletion of electrolytes and muscle glycogen. Weight loss should not exceed 2–3 pounds/week.

PERFORMANCE-ENHANCING DRUGS

The use of performance-enhancing substances among college and high school athletes is on the rise. The incidence of creatine and anabolic steroids use among high school males has been reported to be approximately 5–10%.

TABLE 13-13. Commonly Used Performance-Enhancing Drugs

SUPPLEMENTS	ILLICIT/BANNED SUBSTANCES	OTHER
Androstenedione	Amphetamines	β-blockers/agonists
Antioxidants	Anabolic steroids	Diuretics
Caffeine	DHEA	Local anesthetics
Creatine	Ephedra	
Vitamins, minerals, and amino acids	Erythropoietin (blood doping)	
	γ-hydroxybutyrate	
	Human growth hormone	
	Narcotics	

Tables 13-13 and 13-14 categorize these substances and outline their intended use as well as the side effects with which they are commonly associated.

INFECTIOUS MYOSITIS

Defined as infection of skeletal muscle. In children, it typically has a viral etiology (e.g., HIV, influenza, coxsackieviruses, echoviruses). Other causes include Lyme borreliosis, trypanosomiasis, and cysticercosis.

TABLE 13-14. Use and Side Effects of Common Performance-Enhancing Drugs

DRUG	ROUTE	GOAL OF USE	SIDE EFFECTS
Anabolic steroids	Oral or injected	↑ protein synthesis and enhancement of muscle strength/size. Blocks effect of cortisol to ↓ muscle breakdown.	Acne, aggression/emotional lability/ psychosis, collagen dysplasia, striae, gynecomastia, hirsutism, hypertension, liver tumors, premature growth plate closure, testicular failure, ↓ HDL/↑ LDL, ↓ sexual function, virilization in females.
Androstenedione	Oral	Theoretically acts as a testosterone precursor.	Limited data on side effects; probably similar to those of anabolic steroids.
Creatine	Oral	A naturally occurring tripeptide that is converted to phosphocreatine, which helps regenerate ATP; prolongs the time before anaerobic production of ATP is needed. Anaerobic metabolism means muscle breakdown.	Muscle cramping, vomiting/diarrhea, renal dysfunction (especially in patients with renal disease), weight gain, bloating.
Growth hormone	Injected	Protein anabolism and lipolysis.	Acromegalic features, behavioral changes, cardiovascular disease, diabetes, hypertension, peripheral neuropathy.

SYMPTOMS/EXAM

In viral myositis, fever, myalgias, and weakness may be seen.

DIFFERENTIAL

Rule out rhabdomyolysis.

DIAGNOSIS

CBC, CK, ESR, liver enzymes, BUN, creatinine, urine myoglobin, ECG.

TREATMENT

Bed rest, IV fluids, antipyretics, analgesics.

ACUTE OSTEOMYELITIS

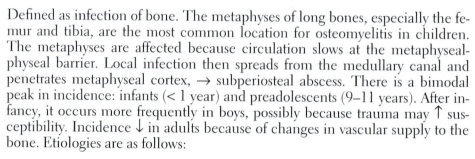

Defined as infection of bone. The metaphyses of long bones, especially the femur and tibia, are the most common location for osteomyelitis in children. The metaphyses are affected because circulation slows at the metaphyseal-physeal barrier. Local infection then spreads from the medullary canal and penetrates metaphyseal cortex, → subperiosteal abscess. There is a bimodal peak in incidence: infants (< 1 year) and preadolescents (9–11 years). After infancy, it occurs more frequently in boys, possibly because trauma may ↑ susceptibility. Incidence ↓ in adults because of changes in vascular supply to the bone. Etiologies are as follows:

- *S. aureus* is the most common cause of osteomyelitis.
- *Streptococcus pneumoniae* and *Haemophilus* spp. are other common pathogens.
- In sickle cell patients, *Salmonella* is a frequent pathogen.
- In neonates, group B strep is a common cause.
- In patients with puncture wounds through tennis shoes, *Pseudomonas aeruginosa* must be considered.

If sickle cell, think Salmonella. If neonate, think group B strep. If foot puncture wound, think Pseudomonas.

Joint motion in osteomyelitis is not limited to the degree seen in septic arthritis.

SYMPTOMS/EXAM

- **Local:** Pain, swelling, tenderness, warmth, erythema, refusal to bear weight.
- **Systemic:** Fever, malaise.

DIAGNOSIS

- CBC, ESR, blood culture (⊕ in only 40–50% of patients).
- Radiographic changes are seen 7–10 days after onset of symptoms. These changes include periosteal elevation and bony destruction (with areas of radiolucency and no surrounding reactive bone).
- Consider a bone scan if the diagnosis is uncertain.
- Bone aspiration is indicated to identify the pathogen and possibly to decompress local infection.

DIFFERENTIAL

Leukemia, rheumatic fever, cellulitis, malignant bone tumors, septic arthritis, stress fracture.

TREATMENT

- Administer a six-week course of antibiotics, with the first week of treatment given IV. May switch to oral antibiotics after at least one week of IV antibiotics if the patient shows clinical improvement.
- All patients should receive an antistaphylococcal agent such as oxacillin or nafcillin. Vancomycin should be given if methicillin-resistant *S. aureus* is suspected.
- In neonates, an aminoglycoside should be added to the antibiotic coverage.
- In children < 5 years of age, cefotaxime should be added to cover *H. influenzae.*
- In sickle cell disease, cefotaxime is needed to cover *Salmonella.*
- For foot punctures, ceftazidime should be given to cover *Pseudomonas.*
- Immobilize the affected bone for three weeks to decrease pain and protect against pathologic fracture.
- Surgical drainage is indicated for patients when fever and symptoms persist despite appropriate antibiotic therapy.

COMPLICATIONS

In children < 1 year of age, bone transphyseal vessels exist that allow infection to spread into joints → 2° septic arthritis. In older children, there are no bridging vessels in the growth plate, which protects the joint and ↓ 2° septic arthritis. The shoulder, hip, and elbow are exceptions because joint capsules extend over the growth plate.

THE MUSCULOSKELETAL SYSTEM AND SPORTS MEDICINE

CHAPTER 14

Neonatology

Albert Chan, MD
Katherine Herz, MD
reviewed by Shannon E. G. Hamrick, MD

First-Trimester Genetic Screening

- Between 10 and 13 weeks' gestation; used to assess risk for trisomies 18 and 21.
- Serum hCG and pregnancy-associated plasma protein A measurements, along with test of nuchal translucency.
- Confirm a suspected diagnosis with chorionic villus sampling (CVS) and ultrasound.

Triple-Screen Test

- Between 15 and 20 weeks' gestation; to assess risk for trisomies 18 and 21 and for neural tube defects.
- Measures maternal serum α-fetoprotein (AFP), β-hCG, and unconjugated estriol.

Prenatal Ultrasound

Ultrasound has numerous diagnostic applications, including the following:
- Single vs. multiple gestation.
- Estimated gestational age (GA):
  - Between 8 and 12 weeks' gestation, use crown-rump length, accurate to within 5–7 days.
  - After the first trimester, use a combination of biparietal diameter (BPD), head circumference (HC), abdominal circumference, and femur length. Accuracy wanes with increased gestation (+/- approximately two weeks in second trimester, +/- approximately three weeks in third trimester).
- Estimated fetal weight and growth, including IUGR and macrosomia diagnosis and monitoring. Accuracy wanes with increased gestation.
- Fetal anatomy:
  - Congenital anomalies may be identified, including anencephaly, hydrocephalus, myelomeningocele, cleft lip and palate, congenital heart defects (CHDs), congenital diaphragmatic hernia (CDH), omphalocele, gastroschisis, renal anomalies, skeletal anomalies.
  - Fetal gender.
- Amniotic fluid volume with amniotic fluid index (AFI) can identify the following:
  - **Oligohydramnios:**
    - Most often 2° to rupture of membranes.
    - Frequently associated with major congenital anomaly.
    - Renal anomalies, bladder outlet anomalies, chromosomal abnormalities, severe congenital heart disease.
  - **Polyhydramnios:**
    - Associated with gestational diabetes mellitus (GDM), multiple gestation.
    - Also associated with a major congenital anomaly.

- Anencephaly, neural tube defects, bowel obstruction, bladder exstrophy.
- Additional applications of ultrasound:
  - Placental location and assessment (placenta previa, abruptio placentae).
  - Assessment of fetal well-being and viability.
  - Biophysical profile (BPP).
  - Doppler study of vessels, especially the umbilical artery.
  - Visual guide for intrauterine procedures (e.g., amniocentesis, CVS).

Amniocentesis

- Ultrasound-guided needle sampling of placental tissue. Usually performed between 16 and 20 weeks' gestation. Associated fetal loss between 0.3% and approximately 0.5%.
- Amniotic fluid tested for bilirubin concentration, evidence of fetal lung maturity, and evidence of chorioamnionitis.

Chorionic Villus Sampling (CVS)

- Ultrasound-guided sampling of placental tissue. Usually performed between 10 and 12 weeks' gestation.
- Associated fetal loss generally < 1%, but varies widely with practitioner.
- Used for first-trimester fetal genetic testing, including karyotyping and fluorescent in situ hybridization (FISH) chromosome analysis.

Percutaneous Umbilical Blood Sampling (PUBS)

- Fetal blood obtained from needle passed into umbilical vein. Used mainly in cases of hydrops fetalis.
- Fetal blood is tested for ABO/Rh typing, hematocrit, viral studies, and chromosomal karyotyping. Also used for in utero transfusion.

PERINATAL ASSESSMENT

Nonstress Testing (NST)

Test of fetal brain stem function. Variations in fetal heart rate (FHR) are monitored.

- **Reactive NST (reassuring):** During 20 minutes of monitoring, two or more episodes of FHR acceleration ≥ 15 bpm above baseline ≥ 15 seconds.
- **Nonreactive NST (nonreassuring):** Failure to meet the above criteria over a prolonged monitoring period. Nonspecific findings should be followed by BPP and/or contraction stress test (CST; see below).

Biophysical Profile (BPP)

NST + ultrasound to asses fetal breathing movements, gross body movements, fetal tone, and amniotic fluid volume.

Contraction Stress Test (CST)

- Evaluates risk of uteroplacental insufficiency through log of contractions and FHR.
- Normal to see FHR accelerations with contractions. Concurrent or late FHR decelerations are concerning.
- Test results may be ⊖ (normal), ⊕ (normal, abnormal immediate delivery recommended), or equivocal (further fetal monitoring is recommended).

Large-for-Gestational-Age (LGA) Infants

- Defined as infants who are 2 SDs above the norm or above the 90th percentile for GA.
- Associated with infants of diabetic mothers (IDMs), Beckwith-Wiedemann syndrome, large parents (genetic predisposition to large size), and hydrops fetalis.

Small-for-Gestational-Age (SGA) Infants

- Infant weight 2 SDs below the norm or below the 10th percentile for GA.
- Associated with large parents (genetics) infants of diabetic mothers (IDMs), Beckwith-Wiedemann syndrome, and hydrops fetalis.

Intrauterine Growth Retardation (IUGR)

Alteration of growth and reduced growth in comparison to the expected pattern. May be symmetric or asymmetric. Risks associated with IUGR are listed in Table 14-1. Causes include:

IUGR is not synonymous with SGA. SGA infants may or may not have IUGR and vice versa.

- **Maternal:** Placental insufficiency (the most common cause in the United States), multiple gestation, severe malnutrition, tobacco or alcohol use, illicit drug use, medications, hypoxemia (e.g., from CHDs), severe malnutrition.
- **Fetal:** Genetic factors, chromosomal anomalies, congenital anomalies, CHDs, congenital infections, inborn errors of metabolism.

SYMPTOMS/EXAM

- **Ponderal index:** Computed as birth weight $\times$ 100/(crown-heel length)^3. An index below the 10th percentile indicates IUGR.
- **Asymmetric IUGR:**
  - "Head-sparing IUGR."
  - Weight is compromised to a greater extent than height or HC.

- Better prognosis; indicates relative preservation of brain growth and development.
- Associated with factors influencing fetal growth later in gestation, including uteroplacental insufficiency, other maternal factors.
- **Symmetric IUGR:**
  - Head circumference, height, and weight are all reduced to the same degree.
  - Worse prognosis.
  - Associated with factors influencing fetal growth starting early in gestation.

Reduced subcutaneous fat leaves IUGR infants more vulnerable to hypothermia.

DIAGNOSIS

- Suspicion based on serial assessment of fundal height, maternal weight gain, and fetal activity.
- Evaluate fetal growth through BPD, abdominal circumference (AC), head circumference (HC), femur length, placental status, AFI.
- Establish diagnosis in neonate through birthweight measurement, physical exam, Ponderal index, Ballard score.

TREATMENT

Specific management recommendations include the following:

- Correct prenatal problems that may cause or exacerbate IUGR.
- Time delivery well and use a skilled resuscitation team (higher risk of birth asphyxia).
- Prevent hypothermia.
- Monitor and sustain appropriate glucose levels.

TABLE 14-1. Risks Associated with IUGR

2° TO HYPOXIA	METABOLIC	HEMATOLOGIC
↑ risk of birth asphyxia.	Hypoglycemia 2° to reduced glycogen stores,	Higher risk of polycythemia/ hyperviscosity 2° to chronic fetal hypoxia.
↑ risk of persistent pulmonary hypertension.	↓ gluconeogenesis, chronic potential	Thrombocytopenia, neutropenia, low
↓ risk of RDS (intrauterine stress promotes earlier lung response).	hyperinsulinism, and ↓ counterregulatory response.	lymphocyte levels. Low IgG levels.
↑ risk of meconium aspiration in infants of later GA.	Hyperglycemia is also possible.Hypocalcemia, especially after birth asphyxia.	Coagulation abnormalities.

- Check hematocrit and treat polycythemia when indicated.
- Screen for TORCH infections.
- Screen for genetic anomalies.

COMPLICATIONS

- Neurodevelopmental disabilities are common.
- Associated with an ↑ risk of adult-onset cardiovascular disease, obesity, and DM.
- Other complications are associated with underlying disorders (e.g., genetic anomalies, TORCH infections).

Fetal Heart Rate (FHR) Monitoring

- Performed via a monitor on the maternal abdomen or by fetal scalp electrode.
- Tachycardia is defined as > 160 bpm and may occur with infection (maternal and/or fetal), hypoxia, thyrotoxicosis, and medications.
- Moderate bradycardia is 90–110 bpm with normal variability; severe bradycardia is defined as < 90 bpm. Bradycardia may occur with hypoxia, heart block, and medications.
- Accelerations are associated with fetal movement and uterine contractions and are considered reassuring.
- Decelerations are defined as late with normal beat-to-beat variability, late with ↓ variability, and variable.
    - **Late with normal variability** indicates an episode of uteroplacental insufficiency with adequate fetal compensation.
    - **Late with ↓ variability** indicates more severe uteroplacental insufficiency and fetal hypoxia.
    - **Variable decelerations** usually indicate umbilical cord compression.

Tests of Fetal Lung Maturity

Performed on a sample of amniotic fluid.

LECITHIN-TO-SPHINGOMYELIN (L/S) RATIO

- L/S ≥ 2:1 indicates mature lungs.
- L/S = 1.5–1.9:1 associated with increased risk of RDS.

PHOSPHATIDYLGLYCEROL

First present at approximately 35 weeks' GA, with a subsequent ↑ in levels.

The pediatric team is called to a forceps-assisted delivery. Late decelerations have been noted. The infant is born and handed to the pediatric team, who note a blue, floppy infant making minimal respiratory effort and having a pulse of 90 bpm. What are the appropriate resuscitation measures, and what Apgar scores should the infant receive? The team initiates simultaneous warming, drying, and stimulating (as in all deliveries) as well as positive-pressure ventilation for suspected 2° apnea. Only then does the infant respond, initiating respiratory effort with a good cry, an ↑ in heart rate to 130 bpm, resolution of central cyanosis, and flexing and movement of all extremities. The initial Apgar score is 3 (0 for appearance, 1 for pulse, 0 for grimace, 1 for activity, 1 for respirations); the five-minute Apgar score is 9 (2 for everything but appearance, 1 off for acrocyanosis).

DELIVERY

Assessment (Apgar Score)

Table 14-2 outlines the manner in which the Apgar score is used to assess a newborn's physical condition.

Neonatal Resuscitation

- The keys to low-risk delivery are **"warm, dry, stimulate."**
- In high-risk deliveries requiring complex resuscitation, key variables are heart rate, respiratory effort, and skin color. These variables should be assessed frequently and together.

> **Assessment of newborns—APGAR**
>
> **A**ppearance (color)
> **P**ulse
> **G**rimace
> **A**ctivity (tone)
> **R**espirations

TABLE 14-2. Apgar Scoring

	SCORE		
SIGN	**0**	**1**	**2**
Appearance (color)	Blue or pale.	Pink body, blue extremities (acrocyanosis).	Completely pink body.
Pulse (heart rate)	Absent.	60–100 bpm.	> 100 bpm.
Grimace (reflex irritability)	No response.	Grimace.	Grimace with cough or sneeze.
Activity (muscle tone)	Floppy.	Some flexion.	Flexion of all extremities; active movement.
Respirations	Absent.	Slow, inconsistent.	Good cry.

Most cardiac failure in newborns is 2° to respiratory failure.

Assume that newborn apnea is 2°.

Never give Narcan to infants of narcotic-addicted mothers, as doing so may potentiate withdrawal symptoms.

Give sodium bicarbonate only after adequate ventilation has been established. Consider tris (hydroxymethyl) aminomethane (THAM) as an alternative (does not produce CO_2).

- 1° apnea implies O_2 deprivation of ≤ 1 minute, and sensory stimuli alone can initiate respiratory effort. 2° apnea implies more prolonged O_2 deprivation, and assisted ventilation is necessary to establish spontaneous respiratory effort.

VENTILATORY RESUSCITATION

- Universal, brief oropharyngeal suctioning with either a bulb syringe or a suction catheter.
- Mechanical ventilation with bag and mask is initiated for poor to absent respiratory effort after an initial (≤ 30-second) trial of sensory stimulation.
- Endotracheal intubation is indicated for prolonged inadequate respiratory effort or in initial resuscitation of infants born through meconium-stained amniotic fluid.

CARDIAC RESUSCITATION

- Begin cardiac compression if HR is < 60 bpm for 30 seconds despite adequate ventilation.
- Initiate compressions at 90 bpm with ventilations at 30 bpm.

MEDICATIONS FOR RESUSCITATION

- Epinephrine IV or ETT.
- Volume expanders (NS, LR, or O-negative whole blood) for infants with obvious blood loss, shock, or those who fail to respond to regular measures.
- Naloxone for infants with poor respiratory effort born to mothers who received narcotic medication within four hours of delivery. Repeat dose may be needed, as the half-life of narcotics exceeds that of naloxone.
- Dextrose for infants at high risk of hypoglycemia (e.g., IDMs and premature infants, infants who suffer birth asphyxia).
- Sodium bicarbonate.

Traumatic Delivery

Acute fetal or placental hemorrhage is a major risk associated with traumatic delivery. Resuscitate with volume expanders, and watch for signs and symptoms of asphyxia.

Multiple Gestation

- Risks 2° to multiple gestation include prematurity, asphyxia, congenital anomalies, IUGR, twin-twin transfusion, and stuck-twin syndrome.
- **Twin-twin transfusion syndrome (TTTS):**
  - 2° to vascular anastomoses between circulations of monozygotic twins.
  - Chronic transfusion starting early in gestation.
  - Seen only in monozygotic, monochorionic twins. Associated mortality approximately 80–100% without treatment; associated with disability in survivors.

NEONATOLOGY

- The donor twin presents with anemia, poor growth, and oligohydramnios; the recipient twin exhibits polycythemia, hypervolemia, ↑ growth, polyhydramnios, and cardiac hypertrophy.
- In cases of acute transfusion, the donor twin suffers anemia and the recipient suffers polycythemia. Large, acute transfusions may result in fetal demise.

Consider partial exchange transfusion in a donor twin with chronic anemia instead to ↑ hematocrit without significantly affecting blood volume.

Very Low Birth Weight (VLBW) and Extremely Low Birth Weight (ELBW)

- VLBW infants are defined as those weighing < 1500 g; ELBW infants are those weighing < 1000 g.
- The conditions are associated with extreme prematurity. Special considerations include:
  - **Assisted ventilation:** Most ELBW infants will require intubation and mechanical ventilation at birth. The need for exogenous surfactant administration is common. Because it is important to maintain lung expansion (i.e., to prevent atelectasis), relatively high PEEP or CPAP will be required.
  - **Oxygenation:** Maintain O_2 saturation in the mid 80% to low 90% range to limit toxicity associated with hyperoxia.
  - **Insensible water loss and temperature maintenance:** Maintain adequate hydration; prevent excessive heat loss and hypothermia with an incubator.

Cyanosis

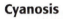

- Seen when > 3 g/dL of hemoglobin in arterial blood or > 5 g/dL in capillary blood is deoxygenated.
- Pahtophysiology and corresponding clinical entities are as follows:
  - **Alveolar hypoventilation:**
    - **Lung parenchyma:** RDS, pulmonary edema, pulmonary hypoplasia, meconium aspiration syndrome.
    - **Space-occupying lesions of the chest:** Pneumothorax, interstitial emphysema, congenital lobar emphysema, CHDs, pleural effusion, abdominal distention.
    - **Obstructive lesions:** Choanal atresia; vocal cord paralysis; vascular rings; stenotic lesions, membranes, and cysts; Pierre Robin syndrome.
    - **CNS:** Infection, hemorrhage, asphyxia, seizures, apnea, malformations, tumors.
    - **Neuromuscular:** Phrenic nerve palsy, thoracic dystrophies.
    - **Metabolic:** Hypoglycemia, hypocalcemia.
    - **Cardiovascular:** Heart failure (PDA or other significant left-to-right shunt, supraventricular tachycardia, congenital AV block).
  - **Right-to-left shunt:**
    - **Intrapulmonary:** Meconium aspiration syndrome, RDS; alveolar hypoventilation may also be seen.

- **Persistent pulmonary hypertension of the newborn (PPHN):** May have alveolar hypoventilation.
  - **Cardiac:** ↓ pulmonary blood flow (tetralogy of Fallot, tricuspid atresia, pulmonary atresia); normal or ↑ pulmonary blood flow (transposition of the great vessels, truncus arteriosus, anomalous pulmonary venous return).
- **Abnormal ventilation-perfusion (V/Q) ratios:**
  - **Lung parenchyma:** Atelectasis, meconium aspiration syndrome, infections, pulmonary hemorrhage.
- **Abnormal diffusion:** Pulmonary interstitial emphysema aspirations, pulmonary hemorrhage.
- **↓ hemoglobin O₂ affinity:** Methemoglobinemia (nitrates, sulfonamides, other drugs, congenital).

  $\downarrow$ **hemoglobin O_2 affinity:** Methemoglobinemia (nitrates, sulfonamides, other drugs, congenital).
- **↓ peripheral circulation (peripheral cyanosis):** Low cardiac output (e.g., hypocalcemia, pneumopericardium, cardiomyopathies), shock of any etiology, polycythemia, hypothermia, hypoglycemia.

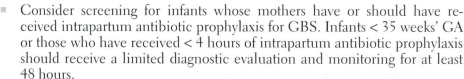

NEONATAL SCREENING AND PROPHYLACTIC MEASURES

Screening

Group B β-Hemolytic Streptococcal (GBS) Sepsis

- Consider screening for infants whose mothers have or should have received intrapartum antibiotic prophylaxis for GBS. Infants < 35 weeks' GA or those who have received < 4 hours of intrapartum antibiotic prophylaxis should receive a limited diagnostic evaluation and monitoring for at least 48 hours.
- A full diagnostic evaluation includes a CBC with differential, blood culture, a CXR if respiratory symptoms are present, and possibly LP.
- A limited evaluation includes a CBC with differential and blood culture, observation for 48 hours, and possibly a C-reactive protein level (CRP).

Any infant with symptoms of sepsis requires a full diagnostic evaluation and empiric therapy for at least 48 hours.

First Urination

- The initial step in management is to differentiate renal failure from urinary retention, usually via urinary catheterization.
- Infants who do not void within 24 hours of birth require evaluation. More than 90% of infants void within the first 24 hours, although a first undocumented micturition often occurs in the delivery room.
- Urinary tract ultrasound can identify abnormalities such as posterior urethral valves (thickened, trabeculated bladder) or ureteropelvic/vesicoureteral junction obstruction.
- **Causes of renal failure** are as follows:
  - **Acute renal failure (ARF):** May be either prerenal or with ATN; most commonly seen in the context of birth asphyxia or shock.
  - **Postpartum medication exposure:**
    - NSAIDs (indomethacin) or nephrotoxic antibiotics can → prerenal or intrinsic renal failure.
    - Opiates, anticholinergics, and paralytics may → functional bladder obstruction.
    - **Intrapartum medication exposure:** ACEIs, NSAIDs, or angiotensin receptor blockers can → renal dysgenesis.

NEONATOLOGY

- **Other:** Additional factors include bilateral renal disease such as polycystic kidney disease, renal agenesis/hypoplasia/dysplasia, and renal vessel thrombosis.

HEARING

- Significant hearing loss affects 0.1–0.3% of well infants.
- Evoked otoacoustic emission (OAE) testing can identify most neonatal hearing problems but may miss problems beyond the cochlea and may be impaired by debris in the ear canal.
- Auditory brain-stem evoked response (ABER) testing should be considered for infants with risk factors for congenital hearing loss, including NICU admission of > 48 hours duration, a family history of permanent childhood hearing loss, craniofacial abnormalities, congenital infection, and stigmata of syndromes with associated hearing loss.

NEWBORN SCREENS

- States vary with respect to the specific disease states for which they test; however, all states test for PKU and hypothyroidism, and most test for galactosemia and hemoglobinopathies.
- Newborn screens may not identify carrier states for many disorders. False ⊖s may occur in the context of prematurity, testing after blood transfusion, and testing too early (before 24 hours of age), and these conditions require that infants be retested.
- **Infants born to HIV-⊕ mothers** should be screened via HIV DNA PCR within the first 48 hours of life and again at 1–2 and 2–4 months of age. Infection can be excluded if two separate tests after one month of age and one test after four months of age are ⊖.

Prophylaxis

OPHTHALMIA NEONATORUM PROPHYLAXIS

Erythromycin or tetracycline is preferred to silver nitrate, as the latter may not protect against chlamydial conjunctivitis.

HEPATITIS B (HBV) IMMUNIZATION

- Recommended at birth for infants weighing > 2000 g who were born to HbSAg-⊖ mothers, but may be delayed until two months of age. Infants weighing ≤ 2000 g should receive the initial dose of HBV vaccine within 30 days.
- If infants are born to mothers whose HbSAg status is unknown, the mothers should be screened. An initial HBV vaccine should then be administered within 12 hours, and hepatitis B immune globulin (HBIG) should be administered within seven days if the mother tests ⊕. For infants weighing ≤ 2000 g, HBIG should be given within 12 hours unless the mother tests ⊖.
- For infants born to HbSAg-⊕ mothers, both HBV vaccine and HBIG should be given within 12 hours of birth. For infants weighing < 2000 g at birth, an additional dose of HBV vaccine must be given between two and three months of age, in between the standard doses at one and six months.

PREVENTION OF HIV TRANSMISSION

Protocols for the prevention of HIV transmission to infants born to HIV-⊕ mothers vary widely but include the following:

- **Predelivery:** Oral maternal antiretroviral drugs.
- **Peripartum:**
  - IV zidovudine (AZT).
  - Consider elective C-section prior to delivery, especially in the presence of a high viral load.
- **Postpartum:** Administration of AZT to the infant for the first six weeks of life.
- Informed consent regarding the risk of transmission via breast-feeding.

FLUIDS, ELECTROLYTES, AND NUTRITION

Fluid Requirements

Neonatal kidneys lack the ability to concentrate urine and retain sodium. Preterm kidneys have a ↓ capacity to resorb filtered bicarbonate and glucose.

- Maintenance fluid requirements vary widely, from 60 mL/kg/day for a relatively well term infant to 200 mL/kg/day for an extremely premature infant on a radiant warmer.
- Risk factors for ↑ insensible losses are as follows:
  - Low birth weight (LBW) due to an ↑ ratio of surface area to volume.
  - Prematurity due to skin H_2O permeability.
  - Gastroschisis or any congenital malformation with exposed abdominal viscera.
  - Environments such as radiant warmers or phototherapy.

Hypoglycemia

- Neonates with symptoms or risk factors (see Table 14-3) should be tested for hypoglycemia.

TABLE 14-3. Causes of Neonatal Hypoglycemia

RISK FACTORS	SYMPTOMS
Prematurity	Irritability
SGA/IUGR	Stupor
Birth weight < 2500 g	Seizures
IDMs	Apnea
Beckwith-Wiedemann syndrome	Cyanosis
Macrosomia	Tachypnea (especially irregular)
Being a discordant, small twin	Hypotonia
Polycythemia	Temperature instability
Hypothermia and cold stress	Feed refusal or poor suck
Suspected sepsis	
Respiratory distress	
Birth asphyxia or hypoxia	
Microphallus or midline defect	
Maternal treatment with terbutaline, propranolol, or oral hypoglycemic agents	

- Management is as follows:
  - Repeat glucose check via serum analysis, as Chemstrips may be unreliable.
  - Give an IV dextrose bolus followed by continuous IV infusion.
  - Treat underlying causes as appropriate.

Hyperglycemia

Can be found in preterm, SGA, or low-birth-weight infants; usually resolves spontaneously after approximately 1–2 weeks. Transiently high glucose can also be found in infants receiving corticosteroids, those receiving exogenous catecholamines, and those with any systemic infection.

Common Electrolyte Abnormalities

Table 14-4 outlines the clinical presentation and treatment of common electrolyte abnormalities.

Hyponatremia, along with poor growth, vomiting, lethargy, and hypotension in the first weeks of life, is suggestive of congenital adrenal hypoplasia.

TABLE 14-4. **Clinical Presentation of Common Electrolyte Abnormalities**

ABNORMALITY	SYMPTOMS	CAUSE	TREATMENT
Hypernatremia	Lethargy, weakness, irritability, seizures, altered mental status.	Dehydration, DI.	Slow replacement with hypotonic fluids; avoid ↓ Na > 15 mEq/dL/24 hours.
Hyponatremia	Lethargy, tremors, seizures.	Dehydration, diuretics, SIADH, cerebral salt wasting, congenital adrenal hyperplasia.	Slow correction with isotonic fluids; hypertonic saline only if seizing.
Hyperkalemia	Weakness, paresthesias, tetany, QRS widening, bradycardia.	Renal failure, acidosis, transfusion of senescent RBCs, endocrinopathy, excess administration of potassium.	Bicarbonate, calcium chloride, insulin/glucose.
Hypokalemia	Arrhythmia, weakness, ileus.	Diuretic use, lack of maintenance intake, renal losses (DKA, Fanconi, Bartter), alkalosis.	Replacement at a rate based on the severity of symptoms.
Hypermagnesemia	Vasodilation, apnea, hypotension.	Maternal treatment of preeclampsia, excess administration.	Calcium, diuretics.
Hypomagnesemia	Weakness, vomiting, hyperreflexia, clonus, tetany.	Lack of maintenance intake, diuretics, GI losses.	Replacement at a rate based on the severity of symptoms.
Hypocalcemia	Tetany, jitteriness, ectopy, seizures.	Prematurity, diuretic use, asphyxia, IDMs, hypoparathyroidism (DiGeorge syndrome/velocardiofacial syndrome), hypomagnesemia.	Calcium gluconate 50–100 mg/kg or calcium chloride 10–20 mg/kg.
Hypophosphatemia	Irritability, paresthesias, apnea, seizures, coma.	Lack of maintenance intake, especially in VLBW children; diuretics, alkalosis.	Replacement.

NEONATOLOGY

Nutrition Pearls

- **Breast-feeding:** Protective against GI pathogens as a result of immune cells, antibodies, enzymes, carrier proteins, glycoproteins, and oligosaccharides; promotes normal flora.
- **High long-chain polyunsaturated fatty acid content (docosahexaenoic acid, arachidonic acid):** May promote neuronal development.
- **Colostrum:**
    - Produced in the first five days postpartum.
    - Twice as rich in protein (~ 2:1 whey to casein) but less fat than mature milk; fewer calories (49 kcal/kg vs. 69 kcal/kg for milk).
    - Insufficient zinc for preterm infants; low in vitamin D; same concentration of minerals.
- Formula protein content: formula—whey < casein; opposite in breast milk—casein < whey.

RESPIRATORY DISORDERS

Meconium Aspiration Syndrome

Always rule out cardiac etiologies in the evaluation of an infant in respiratory distress.

- Typically affects term or near-term infants, often with fetal distress. Meconium may not be present at delivery. Blood aspiration looks similar to that of meconium aspiration.
- **Sx/Exam:** Respiratory distress presents immediately.
- **Dx:** CXR shows coarse irregular infiltrates and hyperexpansion but does not predict clinical severity.
- **Tx:** Tracheal suctioning does not prevent all cases of aspiration, as some aspiration occurs in utero. Significant ventilatory support is often required.
- **Complications:** Pneumothorax, PPHN, shock.

Persistent Pulmonary Hypertension of the Newborn (PPHN)

*Hyperoxia test: A PO_2 > 150–200 after 100% Fio_2 is suggestive **against** cyanotic heart disease (right-to-left shunting).*

- Failure of the physiologic ↓ in pulmonary vascular resistance after birth → poor lung perfusion and right-to-left shunting through the PDA. Uncommon in preterm infants.
- Risk factors include chronic fetal hypoxia, maternal DM, infection, hypoxia (especially RDS), cyanotic heart disease, cold stress, hypoglycemia, and pulmonary hypoplasia (e.g., in CDH).
- **Sx/Exam:** Respiratory distress, shock, postductal < preductal saturations.
- **Tx:** Inspired O_2; mild hyperventilation to a pH of 7.45. Inhaled nitric oxide. May require extracorporeal membrane oxygenation (ECMO).

Transient Tachypnea of the Newborn

- Tachypnea that results from retained fetal lung fluid and lasts 12–24 hours. Requires O_2.
- Generally affects term or near-term infants, with an ↑ risk in infants delivered by C-section or after a short labor.
- **Dx:** CXR shows perihilar streaking and fluid in the fissures.
- **Tx:** O_2, supportive care.

Congenital Pneumonia

- Usually presents in the first 24 hours of life. Caused by GBS, *E. coli*, and *Klebsiella*.
- Affects neonates of all gestational ages, with or without risk factors for intrauterine infection.
- **Dx:** Infiltrates are commonly diffuse on x-ray.
- **Tx:** Antibiotics; oxygenation and ventilation as necessary.

Respiratory Distress Syndrome (RDS)

- Also known as hyaline membrane disease. Caused by a surfactant deficiency that → ↓ lung compliance, atelectasis, and V/Q mismatch.
- The most common cause of respiratory distress in preterm infants, occurring in 14% of all low-birth-weight (< 2500-g) infants.
- Risk is ↑ in IDMs, males, Caucasians, and infants born via C-section without labor as well as those with birth asphyxia, chorioamnionitis, and non-immune hydrops. Has a familial predisposition.
- **Sx/Exam:** Respiratory distress occurs within four hours of birth but worsens over the next 48 hours.
- **Dx:** CXR shows ground-glass appearance with air bronchograms and hypoinflation.
- **Tx:**
    - **Antenatal steroids:** Improve lung maturity. Betamethasone and dexamethasone cross the placenta readily and improve mortality if given > 24–48 hours prior to delivery; however, they are of unknown benefit after 34 weeks' GA. Administration of > 3 courses of antenatal steroids is associated with ↓ neurologic outcome and growth.
    - **Early intubation:** To prevent hypoxemia and acidosis. Maintaining adequate lung volume with PEEP or CPAP ↓ atelectasis and V/Q mismatch.
    - **Endotracheal surfactant administration:** The first dose (prophylactic) is usually given in the delivery room; subsequent doses may improve outcome. Surfactant administration ↓ the degree of ventilation and oxygenation support necessary and improves overall mortality. Associated with a risk of pneumothorax during administration due to an acute change in lung compliance. Prophylactic therapy may play a role in infants < 26–27 weeks old.
    - **Empiric antibiotic therapy:** Sepsis and congenital pneumonia may be indistinguishable from RDS early on.
    - Optimize thermoregulation to reduce further cold stress; optimize nutrition.
- **Complications:**
    - Hypoxemia and hypercarbia may → PPHN and PDA.
    - A severe need for ventilatory support (barotrauma, oxygen toxicity) → pneumothorax/pneumomediastinum, pulmonary interstitial emphysema, and long-term results in bronchopulmonary dysplasia.
    - Tracheal stenosis if prolonged intubation.

Congenital Diaphragmatic Hernia (CDH)

- The most common cause of pulmonary hypoplasia. Often associated with a scaphoid abdomen.

- **Tx:**
    - Immediate intubation and assisted ventilation. Avoid bag-mask positive pressure ventilation.
    - Immediate GI decompression.
    - Limit spontaneous respiration via paralysis.
    - Evaluate for other congenital abnormalities, which are present in up to 40% of infants with CDH.
- **Complications:** Associated with a high risk of pneumothorax and pulmonary hypertension due to abnormal vasculature. Bronchopulmonary dysplasia and chronic lung disease may develop.

Pulmonary Hemorrhage

- Most cases are clinically not evident, with up to 80% of preterm infants having only autopsy evidence. Massive bleeding is clinically evident as respiratory distress and frank blood from the endotracheal tube/upper airway. The mortality rate of clinically evident pulmonary hemorrhage is roughly 30%.
- Aside from prematurity, an ↑ risk is associated with birth asphyxia, maternal toxemia, maternal cocaine use, erythroblastosis fetalis, infection, RDS, and ECMO.
- **Tx:** Endotracheal intubation and suction; maintenance of high mean airway pressure.

Spontaneous Pneumothorax

- Immediate onset of respiratory distress. Occurs in 1% of all deliveries, especially those requiring intubation or positive-pressure ventilation.
- **Sx/Exam:** Unilaterally ↓ breath sounds.
- **Dx:** Diagnose via transillumination and CXR.
- **Tx:** Administration of 100% O_2 may → the rapid resorption of intrapleural air. Needle thoracentesis if the patient is symptomatic with tachypnea, an O_2 requirement, tachycardia, or BP instability.

Airway Obstruction

- Choanal atresia.
- **Symptoms/Exam:**
    - The Pierre Robin sequence presents with micrognathia, glossoptosis, and posterior palatal cleft.
    - May occur in the context of other syndromes (e.g., velocardiofacial syndrome, CHARGE association).
    - Laryngeal malformations, tracheomalacia.

Congenital Cystic Adenomatous Malformation (CCAM)

- A developmental lung anomaly that acts as a space-occupying mass.
- Characterized by overgrowth of terminal bronchioles with persistence of airway communications → single or multiple cysts.
- Respiratory distress usually begins within the first hours of life if the CCAM is of significant size. Additionally, large CCAMs with midline shift of mediastinal structures can → hydrops fetalis.

- **Tx:** Larger cysts (type I) are amenable to resection and have better survival than do those with multiple smaller cysts (type II or III). Type II CCAMs have an ↑ association with other congenital malformations.
- **Complications:** Pneumothorax.

Congenital Lobar Emphysema

- A defect in bronchial cartilage → air trapping from the collapse of bronchi during expiration.
- **Sx/Exam:** Presents as respiratory distress with wheezing. Hyperinflation may → mediastinal shift.
- **Dx:** CXR reveals upper more than lower lobe involvement.

Pulmonary Sequestration

- Abnormal pulmonary tissue that is not continuous with the respiratory tract and is variably supplied by systemic vasculature.
- Some 90% are left sided; 40% of extralobar sequestrations are associated with other congenital abnormalities, including bronchogenic cysts, heart defects, and CDH.
- **Dx:** Angiography is required to determine arterial supply.
- **Tx:** Surgical.

GASTROINTESTINAL DISORDERS

Gastroschisis and Omphalocele

Abnormal development of the abdominal cavity with failure of abdominal contents to return to the abdominal cavity → abdominal wall defects. Table 14-5 contrasts the two conditions.

TABLE 14-5. Gastroschisis vs. Omphalocele

	GASTROSCHISIS	OMPHALOCELE
Location	Right of umbilicus.	Central.
Umbilical cord	Intact.	Umbilical cord elements surround the sac and join above the extrusion.
Protective sac	Full-thickness defect; no protective sac.	Protective sac is preserved.
Liver and spleen	Remain within the abdominal cavity.	Partially extruded in large defects.
Associated congenital anomalies	**Rare.**	**Common.**

GASTROSCHISIS

Associated with concomitant intestinal atresias or malrotation.

SYMPTOMS/EXAM

See Table 14-5.

DIAGNOSIS

Prenatal ultrasound.

TREATMENT

- Temperature regulation (high risk of infant hypothermia due to exposure of large surface area).
- Fluid regulation (high fluid losses are possible; apply protective dressing and wrap the abdomen in cellophane).
- NG decompression, broad-spectrum antibiotics, TPN.
- **The definitive treatment is surgical correction.**

COMPLICATIONS

Impaired peristalsis and intestinal absorption (usually temporary). Risk of necrotizing enterocolitis (NEC).

OMPHALOCELE

SYMPTOMS/EXAM

- Associated congenital anomalies occur in a majority of cases and include the following:
  - Chromosomal abnormalities, including trisomies and Beckwith-Wiedemann syndrome.
  - Congenital heart disease.
  - Pentalogy of Cantrell → omphalocele, anterior diaphragmatic hernia, sternal cleft, ectopia cordis, and intracardiac defects (VSD or left ventricular diverticulum).
- Peristalsis and absorption issues are less frequent than in gastroschisis, as the membrane protects intestines (see also Table 14-5).

DIAGNOSIS

Prenatal ultrasound.

TREATMENT

- **Ruptured sac:** As with gastroschisis, treat with emergent surgical repair.
- **Intact sac:** Treat with urgent, but not necessarily emergent, surgical repair.
- Temperature regulation issues are generally less significant, as the protective membrane allows for heat conservation.

- Associated with prematurity, IUGR. Often related to associated congenital anomalies.

Duodenal Obstruction

SYMPTOMS/EXAM

- Presents with vomiting and a possible history of polyhydramnios together with a large volume of gastric contents at birth.
- Abdominal distention is less prominent (vs. distal obstruction).

DIAGNOSIS

- AXRs (KUB and cross-table lateral) reveal the **double-bubble sign** from gas collection in the distal stomach and duodenum proximal to the obstruction, as well as lack of distal bowel gas.

TREATMENT

NPO and IV fluids; NG decompression; surgical repair.

It is abnormal to have no radiographic evidence of air in the rectum by 24 hours of life.

Pyloric Stenosis

SYMPTOMS/EXAM

- Presents with projectile vomiting and associated feeding intolerance. Onset at 2–8 weeks of life.
- The characteristic duodenal "olive" may be palpated.

DIAGNOSIS

- Labs reveal hypochloremic alkalosis, hyponatremia, and hypokalemia.
- Upper GI contrast studies reveal the characteristic **string sign.**
- Ultrasound allows for definitive diagnosis.

TREATMENT

- NPO with IV fluids to treat dehydration.
- **Correct electrolyte abnormalities:** Replace chloride with NS; replace potassium with KCl.
- Surgical repair (pyloromyotomy) is definitive.

*Pyloric stenosis is considered a **medical, not a surgical, emergency.** Chloride repletion is key, and surgery should be delayed until this is achieved.*

> A three-week-old infant presents to the ER with a recent history of poor feeding followed by the onset of bilious emesis and bloody stools. On examination, the infant is noted to be irritable, crying throughout with little response to his parents' efforts to console him. He is also noted to have a distended, tender abdomen. What is the suspected condition, and what should happen next? This is malrotation with midgut volvulus, and the infant is taken to the OR immediately following diagnosis.

Malrotation with Midgut Volvulus

SYMPTOMS/EXAM

- Obstruction may be chronic intermittent or acute.
- Acute obstruction presents with bilious emesis and bloody, mucoid stools as well as with feeding intolerance, peritonitis, irritability or lethargy, and shock.

DIAGNOSIS

- Upper GI contrast study with small bowel follow-through reveals evidence of duodenal obstruction with a **corkscrew appearance;** abnormal position of the ligament of Treitz; and abnormal position of the cecum (i.e., not in the RLQ).
- Contrast enema reveals abnormal position of the cecum.
- Labs reveal metabolic acidosis and possible thrombocytopenia.

TREATMENT

NPO with IV fluids; correction of dehydration and metabolic acidosis; NG decompression; **emergent surgical correction.**

COMPLICATIONS

Midgut necrosis complicated by short gut syndrome.

Proximal GI Obstruction

SYMPTOMS/EXAM

Vomiting is prominent and distention less prominent.

DIAGNOSIS

AXRs (KUB and cross-table lateral); upper GI contrast study with small bowel follow-through.

TREATMENT

NPO with IV fluids; NG decompression; surgical repair.

Distal GI Obstruction

SYMPTOMS/EXAM

- Abdominal distention is prominent.
- Presents with absence or limited passage of stool as well as with feeding intolerance.
- Vomiting is possible and is most likely bilious.

DIAGNOSIS

- AXRs (KUB and cross-table lateral) reveal multiple dilated loops.
- Contrast enema may reveal clear evidence of colonic atresia, microcolon, a transition zone (proximal dilatation, distal normal caliber) suggesting a diagnosis of Hirschsprung disease, or evidence of meconium plug–hypoplastic left colon syndrome.

- A rectal mucosal biopsy is required for a definitive diagnosis of Hirschsprung disease.

TREATMENT

Treatment depends on the etiology:

- Ileal or colonic atresia requires surgical repair.
- Meconium plug–hypoplastic left colon syndrome requires time, colonic digital exam stimulation, and enemas.
- Hirschsprung disease should be treated with surgical resection of the aganglionic segment.

COMPLICATIONS

Hirschsprung's disease is often complicated by potentially severe enterocolitis.

Imperforate Anus

Lack of an anal opening of appropriate size and/or location. May be high or low (see Table 14-6).

SYMPTOMS/EXAM

Presents with lack of a proper anal opening and no passage of stool.

DIAGNOSIS

- Calibration of the perineal opening if present.
- Plain films of the lumbosacral spine and urinary tract (first-line screen for likely associated dysmorphisms).

TREATMENT

- Surgical correction; exact treatment varies.

COMPLICATIONS

- Incontinence (especially in high lesions).
- Associated with VACTERL as well as with other congenital anomalies, including urologic abnormalities, spinal abnormalities, and uterine and/or vaginal abnormalities.

TABLE 14-6. High vs. Low Imperforate Anus

HIGH IMPERFORATE ANUS	LOW IMPERFORATE ANUS
The rectum terminates above the puborectalis sling.	The rectum develops through the puborectalis sling in the proper location.
No associated perineal fistula.	Imperforate anus with possible associated fistula.
Rectovaginal (female) or rectourinary (male) fistula is possible.	Simple anal stenosis is also possible.

Meconium ileus is the most common neonatal presentation of CF (90% of patients with meconium ileus will be diagnosed with CF).

Meconium Ileus

Obstruction of the terminal ileum with meconium.

SYMPTOMS/EXAM

Signs and symptoms of distal GI obstruction, including abdominal distention, vomiting, passage of few (inspissated meconium) or no stools. Colonic perforation may lead to peritonitis.

DIAGNOSIS

- AXRs (KUB and cross-table lateral) reveal dilated loops of variable caliber and lucency as well as calcifications characteristic of perforation with leakage of meconium into the peritoneal space.
- Barium enema reveals microcolon.

TREATMENT

- Enemas with fluid and electrolyte replacement if necessary.
- Surgical repair if needed.

COMPLICATIONS

Intestinal perforation; complications from CF.

A neonate who does not pass meconium in the first 24 hours of life requires evaluation.

GI Bleeding

SYMPTOMS/EXAM

Hematemesis (with upper GI bleeding) and blood in stool ranging from occult heme-⊕ stool to blood streaking or hematochezia.

DIAGNOSIS

- **Apt test** distinguishes maternal from fetal blood on the basis of differences between hemoglobin F and hemoglobin A. Solution remains pink if fetal blood and turns yellow-brown if maternal blood.
- **Obtain the following labs:**
    - CBC with differential and platelets; coagulation studies (PT/PTT, fibrinogen, platelets); electrolyte panel.
    - ABG to evaluate for metabolic acidosis.
    - Lab workup for suspected NEC.
- **Imaging to obtain** include AXRs, ultrasound to evaluate for pyloric stenosis, and an upper GI contrast study with small bowel follow-through to look for malrotation and other forms of obstruction, endoscopy to confirm ulcers.

TREATMENT

- **Upper GI bleeding:** Gastric lavage, volume replacement (NS), blood transfusion.
- **Stress ulcers:** H_2 blockers.
- **NG trauma:** Prevent by using the smallest tube possible; observation.
- **Anal fissure:** Observation +/– petroleum jelly.
- **Formula intolerance:** Diagnose and resolve through trial of elemental formula.
- **Hemorrhagic disease of the newborn:** Vitamin K.

> A premature infant born at 29 weeks' GA is in the intensive care nursery and is doing well. Enteral feedings were begun five days earlier. The mother is not interested in breast-feeding, so the infant is receiving formula. Overnight, the infant is noted to have an ↑ number of apneic spells (up from four in a 12-hour period to four in one hour) accompanied by ↑ abdominal girth, and before a scheduled feed he is noted to have 1.5 mL of green gastric residual. What steps should be taken next? This is suspected NEC. The infant is made NPO and placed on IV fluids. A baseline KUB is obtained and reveals a mild ↑ in the caliber of intestinal loops but no other abnormalities. A CBC and blood cultures are obtained.

Necrotizing Enterocolitis (NEC)

The most common life-threatening GI disorder of the neonatal period. Involves varying degrees of intestinal necrosis that may be associated with gas accumulation in the submucosal layers (pneumatosis intestinalis), perforation, peritonitis, sepsis, and death. Terminal ileum and colon are most commonly affected. Pathogenesis is not completely understood but is thought to be multifactorial; some combination of a breach in the intestinal mucosal barrier, infection, and immature host defenses. Risk factors include the following:

- **Prematurity** (and associated LBW).
- Enteral feedings (especially when rapidly advanced in volume and concentration); formula feedings.
- Bowel ischemia caused by umbilical artery or umbilical vein catheters, PDA, indomethacin for PDA, polycythemia, birth asphyxia, in utero cocaine exposure, or RDS.

SYMPTOMS/EXAM

- Signs and symptoms:
    - Feeding intolerance with an ↑ in gastric residuals (often bilious); abdominal distention; heme-⊕ stools (ranging from occult to frankly bloody in severe cases).
    - Abdominal wall discoloration; abdominal tenderness; absence of bowel sounds.
    - Apnea; temperature instability.
    - Hypo- or hyperglycemia.
    - Hypotension.
    - Thrombocytopenia.
- Severe disease is associated with peritonitis, sepsis, DIC, and shock.

Criteria for the diagnosis and treatment of NEC are outlined below (see also Table 14-7).

- **Stage 1—suspected NEC:**
  - NPO, IV fluids.
  - Baseline KUB.
  - Test all stools for occult blood.
  - CBC with differential and platelets; blood culture.
  - Urine and CSF cultures if systemic signs and symptoms are present.
  - Serial abdominal exams.
  - Consider NG decompression, antibiotics, and stool culture.
  - Consider slow resumption of feeds in three days if consistent improvement is seen.
- **Stage 2 or 3—definite to advanced NEC:**
  - NPO for at least 7–10 days.
  - IVF with fluid resuscitation PRN; extreme "third spacing" volume loss may occur.
  - NG decompression.
  - Serial AXRs to evaluate for pneumatosis intestinalis, portal venous air, and pneumoperitoneum.
  - Obtain a blood culture and start antibiotics (ampicillin and gentamicin).
  - Follow CBC with differential and platelets to evaluate for falling platelet levels or a shift toward immature WBCs.
  - Follow coagulation studies for evidence of DIC and support with FFP PRN.
  - Follow ABG for evidence of metabolic and/or respiratory acidosis with correction PRN.
  - Follow electrolytes and correct abnormalities; watch for hyperkalemia.
  - Give volume expanders and pressors PRN to maintain adequate SBP.
  - Endotracheal intubation with mechanical ventilation PRN.
  - Surgical consultation.

TABLE 14-7. Diagnosis and Treatment of NEC

DIAGNOSTIC CATEGORY	SUSPECTED NEC	DEFINITE NEC	ADVANCED NEC
Systemic illness	Temperature instability, glucose instability, ↑ episodes of apnea/bradycardia.	Mild to moderate symptoms.	Severe symptoms with possible hypotension and shock.
Abdominal symptoms	↑ gastric residuals, abdominal distention, occult or grossly bloody stools.	↑ abdominal distention, abdominal tenderness, absent bowel sounds.	Marked distention, peritoneal signs.
Labs		Metabolic acidosis, low platelets.	Metabolic and respiratory acidosis, DIC.
Imaging	AXR reveals normal to mild distention, bowel wall thickening, and possibly a fixed, dilated loop.	Pneumatosis intestinalis, portal venous gas.	Pneumoperitoneum if perforation has occurred.

- Intestinal stricture → bowel obstruction, short bowel syndrome, and cholestasis (associated with prolonged TPN).
- Mortality is as high as 20–30%.

HEMATOLOGIC DISORDERS

Physiologic Anemia

Defined as a normal ↓ in infant hemoglobin from 14–20 g/dL at birth (infants > 34 weeks' GA) to a nadir of approximately 11 g/dL between 8 and 12 weeks of age.

DIAGNOSIS

Appropriate timing and degree of hemoglobin nadir may be noted on labs.

Anemia of Prematurity

SYMPTOMS/EXAM

- Premature infants (< 34 weeks' GA) suffer a more rapid and substantial ↓ in their hemoglobin levels. The nadir is usually reached between four and eight weeks of life, with hemoglobin falling to approximately 7–9 g/dL.
- The extent of the drop is related to a ↓ RBC mass at birth, a ↓ birth level of erythropoietin and weaker response, a shorter RBC life span, ↑ iatrogenic loss (blood draws), and ↑ overall infant growth rate.
- Anemia → pallor, tachycardia, tachypnea, apnea, poor feeding and suboptimal weight gain, and ↓ activity.

DIAGNOSIS

Infants born at < 34 weeks' GA exhibit variations in RBC indices that include ↓ hemoglobin (nadir of 7–9 g/dL), ↑ reticulocyte count, and ↑ MCV.

TREATMENT

Iron, Epogen, blood transfusion.

Hemolytic Disease of the Newborn: Erythroblastosis Fetalis

- Maternal antibody against RBC antigens that cross the placenta and coat fetal RBCs → accelerated fetal RBC destruction via extravascular hemolysis.
- Can occur with Rh incompatibility (D antigen on Rh group), ABO incompatibility, and, rarely, minor blood group antigens such as Kell, Duffy, C, and E.
- Associated with early jaundice and anemia.

ISOIMMUNE HEMOLYTIC ANEMIA: ABO INCOMPATIBILITY

SYMPTOMS/EXAM

- Presents with early jaundice (within the first 24 hours).
- True anemia is rare (reticulocytosis usually compensates for hemolysis).

Neonatal anemia is defined as hemoglobin < 13 g/dL (central venous sample) or < 14.5 g/dL (capillary sample).

NEONATOLOGY

411

Type A blood is most antigenic and therefore most often associated with significant hemolytic disease.

*In isoimmune hemolytic anemia, no maternal amnestic response occurs, so birth order is **not** a risk factor.*

Causes of hydrops fetalis—VICTIMS

Vascular abnormalities
Infection (TORCH)
Cardiac (CHD, dysrhythmias)
Thoracic abnormalities (e.g., CCAM)
Isoimmune hemolytic anemia
Many others (e.g., chromosomal, CNS, lymph system abnormalities)
Skeletal abnormalities

Nonimmune causes of hemolytic disease are now more common than immune-mediated causes such as isoimmune hemolytic anemia.

DIAGNOSIS

- CBC with differential and platelets reveals characteristic microspherocytosis, polychromasia, and normoblastosis.
- Reticulocyte count is ↑ to 10–30% (vs. a normal value of 4–5%).
- Direct Coombs' test is **weakly** ⊕.
- LFTs reveal indirect hyperbilirubinemia with an early, rapid ↑ in bilirubin level.

TREATMENT

- Early diagnosis is key. Appropriate treatment must be initiated to prevent complications from hyperbilirubinemia and significant anemia.
- With maternal blood type O, newborn cord blood should be sent for typing and Coombs' testing.
- Treat hyperbilirubinemia with early, aggressive phototherapy and frequent bilirubin levels; initiate exchange transfusion if necessary (rarely needed); consider IVIG in cases of significant hemolysis.

COMPLICATIONS

Anemia is usually mild. The most common complications are those associated with hyperbilirubinemia.

ISOIMMUNE HEMOLYTIC ANEMIA: RH INCOMPATIBILITY

Maternal Rh sensitization usually occurs with delivery, miscarriage, abortion, ectopic pregnancy, or invasive prenatal procedure (chorionic villus sampling, amniocentesis, fetal blood sampling). Risk factors include the following:

- **Birth order:** Anamnestic response to sensitization occurs in this case, with augmented antibody response to each exposure.
- **C-section delivery:** Associated with placental trauma.
- **Male gender:** Associated with an ↑ risk of hemolysis for unknown reasons.
- **Ethnicity:** Rh-⊖ status is most common among Caucasians.

SYMPTOMS/EXAM

- Mild to severe anemia with associated complications, possible pallor, cyanosis, tachycardia, tachypnea, and jaundice with indirect hyperbilirubinemia.
- Hepatosplenomegaly is also seen.
- Hydrops fetalis is seen in severe cases and is characterized by:
    - Hypoproteinemia with associated fluid collections (ascites, pleural effusion, generalized edema).
    - Severe anemia with associated hypoxemia; high-output cardiac failure with CHF.
    - Pulmonary edema; insufficient surfactant.
    - Cardiovascular problems, including hypotension, poor perfusion, and dysrhythmias.
    - Metabolic acidosis.

- Look for an Rh-⊖ mother previously sensitized to Rh (D) antigen and an Rh-⊕ fetus.
- CBC with differential and platelets reveals moderate to severe anemia, polychromasia, and normoblastosis.
- Reticulocyte count ↑ to 10–40%.
- Direct antiglobulin test (DAT) is usually **strongly** ⊕.
- Early (within first 24 hours) indirect hyperbilirubinemia.

TREATMENT

- **Prenatal:**
  - Maternal blood typing.
  - Anti-Rh antibody titer to detect sensitization in Rh-⊖ patients, repeated at 28–34 weeks' gestation.
  - RhoGAM at 28 weeks' gestation if there is no evidence of sensitization.
  - If sensitization has occurred, serial antibody titers, serial amniotic fluid bilirubin concentrations, and serial fetal ultrasounds can all help determine if and when an infant must be delivered early.
  - Consider intrauterine fetal transfusion when severe hemolysis and anemia occur too early in gestation for delivery to be an option.
- **Postnatal** (excluding hydrops fetalis management):
  - Cord blood studies for typing, initial hemoglobin level, initial bilirubin level, direct Coombs' test.
  - Serial bilirubin levels to evaluate both absolute level and rate of ↑.
  - Aggressive phototherapy to treat hyperbilirubinemia.
  - Exchange transfusion if and when necessary. A bilirubin ↑ of > 0.5 mg/dL/hour or > 5 mg/dL over 24 hours within the first 48 hours of life, or projection of a level exceeding the threshold, are indications for exchange transfusion.
  - IVIG to mitigate hemolysis.

HYDROPS FETALIS

- Resuscitation of newborns may be complex and may require assisted ventilation; evacuation of fluid collections (thoracentesis, paracentesis); glucose monitoring and PRN supplementation; and single-volume exchange transfusion just after delivery.
- Tx:
  - **Central arterial and venous catheterization:** Allows for simple and exchange transfusions, ABG monitoring, BP monitoring, and labs.
  - Mechanical ventilation with high PEEP.
  - Exogenous surfactant.
  - **Medical interventions:** Consider diuretics, inotropes, and volume expanders.
  - Cardiac evaluation with ECG and echocardiography when indicated.

RhoGAM should be routinely administered to the mother at 28 weeks' gestation or within 72 hours of any episode associated with a high risk of sensitization.

Appropriate RhoGAM administration at 28 weeks' gestation may result in ⊕ infant DAT (hemolysis and reticulocytosis will be absent).

In utero hemolysis can be monitored via serial determination of bilirubin concentration in the amniotic fluid and MCA with Doppler velocimetry.

An initial hemoglobin < 12 g/dL and a bilirubin > 4 mg/dL are associated with an ↑ risk of severe disease.

NEONATOLOGY

An infant is born at 37 weeks to a mother with a history of preeclampsia. The infant is noted to have a relatively ruddy appearance that deepens during the next few hours. The infant is also noted to have mild tachycardia and tachypnea. A dextrose stick reveals a glucose level of 58. What is the suspected diagnosis? The team suspects polycythemia. A spun hematocrit level is found to be 70, confirming the diagnosis.

Polycythemia/Hyperviscosity

Increased concentration of RBCs often → elevated blood viscosity. Risk factors include:

- High altitude.
- Delayed cord clamping (> 30-second delay).
- High-risk delivery.
- Endocrine disorders (IDMs, GDM, congenital thyrotoxicosis, congenital adrenal hyperplasia, genetic trisomies).
- Recipients of twin-twin transfusion.
- Birth asphyxia.
- Neonatal age (highest hematocrit at 2–4 hours after birth).

SYMPTOMS/EXAM

- Presents with plethora (ruddy, deep red skin color).
- Symptoms include lethargy, irritability, and vasomotor instability; respiratory distress; tachycardia; feeding intolerance; hypoglycemia; hyperbilirubinemia; and other metabolic abnormalities (hypocalcemia, hypomagnesemia).

DIAGNOSIS

- Central venous hematocrit > 65% (above this level, blood viscosity ↑ exponentially).
- Symptomatic infant.

TREATMENT

- Observation alone is adequate for almost all asymptomatic infants.
- Partial exchange transfusion (with saline) is appropriate in symptomatic infants.
- The benefits of partial exchange transfusion are the subject of increasing debate.

COMPLICATIONS

Seizures, pulmonary hypertension, NEC, renal failure.

Hemorrhagic Disease of the Newborn

SYMPTOMS/EXAM

Presents with bleeding (circumcision, mucosal, GI, intracranial) related to vitamin K deficiency.

DIAGNOSIS

- **Early form:** Bleeding on the first day of life; related to maternal medications that suppress fetal vitamin K production. Drugs include INH, rifampin, warfarin, phenytoin, and barbiturates.
- **Classic form:** Bleeding onset between the second and seventh days of life; related to lack of vitamin K supplementation at birth as well as normal but inadequate breast milk combined with lack of gut flora.
- **Late form:** Bleeding onset between two weeks and six months of age; related to inadequate vitamin K intake among breast-feeding infants and/or hepatobiliary disease.

TREATMENT

- IM vitamin K prophylaxis.
- IV/SQ vitamin K treatment (**not IM** 2° to risk of hematoma).
- Vitamin K supplementation to prevent hemorrhage in known deficiency states with repeated doses PRN.

Neonatal Alloimmune Thrombocytopenia

Occurs when there is a mismatch between maternal and paternal platelet antigens, with a fetus inheriting a platelet antigen from the father that the mother does not express. The most common antigen is HPA-1a. Maternal sensitization → antibody formation; antibodies then cross the placenta and attach to fetal platelets with subsequent destruction of fetal platelets by the reticuloendothelial system.

SYMPTOMS/EXAM

- Presents with thrombocytopenia and bleeding.
- Intracranial hemorrhage possible (see the discussion of complications).
- Petechiae (generalized), GI bleeding, and mucosal bleeding are also seen.

DIAGNOSIS

Lack of an appropriate bump in platelet count to random donor platelet transfusion supports the diagnosis.

TREATMENT

- Consider C-section delivery in known cases.
- Treat with transfusion of specific antigen-⊖ platelets when platelet count is < 20,000–30,000.
  - Maternal platelets are preferred where possible.
  - Platelets should be irradiated and washed or plasma reduced.
  - If maternal platelets cannot be harvested, HPA-1a-⊖ platelets are recommended.
- Consider IVIG and steroids.

Intracranial hemorrhage.

HYPERBILIRUBINEMIA

Unconjugated Hyperbilirubinemia

May be physiologic or pathologic. Risk factors for the development of pathologic hyperbilirubinemia include the following:

- **Prematurity** (GA < 37 weeks).
- **↑ RBC breakdown:**
  - **Hemolysis:** ABO incompatibility with ⊕ DAT (direct Coombs' test); Rh or other antigen incompatibility; RBC enzyme defects; RBC membrane defects.
  - **Other:** Cephalohematoma or significant bruising; polycythemia.
- **↑ enterohepatic circulation (reabsorption):** Breast-feeding jaundice (dehydration, inadequate milk intake); bowel obstruction; no enteric feedings 2° to other disorders.
- **↓ hepatic uptake and conjugation of indirect bilirubin:** Immature glucuronyl transferase (normal), Gilbert syndrome, Crigler-Najjar syndrome, pyloric stenosis, hypothyroidism, IDMs, breast milk jaundice.
- East Asian ethnicity (associated with a later, higher peak).

SYMPTOMS/EXAM

- Presents with jaundice and characteristic cephalocaudal progression with rising serum bilirubin levels.
- **Physiologic jaundice:**
  - **Term infants:** The majority of all newborns (50–60%) become jaundiced in the first week of life. Bilirubin level peaks at 3–5 days of life. The average peak total serum bilirubin level is 6 mg/dL.
  - **Preterm infants:** More often become jaundiced; have an earlier rise and a later peak (5–7 days). Associated with a higher risk of bilirubin encephalopathy.
- **Nonphysiologic (pathologic) jaundice:**
  - Jaundice within the first 24 hours of life and > 1 week in duration.
  - Bilirubin rising at a rate of > 5 mg/dL in 24 hours.
  - A direct bilirubin > 2 mg/dL.
  - In healthy, term infants, a total serum bilirubin level > 15 mg/dL at any time (lower absolute levels are found in preterm and sick infants).
- **Acute hyperbilirubin encephalopathy:**
  - **Early phase:** Lethargy, poor suck, hypotonia.
  - **Intermediate phase:** Irritability, hypertonia, fever, high-pitched cry.
  - **Advanced phase:** Hypertonia (specifically retrocollis and opisthotonos); fever, shrill cry, refusal to feed, apnea, severely altered mental status with possible coma, seizures, death.

DIAGNOSIS

- Total and direct serum bilirubin levels.
- Hematocrit.
- Determination of the blood type and Rh factor of both infant and mother.
- Direct antiglobulin test (Coombs' test) on the infant.

- Serial bilirubin level checks q 4–24 h depending on the absolute level and rate of rise.
- **Phototherapy:** Algorithms for initiation vary. Do not let total serum bilirubin exceed 15 mg/dL in an infant < 48 hours old or 20 in an infant 48–72 hours old.
- **Exchange transfusion:**
  - Recommended threshold levels for the decision to perform exchange transfusion vary.
  - In general, the threshold is a total serum bilirubin > approximately 20 mg/dL in full term infants.
  - In premature infants, the threshold is computed as weight (kg) × 10.

Total serum bilirubin should drop 30–40% with phototherapy over the first 24 hours, with the greatest reduction seen in the first 4–6 hours.

COMPLICATIONS

The most significant complication of hyperbilirubinemia is **kernicterus,** or chronic bilirubin encephalopathy. Presents with severe athetoid cerebral palsy, hearing impairment perhaps as severe as deafness, paralysis of upward gaze, and dental enamel dysplasia. Intellectual disability is rare.

Conjugated Hyperbilirubinemia

Occurs 2° to cholestasis. Etiologies are as follows:

- **Hepatocellular disease:**
  - Hepatitis (neonatal idiopathic, viral, bacterial).
  - Neonatal hemochromatosis.
  - TPN (usually prolonged).
  - Hepatic ischemia.
  - Metabolic disorders (galactosemia, hypothyroidism, other).
- **Biliary tree disorders:** Extrahepatic biliary atresia, insufficient bile ducts (Alagille syndrome, nonsyndromic), choledochal cyst.

SYMPTOMS/EXAM

Jaundice appears green rather than yellow.

DIAGNOSIS

- Total and direct bilirubin levels; AST, ALT, GGT.
- Urine-reducing substances.
- Hepatic ultrasound.
- Also consider HBV and HCV serologies; very long chain fatty acid level; HIDA scan; cholangiography.

TREATMENT

Conjugated bilirubin is not toxic and therefore carries no risk of acute or chronic bilirubin encephalopathy. No phototherapy.

COMPLICATIONS

Phototherapy may cause "bronze baby syndrome" and is contraindicated.

A term infant is born to a known GBS-$\oplus$ mother who was found to have ruptured membranes on her arrival at the labor-and-delivery department, and who received antibiotics < 4 hours prior to the delivery of her infant. How should the nursery team treat this patient? A CBC and blood cultures are obtained, and the infant is placed on ampicillin and gentamicin.

Neonatal Sepsis

May be early or late onset (see Table 14-8).

EARLY-ONSET NEONATAL SEPSIS

The first signs and symptoms may be subtle and may include feeding intolerance, ↑ need for supplemental O_2, and tachycardia. Risk factors are as follows **(think vertical transmission):**

- **Prematurity** (risk is inversely related to GA and birth weight).
- Premature ROM; prolonged ROM.
- Maternal GBS-$\oplus$ status (colonization).
- Maternal intrapartum fever.
- Chorioamnionitis.
- Multiple gestation.
- Neonatal resuscitation.
- Invasive procedures or instrumentation.

DIAGNOSIS

- **CBC with differential and platelet count:**
    - Absolute neutrophil count may be ↑.
    - The ratio of immature to total neutrophils (I/T ratio) > 0.3.
    - Neutropenia and thrombocytopenia are late signs.

TABLE 14-8. Characteristics of Early- and Late-Onset Neonatal Sepsis

CHARACTERISTIC	EARLY ONSET	LATE ONSET
Timing	First 5–7 days of life.	After the first week of life.
Symptoms	Nonspecific, systemic illness. Respiratory symptoms may be prominent.	Less frequently systemic; meningitis is common.
Transmission	Vertical.	Horizontal.
Causative organisms	Gram $\ominus$s now predominate (recent change): *E. coli*, GBS.	Gram $\oplus$s predominate: coagulase-$\ominus$ staph, *E. coli*, *Klebsiella*, *Pseudomonas*, *Candida*.

- Blood culture; LP for any symptomatic infant or for those with a ⊕ blood culture.
- Serial acute-phase reactant measures, especially serial serum CRP:
  - Rules out sepsis in patients > 28 weeks' GA if the level at 12 and 36 hours of life is < 1.0 mg/dL.
  - Does not rule in disease.
- Obtain a CXR for any infant with respiratory symptoms.
- Obtain a tracheal aspirate in the presence of any signs or symptoms of respiratory disease.
- Consider a urine culture.
- Examine the placenta and fetal membranes to evaluate for evidence of chorioamnionitis.

TREATMENT

- **Asymptomatic term infants:**
  - **One risk factor:** Minimum of careful exam plus a CBC with differential and platelet count.
  - **More than one risk factor:** Exam, CBC, blood culture, antibiotics.
- **Symptomatic and/or preterm infants:** CBC plus blood culture plus antibiotics. Antibiotics include ampicillin plus gentamicin or IV cefotaxime at meningitic doses.

LATE-ONSET (VS. NOSOCOMIAL) NEONATAL SEPSIS

Infants may become critically ill **soon** after the initial symptoms. Meningitis is more common with this presentation. Risk factors are as follows (**think horizontal transmission**):

- Prematurity.
- Term infants with medical or surgical conditions.
- Endotracheal intubation.
- Indwelling catheters (urinary, venous).
- Prior exposure to broad-spectrum antibiotics.

DIAGNOSIS

- CBC with differential and platelet count plus blood culture plus LP plus urine culture.
- CRP levels (in infants of any GA) at 12 and 36 hours after onset of symptoms.
- If levels are < 1.0 mg/dL at each sampling, the risk of sepsis is low.

TREATMENT

- Ampicillin + gentamicin or IV cefotaxime at meningitic doses.
- Supportive care.

Neonatal Candidiasis

SYMPTOMS/EXAM

Presentation is the same as that of neonatal sepsis. Usually late onset.

DIAGNOSIS

When blood culture is $\oplus$ (documented candidemia), evaluation for disseminated disease should also include the following:

- Urine and CSF cultures.
- Ophthalmologic exam (to rule out endophthalmitis).
- Echocardiogram (to rule out endocarditis).
- Renal ultrasound (to rule out fungus balls and abscesses).
- Radiographic skeletal survey (if any evidence of arthritis or osteomyelitis). Also consider diagnostic aspirate.

TREATMENT

Options include amphotericin B, fluconazole, and flucytosine (5-FC).

COMPLICATIONS

Invasive/disseminated disease is associated with particularly high mortality (25–35%).

An infant born at 37 weeks' GA is noted on initial well-baby exam to be SGA and have hepatosplenomegaly. The infant is carefully monitored and soon develops other signs and symptoms of illness, including jaundice and petechiae. Along with a sepsis workup, what other infections should be ruled out in this case? TORCH infections.

TORCH Infection

Consists of the following:

- Toxoplasmosis
- Other (HBV, syphilis, VZV, EBV, coxsackievirus, parvovirus)
- Rubella
- Cytomegalovirus (CMV)
- Herpes simplex virus (HSV)

Signs and symptoms common to the TORCH infections are discussed below.

TOXOPLASMOSIS (TOXOPLASMA GONDII)

Classic triad is obstructive hydrocephalus, chorioretinitis, and intracranial calcifications. Generally includes disseminated disease +/– CNS disease +/– ocular disease. The most significant risk factor is **maternal 1° infection during pregnancy.** The highest risk of transmission with infection occurs during the third trimester, and the most severe sequelae are associated with infection during the first trimester. Maternal infection risk factors include contact with cat feces (after contact with soil, litter boxes, etc.), ingestion of undercooked meat (especially pork) or eggs, and consumption of unpasteurized milk.

- **Disseminated disease:** Fever, hepatosplenomegaly, lymphadenopathy, eosinophilia, anemia, bleeding diathesis, rash, pneumonitis, direct hyperbilirubinemia.
- **CNS disease:** CSF abnormalities ($\uparrow$ protein), seizures, intracranial calcifications, microcephaly, hydrocephalus.
- **Ocular disease:** Chorioretinitis.
- Subclinical disease is thought to be most common and is followed by subsequent identification of visual/neurologic disease or learning disabilities; may lead to visual/neurologic disease or learning disabilities identified later in life.

DIAGNOSIS

- Serologic studies for:
    - $\uparrow$ **toxoplasma IgM:** $\oplus$ 1–2 weeks after infection; present for months to years.
    - $\uparrow$ **toxoplasma IgG:** Specific.
    - $\uparrow$ **toxoplasma IgA:** $\oplus$ in > 95% of patients with acute infection.
    - $\uparrow$ **toxoplasma IgE:** $\oplus$ in nearly all women who seroconvert during pregnancy.
- PCR gene amplification from amniotic fluid.
- Direct isolation of the organism (not usually available).
- CSF studies: IgM to toxoplasmosis.
- Head CT or cranial ultrasound reveals intracranial calcifications.
- Long-bone films show metaphyseal lucency and irregular epiphyseal calcification.
- Ophthalmologic exam reveals chorioretinitis.

TREATMENT

- Treatable but **not curable.**
- Give pyrimethamine + sulfadiazine + leucovorin calcium supplements.
- Spiramycin may be included in the regimen after six months of initial treatment with the above.

COMPLICATIONS

- Remember the classic triad of obstructive hydrocephalus, chorioretinitis, and intracranial calcifications.
- Abortion, stillbirth, and $\uparrow$ teratogenicity are associated with infection earlier in gestation.

RUBELLA

Risk factors include lack of maternal immunity to rubella, 1° maternal infection, maternal reinfection, and maternal viremia in **either the first or the last trimester.** Fetal infection essentially inevitable with maternal viremia in the ninth month of gestation. Seasonal pattern, with $\uparrow$ prevalence in the spring.

SYMPTOMS/EXAM

- The majority of infants with congenital rubella syndrome (CRS) are normal at birth, with the disease manifesting later in life as immunologic dyscrasias, hearing deficits, endocrinopathies (DM, thyroid disease). Man-

ifestations appear later in life as hearing deficits, endocrinopathies (DM, thyroid disease), psychomotor retardation, and other CNS effects.
- **Teratogenic effects:** IUGR, CHD (PDA, peripheral pulmonary artery stenosis), hearing deficits (sensorineural hearing loss), ocular deficits (glaucoma, cataracts), neonatal purpura, "blueberry muffin" rash.
- **Systemic effects:** Hepatosplenomegaly, hepatitis, jaundice, thrombocytopenia, encephalitis, meningitis, bony lesions ("celery-stalking" images on long bone).

DIAGNOSIS

CRS can be diagnosed through serologic studies and viral culture (from a nasopharyngeal swab, a conjunctival swab, urine, and CSF).

TREATMENT

There is no treatment for infection, only 2° treatment for complications.

PREVENTION

Prevent by **immunizing** young children (susceptible population, reservoir of infection). **Do not immunize nonimmune pregnant women** (live-virus vaccine is contraindicated).

CYTOMEGALOVIRUS (CMV)

More than 90% of neonates infected with CMV are asymptomatic. Symptomatic infants have a 20–30% mortality rate. Risk factors include 1° maternal infection, maternal reinfection or viral reactivation, prematurity, low socioeconomic status, maternal drug abuse, and a high number of maternal sexual partners.

SYMPTOMS/EXAM

Classic CMV inclusion disease presents with the following:

- IUGR.
- Hepatosplenomegaly, jaundice, abnormal LFTs.
- Thrombocytopenia +/– purpura.
- CNS effects (microcephaly, intracerebral [subependymal] calcifications, chorioretinitis, sensorineural hearing loss).
- Pneumonitis.
- Hemolytic anemia.

DIAGNOSIS

- Urine and/or saliva culture of organism (gold standard), PCR.
- Radiology studies (head CT or skull films) may reveal intracranial calcifications.
- Ophthalmologic exam; ABER for hearing exam.
- **Labs:** CBC, liver enzymes, bilirubin levels. CSF for regular indices, CSF CMV culture and/or DNA test.

TREATMENT

Consider ganciclovir.

COMPLICATIONS

Sensorineural hearing loss, ocular abnormalities, mental retardation, learning disabilities.

HERPES SIMPLEX VIRUS (HSV)

Risk factors for HSV transmission include maternal HSV-2 (more common than HSV-1), 1° maternal infection, reactivation of maternal infection, ROM, and delivery through the birth canal with active lesions and/or cervical shedding.

SYMPTOMS/EXAM

- There are three major categories of disease:
    - Mucocutaneous symptoms (skin, eyes, mouth [SEM]) are as follows: vesicular lesions, keratoconjunctivitis, chorioretinitis.
    - **CNS** (+/– SEM disease) usually present at approximately two weeks of age. Full fontanelle, irritability, poor feeding, temperature instability, encephalitis, seizures, tremors.
    - **Disseminated disease** (+/– SEM and CNS manifestations) include jaundice with abnormal liver enzymes, respiratory distress, lethargy and poor feeding, rash or purpura, bleeding, apnea, and shock; occurs early. Hepatosplenomegaly, jaundice with abnormal liver enzymes, rash or purpura, respiratory distress, apnea, lethargy and poor feeding, bleeding, shock.

DIAGNOSIS

- Viral culture (conjunctiva, nasopharynx, throat, urine, feces, CSF).
- Immunologic assays.
- Tzanck smear.
- CSF reveals ↑ RBCs, WBCs, and protein; sample for PCR.
- Head CT/MRI; EEG; characteristic localization of disease in temporal lobes.

TREATMENT

- **Antenatal:**
    - Consider acyclovir for women with 1° or 2° infection just before or at the time of delivery.
    - Deliver by C-section if there is clear evidence of 1° or 2° disease.
    - If there are no visible lesions and no prodromal symptoms, vaginal delivery is acceptable.
- **Neonatal:**
    - Isolation; high-dose acyclovir × 21 days.
    - Prophylaxis in infants born to mothers with active lesions should be given for 1° infection. For 2° infection, consider prophylaxis +/– surface cultures.
    - Breast-feeding is acceptable.
    - Parents with oral lesions should wear masks and should not kiss their infants.

COMPLICATIONS

- Psychomotor retardation and other neurologic problems.
- Mortality is highest in cases of disseminated disease.

> An infant is born to a known HBV (HBsAg)-⊕ mother who wishes to breast-feed. How should the infant be treated, and what do you tell the mother? The infant should receive HBIG within 12 hours after delivery as well as the HBV vaccine. Breast-feeding is acceptable, as the HBIG and vaccine protect the infant against infection.

Hepatitis (A, B, C, D, E)

HAV and HEV are likely to be transmitted only **rarely** because they have no associated carrier state. HDV occurs only as a coinfection with HBV, and management is therefore essentially the same. HBV, HCV, and HDV (delta) are more likely to be transmitted as a result of persistent infectious states.

HEPATITIS A (HAV)

- IVIG should be given to infants of infected mothers who became symptomatic two weeks before to one week after delivery.
- Isolation is indicated, but breast-feeding is acceptable.

HEPATITIS B (HBV)

Risk factors for HBV include the following:

- ⊕ HBe antigen and ⊖ anti-HBe in maternal blood test.
- High titer of maternal HBsAg.
- Maternal acute hepatitis in the third trimester or early postpartum period.
- Asian ethnicity.

SYMPTOMS/EXAM

Presentation varies and may include the following:

- Mild acute infection that is cleared.
- Chronic active hepatitis.
- Chronic persistent hepatitis.
- Chronic asymptomatic carriage.
- Fulminant hepatitis.

DIAGNOSIS

- Liver transaminases (AST, ALT) may be ↑.
- Bilirubin (conjugated and unconjugated) may also be ↑.
- Obtain a hepatitis panel both in the mother (HBsAg, HBeAg, anti-HBe, anti-HBc) and in the infant (HBsAg, anti-HBc IgM).

TREATMENT

- **In the presence of a mother who is known to be ⊕:**
  - HBIG within the first 12 hours of life.
  - HBV vaccine at birth and at one month and six months of age. (In premature infants weighing < 2 kg, the dose given at birth should not be counted in the series of three vaccines; give the "first" of three doses when the infant weights > 2 kg.)

- **If maternal status is unknown:**
  - Test the mother as soon as possible.
  - Give the infant HBV vaccine within the first 12 hours of life.
  - If the mother is found to be ⊕, give the infant HBIG within the first seven days of life.
  - Preterm infants should be given both vaccine and HBIG.
- Breast-feeding is acceptable if proper treatment is given.

COMPLICATIONS

Hepatocellular carcinoma is associated with a chronic carrier state.

HEPATITIS C (HCV)

SYMPTOMS/EXAM

- Long incubation period.
- The majority of infected infants have mild acute illness.
- Majority of infected infants have mild acute illness, but most go on to suffer chronic hepatitis.

DIAGNOSIS

- PCR diagnosis at 1–2 months of age.
- Serologic testing for anti-HCV antibody at > 2 years of age to allow for adequate clearance of maternal antibody.

COMPLICATIONS

Hepatocellular carcinoma is associated with chronic carrier state.

Varicella-Zoster (VZV) Infection

May be fetal/congenital, perinatal, or neonatal.

SYMPTOMS/EXAM

- **Fetal varicella-zoster syndrome:**
  - Occurs with 1° infection during pregnancy.
  - CNS manifestations include microcephaly, encephalitis, seizures, mental retardation, and intracranial calcifications.
  - Ophthalmologic manifestations include microphthalmos, chorioretinitis, cataracts, optic nerve atrophy, and Horner's syndrome.
  - Cicatricial skin lesions.
  - Symptoms of the limbs and fingers may include atrophy, hypoplasia.
- **Perinatal varicella-zoster syndrome:**
  - Occurs when the mother is infected during the last 21 days of pregnancy or within the first few days after delivery. The neonate typically shows signs and symptoms within the first 10 days of life.
  - Mild disease is possible.
  - Centripetal rash.
  - Possible fever, cyanosis, pulmonitis with diffuse nodular-miliary pattern on CXR.
  - Severe cases with multi-organ involvement.

- **Neonatal varicella-zoster syndrome:**
    - Infants usually present between 10 and 28 days of life.
    - Transmission occurs via droplets.
    - Disease is usually mild, with partial protection from maternal antibody.
    - Characteristic rash is present.
    - May be complicated by pneumonitis.

DIAGNOSIS

- Serologic evidence of VZV IgM antibody.
- PCR of DNA from tissue samples.
- VZV culture from vesicular lesions.

TREATMENT

- **If the mother was exposed during first or second trimester:**
    - Treat with varicella-zoster immune globulin (VZIG).
    - Consider acyclovir if the mother is diagnosed with active disease.
- **Perinatal exposure to mother with VZV infection 5–7 days before or 2–3 days after delivery:**
    - Give the infant VZIG and institute respiratory isolation.
    - Infants of mothers with rash > 7 days before delivery do not need VZIG; maternal antibody is protective.
    - Consider acyclovir in symptomatic infants.
    - Antibiotics for any superinfected skin infections.
- **Postnatal infection:** Treatment is the same as that for infants with perinatal exposure.

COMPLICATIONS

Fetal syndrome is the most significant complication and usually involves severe neurologic impairment.

Syphilis (*Treponema pallidum*)

Caused by spirochete.

SYMPTOMS/EXAM

- **Early congenital syphilis:** Hemolytic anemia, jaundice, rash (including palms and soles), osteochondritis, pneumonitis, snuffles.
- **Late congenital syphilis:** Hutchinson's teeth, healed retinitis, hearing impairment (2° to CN VIII nerve damage), saddle nose, saber shins, hydrocephalus, mental retardation.

DIAGNOSIS

- **Nonspecific antibody tests:**
    - VDRL, RPR.
    - Monitor titers; if ↓ within the first eight months, the infant is likely not infected.

- Specific treponemal tests:
  - FTA-ABS; if ⊕ beyond 6–12 months of age, the infant is likely infected.
  - Microhemagglutination test for *T. pallidum* (MHTPA).
  - IgM FTA-ABS (limited specificity).
- Microscopic dark-field examination of tissue specimens.
- CBC with differential and platelets.
- CNS indices plus VDRL and possible PCR/dark-field examination.

TREATMENT

- Treat the mother with penicillin; effective treatment should result in ↓ titers.
- Treat VDRL-⊕ infants.
  - The drug of choice is aqueous crystalline penicillin G × 10–14 days.
  - Monitor titer levels at 3, 6, and 12 months (should ↓).

Gonorrhea

Caused by gram-⊖ diplococci.

SYMPTOMS/EXAM

- **Ophthalmia neonatorum** is the most common presentation.
- **Gonococcal arthritis** usually occurs at the knees and/or ankles, but all joints are at risk. Symptom onset is 1–4 weeks after birth.
- Meningitis, sepsis also possible.

DIAGNOSIS

- **Maternal:** Obtain an endocervical culture.
- **Infant:**
  - Gram stain of exudates.
  - Obtain cultures of the eye, nasopharynx, orogastric area, and anorectal area. Obtain CT cultures as well as GC cultures.
  - Blood culture; CSF indices and culture.
  - Consider LCR.

TREATMENT

- Treat infants of infected mothers with single dose of ceftriaxone.
- Treat nondisseminated infection (e.g., ophthalmia neonatorum) with a single dose of ceftriaxone or cefotaxime plus saline eye irrigation; no topical treatment.
- Prophylaxis against ophthalmia neonatorum with erythromycin eye ointment.
- Disseminated infection (arthritis, sepsis) should be treated with ceftriaxone or cefotaxime × 7 days; treat meningitis × 10–14 days.
- Isolation for 24 hours.

COMPLICATIONS

Corneal perforation and blindness.

Chlamydia

Caused by *Chlamydia trachomatis*.

SYMPTOMS/EXAM

- Patients are usually afebrile, but present with:
  - Conjunctivitis.
  - Pneumonia (later presentation, at 3–11 weeks of age; symptoms worsen over time).
  - Rhinorrhea and cough (impair sleeping and eating) with otitis media.

DIAGNOSIS

- Tissue and sputum cultures, direct fluorescent antibody (DFA) staining, ELISA, PCR/LCR.
- Serologic studies to identify IgM.
- Gram stain of ocular discharge.
- CXR with hyperinflation and diffuse interstitial or alveolar infiltrates.

TREATMENT

- **Conjunctivitis:**
  - Prophylaxis with erythromycin ophthalmic ointment.
  - Erythromycin PO × 14 days. A repeat course may be necessary.
- **Pneumonia:** Treat with erythromycin × 14 days. No isolation is necessary.

COMPLICATIONS

Reactive airway disease may develop after pneumonia. Blindness may result if conjunctivitis is not treated.

> A healthy, term infant is born to a known HIV-⊕ mother on highly active antiretroviral therapy (HAART) with an undetectable viral load. How should the infant be treated and monitored? Administer AZT at a 2 mg/kg/dose q 6 h starting at 8–12 hours of life and continuing for six weeks. Virologic assay (HIV DNA PCR) on blood samples should be taken within the first 48 hours of life as well as at 14 days, 1–2 months, and 3–6 months. ELISA should be obtained twice at 6–18 months or once at 18–24 months. If all are ⊖, the child is considered ⊖.

Human Immunodeficiency Virus (HIV)

Children who are infected by vertical transmission of HIV tend to manifest signs and symptoms earlier (shorter latency period), with AIDS-defining conditions evident in many patients by four years of age.

SYMPTOMS/EXAM

- **General:** LBW, failure to thrive.
- **Nonspecific:** Fever, lymphadenopathy, hepatosplenomegaly, thrombocytopenia.
- **Infectious:** Recurrent thrush and candidal esophagitis; invasive bacterial infections, especially *Pneumococcus*; PCP, GI infections, VZV, CMV.
- **Respiratory:** Recurrent UTI, otitis media, sinusitis, bacterial infections, PCP.

Erythromycin treatment at < 6 weeks of age is associated with an ↑ risk of infantile hypertrophic pyloric stenosis.

Gonococcal conjunctivitis is usually more severe and tends to present earlier than chlamydial.

- **Cardiac:** Myocardial dysfunction, dysrhythmias, cardiomyopathies.
- **Neurologic:** Progressive encephalopathy, failure to achieve milestones, basal ganglia calcification, cortical atrophy.

DIAGNOSIS

- **Virology:** HIV DNA PCR should be performed within the first 48 hours of life and at 14 days, 1–2 months, and 3–6 months. Confirm $\ominus$ status with serial HIV ELISA between 6 and 24 months.
- **Markers of disease:** Low CD4 count or percentage; hypergammaglobulinemia.
- **Characteristic diseases:** Include candidiasis, PCP, cryptococcosis, *Mycobacterium avium–intracellulare*, EBV, and Kaposi's sarcoma.

TREATMENT

- **To prevent vertical transmission:**
  - Give zidovudine (AZT) during pregnancy, delivery, or HAART.
  - Deliver by C-section.
  - Treat the newborn with prophylactic AZT.
- **Supportive care of infected infants:**
  - Regular IVIG prophylaxis.
  - Vaccines should be given routinely, including live vaccines such as MMR and varicella, unless the patient is severely immunocompromised.
  - Nutritional optimization and support.
  - Prophylaxis (TMP-SMX for PCP; antivirals for VZV, HSV).

NEUROLOGIC DISORDERS

Seizures

Seizures have a variety of etiologies and can be distinguished as follows:
- **Bacterial meningitis** accounts for 5–10% of neonatal seizures, and such seizures are more delayed in onset (occurring in the first week).
- Neonatal seizures may result from subdural or subarachnoid hemorrhage 2° to birth trauma. The diagnosis often requires CT, as ultrasonography does not effectively visualize the periphery of the cranial vault.
- Venous sinus thrombosis commonly presents with neonatal seizures.
- Hypoglycemic seizures are more common in preterm infants, IDMs, and ill infants.
- Seizures from electrolyte abnormalities tend to be refractory to treatment with anticonvulsants and require treatment of the underlying abnormality.
- Hypocalcemic seizures are rare but more common in IDMs, preterm neonates, and those with hypoxic-ischemic encephalopathy (HIE) and are associated with tetany, laryngospasm, and weakness.
- Hypomagnesemic seizures may be associated with hypocalcemia resulting from functional hypoparathyroidism.
- Hyponatremic seizures may require hypertonic saline.
- Benign familial neonatal seizures classically begin during the first days of life and resolve by six months of life.
- AVMs may present with cranial bruits.
- Infants with a small HC may have congenital infection or structural abnormalities such as cortical dysgenesis.

The most common cause of seizures in preterm and term neonates is HIE from perinatal asphyxia. The seizures usually occur within the first 24 hours of life.

Physiologic neonatal jitteriness tends to have faster movements, involves all extremities, and can be stimulated by startle and stopped by restraint. It typically does not involve eye movements or autonomic instability.

"Fifth-day fits" are in the spectrum of benign familial neonatal seizures.

- Narcotic withdrawal, cerebral dysgenesis, pyridoxine deficiency, and inborn errors of metabolism (IEMs) are uncommon causes of neonatal seizures.
- Infants with particular odors can be diagnosed as follows:
  - **Maple syrup:** Branched-chain ketonuria.
  - **Musty:** PKU.
  - **Sweaty feet:** Isovaleric acidemia.

TREATMENT

The treatment of neonatal seizures involves management of ABCs and anti-convulsant therapy (lorazepam and phenobarbital). The prognosis depends on the underlying etiology, but mortality is four times greater in preterm than term infants.

Hypoxic-Ischemic Encephalopathy (HIE)

Ischemia due to global hypoxia or localized stroke. May be mild, moderate, or severe (see Table 14-9). Complications include cerebral palsy, seizures, hearing loss, and visual impairment.

Neural Tube Defects

- Folate deficiency during pregnancy ↑ the risk of spinal dysraphism. Zinc deficiency also ↑ that risk. Associated with high maternal serum AFP, but sensitivity and specificity are low.
- Spina bifida occulta can be missed in infancy and may present with subtle findings later in life (UMN signs; constipation or urinary incontinence).
- Myelomeningoceles are most often associated with Chiari II malformations and obstructive hydrocephalus, requiring ventriculoperitoneal shunting. Ultrasound in the second trimester is the best test to identify myelomeningocele. Treatment is required within the first few days of life. Long-term complications include abnormalities of spinal curvature, bladder function, growth, and lower extremity function.
- Other presentations include lumbosacral dimple, hypertrichosis, tail or pseudotail, lipoma, hemangioma, aplasia cutis, dermoid cyst, or dermoid sinus.

TABLE 14-9. Presentation of Hypoxic-Ischemic Encephalopathy

SEVERITY	SYMPTOMS	PROBABILITY OF NORMAL LONG-TERM OUTCOME (%)
Mild	Hyperalertness.	100
Moderate	Proximal hypotonia, impaired consciousness, seizures (easy to control).	50–80
Severe	Weakness, global hypotonia, coma, refractory seizures.	0

- **Dx:**
  - Ultrasound will demonstrate incomplete closure of lumbosacral verte-brae and is the test of choice in infants < 6 months of age.
  - Plain radiography is insensitive, and CT scan may show bony defects.
  - MRI offers the most definitive evaluation of spinal dysraphism.

Hydrocephalus

- Most commonly due to obstruction in the ventricular system, usually aqueductal stenosis or fourth ventricle abnormality.
- Nonobstructive hydrocephalus is uncommon in infancy but may be due to CNS infection or hemorrhage.
- Other causes of high ICP include cerebral infection, mass, hemorrhage, or metabolic derangement (acid-base or electrolytes)
- **Sx/Exam:** Hydrocephalus manifests as a rapid ↑ in HC, a bulging fontanelle, split sutures, papillary dilation, vomiting, and lethargy. Down-ward gaze ("setting-sun" sign), anisocoria, hypopnea, impaired EOMs, and papilledema are rare in infants.
- **Tx:** Ventriculoperitoneal shunting.

Intracranial Hemorrhage (ICH)

- In **term neonates,** ICHs are most commonly subarachnoid and are associ-ated with asphyxia or birth trauma from a difficult delivery.
  - **Sx/Exam:** Symptoms include irritability, apnea, bradycardia, cyanosis, and seizures (usually around the second day of life).
  - **Dx:** CT is the best modality for diagnosis in term newborns; cranial ul-trasonography is less sensitive. ↑ CSF RBCs and xanthochromia are confirmatory.
- Subdural hemorrhages usually present more slowly owing to expanding in-tracranial mass effect. Associated seizures usually occur on the second to third day of life. Other symptoms include bulging fontanelle, megalo-cephaly, and anemia.
- In **preterm infants,** intraventricular and periventricular hemorrhages of the subependymal germinal matrix are the most common ICHs. They oc-cur in 20–30% of infants born at < 31 weeks' gestation, and almost all oc-cur within the first four days of life.

All infants born at < 32 weeks' gestation require screening cranial ultrasound.

Periventricular Leukomalacia (PVL)

- A spectrum of white matter injury classically seen in preterm infants.
- Cystic PVL is the most severe form and → coagulation necrosis and lique-faction in the periventricular white matter. Lesions are usually bilateral, small, multiple, fairly symmetric, and well detected by ultrasonography.
- The pathophysiology is unclear. In addition to vascular boundary zones, one proposed etiology is selective vulnerability to specific cell types pre-sent in the developing brain to hypoxia-ischemia. In preterm infants, there may be selective vulnerability of certain cell types to hypoxia-ischemia.

Congenital Brachial Plexus Injury

- Presents with asymmetric Moro reflex. Occurs in approximately 0.1% of births; 90% recover spontaneously. Some 10% are bilateral.

- **Erb's palsy:** Due to upper brachial plexus injury (C5, C6). Symptoms include "headwaiter's tip hand," shoulder adduction, elbow extension, forearm pronation, and wrist flexion. **Grasp is present.**
- **Klumpke's paralysis:** Due to lower brachial plexus injury (C8, T1). Symptoms include hand weakness with **impaired grasp.** Most have Erb's palsy, and 30% have associated Horner's syndrome.

Normal Neonatal Vision

At birth, term neonates can fixate and respond to light, and acuity is roughly 20/400. Focal length is best at 8–15 inches. On average, horizontal tracking begins at one month of age, vertical tracking at two months, and circular tracking at three months.

Conjunctivitis

- **Chlamydia:** Some 60–70% of cases are transmitted via vaginal delivery. Watery discharge progresses to purulence and erythema. Silver nitrate is insufficient prophylaxis.
- *Neisseria gonorrhoeae:* Presents with sudden onset of purulent discharge; can be complicated by corneal ulceration.
- **Chemical conjunctivitis:** May result from antibiotic ointment.

Dacryostenosis

- Nasolacrimal duct obstruction occurs in roughly 6% of infants; 30% of cases are bilateral.
- **Sx:** Presents with mucoid discharge with tearing and crusting. Conjunctival or corneal injection is absent, as are photophobia and blepharospasm.
- **Tx:**
  - Spontaneous resolution occurs in 95% of cases by 12–13 months of age.
  - The efficacy of nasolacrimal duct massage is debatable. Nasolacrimal duct probing is 80% effective.
- **Complications:** Dacryocystitis (inflammation, erythema, and tenderness of the lacrimal sac); may require systemic antibiotics.

Congenital Glaucoma

- Sturge-Weber syndrome and other causes of port-wine stains involving the eyelids may be accompanied by glaucoma.
- Other diseases associated with infantile glaucoma are neurofibromatosis, retinoblastoma, trisomy 21, congenital rubella, and syphilis.
- **Sx/Exam:** Presents with a large iris rather than with pain or vision loss. Other symptoms include blepharospasm, tearing, and photophobia.

Leukocoria

- Defined as impairment of the red reflex. May be due to a variety of causes, including the following:

- **Retinoblastoma:** Bilateral in 30% of cases; associated with the autosomal-dominant Rb gene (chromosome 13). Can invade the brain via the optic nerve. Treatment (radiation, chemotherapy, enucleation) ↑ the risk of 2° osteosarcoma.
- **Cataracts:** Not all congenital cataracts require surgical intervention, but those that do have the best outcome with very early surgical intervention.
    - In the context of congenital infection, most commonly congenital rubella, can be associated with microphthalmia. More rarely seen with toxoplasmosis, HSV, CMV, EBV, hepatitis, and VZV.
    - Can be associated with trisomy 21, 18, and 13 and with other genetic syndromes as well as with metabolic and systemic disorders such as galactosemia and Alport's syndrome.
    - Inherited cataracts are most commonly autosomal dominant. Rarely, they may be autosomal recessive, X-linked, or sporadic.
- **Persistent hyperplastic primary vitreous (PHPV):** A persistence of fetal vascular and fibrotic tissue. Usually unilateral and associated with microphthalmia.
- Other causes of retinopathy or retinal detachment.
- Congenital infections that can → vision loss, usually via retinopathy, include CMV, toxoplasmosis, varicella, and HSV.
- Congenital infections less likely associated with vision loss include rubella and syphilis.

After the neonatal period, retinoblastoma commonly presents with strabismus.

Retinopathy of Prematurity (ROP)

- Defined as abnormal neovascularization with subsequent scarring, retinal retraction, and detachment.
- Preterm infants should receive a first ROP exam between 31 and 33 corrected GA, when the retinal vessels are sufficiently developed, and should be reexamined at one- to two-week intervals until full retinal vessel development at 44 weeks' corrected GA.
- LBW and early GA at delivery are the strongest risk factors for ROP. Other risk factors for developing ROP include hyperoxia, shock, asphyxia, hypothermia, and light exposure.

> **CHARGE syndrome:**
>
> **C**oloboma
> **H**eart defect
> **A**tresia (choanal)
> **R**etardation (mental and growth)
> **G**enital anomaly
> **E**ar anomaly

Coloboma

- A defect of the iris due to improper closure of the anterior embryonal fissure.
- May be an isolated defect that may be sporadic or may be inherited either in an autosomal-dominant fashion or in conjunction with a variety of genetic syndromes, including trisomy 13, trisomy 18, and CHARGE, genital anomaly, ear anomaly), Marfan's, Rubinstein-Taybi, Sturge-Weber, basal cell nevus, and cat-eye syndromes.

Aniridia

- Usually involves bilateral absence of most or all of both irises.
- The autosomal-dominant or sporadic form is associated with Wilms' tumor. The 11p deletion includes aniridia, GU abnormalities, and mental retardation.
- **Sx/Exam:** Presents with photophobia and nystagmus. Associated with cataracts, glaucoma, and corneal changes.

Infants of Diabetic Mothers (IDMs)

- IDMs are at ↑ risk for a variety of disorders.
- These include hypoglycemia (due to hyperinsulinemia from in utero hyperglycemia), polycythemia, hypocalcemia, hypomagnesemia, hyperbilirubinemia, RDS, macrosomia (birth trauma), organomegaly, caudal regression anomalad (sacral agenesis with lower extremity, bowel, and bladder dysfunction), hypertrophic cardiomyopathy, TGA, ASD, VSD, small left colon syndrome, CNS abnormalities, neural tube defects, renal vein thrombosis, and other congenital abnormalities.

Maternal Hypertension

- Results in growth failure from placental insufficiency. Associated with an ↑ risk of birth asphyxia as well as with polycythemia and hypoglycemia.
- Maternal treatment with magnesium or delivery of the fetus for pregnancy-induced hypertension → hypermagnesemia and complications of prematurity.
- HELLP syndrome (hemolysis, elevated liver function tests, low platelets) may → isolated neonatal thrombocytopenia.

Advanced Maternal Age

Associated with an ↑ risk of chromosomal abnormalities, including trisomy 13, trisomy 21, and neural tube defects.

Teenage Pregnancy

Associated with an ↑ risk of LBW, GBS exposure, and neural tube defects. Later, it may ↑ risk of asthma, affect school performance, and → behavioral problems.

Maternal SLE

Associated with heart block.

Maternal PKU

Associated with spontaneous abortion, microcephaly, and mental retardation.

Maternal ITP

Some 70% of cases → thrombocytopenia in the infant, peaking at 4–6 weeks and resolving at roughly 2–3 months.

Intrauterine Constraint

Associated with clubfeet, limb reduction defects, muscle and skin aplasia, anterior midline and neural tube closure defects, and craniofacial and ear abnormalities.

NEONATOLOGY

Exposure to Intrapartum Drugs of Abuse

- **Fetal alcohol syndrome:** Characterized by IUGR and poor growth in infancy as well as cardiac defects. Neurologic sequelae include microcephaly, mental deficiency, irritability, hyperactivity, and developmental delay. Characteristic facies include midface hypoplasia with flat philtrum and a long upper lip; a flat nasal bridge with epicanthal folds; microphthalmia with short palpebral fissures; micrognathia; and a small upturned nose.
- **Toluene:** IUGR; microcephaly; CNS, craniofacial, and limb abnormalities.
- **Opiates:** Preterm abruption, preterm labor, IUGR. Postnatally, opiate withdrawal presents with tremulousness, convulsions, seizures, ↑ DTRs, irritability, a harsh and shrill cry, vomiting, diarrhea, and autonomic instability. Symptom onset depends on the timing and half-life of the last maternal dose of opiate and can be delayed up to one week (e.g., if the infant was born to a mother on methadone who took a dose shortly before delivery). Treatment is with long-acting opiates, weaned over weeks.
- **Cocaine:** Toxicity primarily affects the CNS, but fetal growth is also affected as a result of vasoconstriction of the placenta. In utero hemorrhagic and ischemic insults → periventricular leukomalacia Also associated with an ↑ risk of placental abruption and preterm labor as well as with an ↑ risk of SIDS and long-term neurobehavioral problems.
- **Amphetamines:** Associated with ↓ birth weight, preterm labor, and possibly congenital malformations; may have other effects similar to those of cocaine.
- **Tobacco:** IUGR is the most common complication. Placental insufficiency and placenta previa may be seen as well. Also associated with an ↑ risk of asthma, otitis media, hypertension, SIDS, preterm birth cleft lip/palate, and cardiovascular defects.

Teratogenic Medications

- **Warfarin:** IUGR, mental retardation, seizures, nasal hypoplasia, stippled epiphyses of the axial skeleton. The highest risk occurs between the sixth and ninth gestational weeks.
- **Lithium:** Ebstein's anomaly.
- **Phenytoin:** Fetal hydantoin syndrome, which may include IUGR, craniofacial abnormalities (hypertelorism with low nasal bridge, low-set ears, wide mouth, cleft lip/palate, and microcephaly), short fingers with nail hypoplasia, and hip dislocation. Roughly 10% of infants exposed have the entire syndrome, with approximately 30% having only some features.
- **Carbamazepine:** Craniofacial abnormalities, growth delay.
- **Valproic acid:** Myelomeningocele, heart defects, characteristic facies (narrow bifrontal diameter, high forehead with epicanthal folds, midface hypoplasia with small mouth, risk of cleft lip, eye problems).
- **Barbiturates:** Similar to fetal hydantoin syndrome.
- **Systemic retinoids/vitamin A toxicity:** CNS abnormalities; ear and clefting abnormalities; branchial and aortic arch abnormalities, including thymic and cardiac abnormalities.
- **DES:** Reproductive tract abnormalities; ↑ risk of developing vaginal and cervical adenocarcinoma.
- **ACEIs:** Renal tubular dysplasia, IUGR, PDA, hypo-ossification of the skull.
- **Tetracyclines:** Staining of bone and teeth.
- **Thalidomide:** Limb reduction/phocomelia, ear hypoplasia/deafness, GI atresias.
- **Thyroid medications:** PTU and iodine deficiency → goiter; methimazole causes aplasia cutis.

CHAPTER 15

Neurology

Rebecca Blankenburg, MD, MPH
reviewed by Jonathan B. Strober, MD

Seizures are classified as follows:

- **Partial seizures:**
  - **Simple partial seizures:**
    - **Sx/Exam:** Brief (10–20 seconds); no alteration in consciousness. Characterized by tonic or clonic movements that tend to involve the face, neck, and extremities. May have preictal aura.
    - **Tx:** Carbamazepine (Tegretol), oxcarbazepine (Trileptal).
  - **Complex partial seizures:**
    - **Sx/Exam:** Average length is 1–2 minutes; involves alteration of consciousness. May begin as simple partial seizure and then progress.
    - **Tx:** Carbamazepine, oxcarbazepine.
  - **Partial seizures evolving into secondarily generalized seizures.**
- **Generalized seizures:**
  - **Absence seizures:**
    - Seen in females more often than males; rarely occurs before five years of age.
    - **Sx/Exam:** Brief lapses in awareness without postictal impairment; average length is 30 seconds. Patients may experience countless seizures daily. EEG shows characteristic 3-Hz spike-and-wave discharges.
    - **Tx:** Ethosuximide, valproic acid, lamotrigine (Lamictal).
  - **Atonic seizures:** Abrupt loss of muscle tone.
  - **Myoclonic seizures:** Rapid, brief, symmetric muscle contractions.
  - Seizures that may be partial or generalized.
  - **Clonic seizures:** Rhythmic jerking; flexor spasm of the extremities.
  - **Tonic seizures:** Sustained muscle contraction.
  - **Tonic-clonic seizures:**
    - Very common; may begin with a partial seizure.
    - **Sx:** Prodromal symptoms include apprehension, mood change, insomnia, and loss of appetite; incontinence is commonly seen.
    - **Tx:** Valproic acid, lamotrigine.

DIAGNOSIS

- Diagnosis depends greatly on the history and physical.
- **Labs:**
  - Dextrose stick.
  - In infants < 6 months of age, check sodium, calcium, and magnesium; in those > 6 months of age, there is no need to check electrolytes unless the history and physical suggests electrolyte abnormalities.
  - Consider CBC, blood culture, UA, urine culture, urine tox screen, serum ammonia, and urine/serum amino and organic acids.
- LP should be considered if fever is present or if the child is < 6 months of age.
- **Imaging:**
  - **Neurologic imaging (head CT or MRI):** Obtain for patients with partial seizure or in infants < 6 months of age; otherwise, not needed for a first seizure unless the history and physical suggests it.
- **EEG.**

TREATMENT

- Treatment should be directed at the specific cause if an etiology can be identified.
- Antiepileptic medications should not be prescribed to a previously healthy child with a first afebrile seizure if there is no family history of seizures, the examination is normal, lab studies are normal, EEG is normal, and the family is compliant.
- Monitor for specific side effects of antiepileptic medicines, including the following:
  - **Cytopenia, aplastic anemia:** Carbamazepine, ethosuximide, valproic acid.
  - **Liver dysfunction and/or failure:** Carbamazepine, valproic acid, phenytoin, phenobarbital.
  - **Stevens-Johnson syndrome:** Phenytoin, phenobarbital, lamotrigine.

Epileptic Seizures

- Defined as two or more unprovoked seizures.
- Has a baseline prevalence of 0.5–1.0%.
- **Dx/Tx:** As above, based on underlying seizure type.

Epileptic Syndromes

BENIGN ROLANDIC EPILEPSY

- Found in school-age, otherwise healthy children. Seizures usually abate by puberty.
- **Sx/Exam:** Seizures have a focal onset and may generalize, but consciousness is preserved. Often occur at night.
- **Dx:**
  - EEG shows sharp, slow discharges localized to rolandic (central, mid-temporal, or sylvian) regions.
  - Other tests are normal.
- **Tx:** Not necessary to treat everyone, but usually well controlled with carbamazepine.

JUVENILE MYOCLONIC EPILEPSY (OF JANZ)

- A disorder of autosomal-dominant inheritance. Patients are of normal intelligence and typically have a ⊕ family history.
- **Sx/Exam:**
  - Morning myoclonic jerks; generalized tonic-clonic seizures upon awakening.
  - Seizures are often precipitated by sleep deprivation or alcohol.
- **Dx:** EEG shows fast, 3- to 5-Hz spike-and-wave discharges → "impulsive petit mal."
- **Tx:** Valproic acid or lamotrigine is usually effective.

LENNOX-GASTAUT SYNDROME

- Slow spike-and-wave activity on EEG accompanied by mental retardation and seizures that usually begin in the first three years of life.

- **Sx/Exam:**
  - Seizures may be atonic, tonic, or atypical absence. Affected patients often have > 2 kinds of seizures, usually on a daily basis.
  - Other neurologic abnormalities, usually motor abnormalities (e.g., hemiparesis, spastic diplegia), are also seen.
  - Mental retardation is seen in most patients.
- **Tx:** Topiramate may be beneficial but seizures are often refractory.
- **Complications:** Has a poor prognosis, with seizures often continuing into adulthood.

Rasmussen syndrome (a pediatric form of epilepsia partialis continua) consists of sudden, profound, intractable unilateral seizures associated with cerebral inflammation of one hemisphere and progressive neurologic deterioration.

LANDAU-KLEFFNER SYNDROME

- Progressive aphasia, seizures, and behavioral disorders.
- Symptoms begin before seven years of age.
- **Sx/Exam:**
  - Presents with a progressive decline in language skills.
  - Seizures are usually simple partial or generalized tonic-clonic.
  - Behavioral problems are common, especially hyperactivity, poor attention, depression, and irritability.
- **Dx:** EEG shows diffuse or multifocal spike-and-wave discharges that are most prominent in the anterior and midtemporal regions.
- **Tx:** Seizures are responsive to valproic acid.
- **Complications:** Language recovery may not occur.

Infantile Spasms

- Defined as sudden, rapid, tonic contractions of the trunk and limbs that gradually relax over several seconds and usually occur in clusters. Subtypes include flexor, extensor, and mixed. Etiologies are as follows:
  - **Perinatal:** Hypoxic-ischemic encephalopathy (HIE), tuberous sclerosis, intrauterine infections, brain malformations, inborn errors of metabolism.
  - **Postnatal:** Herpes encephalitis, HIE, head trauma.
- **Tx:** ACTH.

The classic triad of infantile spasms consists of spasms, hypsarrhythmia on EEG (slow, disorganized brain waves with multifocal spike activity), and developmental delay.

> A two-year-old boy experiences a single generalized tonic-clonic seizure that lasts for roughly three minutes during a febrile illness without any residual neurologic deficits. He recovers from his illness without experiencing any further seizures. Compared to the general pediatric population, his risk for developing epilepsy is ↑ how many times? Two to four times.

Febrile Seizures

Seizure activity associated with a fever occurring in a previously healthy child six months to five years of age who has no evidence of intracranial infection or other defined cause. Affects approximately 3–5% of children; average age at onset is 23 months. Subtypes are listed in Table 15-1.

TABLE 15-1. Febrile Seizure Subtypes

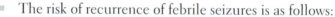

SIMPLE FEBRILE SEIZURES[a]	COMPLEX FEBRILE SEIZURES[b]
Single	Multiple episodes (in 24 hours)
Lasting ≤ 15 minutes	Lasting > 15 minutes
Generalized seizure	Focal seizure
No residual neurologic deficits	Focal neurologic deficits remain (e.g., Todd's paralysis)

[a] Must include all of the variables in column one.
[b] Includes any of the variables in column two.

DIAGNOSIS

- If there is any evidence of a complex febrile seizure, a prolonged postictal state, or an abnormal neurologic exam, do an LP for CSF cell count, glucose, protein, and culture.
- No radiologic imaging or EEG is needed in patients with simple febrile seizures, but imaging is recommended for those with complex febrile seizures.

TREATMENT

Anticonvulsants are rarely needed.

COMPLICATIONS

Most febrile seizures occur during the first 24 hours of illness; thus, the seizure is the first sign of illness in approximately 25–50% of cases.

- The risk of recurrence of febrile seizures is as follows:
  - **Children with a history of simple febrile seizures: 30%.**
  - **Children with a history of complex febrile seizures: 50%.**
  - Recurrence risk is higher in children < 1 year of age and in those with a ⊕ family history of seizures.
  - Around-the-clock antipyretics do not ↓ the risk of recurrence.
- The risk of epilepsy is as follows:
  - **Baseline risk for all children: 0.5–1.0%.**
  - **Children with a history of simple febrile seizures: 2–4%.**
  - **Children with a history of complex febrile seizures: 6%.**

Status Epilepticus

- Affects 60,000–120,000 children annually in the United States. One-third of cases are an initial event in children with new-onset epilepsy; one-third occur in children with established epilepsy.
- Other etiologies include complex febrile seizures, electrolyte abnormalities, hypoglycemia, meningitis, encephalitis, trauma, tumor, stroke, intoxication, and degenerative or progressive neurologic conditions.
- The mortality rate due to prolonged seizure in children is 1–3%.
- Tx:
  - **Anticonvulsants:** Best administered IV/PO; if this is not possible, give rectally or IM.
    - First give lorazepam (preferred) or diazepam (may be repeated two more times).

- Then give fosphenytoin for children or phenobarbital for infants.
    - Then administer continuous pentobarbital, midazolam, or propofol.
- **IV fluids:** NS bolus.
    - Correct any electrolyte abnormalities; give O_2 and antibiotics if necessary.

PAROXYSMAL DISORDERS (NONSEIZURES)

Table 15-2 outlines the differential of disorders that mimic epilepsy in the pediatric population.

TABLE 15-2. Disorders That Mimic Epilepsy in Children

EVENT	EPIDEMIOLOGY	SYMPTOMS/EXAM	DIAGNOSIS	TREATMENT
Benign paroxysmal vertigo	Affects toddlers; rare after three years of age.	Sudden onset; the child falls, refuses to walk, or chooses to sit. The child is frightened. May present with nausea/vomiting. Consciousness and verbalization are not changed. No drowsiness or lethargy is seen afterward. In the long term, may be associated with motion sickness and migraines.	Neurologic exam is normal except that abnormal vestibular function may be elicited by ice-water caloric testing.	Acetazolamide (Diamox).
Breath-holding spells	Peaks at two years of age; rare before six months and after five years of age.	Loss of consciousness; pallor or cyanosis. May be associated with generalized clonic jerks. Always provoked by scolding or other upsetting events.	Classic history; examination is normal. May be associated with iron deficiency anemia.	Reassure parents and advise them not to reinforce the child's actions.
Syncope	Affects adolescents; rare before 10 years of age. Girls are affected more often than boys.	Loss of consciousness; dizziness and clouded vision. Precipitated by fear, pain, excitement, and long periods of standing (especially in warm environments). Usually due to systemic hypotension.	EEG shows transient slowing but no seizure spikes. Tilt test may be ⊕.	β-blockers may be used if syncope is vasovagal and recurrent.

TABLE 15-2. **Disorders That Mimic Epilepsy in Children** *(continued)*

EVENT	EPIDEMIOLOGY	SYMPTOMS/EXAM	DIAGNOSIS	TREATMENT
Cough syncope	Affects asthmatics.	Prolonged cough spasm in asthmatics → unconsciousness. Urinary incontinence is common. Recovery begins within seconds, with patients returning to consciousness within minutes.	Classic history; examination is normal.	Prevention of bronchoconstriction.
Cardiogenic syncope	The incidence of prolonged QT syndrome is 1 in 10,000–15,000.	Sudden loss of consciousness during exercise or during an emotional or stressful event. Associated with prolonged QT or other arrhythmias.	ECG; exercise testing or Holter monitor may be necessary.	β-antagonists. It may be necessary to place a pacemaker or do a left cervicothoracic sympathectomy.
Night terrors	Most commonly affects children 4–6 years of age, with boys affected more frequently than girls. Approximately 1–3% of children are affected.	Sudden onset; occurs during sleep stage 3 or 4. The child screams and appears frightened. Dilated pupils, tachycardia, and hyperventilation may be seen. Lasts a few minutes, during which the child cannot be consoled, but the child falls back to sleep afterward and has no memory of the event the next day.	Classic history; examination is normal.	No treatment is needed if the course is not protracted. If protracted, rule out any underlying emotional problems in the child's life. A short course of diazepam or imipramine may be tried for protracted cases.
Narcolepsy	Rarely occurs before adolescence. Incidence is 1 in 2000.	Paroxysmal attacks of irrepressible daytime sleep. May be associated with loss of muscle tone (cataplexy). No postictal state is seen.	EEG shows recurrent REM sleep attacks.	Scheduled naps; stimulants and antidepressants.
Nonepileptic events (aka pseudoseizures or psychogenic seizures)	Most likely to occur in children with a history of seizures. Usually affects children 10–18 years of age, with girls affected more frequently than boys.	Movements are thrashing rather than clonic. Short or absent postictal state; no loss of sphincter tone.	EEG shows excess of muscle artifact but no underlying seizure activity.	Evaluate for underlying psychosocial problems.

Lifetime prevalence in children 7–9 years of age is 60–69%; lifetime prevalence in children 15 years of age is 75%. Subtypes and their differentials are listed in Table 15-3. Indications for imaging are outlined in Table 15-4.

Migraine Headaches

Chronic, recurrent headaches that are unilateral in teens and adults but may be bilateral in children. Triggers include caffeine, sleep disturbances, stress, diet, and menses. Often associated with a $\oplus$ family history, car sickness, and "ice cream headaches."

SYMPTOMS/EXAM

- Presents with throbbing +/– aura.
- Associated with nausea, vomiting, abdominal pain, photophobia, and phonophobia.
- Relieved by sleep.

TABLE 15-3. Differential Diagnosis of Headache

ACUTE HEADACHE	RECURRENT OR CHRONIC HEADACHES	CHRONIC PROGRESSIVE HEADACHES
↑ ICP	Migraine	Hydrocephalus
↓ ICP	Tension	Brain tumors
Meningeal inflammation	Analgesic rebound	Malformations (Arnold-Chiari, Dandy-Walker)
Vascular disorders	Caffeine withdrawal	
Bone/soft tissue referred pain	Sleep deprivation	Infection (abscess, chronic meningitis)
Infection	Brain tumor	Subdural hematoma
	Psychogenic factors	Pseudotumor cerebri
	Cluster (rare in children and teens)	Aneurysm/vascular malformation
		Hypertension
		Medications

TABLE 15-4. Indications for Imaging Children with Headache

IMAGING STRONGLY INDICATED	CONSIDER IMAGING
Chronic progressive headaches	Headache or vomiting on awakening
"Worst headache of my life"	Unvarying location of headaches (especially occipital)
Abnormal neurologic exam	
Meningeal signs + focal neurologic findings/altered mental status	Persistent headache and no family history of migraines
Ventriculoperitoneal (VP) shunt	Neurocutaneous syndrome
Significant head trauma	

445

DIAGNOSIS

Normal neurologic exam; rule out more significant pathology.

TREATMENT

- Supportive (provide a dark, quiet room; encourage sleep); NSAIDs, triptans.
- If migraines continue > 3–4 times a month or interfere with school, consider β-blockers, calcium channel blockers, TCAs, SSRIs, or anticonvulsants.
- Nonpharmacologic treatments including biofeedback and acupuncture may be useful.

PREVENTION

Avoidance of triggers.

Tension Headaches

- Chronic, recurrent headaches that often occur during or after a stressful situation.
- **Sx/Exam:** Throbbing; no nausea or vomiting.
- **Dx:** Normal neurologic exam; rule out more significant pathology.
- **Tx:** Supportive; NSAIDs, counseling.

Pseudotumor Cerebri

Etiologies include the following:

- **Drugs:** Tetracyclines, corticosteroids, nitrofurantoin, vitamin A toxicity.
- **Endocrine disorders:** Hyperthyroidism, Cushing's syndrome, hypoparathyroidism.
- **Other:** Obesity, thrombosis of dural venous sinuses 2° to otitis media, mastoiditis, head trauma, jugular vein obstruction, dehydration.

Patients with pseudotumor cerebri may complain of loss of vision that worsens with standing or with Valsalva owing to reduction in blood flow to the optic nerve.

SYMPTOMS/EXAM

- Presents with headache, stiff neck, and diplopia from ↑ ICP.
- May lead to vision loss.
- The remainder of the neurologic exam is normal except for possible papilledema or CN III/VI nerve palsy.

DIAGNOSIS

- CT scan is normal except for the possible finding of small ventricles.
- CSF is normal except for ↑ opening pressure.

TREATMENT

- Removal of the precipitant.
- Acetazolamide, furosemide, HCTZ, corticosteroids.
- In severe cases, lumboperitoneal shunt, ventriculoperitoneal shunt, or optic nerve decompression may be tried.

Meningitis

Diffuse CNS infection involving the meninges. May be bacterial, viral, fungal, or aseptic.

SYMPTOMS/EXAM

- Historical exam findings:
  - **Children > 12 months of age:** Headache, neck pain, back pain, nausea, vomiting, irritability.
  - **Children < 12 months of age:** Nonspecific complaints.
- Physical exam findings:
  - **Children > 12 months of age:** Nuchal rigidity.
  - **Kernig's sign:** Flex the patient's leg at both the hip and the knee and then extend the leg. The sign is ⊕ when this maneuver causes neck pain and flexion.
  - **Brudzinski's sign:** Passively flex the neck; the sign is ⊕ when the legs flex.

> **Kernig's sign: K** is for **K**ernig and **K**nee.

DIAGNOSIS

The gold-standard diagnosis is via CSF analysis (see Table 15-5) following an LP (↑ ICP must first be ruled out).

BACTERIAL MENINGITIS

- Associated with the highest morbidity and mortality; results in 500–1000 deaths per year in the United States. Etiologies are listed in Table 15-6.
- **Tx:** Steroids followed 30 minutes later with antibiotics (see Table 15-6).

TABLE 15-5. CSF Analysis in Meningitis

	NORMAL LEVELS	BACTERIAL	VIRAL	FUNGAL
Pressure (mmHg)	50–80	Usually ↑ (100–300)	Normal or slightly ↑ (80–150)	Usually ↑
Leukocytes (mm³)	< 5	> 1000	100–500	10–500
% neutrophils	0	> 50	< 20	Varies
Protein (mg/dL)	20–45	100–500	50–200	25–500
Glucose (mg/dL)	> 50 or 75% serum glucose	↓ < 40 or < 66% serum	Generally normal	< 50; continues to ↓ if untreated
Lab cultures		Gram stain of CSF	CSF PCR may show HSV or enteroviruses	Budding yeast may be seen; serum and CSF cryptococcal antigen

TABLE 15-6. Common Causes of Bacterial Meningitis

Age	Bacteria	Treatment
Neonates (< 1 month of age)	Group B streptococcus, gram-⊖ enteric bacilli, *Listeria monocytogenes*, *E. coli*.	Ampicillin and gentamicin or ampicillin and cefotaxime.
Infants (1–24 months of age)	*Streptococcus pneumoniae*, *Neisseria meningitidis*, *Haemophilus influenzae* type b.[a]	Third-generation cephalosporin; add vancomycin until sensitivities are known.
Children (> 24 months of age)	*S. pneumoniae*, *N. meningitidis*, *H. influenzae* type b.[a]	Same as above.

[a] Note that *H. influenzae* type b is becoming much less common as a result of the Hib vaccine.

- Complications:
  - Acute: SIADH, seizures (approximately 15–20%).
  - Long term: Neurologic sequelae, including mental retardation; hearing defects.

VIRAL MENINGITIS

- Roughly 80% of cases are caused by enterovirus, echovirus, coxsackievirus, and nonparalytic poliovirus.
- Tx:
  - Enterovirus: Supportive care.
  - HSV: Acyclovir.
- Complications:
  - The prognosis is good, but acute complications include SIADH (occurs in 10% of cases).
  - Long-term complications are rare.

FUNGAL MENINGITIS

- *Cryptococcus neoformans* is a relatively uncommon but classic cause of fungal meningitis. *Candida* is also a cause in premature neonates.
- Primarily found in immunocompromised patients, but 30% of cases arise in immunocompetent children.
- Can be rapidly fatal or evolve over months to years.
- Tx: Amphotericin B.
- Complications: Hydrocephalus (due to direct lymphatic obstruction).

ASEPTIC MENINGITIS

- Caused by agents that are not easily cultured in a viral or bacterial medium, including *Borrelia burgdorferi* (Lyme disease) and *Treponema pallidum* (syphilis).
- Also includes tuberculous meningitis, whose incidence is ↑; most commonly seen in children six months to six years of age.

- The prognosis of Lyme disease is good with appropriate diagnosis and treatment.
- The prognosis of tuberculous meningitis depends on the stage of disease in which treatment is initiated. Complete recovery is achieved in 90% of patients whose treatment was initiated in the first stage; approximately 20% fully recover when treatment is started in the third stage.
- **Complications:** Acute complications with tuberculous meningitis include cranial nerve findings, especially those attributable to CN VI, which → eye palsy.

Encephalitis

A disease process that primarily affects the brain parenchyma. Usually caused by infectious organisms, but may also be associated with chemical or neoplastic spread.

CHRONIC BACTERIAL MENINGOENCEPHALITIS

- **Tuberculosis and mycobacterioses:**
  - Caused by TB and mycobacteria.
  - *Mycobacterium avium–intracellulare* is common among AIDS patients.
  - **Sx/Exam:** Headaches, malaise, confusion, and vomiting are common.
  - **Complications:** Serious complications include arachnoid fibrosis → hydrocephalus and arterial occlusion → infarcts.
- **Neurosyphilis:**
  - Caused by *Treponema pallidum.*
  - **Sx/Exam:**
    - **Congenital syphilis:** Mucopurulent rhinitis ("snuffles"), maculopapular rash, lymphadenopathy.
    - **3° syphilis (late stage):** Neurologic, cardiovascular, and granulomatous disease; usually not seen in children/adolescents because it takes 10–20 years to progress to this stage.
  - **Dx:** Screen with RPR or VDRL; confirm with antitreponemal antibody test.
  - **Tx:** IV penicillin G.

VIRAL MENINGOENCEPHALITIS

- **HSV meningoencephalitis:**
  - Caused by HSV-1 in children and adults and by HSV-2 in neonates.
  - **Sx/Exam:** Irritability, seizures, ↓ mental status.
  - **Dx:** CSF is HSV PCR ⊕.
  - **Tx:** IV acyclovir.
- **HSV-2 encephalitis:**
  - Most common among sexually active teens.
  - **Sx/Exam:** May have a mild course characterized by changes in mood, memory, and behavior.
  - **Dx:** CSF is HSV PCR ⊕.
  - **Tx:** Self-limiting; no treatment is necessary.
- **Rabies encephalitis:**
  - Caused by a bite from an infected animal, most frequently bats (more common than dogs).

- **Sx/Exam:**
  - Early symptoms include malaise and fever.
  - The pathognomonic feature is paresthesia around the bite.
- **Dx:** Establishment of a known rabies contact.
- **Tx:**
  - If treated immediately following exposure, rabies immunoglobulin and vaccine are given.
  - Supportive care.
- **Complications:**
  - The prognosis is poor if medical attention is first sought at the time of clinical presentation of rabies in the patient.
  - Severe encephalitis and coma can → death from respiratory failure.

ACUTE DISSEMINATED ENCEPHALOMYELITIS

A postviral or parainfectious autoimmune process targeted against CNS myelin and → inflammation of white matter in the brain and spinal cord. May be idiopathic or associated with viral or bacterial infections as a complication of immunizations.

ADEM lesions are most often found at the junction of deep cortical gray and subcortical white matter. Multiple sclerosis lesions are typically periventricular.

SYMPTOMS/EXAM

- Presents with sudden-onset headache, delirium, lethargy, coma, seizures, stiff neck, fever, ataxia, optic neuritis, transverse myelitis, monoparesis, and hemiplegia.
- Bladder/bowl dysfunction is also seen.

DIAGNOSIS

- MRI shows ↑ T2 signal intensity.
- CSF reveals mildly ↑ opening pressure and ↑ lymphocytes.

TREATMENT

- Corticosteroids.
- The prognosis varies but is good overall if the condition is promptly diagnosed and treated.

 A five-year-old girl is involved in a motor vehicle accident and suffers head trauma with a penetrating wound. She later develops a ring-enhancing lesion in her brain that is detected with MRI. What is her most likely diagnosis? Brain abscess.

Brain Abscess

Most commonly found in children 4–8 years of age. Etiologies are as follows:

- **S. aureus:** Almost always the cause in the presence of a penetrating wound. Also found in some septic emboli.
- Streptococci.
- **Anaerobic organisms:** Gram-⊕ cocci, *Bacteroides, Fusobacterium, Prevotella, Actinomyces, Clostridium.*
- **Gram-⊖ aerobic bacilli:** Enteric rods, *Proteus, Pseudomonas aeruginosa, Citrobacter diversus, Haemophilus.*

- The number of organisms cultured from abscess is one organism in 70% of cases, two organisms in 20% of cases, and ≥ 3 organisms in 10% of cases.

DIAGNOSIS

- **Head CT/MRI with contrast:** The best test; shows ring-enhancing lesion.
- WBC count may be normal or ↑.
- Blood culture is ⊕ in only 10% of cases.
- CSF cultures are rarely ⊕.

TREATMENT

- Antibiotic regimen should include coverage for the most likely organism and should usually be given for 4–6 weeks.
- If the organism is unknown, vancomycin, a third-generation cephalosporin, and metronidazole are often used.
- Surgical intervention is rarely necessary.

COMPLICATIONS

- The mortality rate is 5–10% (the rate has greatly ↓ as a result of CT).
- Some 50% of survivors have long-term sequelae, including behavior and learning problems, seizures, hydrocephalus, cranial nerve abnormalities, and hemiparesis.

DISORDERS OF HEAD GROWTH

Craniosynostosis

Defined as premature closure of cranial sutures. Incidence is 1 in 2000 live births. The majority of cases are idiopathic, but other etiologies are as follows:

- Some 10–20% of cases having a genetic cause, including Crouzon, Apert, Carpenter, Chotzen, and Pfeiffer syndromes.
- All of the genetic syndromes are associated with an ↑ risk of other anomalies.

TREATMENT

Craniectomy may be done for cosmetic purposes and is mandatory for the management of ↑ ICP.

Microcephaly

Defined as a head circumference ≥ 3 SDs below the mean for age and gender. Etiologies are as follows:

- 1° (genetic):
  - **Familial (autosomal recessive):** Severe mental retardation.
  - **Autosomal dominant:** Mild mental retardation.
  - **Chromosomal syndromes:** Down syndrome; trisomy 18; cri-du-chat syndrome; Cornelia de Lange, Rubinstein-Taybi, and Smith-Lemli-Opitz syndromes.
- 2° (nongenetic): Radiation, congenital infection (CMV, rubella, toxoplasmosis), drugs (alcohol, hydantoin), meningitis/encephalitis, malnutrition, metabolic factors, hyperthermia, HIE.

DIAGNOSIS

- ⊕ family history.
- Karyotype if there is a suspected chromosomal anomaly.
- Obtain TORCH titers.
- Head CT/brain MRI.

TREATMENT

- Offer appropriate genetic counseling.
- Follow for possible mental retardation and connect the family with appropriate services.

Macrocephaly

Defined as a head circumference ≥ 3 SDs above the mean for age and gender. Etiologies include the following:

- ↑ ICP with hydrocephalus (most common).
- **Megalencephaly (abnormally large and heavy brain):** May be 1° (sporadic or associated with neurofibromatosis, tuberous sclerosis, myelomeningocele, or achondroplasia) or 2° (metabolic).
- Thickening of the skull.
- Hemorrhage into the subdural or epidural spaces.

DIAGNOSIS

Benign extra-axial space thickening is often a familial condition that can → macrocephaly. A family history can help render the diagnosis; a head CT/MRI will demonstrate the condition conclusively.

- ⊕ family history.
- Evaluate for ↑ ICP.
- If no ↑ ICP or neurologic abnormalities are found, the presumed diagnosis is benign familial megalencephaly, and further workup is unnecessary.
- If any ↑ ICP or neurologic abnormalities are found, consider skull x-rays, head CT, brain MRI, and EEG.

TREATMENT

- Treat the underlying disorder.
- Follow for possible mental retardation, and connect the family with appropriate services.

Hydrocephalus

An abnormal accumulation of CSF within the ventricles of the brain. Etiologies are as follows:

- **Obstructive (noncommunicating) hydrocephalus:**
  - Most commonly due to stenosis of the aqueduct of Sylvius.
  - May also be caused by obstruction in the fourth ventricle resulting from posterior fossa tumors, type II Arnold-Chiari malformations, Dandy-Walker syndrome, and expanding vein of Galen malformations.
- **Nonobstructive (communicating) hydrocephalus:**
  - Occurs after an SAH, usually following intraventricular hemorrhage in a preemie (most common), meningitis, intrauterine infections, or leukemia.
  - Blood or infectious, viscous fluid may obliterate the cisterns or arachnoid villi and obstruct CSF flow.
- **Hydrocephalus ex vacuo:** ↓ brain parenchyma → hydrocephalus.

SYMPTOMS/EXAM

- Obtain a detailed history and physical exam, and look for a family history of aqueductal stenosis (recessive X-linked cases have been reported).
- Examination may reveal irritability, a bulging anterior fontanelle, widened sutures, eyes that deviate downward (sunset sign), papilledema, and ↑ tone/reflexes. Presentation by age group is as follows:
  - **Infants:** Head circumference ↑ at an accelerated rate → a bulging anterior fontanelle; signs of ↑ ICP include ↓ feeding, vomiting, ↓ mental status, and lethargy.
  - **Children/adolescents:** Signs of ↑ ICP include vomiting, headache, and ↓ mental status.

DIAGNOSIS

- Ultrasound may be helpful in infants.
- Head CT/MRI (in infants, children, and adolescents).

TREATMENT

- Where possible, treat the underlying cause.
- Medical management with acetazolamide (to ↓ CSF production) and furosemide (Lasix) may provide some relief.
- It may be necessary to place an external ventricular drainage or VP shunt if the cause is permanent.

MALFORMATIONS OF THE BRAIN

Arnold-Chiari Malformation

ARNOLD-CHIARI MALFORMATION TYPE I

Defined as cerebellar tonsillar herniation through the foramen magnum into the cervical canal (as seen in Figure 15-1). Produces symptoms during adolescence or adult life; syringomyelia is associated with 40–75% of cases. Not associated with hydrocephalus.

SYMPTOMS/EXAM

Recurrent headache, neck pain, urinary frequency, progressive lower extremity spasticity.

TREATMENT

- Close observation; serial MRIs to evaluate progress.
- Surgery as necessary.

ARNOLD-CHIARI MALFORMATION TYPE II

Defined as cerebellar tonsillar and lower medullary herniation through the foramen magnum (as seen in Figure 15-1). The most common type of Arnold-Chiari malformation; also associated with progressive hydrocephalus in almost all cases and with myelomeningocele in > 95% of cases.

SYMPTOMS/EXAM

- Some 10% present in infancy with stridor, weak cry, and apnea.
- The more indolent form presents with gait abnormalities, spasticity, and ↑ incoordination.

Normal

Chiari I

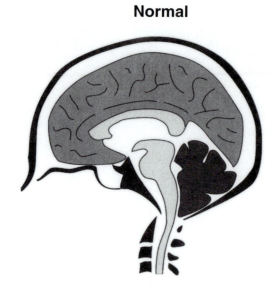
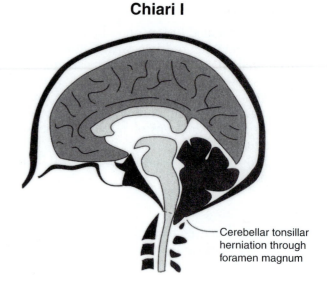

Cerebellar tonsillar
herniation through
foramen magnum

Chiari II

Cerebellar tonsillar
and lower medullary
herniation, with
kinking of the medulla

Cervical
meningomyelocoele

FIGURE 15-1. Arnold-Chiari malformations.

(Reproduced, with permission, from Stead LG et al. *First Aid for the Pediatrics Clerkship.* New York: McGraw-Hill, 2004:315.)

- Skull and cervical spine x-rays show a small posterior fossa and widened cervical canal.
- Head CT with contrast/brain MRI show cerebellar tonsils protruding downward into the cervical canal and hindbrain abnormalities.

TREATMENT

- Close observation; serial MRIs to evaluate progress.
- Surgical decompression as necessary.

Lissencephaly

- Defined as a cerebrum that lacks all sulci. Caused by disordered migration of the cortical neuroblasts → poor sulcation of the cerebrum.
- **Sx/Exam:** Presents with neurologic impairment.
- **Dx:** Head CT or brain MRI.
- **Tx:** Supportive care.

Polymicrogyria

- Defined as numerous small sulci on the cerebral surface. Caused by disordered migration of the cortical neuroblasts → excessive sulcation of the cerebrum.
- **Sx/Exam:** Presents with neurologic impairment.
- **Dx:** Head CT or brain MRI.
- **Tx:** Supportive care.

Agenesis of the Corpus Callosum

Agenesis or hypoplasia of the corpus callosum occurs if the nerve fibers fail to grow out, are destroyed, or are prevented from crossing the interhemispheric midline. Causes include teratogens (alcohol), chromosomal mutations (8, 9, 13, 18), heredity (X-linked, recessive, and dominant forms), and inborn errors of metabolism (nonketotic hyperglycemia, organic acidurias, peroxisomal disorders).

SYMPTOMS/EXAM

- Hypo- or hypertelorism; organic acidurias.
- Retinal and vertebral anomalies and infantile spasms in females (Aicardi syndrome).
- Recurrent hypothermia (Shapiro syndrome).
- Neurodevelopmental delay, especially if other malformations are present (e.g., destructive lesions, heterotrophias, holoprosencephaly).
- Development may be relatively normal if it is the only neurologic malformation.

DIAGNOSIS

- Head CT or brain MRI.
- Coronal radiographs show a pathognomonic bat-wing ventricular pattern (in full agenesis of the corpus callosum).

TREATMENT

Supportive care.

Dandy-Walker Malformation

Defined as cystic expansion of the fourth ventricle in the posterior fossa.

SYMPTOMS/EXAM

- Some 90% of affected children have hydrocephalus.
- A significant number have related anomalies such as agenesis of the posterior cerebellar vermis and corpus callosum.

DIAGNOSIS

- Rapid ↑ in head circumference; prominent occiput.
- Cerebellar ataxia.
- Delayed motor and cognitive development.
- Transillumination of the posterior brain may be ⊕.
- Brain MRI shows a cystic structure of the posterior fossa.

TREATMENT

A VP shunt is placed to shunt the cystic cavity.

SPINAL CORD DISEASES

A four-month-old baby is brought to your clinic for the first time, and you observe a midline hair tuft overlying the spine. What diagnostic study would you do next? Ultrasound.

Tethered Cord

In the fetus, the spinal cord is the same length as the spinal column. Because of differential growth, however, the conus medullaris in a child is around L1. Normally, the distal embryonic spinal cord regresses and only a thin, thread-like filum terminale is left attached to the coccyx. Tethered cord occurs when a thickened, ropelike filum terminale anchors the conus medullaris at L2 or below.

Some 70% of patients with tethered cord have an overlying skin malformation such as hair tuft, hyperpigmentation, dermal pit, lipoma, or cutaneous hemangioma.

SYMPTOMS/EXAM

- Some 70% of patients have an overlying skin malformation such as hair tuft, hyperpigmentation, dermal pit, lipoma, or cutaneous hemangioma.
- Clinical presentation varies, and the disorder may be diagnosed from birth to adulthood.
- Infants may have asymmetric foot or leg growth.
- Children may have bladder abnormalities, progressive scoliosis, or distal pain in the lower extremities.

DIAGNOSIS

MRI shows the level of the conus medullaris and filum terminale.

TREATMENT

Surgical transection of the thickened filum terminale.

Neural Tube Defects

Conditions in which the neural tube fails to close between the third and fourth week of gestation. Account for most congenital anomalies of the CNS. Causes include malnutrition (especially ↓ folate), radiation, drugs, chemicals, and genetic factors involving folate-dependent pathways.

DIAGNOSIS

- α-fetoprotein (AFP) testing at 16–18 weeks' gestation shows a high AFP.
- More severe defects may also be seen on ultrasound.

Spina Bifida Occulta

A midline defect of the vertebral bodies without protrusion of the spinal cord and meninges.

SYMPTOMS/EXAM

- Most patients are asymptomatic, and neurologic examination is normal.
- Physical exam may reveal a tuft of hair, discoloration of the skin, lipoma, or a pit in the lower midline back.
- May occasionally be associated with more significant abnormalities of the spinal cord, including tethered cord, syringomyelia, and diastematomyelia.

DIAGNOSIS

Spinal x-ray will show a defect in the closure of the posterior vertebral arches and laminae, usually involving L5–S1.

Meningocele

Forms when the meninges herniate through a defect in the posterior vertebral arches.

SYMPTOMS/EXAM

- The spinal cord is usually normal. However, the condition can be associated with tethered cord, syringomyelia, and diastematomyelia.
- Physical examination reveals a fluctuant midline mass along the spinal column in the lower back.
- Most meningoceles are covered with skin.
- A thorough neurologic examination is warranted.

DIAGNOSIS

- Head CT is recommended because of the association with hydrocephalus.
- Lumbar spine x-ray/ultrasound/MRI can delineate the extent of the meningocele and help determine if other neural tissue is involved and if there are other anomalies.
- Occasionally, anterior meningoceles protrude into the pelvis through a defect in the sacrum. Children may have constipation or bladder dysfunction due to the ↑ size of the meningocele; females may have associated GU abnormalities. X-rays show a defect in the sacrum, and CT/MRI can show the extent of the meningocele.

TREATMENT

- If thin skin covers the meningocele or CSF is leaking, surgery must be done immediately to prevent meningitis.
- If thick skin covers the meningocele and the child has a normal neurologic exam, surgery can be delayed.

Myelomeningocele

Forms when the meninges and underlying spinal cord herniate through a defect in the posterior vertebral arches. Incidence is 1 in 4000 live births. The recurrence risk if one child is affected is 3–4%. If two children are affected, the risk is 10%.

Symptoms/Exam

- May be located anywhere along the spinal cord, but 75% are in the lumbosacral area.
- Some 80% of patients have hydrocephalus in association with a type II Arnold-Chiari malformation.
- The lower the myelomeningocele, the lower the likelihood of hydrocephalus.

Diagnosis

- May be diagnosed clinically.
- MRI can further evaluate the extent of the defect.
- The GU tract must be carefully evaluated and reassessed.

Myelomeningocele is the most severe type of neural tube defect involving the spinal column.

Treatment

- Involves a multidisciplinary approach with surgeons, physicians, and therapists.
- Surgery may be delayed for a few days after birth as long as there is no CSF leak.
- Regular bladder cauterization has greatly ↓ morbidity and mortality.

Complications

- For children who are managed aggressively, there is a 10–15% risk of mortality, and death usually occurs before four years of age.
- At least 70% of patients have normal intelligence, but learning disabilities and seizures are more prevalent than in the normal population.
- Almost all children who have a lumbosacral or sacral lesion learn to walk; approximately half of other children with higher lesions learn to walk with the aid of canes and braces.

PERIPHERAL NEUROPATHIES

 A 13-year-old girl presents with progressive weakness that began in her legs and is now involving her trunk. What CSF finding would be most classic with a diagnosis of Guillain-Barré syndrome? Increased protein.

Guillain-Barré Syndrome

A postinfectious neuropathy that leads to muscle weakness and paresthesias; the most common pediatric peripheral neuropathy. Occurs in healthy individuals days to weeks after an antecedent illness, typically beginning in the legs and progressing in an ascending fashion to the trunk, arms, and bulbar muscles. From birth to 30 years of age, the annual incidence is 1.3–1.9 in

100,000. It can occur in all ages, although there is a peak in adolescence/early adulthood and again in later adulthood. Males and females are affected equally. Causes include the following:

- Autoimmune conditions of the peripheral nervous system.
- *Campylobacter jejuni* and *Mycoplasma pneumoniae* are the most common causes.
- Other antecedent infections include the following:
  - **Viral:** CMV, EBV, other herpesviruses, HIV.
  - **Bacterial:** More rarely, typhoid, *Listeria*, tularemia, and TB.
  - Other antecedent events have included surgery and vaccination.
  - In the majority of cases, the agent responsible for the prodromal illness cannot be identified.

SYMPTOMS/EXAM

- Diagnosed primarily on the basis of clinical appearance.
- Features required for diagnosis include progressive motor weakness of > 1 limb and areflexia (loss of ankle jerks and diminished knee and biceps reflexes will suffice if other features are consistent with the diagnosis).
- The syndrome progresses over hours, days, or weeks, with 50% of patients having complete progression in two weeks, 80% in three weeks, and 90% in four weeks.

DIAGNOSIS

- CSF generally shows ↑ protein after the first week but may be normal in 20% of children; WBC count is normal.
- EMG can take up to three weeks to demonstrate ⊕ findings; the first abnormality is in the F wave.
- Nerve conduction studies are slow.

TREATMENT

- Monitoring and supportive care.
- IVIG and plasmapheresis have been shown to shorten the disease course.
- Rehabilitation may be needed to effect a full recovery.

COMPLICATIONS

- Respiratory compromise may result in death. With better respiratory monitoring, the risk of mortality has greatly improved, but mortality is still 3–5%.
- Some 7–10% relapse.

Familial Dysautonomia (Riley-Day Syndrome)

An inherited neuropathy affecting sensory and autonomic nerves.

SYMPTOMS/EXAM

- Infants have difficulty feeding → aspiration.
- Vomiting and sweating spells and seizures are also seen.
- Temperature dysregulation and insensitivity to pain are additional features.

The Miller Fisher variant of Guillain-Barré syndrome is characterized by gait ataxia, areflexia, and ophthalmoparesis.

Charcot-Marie-Tooth is the most common inherited peripheral neuropathy.

A 17-year-old girl newly diagnosed with myasthenia gravis is noted to have titers of anti–ACh receptor antibodies. What surgery should be considered for this patient? Thymectomy.

Ocular myasthenia gravis is the most common form. May "burn out," generalize, or stay purely ocular.

Congenital myasthenia gravis is a nonimmunologic process that may be due to a defect in ACh synthesis, an excess of acetylcholinesterase, or an endplate ACh receptor deficiency that presents at birth.

Neonatal myasthenia gravis is due to passive transplacental transfer of antibodies in neonates born to mothers with myasthenia gravis. It presents at birth and resolves over several weeks.

Myasthenia Gravis

Autoimmune degradation of the postsynaptic ACh receptors leading to muscle fatigue. Generally nonhereditary; usually occurs after 10 years of age, but can affect children as young as six months of age. In prepubertal children, males are affected more often than females; in postpubertal children, the opposite is the case. If left untreated, the disease can progress and respiratory compromise may occur. Etiologies are as follows:

- Immune-mediated neuromuscular blockade.
- May occasionally be associated with hypothyroidism (Hashimoto's thyroiditis).
- Infants born to myasthenic mothers may have a transient form called transient neonatal myasthenia gravis, which lasts days to weeks (until ACh receptor antibodies disappear) and should be distinguished from a rare and often hereditary form called congenital myasthenia gravis.

SYMPTOMS/EXAM

- Ptosis and extraocular eye weakness are the earliest symptoms.
- Dysphagia and facial weakness are also common.
- Rapid fatigability of muscles is a hallmark and is the feature that distinguishes myasthenia gravis from most other neuromuscular disorders.

DIAGNOSIS

- Diagnosis is based on two of three ⊕ findings: EMG, edrophonium (Tensilon) test (or response to Mestinon), and/or antibodies.
- Decremental response is seen on EMG with repetitive nerve stimulation; motor nerve conduction remains normal.
- ACh receptor–binding or –blocking antibodies are detected in seropositive forms.
- Other labs include ANA and abnormal immune complexes, TSH, and FT_4.

TREATMENT

- Cholinesterase-inhibiting drugs (neostigmine, pyridostigmine) are the mainstays of treatment.
- Give oral steroids as needed for immunosuppression.
- Steroid-sparing medications (e.g., azathioprine) may also be used.
- IVIG and plasmapheresis may be tried when steroids are ineffective.
- Thymectomy should be considered and is most effective in children with high titers of anti–ACh receptor antibodies who are symptomatic and < 2 years of age.
- Immunosuppression, thymectomy, or treatment of associated hypothyroidism may effect a cure.

COMPLICATIONS

- The prognosis varies, with some children going into spontaneous remission and others remaining symptomatic into adulthood.
- Congenital myasthenia gravis is almost always a permanent disorder without spontaneous remission and has a poor prognosis.

A six-month-old boy presents with hypotonia and constipation. He is later found to have *Clostridium botulinum* toxin in his stool. What are two common sources of exposure? Honey and soil.

Botulism

- Sx/Exam:
  - The first sign of infant botulism is lack of defecation.
  - In children, it usually presents with bilateral symmetric descending flaccid paralysis of the cranial nerves and weak cry.
- **Dx:** EMG shows decremental response on repetitive nerve stimulation. *C. botulinum* toxin may be detected in stool.
- **Tx:** Human botulinum immunoglobulin in an acute setting; supportive care.
- **Complications:** Many cases progress to respiratory paralysis, with 50% of patients requiring intubation.

MUSCLE DISEASES

Duchenne Muscular Dystrophy

An X-linked disorder that is the most common hereditary neuromuscular disease. Incidence is 1 in 3600 live male births. Some 30% of cases are new mutations.

SYMPTOMS/EXAM

- Rarely symptomatic at birth or early infancy, although patients may be slightly hypotonic.
- Children typically start walking at a normal age.
- Pelvic girdle weakness may be seen as early as two years of age.
- Proximal strength is affected more often than distal strength.
- Gowers' sign is seen as early as three years of age and is fully expressed by 5–6 years of age.
- Patients are usually unable to walk (even with assistance) past 12 years of age.
- Weakness relentlessly progresses into the second decade.
- Other systemic involvement includes the following:
  - Pulmonary involvement in the form of weak cough and ↓ respiratory reserve.
  - Pharyngeal weakness.
  - Cardiomyopathy; pharyngeal weakness.
  - Incontinence is uncommon and is a late event.
  - Mild intellectual impairment (only 20–30% have an IQ < 70).
  - Scoliosis.

DIAGNOSIS

- ⊕ Gowers' sign; pseudohypertrophy of the calves and wasting of the thigh muscles.

In Duchenne muscular dystrophy, proximal strength is affected to a greater degree than distal strength.

Gowers' sign is a maneuver in which a child uses the hands to "climb up" the legs in order to assume an upright position.

- Genetic testing for dystrophin gene.
- Muscle biopsy is diagnostic.
- ↑ CK is also seen.
- Echocardiography, ECG, and CXR to evaluate cardiac function.
- EMG shows characteristic myopathic features.
- Motor and sensory nerve conduction velocities are normal.

TREATMENT

- Steroids (prednisone and deflazacort) are sometimes recommended.
- Supportive care; physical therapy.

COMPLICATIONS

Death usually occurs by approximately 18 years of age.

Becker Muscular Dystrophy

Becker muscular dystrophy presents as a milder form of Duchenne muscular dystrophy.

A genetic defect at the same locus as Duchenne muscular dystrophy, but patients have a milder course.

SYMPTOMS/EXAM

- Onset of weakness is later than that of Duchenne muscular dystrophy.
- Patients are ambulatory until late adolescence/early adulthood but have the same rates of cardiomyopathy.
- Pseudohypertrophy of the calves and wasting of the thigh muscles are characteristic.
- ↓ frequency of learning disabilities (compared to Duchenne muscular dystrophy).

DIAGNOSIS

- Genetic testing for dystrophin gene.
- Muscle biopsy is diagnostic.
- ↑ CK is seen (the same levels as those found in Duchenne muscular dystrophy).

TREATMENT

Supportive care; physical therapy.

COMPLICATIONS

Death usually occurs in the 30s to 40s.

Myotonic Dystrophy

Amplification of the CTG triplet repeat of the myotonic dystrophy gene on chromosome 19, which codes for a protein kinase found in skeletal muscle. Symptoms usually become more severe with each successive generation.

SYMPTOMS/EXAM

- **Congenital myotonic dystrophy:** Presents in the newborn period with hypotonia, facial diplegia, tenting of the upper lip, feeding problems, and intercostal and diaphragmatic weakness leading to respiratory distress.
- **Juvenile myotonic dystrophy:** Presents in the first decade of life with progressive weakness; atrophy of temples, hands, and sternocleidomastoid muscles; impaired speech and hearing; and mental retardation.

TREATMENT

Supportive care; physical therapy.

COMPLICATIONS

Symptoms worsen over time; joint contractures and cardiomyopathy may develop.

VASCULAR ANOMALIES

Aneurysms

Affects males more than females (2:1); familial occurrence is common. Most often related to a congenital disease—e.g., Ehlers-Danlos syndrome, AVMs, coarctation of the aorta, or polycystic kidney disease (berry aneurysms). Acquired aneurysms are most likely due to bacterial endocarditis.

SYMPTOMS/EXAM

- Most often present with subarachnoid hemorrhage (intense headache, nuchal rigidity, progressive loss of consciousness).
- May present with headache and focal neurologic deficits due to cranial nerve compression.
- More likely to rupture in children < 2 years or > 10 years of age.

Acquired aneurysms are most often due to bacterial endocarditis.

DIAGNOSIS

Angiography is the preferred diagnostic modality.

TREATMENT

- **Not ruptured:** Surgical resection or embolization.
- **Ruptured:** Surgical clipping or endovascular coiling within two days of hemorrhage.

> A two-week-old girl presents with feeding intolerance and respiratory distress and is noted to have a 2/6 systolic murmur and hepatomegaly on physical exam. After ruling out primary cardiac and respiratory causes, you consider an AVM as a possible etiology. What additional physical exam finding would support this diagnosis? Hearing a bruit when listening to the anterior fontanelle.

Arteriovenous Malformations (AVMs)

- Sx/Exam:
    - Most often present with hemorrhage (either subarachnoid or intracerebral bleed).
    - If small but unruptured, may present with headache or seizures.
    - If larger but unruptured, may also present with progressive neurologic deficit.
    - In infants, may present with CHF from high-output heart failure.
    - A high-pitched bruit may be auscultated over the head in 50% of cases.

- **Dx:**
  - Angiography is the preferred test.
  - MRI/CT with contrast can demonstrate AVM.
- **Tx:** Surgical resection or embolization.

VEIN OF GALEN MALFORMATIONS

- A common AVM variant consisting of a large shunt between the cerebral arteries and the vein of Galen. Mortality is 50%.
- **Sx/Exam:** Usually presents in infancy with high-output CHF and failure to thrive.
- **Tx:** Surgical resection is the standard of care, although it remains difficult.

CAVERNOUS HEMANGIOMAS

- Low-flow AVMs that have a tendency to leak but do not cause large intracranial hemorrhage. May be familial.
- **Sx/Exam:** Most commonly presents as seizure.
- **Dx:** Brain MRI has a "popcorn" appearance.
- **Tx:** Surgical resection if symptomatic.

VENOUS ANGIOMAS

- **Sx/Exam:** Rarely symptomatic; most commonly present as seizure.
- **Tx:** Surgical resection is not indicated unless complications arise.

Stroke

Some 1–3 in 100,000 children are affected by a clinically significant stroke each year. The cause is known in 75% of cases and may include congenital heart disease, sickle cell disease, coagulation disorders, endocarditis, other infections (meningitis, systemic infection), autoimmune disease, rheumatic disease, metabolic disease, leukemia, lymphoma, polycythemia, intracerebral vascular processes, trauma, and drugs (cocaine). Types of stroke in children include the following:

- **Arterial thrombosis:** May be caused by blunt trauma of the posterior pharynx → intimal tear, dissection, and shedding of emboli.
- **Venous thrombosis:** May have septic causes (e.g., bacterial meningitis, otitis media, mastoiditis) or aseptic causes (e.g., congenital heart disease, leukemia, dehydration, hypercoagulable states).
- **Arterial embolism:** May be caused by cardiac anomalies, including paradoxical emboli through a patent foramen ovale, septic emboli from bacterial endocarditis, arrhythmias, and myxoma.
- Other causes include intracranial hemorrhage.

DIAGNOSIS

- History and physical.
- Head CT/brain MRI; angiogram if necessary.
- Echocardiography to rule out congenital heart disease.
- Hypercoagulable workup if indicated.

TREATMENT

- Treatment depends on the type and cause of stroke.
- Treat the underlying cause.
- Aspirin has a modest effect on ischemic strokes.
- Anticoagulants remain controversial.

CEREBRAL PALSY (CP)

A nonprogressive disorder of movement and posture caused by injury to the immature brain before, during, or after birth. Incidence is 2–3 in 1000 live births. Causes include intrauterine growth retardation; prematurity (especially in infants weighing < 1000 g); prenatal, peripartum, or other asphyxia; early infection; and kernicterus.

Some 80% of instances of asphyxia associated with CP are antenatal, with only 10% occurring peripartum.

SYMPTOMS/EXAM

- A thorough history should be taken of pregnancy, delivery, and the post-partum period.
- Physical examination reveals hypertonia and hyperreflexia.
- Patients do not lose skills previously learned.
- Subtypes of CP and their clinical presentation are listed in Table 15-7.

TABLE 15-7. Types of Cerebral Palsy

MOTOR SYNDROME	CLINICAL FINDINGS	NEUROPATHOLOGY
Spastic diplegia	Bilateral spasticity of the legs more than the arms. Often first noticed when the infant is learning to crawl. If severe, spasticity may make it difficult to put on diapers. Scissoring of the legs. Usually associated with normal intellectual development and a low risk of seizures.	PVL.
Spastic quadriplegia	The most severe form, affecting all extremities. Has a strong association with mental retardation and seizures. Evidence of athetosis is often seen; may be diagnosed with mixed CP.	PVL, multicystic encephalomalacia.
Spastic hemiplegia	One-sided CP; arms are more frequently affected than the legs. Hand preference at an early age. Delayed walking. Patients often walk on tiptoes owing to ↑ tone. Associated with a ⊕ family history of thrombophilic states or strokes.	Stroke.
Dyskinesia/ataxia	Less common than spastic CP. Infants are hypotonic with poor head control; feeding and speech are affected. Intellectual problems and seizures are uncommon.	Basal ganglia pathology involving the putamen, globus pallidus, and thalamus.

DIAGNOSIS

MRI can show periventricular leukomalacia (PVL), multicystic encephaloma-lacia, stroke, and any pathology in the basal ganglia.

TREATMENT

- Warrants a multidisciplinary approach involving neurology, pediatrics, physical/occupational/speech therapy, and educational support.
- Use braces and physical therapy to ↓ contractures.
- Provide adaptive equipment (e.g., walkers, canes, poles).
- Spasticity has been treated with varying success with a number of medications, including baclofen, dantrolene sodium, and benzodiazepines.
- Baclofen pumps may be useful.
- Occasionally, surgical procedures such as rhizotomies and tenotomies have been helpful.

NEURODEGENERATIVE DISORDERS

Progressive neurologic deterioration with loss of speech, vision, hearing, or motor function. Subtypes are listed in Table 15-8.

- **Sx/Exam:**
  - History confirms the loss of developmental milestones.
  - Physical examination localizes the process within the nervous system.
- **Dx:** Biochemical molecular testing; brain MRI.
- **Tx:**
  - Genetic counseling.
  - Bone marrow transplantation may be helpful in some cases.
- **Complications:** Few treatment options have been successful; the outcome is usually fatal.
- **Prevention:** Possible with prenatal diagnosis.

Think Rett syndrome with hand wringing and nonpurposeful movement of the hands in a two-year-old girl.

Rett Syndrome

- An X-linked disorder that primarily affects females, although some males are diagnosed with severe forms. Incidence is 1 in 15,000–22,000.
- **Sx/Exam:**
  - Development is normal until 12–18 months of age, after which regression of motor and language abilities is seen.

TABLE 15-8. Types of Neurodegenerative Disorders

INHERITED	BASAL GANGLIA	SPINOCEREBELLAR	MISCELLANEOUS
Sphingolipidoses:	Huntington's disease	Friedreich's ataxia	MS
◾ Niemann-Pick disease	Dystonia musculorum	Ataxia-telangiectasia	Pelizaeus-Merzbacher disease
◾ Gaucher disease	deformans	Olivopontocerebellar	Alexander disease
◾ GM1 and GM2 gangliosidosis	Wilson disease	atrophy	Canavan's spongy degeneration
◾ Krabbe disease	Hallervorden-Spatz	Abetalipoproteinemia	Kinky hair disease
◾ Metachromatic leukodystrophy	disease		Rett syndrome
Neuronal ceroid lipofuscinoses			Subacute sclerosing panencephalitis
Adrenoleukodystrophy			
Sialidosis			

- Hand wringing and nonpurposeful movement of the hands are hall-marks.
- Other symptoms include ataxia and episodes of hyperventilation.
- Acquired microcephaly with ↓ brain growth is seen after the first year of life.
- Most patients have generalized tonic-clonic seizures.
- **Tx:** Anticonvulsants.
- **Complications:**
  - After initial regression, the disease plateaus.
  - Death may occur during adolescence or early adulthood.

ATAXIA

Defined as inability to coordinate motor activity. Etiologies are listed in Table 15-9.

Acute cerebellar ataxia most commonly occurs after varicella infection.

Acute Cerebellar Ataxia

- Thought to be an autoimmune response against a virus targeted to the cerebellum. Usually affects children 1–3 years of age.
- **Dx:**
  - A diagnosis of exclusion that often follows a virus by 2–3 weeks.
  - Presents with severe truncal ataxia.
  - Horizontal nystagmus is seen in 50% of cases.
- **Tx:** No treatment is necessary; patients recover within two months.

 A six-year-old girl presents with progressively worsening ataxia, worsening visual acuity, absent DTRs, and a low ejection fraction on echocardiogram. What is her most likely diagnosis? Friedreich's ataxia.

TABLE 15-9. Etiologies of Ataxia

ACUTE OR RECURRENT ATAXIA	CHRONIC OR PROGRESSIVE ATAXIA
Drug ingestion	Hydrocephalus
Infection	Hypothyroidism
Postinfectious	Brain tumor
Head trauma	Paraneoplastic syndrome
Basilar migraine	Low vitamin E
Benign paroxysmal vertigo	Wilson disease
Brain tumor	Inborn errors of metabolism
Hydrocephalus	Inherited ataxias
Seizure	
Vascular events	
Guillain-Barré syndrome, Miller Fisher variant	
MS	
Inborn errors of metabolism	
Conversion reaction	
Inherited ataxias	

Friedreich's Ataxia

- Caused by an autosomal-recessive mutation, usually a triplet expansion, on chromosome 9 → degeneration of dorsal columns and roots, spinocerebellar tracts, pyramidal tracts, and cerebellar hemispheres. Onset occurs before 10 years of age.
- Sx/Exam:
    - Slow progressive ataxia, with the legs more severely affected than the arms.
    - Severe hypotonia; peripheral nerve sensory dysfunction.
    - Romberg test is ⊕.
    - DTRs are ↓ to absent.
    - Skeletal abnormalities, cardiomyopathy, and optic atrophy are also seen.
- Tx: Genetic counseling.

> A two-year-old girl previously diagnosed with several cases of conjunctivitis now presents with ataxia. What diagnosis do you consider? Ataxia-telangiectasia. On the exam, be aware of a two-year-old patient with "conjunctivitis" and ataxia. Conjunctival telangiectasias are often initially misdiagnosed as conjunctivitis.

Ataxia-Telangiectasia = Absent Thymus.

Ataxia-Telangiectasia

- The most common degenerative ataxia. Caused by an autosomal-recessive mutation. Onset is at approximately two years of age.
- Sx/Exam:
    - Oculomotor apraxia is common.
    - Telangiectasia starts at 4–6 years of age and most commonly affects the nose, the conjunctiva, and exposed surfaces of the extremities.
    - Also associated with a 50- to 100-fold ↑ in brain tumors and lymphoid tumors.
- Tx: Genetic counseling.

MOVEMENT DISORDERS

Tics

Involuntary, brief, repetitive, stereotyped, purposeless movements or vocalizations commonly involving the face, mouth, eyes, head, and neck. Affect 10% of children < 10 years of age; often precipitated by anxiety, stress, fatigue, and excitement. Can be motor or vocal as well as simple or complex.

SYMPTOMS/EXAM

Presentation varies by subtype.

- **Motor:**
    - **Simple:** Involve one muscle group and → eye blinking, jaw snapping, head twitching, shoulder shrugging, and tongue movements.
    - **Complex:** Combination of simple motor tics, or may involve multiple muscles → facial grimacing, touching, spitting, and gesturing.

- **Vocal:**
  - **Simple:** Involve sounds made by moving air through the nose or mouth, including grunting, barking, hissing, sniffing, snorting, or throat clearing.
  - **Complex:** May involve words, phrases, and sentences and may include repetition of patient's own words (palilalia), repetition of other people's words (echolalia), or obscene words (coprolalia).
- Associated with the following:
  - **Genetic syndromes:** Down syndrome, fragile X syndrome, Rett syndrome.
  - **Developmental problems:** Pervasive developmental disorder; autism.
  - **Drugs:** Antiepileptic medications; stimulants (amphetamines, methylphenidate).
  - **Infections:** Encephalitis, rubella.

TREATMENT

- Medication is generally not required.
- Relaxation techniques can be used to minimize stress.
- Most simple tics resolve within one year.

Tourette Syndrome

Incidence is 10–30 in 10,000 children, with males affected more often than females (10:1 to 2:1) and children affected more frequently than adults. Onset is before 18 years of age. Etiologies are as follows:

- **Genetic:** Has a 50% concordance in monozygotic twins and 8% in dizygotic twins.
- **Neurochemical:** Associated with impaired dopamine regulation in the caudate nucleus.

DIAGNOSIS

- Multiple motor and vocal tics occur multiple times per day almost daily for > 1 year.
- No tic-free period is seen for > 4 months
- Impairment in social functioning may be seen but is not essential for diagnosis.
- Comorbidities include OCD, ADHD, conduct disorder, depression, anxiety disorders, and learning disabilities.

TREATMENT

- Provide education and reassurance about tics.
- If tics are severe, haloperidol, risperidone, clonidine, or pimozide may be needed.
- Psychotherapy may be beneficial.

Sydenham Chorea

A subacute movement disorder that appears weeks to months after group A streptococcal infection and remits over weeks to months. Average age at onset is 8–12 years; females are affected more often than males.

Coprolalia is seen in 20–40% of patients with Tourette syndrome but is not required for diagnosis.

SYMPTOMS/EXAM

- Clinical features include general chorea, hypotonia, dysarthria, muscle weakness, and restlessness.
- Movement disorder disappears during sleep.
- Associated emotional and behavioral disturbances are seen.
- Writing difficulties are common.

DIAGNOSIS

With Sydenham chorea, think of strep and treatment of strep (penicillin).

- Conduct a careful history and physical exam to assess for any other major manifestations of rheumatic fever and recent streptococcal infection.
- Recent strep culture or current ASO or anti-DNase B.
- Obtain serum electrolytes, calcium, glucose, TSH, FT_4, CBC, ESR, copper, ceruloplasmin, ANA, and anticardiolipin antibodies.
- MRI is normal.

TREATMENT

- Penicillin.
- Treatment of actual chorea should be reserved for more severely affected individuals and is usually either symptomatic or immunomodulatory.
    - **Symptomatic:** Neuroleptics (haloperidol), benzodiazepines, valproic acid.
    - **Immunomodulatory:** Steroids.

COMPLICATIONS

Although spontaneous resolution occurs in weeks to months, the recurrence rate may be as high as 20%.

NEUROCUTANEOUS DISORDERS

Neurofibromatosis

An autosomal-dominant disorder involving spontaneous mutations of chromosome 17 (type 1) or chromosome 22 (type 2). Type 1 is the most common (90%) and has an incidence of 1 in 4000; type 2 is responsible for 10% of cases and has an incidence of 1 in 50,000.

EXAM/DIAGNOSIS

NF1 is characterized by café-au-lait spots, axillary/inguinal freckling, Lisch nodules, and neurofibromas; NF2 is characterized by acoustic neuromas.

- **Type 1 (NF1):**
    - Onset is in childhood.
    - Diagnosis is made by two or more of the following:
        - Six or more café-au-lait spots (0.5 cm in prepubertal and 1.5 cm in pubertal children) are the hallmark of NF1 (present in nearly 100% of cases).
        - Axillary or inguinal freckling.
        - Two or more iris Lisch nodules (melanocytic hamartomas).
        - Two or more neurofibromas or one plexiform neurofibroma.
        - Distinctive osseous lesions (sphenoid dysplasia, thinning of the long bone cortex).
        - Optic glioma.
        - A first-degree relative with confirmed NF1.
    - Also common are learning disabilities, migraines, and seizures.
    - Patients are at ↑ risk for other CNS tumors (meningiomas and astrocytomas).

- **Type 2 (NF2):**
  - Onset is in adolescence.
  - Diagnosis is made when one of the following is present:
    - Bilateral CN VIII masses consistent with acoustic neuromas, or
    - A first-degree relative with the disease **and** a patient with neurofibroma, meningioma, glioma, or schwannoma.
  - Patients are at greater risk for CNS tumors than in NF1 and often have multiple tumors.

TREATMENT

- Genetic counseling on future pregnancies.
- Treatment should be aimed at preventing future complications and early detection of malignancies.

Tuberous Sclerosis

An autosomal-dominant disorder associated with chromosome 9 or 16. More than half of all cases are spontaneous mutations. Incidence is 1 in 6000.

SYMPTOMS/EXAM

- Presentation varies widely, ranging from severe mental retardation and incapacitating seizures to normal intelligence and no seizures.
- Generally, the earlier the presentation, the more severe the disease.
  - May present with infantile spasms during infancy or with seizures and pathognomonic skin lesions during childhood (see Table 15-10).
  - Retinal lesions include phakomas (round, flat gray lesions near the optic disk) and mulberry tumors (arise from the nerve head).

DIAGNOSIS

- Do a careful search for skin and retinal lesions in all patients with seizure disorders.
- Head CT or MRI shows calcified tubers in the periventricular area (which may not arise until patients are 3–4 years of age).

TABLE 15-10. Skin Lesions of Tuberous Sclerosis

LESION	DESCRIPTION	PERCENTAGE
Ash leaf spot	Hypopigmented macules seen best with Wood's lamp.	90%
Sebaceous adenoma	Begin as tiny red nodules over the nose and cheeks and then grow, coalesce, and become flesh colored (in adolescents).	75%
Shagreen patch	Roughened patch of skin located in the lumbosacral region.	25% (< 5 years), 50% (> 5 years)
Ungual fibromas	Red to flesh-colored benign tumors located underneath or adjacent to the nails, more frequently affecting the toes than the fingers.	15–20%

The classic triad of tuberous sclerosis consists of seizures, mental retardation, and facial angiofibromas (adenoma sebaceum).

- Genetic testing is available.
- Baseline studies include echocardiogram, CXR, and renal ultrasound.

TREATMENT

Seizure control.

COMPLICATIONS

- A large number of young patients with tuberous sclerosis and infantile spasms have mental retardation.
- Rhabdomyomas of the heart, which are found in 50% of cases, may resolve spontaneously but may also → CHF.
- In most patients, the kidneys are affected by hamartomas or polycystic disease.
- Angiomyolipomas may → generalized pulmonary cystic or fibrous changes as well as pneumothorax.
- Occasionally a tuber differentiates into a malignant astrocytoma.

Sturge-Weber Syndrome

A spontaneous mutation with an incidence of 1 in 50,000.

SYMPTOMS/EXAM

- **Facial port-wine stain:** Unilateral distribution of the ophthalmic branch of the trigeminal nerve.
- **Variable neurologic involvement:** Seizures, mental retardation, contralateral hemiparesis, hemiatrophy, homonymous hemianopsia.
- **Ocular defects:**
    - Glaucoma is seen in 50% of patients and is almost always ipsilateral.
    - Other ocular defects include hemangiomas of the choroids, conjunctiva, and episclera; retinal detachment; vascular tortuosity; and buphthalmos.

DIAGNOSIS

- Skull x-ray/head CT show calcification of the cortex underlying the angioma.
- Head CT with contrast/brain MRI show atrophy of the underlying hemisphere.

TREATMENT

- Antiepileptic drugs are effective in only 40% of cases.
- Surgical intervention may be necessary to treat intractable seizures.

HEARING

Hearing Loss

It is estimated that 1–2 newborns in 1000 live births have moderate, severe, or profound bilateral sensorineural hearing loss (50% of whom have profound bilateral hearing loss > 75 dB); 1–2 newborns in 1000 live births have mild or unilateral sensorineural hearing loss. By 19 years of age, the prevalence doubles. In school-age children, 3 in 1000 have unilateral hearing loss of ≥ 26 dB and 13 in 1000 have unilateral hearing loss of ≥ 45 dB. Types of hearing loss are as follows:

- **Peripheral hearing loss:** Conductive or sensorineural hearing loss. Caused by dysfunction in the transmission of sound through the external or middle ear or by abnormal transduction in the inner ear and CN VIII.
  - **Conductive hearing loss:** Sound is physically impeded in the external and/or middle ear. More common than sensorineural hearing loss.
    - **Common causes in the ear canal:** Foreign body, impacted cerumen, atresia or stenosis.
    - **Common causes in the middle ear:** Otitis media with effusion, perforated tympanic membrane, discontinuity of the ossicular chain, otosclerosis, cholesteatoma.
  - **Sensorineural hearing loss:** Damage to or incorrect development of structures in the inner ear. Common causes include hair cell destruction from disease, noise, or ototoxic medicines; cochlear malformation; perilymphatic fistula of the round or oval window membrane; and lesions of the acoustic division of CN VIII.
- **Central hearing loss:** Caused by hearing deficits along the central auditory nervous system from the proximal CN VIII to the cerebral cortex.
  - Tumors or demyelinating disease of CN VIII and the cerebellopontine angle are very rare in children.
  - Central auditory processing disorders make it difficult for children to listen selectively and to process and integrate auditory information.

SYMPTOMS/EXAM

Risk factors for hearing loss include the following:

- A family history of hereditary childhood sensorineural hearing loss.
- In utero CMV, rubella, syphilis, HSV, toxoplasmosis.
- Craniofacial abnormalities, including abnormalities of the pinna or ear canal.
- Birth weight < 1500 g.
- Apgar scores of 0–4 at one minute and 0–6 at five minutes.
- Hyperbilirubinemia at levels requiring exchange transfusion.
- Ototoxic medications.
- Bacterial meningitis.
- Mechanical ventilation of ≥ 5 days.
- Head trauma.
- Recurrent or persistent otitis media for ≥ 3 months.
- Parent or caregiver concern about hearing, speech, or generalized development.

DIAGNOSIS

Universal hearing screening at birth is recommended by the American Academy of Pediatrics (AAP).

- Screening is most effective if moderate to profound hearing loss is diagnosed by six months of age.
- Study types are as follows:
  - **Otoacoustic emissions (OAEs):** Can diagnose hearing loss of ≥ 30–40 dB; if hearing loss is diagnosed, auditory brain-stem evoked response (ABER) is recommended.
  - **ABER:** Can differentiate types of hearing loss; the most definitive type of testing.
  - **Audiometry:** Gives a fundamental description of hearing sensitivity.
  - **Tympanometry:** Measures the ability of the middle ear to transmit sound energy as a function of air pressure in the external ear canal.

Hearing loss is the most common cause of isolated language delay.

TREATMENT

- Speech and language evaluation.
- **Conductive hearing loss:** Consider tympanostomy tubes if appropriate or correction of underlying pathology.
- **Sensorineural hearing loss:** Hearing aids.
- Treatment of severe hearing loss is controversial; options include sign language, lip reading, hearing aids, and cochlear implants.

VISION

Strabismus

The literal definition is "to squint or look obliquely." Affects approximately 4% of children < 6 years of age; 30–50% of these children will develop amblyopia.

Strabismus = "to squint."

DIAGNOSIS

- **Corneal light reflex:** Have the child look directly into a light source and observe where the reflection lies in both eyes. If light is off center in one pupil or asymmetric, strabismus exists.
- **Cover-uncover test:** Have the child stare at a distant object, and then cover and uncover each of the eyes in turn; if there is movement of the uncovered eye once the other eye is covered, strabismus exists.

TREATMENT

- Prescription glasses may help if the condition is due to refraction.
- Eye muscle surgery may be necessary.

Amblyopia

Defined as a ↓ in visual acuity in one or both eyes caused by an unclear retinal image, which → improper development of the visual cortex. Caused by strabismus (most common), refractive errors, or opacity in the visual field (e.g., cataract).

DIAGNOSIS

Visual acuity testing. Best if diagnosed and treated early (by four years of age).

TREATMENT

- Removal of any potential pathology (cataract).
- Prescription glasses may help if the condition is due to refraction.
- Patching of the good eye until amblyopia has resolved in the bad eye.

PRIMITIVE REFLEXES

Table 15-11 outlines primitive reflexes.

TABLE 15-11. Primitive Reflexes

REFLEX	TIMING	ELICIT	RESPONSE
Moro	Birth to 3–6 months.	While supine, allow the head to suddenly fall back approximately 3 cm.	Symmetric extension and adduction, then flexion, of limbs.
Startle	From when Moro disappears to 1 year.	Startle.	Arms and legs flex immediately.
Galant	Birth to 2–6 months.	While prone, stroke the paravertebral region of the back.	Pelvis will move in the direction of the stimulated side.
Sucking	Becomes voluntary at 3 months.	Stimulate lips.	Sucks.
Babinski	Birth to 12 months.	Stroke from toes to heel.	Extension of the great toe and fanning of the other toes.
Tonic neck	Birth to 4–6 months.	While supine, rotate the head laterally.	Extension of limbs on the chin side, and flexion of limbs on the opposite side (fencing posture).
Rooting	Birth to 4–6 months.	Stroke the finger from mouth to earlobe.	Head turns toward the stimulus and mouth opens.
Palmar/plantar grasp	Birth to 4–9 months	Stimulation of palm or plantar surface of foot.	Palmar grasp/plantar flexion.
Parachute	Appears at 9 months.	Horizontal suspension and quick thrusting movement toward surface.	Extension of the extremities.

Reproduced, with permission, from Stead LG et al. *First Aid for the Pediatrics Clerkship.* New York: McGraw-Hill, 2004:40.)

CHAPTER 16

Oncology

Wilbur Lam, MD
Debbie Sakaguchi, MD
reviewed by Robert E. Goldsby, MD

A three-year-old boy with fever and petechiae has a WBC count of 1000, a hemoglobin level of 12.0, and a platelet count of 9000. What is his most likely diagnosis? Any patient with at least two ↓ cell lines on a CBC (in this case, leukopenia and thrombocytopenia) should be given a presumptive diagnosis of acute leukemia until proven otherwise.

Acute Lymphoblastic Leukemia (ALL)

The most common malignancy in children; peak incidence is at 2–5 years of age. Risk factors include ataxia-telangiectasia, Bloom syndrome, Klinefelter syndrome, trisomy 21, neurofibromatosis, Fanconi anemia, and Wiskott-Aldrich syndrome. Poor prognostic factors include a WBC count > 50,000/mm³, age < 1 year or > 10 years, cytogenetics with lower ploidy, ⊕ Philadelphia chromosome, male gender, T-cell lineage, and inability to achieve complete remission 4–6 weeks after induction.

SYMPTOMS/EXAM

Pallor, fever, bruising/purpura, bone pain, fatigue, lymphadenopathy, hepatosplenomegaly, CNS disease → headache, cranial nerve palsies.

DIFFERENTIAL

Chronic EBV, CMV, immune-mediated thrombocytopenic purpura (ITP), juvenile rheumatoid arthritis.

DIAGNOSIS

- Abnormal WBC count, neutropenia, blasts.
- Anemia (normocytic, low reticulocyte count), thrombocytopenia.
- ↑ uric acid, ↑ potassium, ↓ calcium, ↑ phosphorus, ↑ LDH.
- Bone marrow aspirate shows a minimum of 25% blasts.
- Testicular exam.
- **Metastatic evaluation:** CSF cytology, CXR.

TREATMENT

- Chemotherapy consisting of prednisone, L-asparaginase, vincristine, cyclophosphamide, cytarabine, 6-mercaptopurine, methotrexate, and daunorubicin (if high risk).
- The specific chemotherapy regimen should be dictated by the prognostic risk factors of the individual patient.

Acute Myelogenous Leukemia (AML)

Accounts for 20% of newly diagnosed leukemia. Shows an ↑ incidence in the neonatal period and adolescence. Poor prognostic factors include a WBC count > 100,000/mm³, age < 1 year or > 15 years, and the chromosomal abnormalities del (7) or del (11). Risk factors are as follows:

- **Environmental:** Ionizing radiation, chemical exposure (pesticides, benzene, chemotherapy).

Risk factors for ALL—ABCDEFW

Ataxia-telangiectasia
Bloom syndrome
C(K)linefelter syndrome
Down syndrome
N**E**urofibromatosis
Fanconi anemia
Wiskott-Aldrich syndrome

The 4 P's of ALL:

Pallor
Pyrexia
Purpura
Pain

ONCOLOGY

- **Genetic:** Ataxia-telangiectasia, Bloom syndrome, Klinefelter syndrome, Kostmann syndrome, trisomy 21, neurofibromatosis, Fanconi anemia, Schwachman-Diamond syndrome.
- **Nongenetic:** Aplastic anemia, paroxysmal nocturnal hemoglobinuria.

SYMPTOMS/EXAM

Pallor, fever, bruising/purpura, pain, gingival hypertrophy, CNS symptoms (headache, vomiting, photophobia, papilledema, cranial nerve palsy), lymphadenopathy, hepatosplenomegaly.

DIAGNOSIS

- Leukocytosis, blasts.
- Anemia (normocytic; low reticulocyte count), thrombocytopenia.
- ↑ uric acid, ↑ potassium, ↓ calcium, ↑ phosphorus, ↑ LDH.
- ↑ PT, ↑ PTT, ↓ fibrinogen.
- Bone marrow aspirate shows a minimum of 25% blasts.
- **Metastatic evaluation:** CSF cytology and immunophenotyping; CXR.

TREATMENT

- **Induction:** Daunorubicin, cytarabine, thioguanine, etoposide, dexamethasone.
- If the patient has a sibling match, bone marrow transplantation after remission is achieved. All-*trans*-retinoic acid should be given for acute promyeloblastic leukemia.

In most cases of CML, leukemic cells are ⊕ for the Philadelphia chromosome (bcr-abl oncogene).

Chronic Myelogenous Leukemia (CML)

Rare in childhood (< 5% of childhood leukemias). More than 80% of cases are diagnosed after the age of four. Exposure to ionizing radiation is a risk factor.

SYMPTOMS/EXAM

Table 16-1 outlines the presentation and diagnosis of CML.

TABLE 16-1. Course of CML

PHASE	PATHOPHYSIOLOGY	SYMPTOMS/EXAM	DIAGNOSIS
Chronic	Expansion of mature cells with abnormal function. Lasts roughly three years.	Fever, night sweats, weakness, abdominal pain, bruising, hepatosplenomegaly.	↑ WBC count, mild anemia, ↑ platelets, ↑ uric acid, ↑ LDH, ↑ vitamin B_{12}, ↑ transcobalamin, bone marrow hypercellular with granulocytes.
Accelerated	Progressive abnormalities in cell differentiation; changes in karyotype. Variable duration.	Progressive constitutional symptoms.	Karyotype changes: duplication of Philadelphia chromosome, isochromosome 17, trisomy 8.
Blast	Loss of differentiation.	Pallor, petechiae, hyperhistaminemic symptoms (pruritus, cold urticaria).	Blasts, basophilia, ↓ hemoglobin, ↓ platelets.

TREATMENT

Imatinib mesylate, busulfan, hydroxyurea, interferon-α, bone marrow transplantation (the only curative option).

Hodgkin's Disease

Because of its bimodal age distribution (peaks in early adulthood and after 50 years of age), most pediatric cases of Hodgkin's disease occur in adolescents; it is rarely seen in children < 5 years of age. Risk factors include congenital or acquired immunodeficiencies (Wiskott-Aldrich syndrome, ataxia-telangiectasia, hypogammaglobinemia, HIV, immunosuppressive therapy for organ transplantation). Poor prognostic factors include extensive spread of disease (supra- **and** infradiaphragmatic disease; involvement of extranodal organs such as liver, lungs, or bone) and the presence of B symptoms (fever, night sweats, and weight loss).

SYMPTOMS/EXAM

- **Lymphadenopathy:**
  - Painless, firm, rubbery supraclavicular or cervical adenopathy is seen in most cases.
  - Mediastinal adenopathy may → persistent cough and to bronchial or tracheal compression.
  - Adenopathy tends to arise in a single group of nodes and slowly spreads in an orderly and sequential fashion.
- Constitutional symptoms include B symptoms, fatigue, weakness, and anorexia.
- Pruritus is common.
- Pain with alcohol ingestion.

DIFFERENTIAL

Chronic inflammatory disorders or infections (atypical mycobacterial infections, toxoplasmosis, infectious mononucleosis), non-Hodgkin's lymphoma, metastatic lymphadenopathy (soft tissue sarcoma, nasopharyngeal carcinoma), leukemia.

DIAGNOSIS

- Definitive diagnosis is with lymph node biopsy that reveals **Reed-Sternberg cells**—giant multinucleated cells with nucleoli that have an "owl's eye" appearance on staining (pathognomonic of Hodgkin's disease).
- **Anemia:** Impaired iron mobilization or Coombs-⊕ hemolytic anemia.
- Immune-mediated thrombocytopenia.
- Neutrophilia, lymphopenia, eosinophilia, monocytosis.
- **Acute-phase reactants:** ↑ ESR, fibrinogen, serum copper, ferritin, and alkaline phosphatase.
- Nephrotic syndrome.
- **Metastatic evaluation:** CXR; CT/MRI of the chest/abdomen/pelvis; bone marrow biopsy.

B symptoms, which adversely affect the prognosis of Hodgkin's disease, include a fever of > 38°C for three consecutive days, night sweats, and > 10% weight loss in the six months prior to admission.

ONCOLOGY

In Hodgkin's disease, constitutional symptoms, elevation of acute-phase reactants, and a typically indolent course often → a misdiagnosis of an inflammatory disorder or chronic infection.

Altered cell-mediated immunity in Hodgkin's disease → autoimmune hemolytic anemia and an ITP-like thrombocytopenia.

TREATMENT

- Chemotherapy consisting of combinations of doxorubicin, bleomycin, vinblastine, vincristine, dacarbazine, procarbazine, cyclophosphamide, mechlorethamine, and prednisone.
- Additional radiation therapy for high-risk and relapsed patients.

> A six-year-old boy is diagnosed with intussusception of the ileocecal junction that is subsequently found to be caused by a malignant process. This clinical scenario best describes which 1° abdominal tumor? Burkitt's lymphoma affecting the ileocecal lymph nodes classically presents as intussusception.

Non-Hodgkin's Lymphoma

A diverse group of malignancies that accounts for < 15% of pediatric cancers in the United States but is responsible for > 50% of such cancers in equatorial Africa. Incidence ↑ with age; most pediatric cases occur in adolescents and are extremely rare in children < 5 years of age. Pediatric non-Hodgkin's lymphomas are generally aggressive, rapidly proliferating, diffuse malignancies. Risk factors include congenital or acquired immunodeficiencies (Wiskott-Aldrich syndrome, X-linked lymphoproliferative syndrome, hypogammaglobulinemia, HIV, immunosuppressive therapy for organ/marrow transplantation). A viral contribution has been postulated, as EBV DNA is often detected in biopsy samples. Classification of pediatric non-Hodgkin's lymphoma is as follows:

- **Burkitt's lymphoma (small noncleaved cell lymphoma):** Histology shows many B cells with large nuclei along with basophilic cytoplasm and few histiocytes → the classic "starry sky" pattern.
- **Lymphoblastic lymphoma:** Usually indistinguishable from ALL lymphoblasts; generally associated with immature T cells.
- **Large cell lymphoma:** Large cells of B-cell, T-cell, or histiocyte origin.

SYMPTOMS/EXAM

Because tumors are aggressive, the duration of symptoms may be days to weeks. Symptoms according to subtype are as follows:

- **Burkitt's lymphoma:**
  - **Sporadic form:** Seen primarily in the United States, with 90% of cases presenting with abdominal pain, distention, an RLQ mass, or intussusception; marrow and CNS involvement; and rapid growth → tumor lysis syndrome
  - **Endemic form:** Seen in equatorial Africa, with most cases involving the jaw, orbit, CNS, and paraspinal areas.
- **Lymphoblastic lymphoma:** Mediastinal disease commonly → airway compression or SVC syndrome.
- **Large cell lymphoma:** Characterized by abdominal involvement, but may also affect unusual sites such as the lungs/pleura, face, brain, skin, testes, and muscle.

DIAGNOSIS

- Biopsy with histology, immunophenotyping, and cytogenetic analysis.
- LDH reflects tumor burden risk for tumor lysis syndrome.
- LFTs, metabolic panel to evaluate for tumor lysis syndrome.
- **Metastatic evaluation:** CSF and bone marrow examination; CXR; CT/MRI of the chest/abdomen/pelvis.

TREATMENT

- **Burkitt's lymphoma and large cell lymphoma:** Intensive chemotherapy for 6–9 months.
- **Lymphoblastic lymphoma:** Milder ALL-like chemotherapy for 15–18 months.

Burkitt's lymphoma is the most rapidly proliferating tumor known, with a doubling rate of ~ 24–48 hours → a high risk of tumor lysis syndrome.

BRAIN TUMORS

Tumors are the most common intracranial mass lesions in childhood. Risk factors include neurofibromatosis, tuberous sclerosis, and CNS irradiation.

SYMPTOMS/EXAM

Presentation depends on age and tumor location.

- **Age < 2 years, infratentorial mass:** Vomiting, unsteadiness, lethargy, irritability.
- **Age > 2 years, supratentorial mass:** Headache, visual changes, seizures, focal neurologic deficit, personality changes.

DIAGNOSIS

CT/MRI (better definition, especially the posterior fossa) with and without contrast; biopsy.

TREATMENT

Surgical resection (tissue diagnosis, reduction of tumor burden), radiation therapy, chemotherapy (nitrosoureas, vincristine, cisplatin, carboplatin, etoposide, cyclophosphamide).

Infratentorial Brain Tumors

Table 16-2 outlines the presentation and treatment of infratentorial brain tumors.

Supratentorial High-Grade Astrocytoma

An aggressive tumor with metastases to the lung, lymph nodes, liver, and bone. Associated with gene mutation of protein 53 (p53), which normally leads to apoptosis.

SYMPTOMS/EXAM

Headache, vomiting, seizures, focal motor symptoms, behavioral changes.

TABLE 16-2. Clinical Manifestations of Infratentorial Brain Tumors

	MEDULLOBLASTOMA	LOW-GRADE ASTROCYTOMA	EPENDYMOMA	BRAIN STEM GLIOMA
Incidence in posterior fossa	30–40%.	30–40%.	10–20%.	10–20%.
Symptoms/ exam—early	Headache, vomiting, diplopia, imbalance.	Unilateral dysmetria; gait disturbance.	Similar to medulloblastoma, but slower onset; hoarseness.	Diplopia, facial weakness, difficulty swallowing.
Symptoms/ exam—late	Extremity dysmetria, coma.	Headache, vomiting.	Similar to medulloblastoma, but slower onset; cranial nerve palsies.	Cranial nerve palsies, weakness.
Symptom duration prior to diagnosis	2–4 months.	3–6 months.	3–6 months.	0–3 months.
Diagnosis	**CT/MRI:** Enhancing isodense/hyperdense lesion; hydrocephalus. **Biopsy:** Undifferentiated cells.	**CT:** Enhancing cystic mass.	**CT:** Variable appearance, calcifications, cysts, hemorrhage. **Biopsy:** Ependymal rosette.	**MRI:** Diffusely infiltrating glioma. **Biopsy:** Usually not indicated.
Treatment	Surgical resection, radiation, chemotherapy (CCNU, vincristine, cisplatin).	Surgical resection, radiation if recurrent tumor.	Surgical resection, radiation.	Radiation.

Adapted, with permission, from Rudolph CD et al. *Rudolph's Pediatrics,* 21st ed. New York: McGraw-Hill, 2002:2210.

DIAGNOSIS

- CT/MRI with contrast reveals an enhancing mass.
- Biopsy reveals hypercellularity, atypical nuclei, mitoses, endothelial proliferation, and anaplasia.

TREATMENT

Surgical resection, radiation. Chemotherapy (in trials) has little impact on survival.

Craniopharyngioma

Cells are derived from squamous epithelial cells in the suprasellar area.

SYMPTOMS/EXAM

Headache, vomiting, ↓ visual acuity and visual fields, hypopituitarism (growth delay, diabetes insipidus [DI]).

ONCOLOGY

DIFFERENTIAL

Intrinsic hypothalamic gliomas, large chiasmal gliomas, Rathke's cleft cyst, suprasellar germ cell tumor.

DIAGNOSIS

CT/MRI with and without contrast reveals a partially cystic, enhancing lesion with calcifications.

TREATMENT

Surgical resection, radiation.

NEUROBLASTOMA

A tumor of neural crest cells of the sympathetic ganglia or adrenal medulla. Located in the adrenal medulla, neck, chest, and abdomen (paravertebral ganglia, organ of Zuckerkandl). Metastasis occurs in the bones, bone marrow, liver, and skin. Poor prognostic features include disseminated disease, N-*myc* amplification, 1p deletion, 17q gain, and normal diploidy.

SYMPTOMS/EXAM

Constitutional symptoms (fever, weight loss, irritability), abdominal mass (irregular shape; crosses midline), neck mass, Horner's syndrome, weakness, bowel/bladder dysfunction, bone pain, orbital ecchymosis, bluish subcutaneous nodules, hepatomegaly, intractable watery diarrhea (due to VIP secretion), opsoclonus-myoclonus (a paraneoplastic syndrome → dancing eyes and dancing feet).

DIFFERENTIAL

Wilms' tumor, rhabdomyosarcoma, Ewing's sarcoma, lymphoma.

DIAGNOSIS

Diagnosis is as follows (see also Table 16-3):

- ↑ urinary VMA and HVA.
- Biopsy reveals a small, round blue-cell tumor and may show N-*myc* amplification.
- **Metastatic evaluation:** CXR, CT of the chest/abdomen/pelvis, MRI of the spinal cord, MIBG scintigraphy, bone marrow aspirate and biopsy.

TREATMENT

Treatment depends on staging, age, and biological factors but may include surgery, radiation, chemotherapy (cyclophosphamide, doxorubicin, etoposide, cisplatin, vincristine), and autologous stem cell transplantation.

WILMS' TUMOR

The second most common malignancy arising in the abdomen. Associated with aniridia, GU malformation (cryptorchidism, hypospadias), mental retardation, hemihypertrophy, and Beckwith-Wiedemann syndrome (macroglossia, omphalocele, visceromegaly).

Neuroblastoma may metastasize to the orbits, giving a raccoon-eye appearance, and may be mistaken for physical abuse.

In general, disseminated neuroblastoma has a poor prognosis. Stage 4S, which has a good prognosis in children < 1 year of age, is the exception to this rule.

Observation is sufficient therapy for stage 1 or 4S neuroblastoma.

TABLE 16-3. International Neuroblastoma Staging System

STAGE	CHARACTERISTICS
1	Local tumor; complete removal.
2A	Local tumor; incomplete removal.
2B	Local tumor with $\oplus$ ipsilateral lymph nodes.
3	Unilateral tumor that crosses the midline or tumor with $\oplus$ contralateral lymph nodes **or** midline tumor.
4	Disseminated to distant lymph nodes, bone, bone marrow, liver, or skin.
4S	Local tumor with dissemination to skin, liver, or bone marrow; must be < 1 year of age.

Adapted, with permission, from Rudolph CD et al. *Rudolph's Pediatrics,* 21st ed. New York: McGraw-Hill, 2002:1619.

SYMPTOMS/EXAM

Often presents as an asymptomatic abdominal mass (rarely crosses the midline), or may present with gross or microscopic hematuria, fever, and hypertension.

DIFFERENTIAL

Neuroblastoma, splenomegaly, hydronephrosis.

DIAGNOSIS

Diagnosis is as follows (see also Table 16-4):

- CT of the abdomen with contrast reveals an intrarenal lesion.
- Biopsy to determine cell types.
  - **Favorable histology:** Blastemal, stromal, epithelial.
  - **Unfavorable histology:** Anaplasia, clear cell sarcoma, rhabdoid.
- **Metastatic evaluation:** CXR.

TREATMENT

Surgical removal, radiation (except stages I and II), chemotherapy (stage I and II—vincristine, actinomycin D; stage III and IV—vincristine, actinomycin D, doxorubicin).

OSTEOSARCOMA

The most common malignant bone tumor. Peaks in adolescence; irradiation is a risk factor. Poor prognostic features include a 1° tumor that is in the spine, the pelvis, or a site that is difficult to resect; a large tumor; metastasis; and poor histologic response to chemotherapy

SYMPTOMS/EXAM

Pain and swelling at the tumor site; location at the ends of bone (distal femur, proximal tibia, proximal humerus); no systemic symptoms.

Wilms' tumor presentation—WAGR

Wilms
Aniridia
GU malformation
Retardation

ONCOLOGY

TABLE 16-4. **National Wilms' Tumor Study Group Staging System**

STAGE	CHARACTERISTICS
I	Tumor limited to the kidney; completely removed.
II	Tumor beyond the kidney; completely removed.
III	Residual tumor present in the abdomen. **1:** Lymph nodes involved. **2:** Tumor penetrated through the peritoneum. **3:** Tumor implanted on the peritoneum. **4:** Tumor remained postoperatively.
IV	Hematogenous metastasis (lung, liver, bone, brain) or lymph node metastasis outside the abdomen/pelvis.
V	Bilateral renal involvement at diagnosis.

Adapted, with permission, from Rudolph CD et al. *Rudolph's Pediatrics,* 21st ed. New York: McGraw-Hill, 2002:1615.)

DIAGNOSIS

- Soft tissue mass with radial calcifications ("sunburst" pattern).
- Biopsy reveals sarcoma cells with malignant osteoid.
- **Metastatic evaluation:** CT of the chest; bone scan.

TREATMENT

Surgical resection, chemotherapy.

EWING'S SARCOMA

The second most common malignant bone tumor; peaks at 10–20 years of age. Poor prognostic features include metastasis and older age.

SYMPTOMS/EXAM

Pain and swelling at the tumor site; location at the midshaft of long bones, flat bones of the ribs, and pelvis; ⊕ systemic symptoms (fever, weight loss).

DIFFERENTIAL

Rhabdomyosarcoma, lymphoma, neuroblastoma.

DIAGNOSIS

- Multiple layers of periosteum around the tumor site ("onion-skinning" pattern).
- Biopsy reveals small, round blue cell; ⊕ MIC2 (CD99) and t(11;22) translocation.
- **Metastatic evaluation:** CT of the chest, bone marrow aspirate, bone scan.

TREATMENT

Surgical resection, radiation, chemotherapy.

Diagnosis of osteosarcoma—SENS

Sunburst
Ends of bone
No **S**ystemic symptoms

Diagnosis of Ewing's—MOSS

Midshaft
Onion skinning
Systemic
Symptoms

The most common soft tissue tumor of childhood; accounts for 5–8% of childhood cancers. Peak incidence is at 2–5 years of age; then a second, smaller peak occurs in adolescence (extremity tumors). Genetic predisposition is associated with Li-Fraumeni syndrome (a familial germ line mutation of the *p53* tumor suppressor gene that also predisposes to other soft tissue and bone sarcomas as well as to leukemias, brain tumors, adrenocortical carcinomas, and early-onset breast carcinomas), Beckwith-Wiedemann syndrome, and neurofibromatosis type 1. Tumors are derived from muscle precursor cells (see Table 16-5). Classified according to pathology:

Botryoid rhabdomyosarcoma appears as a "cluster of grapes," often in the bladder or vagina.

- **Embryonal (63%):**
  - Botryoid is a variant subtype that usually occurs in hollow organs.
  - More likely in younger patients with head, neck, or GU tumors.
- **Alveolar (19%):**
  - An aggressive subtype that is often seen with metastatic disease at diagnosis.
  - More likely in adolescents with extremity tumors.
- **Pleomorphic (1%):** Usually seen in adults.
- **Undifferentiated sarcoma (10%).**
- **Other (7%).**

SYMPTOMS/EXAM

- Symptoms result from the mass effect of tumor growth onto adjacent organs or tissues and can occur anywhere in the body.
  - Orbital rhabdomyosarcoma → proptosis.
  - Bladder rhabdomyosarcoma → urinary obstruction, constipation, hematuria.
- Chronic drainage (nasal, aural, sinus, vaginal) is also seen.

TABLE 16-5. Characteristics of Rhabdomyosarcoma

1° SITE	FREQUENCY (%)	SYMPTOMS AND SIGNS	PREDOMINANT PATHOLOGIC SUBTYPE
Head and neck	**35**		Embryonal.
Orbit	9	Proptosis.	
Parameningeal	16	Cranial nerve palsies; aural or sinus obstruction +/– drainage.	
Other	10	Painless, progressively enlarging mass.	
Genitourinary	**22**		Embryonal (botryoid variant in bladder and vagina).
Bladder and prostate	13	Hematuria, urinary obstruction.	
Vagina and uterus	2	Pelvic mass, vaginal discharge.	
Paratesticular	7	Painless mass.	
Extremities	**18**	Affects adolescents; swelling of affected body part.	Alveolar (50%), undifferentiated.
Other	**25**	Mass.	Alveolar, undifferentiated.

Reproduced, with permission, from Hay WW et al. *Current Pediatric Diagnosis & Treatment,* 17th ed. New York: McGraw-Hill, 2005:935.

DIAGNOSIS

- Open biopsy; CT/MRI to determine the extent of 1° tumor and regional lymph node involvement.
- Skeletal survey or bone scan to evaluate for bony metastasis.
- Bilateral bone marrow aspirates/biopsies to evaluate for marrow metastasis.
- Parameningeal rhabdomyosarcoma also requires LP to evaluate for tumor cells in the CSF.

TREATMENT

A combination of surgery, chemotherapy, and radiation therapy.

With rhabdomyosarcoma, a chest CT is mandatory to rule out pulmonary metastasis, the most common site of metastatic disease at diagnosis.

RETINOBLASTOMA

The most common intraocular malignancy; derived from embryonal retinal cells. Bilateral disease presents earlier (average age 14 months) than unilateral disease (average age 23 months). Ten percent of cases are autosomal dominant (*RB1* tumor suppressor gene mutation); 90% are sporadic.

SYMPTOMS/EXAM

Leukocoria (white papillary reflex), strabismus, painful red eye, proptosis.

DIFFERENTIAL

Toxocara canis granuloma, astrocytic hamartoma, retinopathy of prematurity, persistent hyperplastic 1° vitreous.

DIAGNOSIS

- A white mass is seen protruding into the vitreous.
- CT of the orbits shows intraocular calcification and local extension.
- **Metastatic evaluation:** Bone marrow biopsy, aspirate, CSF cytology, bone scan, CT of the liver.

TREATMENT

- Radiotherapy; local control (cryotherapy, photocoagulation, radioactive plaques); enucleation.
- Chemotherapy for metastatic disease; also used up front in high-risk patients in an attempt to spare vision.

COMPLICATIONS

Intracranial spread; risk of second malignancy (in heritable retinoblastoma), especially osteosarcoma.

GERM CELL TUMORS

Account for 3% of pediatric neoplasms. Anatomic locations are gonadal (ovarian/testicular) and extragonadal (intracranial, sacrococcygeal, thoracic [usually the anterior mediastinum]). In general, girls have a higher overall incidence, but boys are at ↑ risk of malignant tumors. Classified as follows:

- **Teratoma:** Mature, immature, malignant.
- **Germinoma:** Seminoma (also known as testicular germinoma), dysgerminoma (also known as ovarian germinoma).

Therapy for benign sacrococcygeal teratomas consists of early and complete excision of tumor, including the coccyx. Risk of recurrence is high if the coccyx is not removed. Therapy for malignant tumors includes excision and chemotherapy.

Patients with cryptorchidism have a 30-fold ↑ chance of developing testicular cancer, usually seminomas or embryonal carcinomas in adulthood.

The use of α-fetoprotein (AFP) in infants with possible germ cell tumors is limited because AFP levels are elevated in the first six months of life. In addition, the half-life of AFP is 8–10 days, so levels may remain ↑ several days after treatment.

- Embryonal carcinoma.
- Endodermal sinus tumor (also called yolk sac tumor).
- Choriocarcinoma.
- Gonadoblastoma.
- Polyembryonal.

Risk factors are as follows:

- **Infants/young children:**
  - Teratomas predominate in infancy.
  - Germ cell tumors are more likely to be extragonadal.
  - In the first years of life, the overall incidence of germ cell tumors ↓ with the exception of endodermal sinus tumors, which have a relatively higher incidence in toddlers.
- **Adolescents/young adults:**
  - The incidence of gonadal tumors, mainly seminomas and dysgerminomas, ↑ with the onset of puberty.
  - In young men, germ cell tumors represent the most common malignant tumor.
- **Sacrococcygeal teratomas:** The most common pediatric germ cell tumor; have a male-to-female ratio of 3:1. Often present at birth.

SYMPTOMS/EXAM

- **Ovarian tumors:**
  - Acute or chronic abdominal pain (80% of patients), a palpable abdominal mass, and abdominal distention.
  - Less commonly presents with precocious puberty, constipation, enuresis, vaginal bleeding, amenorrhea, and ovarian torsion.
- **Testicular tumors:** Painless scrotal masses that may be accompanied by hydroceles or inguinal hernias.
- **Anterior mediastinal tumors:** In adolescents, usually asymptomatic; in infants, present with cough, dyspnea, and hemoptysis.
- **Intracranial tumors:** Visual disturbances, nystagmus, anorexia, precocious puberty, hypopituitarism, Parinaud's syndrome, signs of ↑ ICP.

DIAGNOSIS

Table 16-6 outlines the characteristics of common germ cell tumors.

TREATMENT

Chemotherapy for malignant germ cell tumors; radiation therapy for intracranial germ cell tumors.

HEPATIC TUMORS

Hepatoblastoma

The most common malignant liver tumor in infants < 3 years of age. Involves immature liver tissue. Associated with hemihypertrophy, Beckwith-Wiedemann syndrome, and familial adenomatous polyposis.

SYMPTOMS/EXAM

Painless abdominal mass; osteopenia.

	HISTOLOGIC GRADING	AFP	β-hCG
Germinoma/seminoma/ dysgerminoma	Malignant		↑
Embryonal carcinoma	Malignant		
Endodermal sinus tumor	Malignant	↑↑↑	
Choriocarcinoma	Malignant		↑↑↑
Teratoma, mature	Benign		
Teratoma, immature	Potentially malignant	↑	

Choriocarcinoma is often misdiagnosed as an ectopic pregnancy because this germ cell tumor presents with an abdominal mass with high β-hCG levels.

DIAGNOSIS

- ↑ AFP, ↑ bilirubin.
- Liver biopsy reveals fetal/embryonal cells and mesenchyme.
- **Metastatic evaluation:** CT of the chest.

TREATMENT

Surgical resection; chemotherapy (cisplatin, 5-FU, doxorubicin); liver transplant can be considered if disease is confined to the liver but unresectable

Hepatocellular Carcinoma

The most common malignant liver tumor in older children and adolescents. Associated with HBV, cirrhosis, and α_1-antitrypsin deficiency.

SYMPTOMS/EXAM

Painful abdominal mass; **anorexia, weight loss, vomiting.**

DIAGNOSIS

- ↑ AFP, ↑ bilirubin, abnormal LFTs.
- Liver biopsy shows pleomorphic tumor cells and giant cells.

TREATMENT

Surgical resection is the only curative option. Responds poorly to chemotherapy.

LANGERHANS CELL HISTIOCYTOSIS (LCH)

A rare spectrum of disorders that are not malignancies but rather a reactive proliferation of histiocytic cells that may be due to an immunoregulatory defect. The male-to-female ratio is 2:1, and the peak age of onset is one year. There is an inverse relationship between age and degree of involvement.

ONCOLOGY

Birbeck granules on electron microscopy plus ⊕ CD1a expression = LCH.

LCH lesions of the skin may mimic seborrheic dermatitis or eczema of the scalp or perineal areas.

LCH lesions of the ear may present with chronic draining and may be mistaken for chronic otitis externa.

Age and degree of organ involvement are the most important prognostic factors in LCH.

SYMPTOMS/EXAM

Clinical syndromes are as follows:

- **Solitary lesion:**
    - Formerly called eosinophilic granuloma; the most benign form of LCH.
    - Usually presents as one or more well-circumscribed lesions of the skull accompanied by pain and swelling.
    - Any bone may be involved, but other common sites are the femur, pelvis, vertebrae, and mandible.
    - Children tend to be older, with 50% > 5 years of age at diagnosis (range 1–9 years).
- **Multiple lesions:**
    - More prevalent in children < 5 years of age.
    - The prognosis depends on age of presentation (younger children have a worse prognosis) and on the degree of organ involvement.
    - Organ systems involved include bone, skin, liver, lung, ears, gums, lymph nodes, spleen, pituitary, bone marrow, and CNS.
    - The triad of DI, exophthalmos, and skull lesions due to LCH was formerly called Hand-Schüller-Christian disease, which usually occurs between two and five years of age.
    - Disseminated LCH, formerly called Letterer-Siwe disease, typically involves fever, weight loss, skin rash, lymphadenopathy, hepatosplenomegaly, and hematologic abnormalities. It usually occurs in children < 2 years of age.

DIAGNOSIS

Distinctive features of Langerhans histiocytes are as follows:

- On light microscopy, nuclei are deeply indented (coffee bean shaped) and elongated, with abundant, pale cytoplasm.
- Birbeck granules are seen on electron microscopy.
- ⊕ CD1a expression on the cell surface.
- ⊕ immunostaining for S-100 protein.

TREATMENT

- Isolated lesions may resolve spontaneously and require no therapy at all; if necessary, intralesional cortical steroids, curettage, or low-dose radiation may be used.
- Multifocal disease is less predictable and is often treated with single or multiagent chemotherapy,
- Localized disease has a favorable prognosis.
- Infants with disseminated disease have a 50% mortality.

CHEMOTHERAPY BASICS AND SIDE EFFECTS

 A patient diagnosed with Hodgkin's disease is scheduled for a pretreatment echocardiogram. Why is this the case? Echocardiography allows for the evaluation of cardiotoxicity due to anthracyclines (daunorubicin, doxorubicin).

Strategy

BLeomycin BLows → pulmonary toxicity.

- The goal is to exploit differences between cancer cells and normal host cells.
- **Combination chemotherapy:** Prevents resistance to individual drugs; generates synergistic activity; combines drugs with different toxicity profiles.
- **Adjuvant chemotherapy:** Prevents recurrences. Administered to patients after the tumor has been removed or treated with radiation and there is no evidence of residual disease.
- **Neoadjuvant chemotherapy:** Chemotherapy that is given prior to surgical tumor removal to shrink the cancer so that the surgical procedure may not need to be as extensive.

Mechanism of Action

Disrupts the synthesis or function of DNA, RNA, or nucleotide precursors.

Toxicity

Results from unintended cell death of actively dividing normal host cells. Common toxicities include myelosuppression, nausea, vomiting, alopecia, mucositis, liver function abnormalities, and allergic reactions (see Table 16-7).

TABLE 16-7. Side Effects of Chemotherapeutic Agents

DRUGS	SPECIFIC TOXICITIES
Alkylating agents	
Cyclophosphamide	Hemorrhagic cystitis.
Ifosfamide	Hemorrhagic cystitis, neurotoxicity, Fanconi's syndrome.
Busulfan	Seizures, pulmonary toxicity, hepatic veno-occlusive disease.
Cisplatin	Nephrotoxicity, ototoxicity.
Carboplatin	Severe marrow suppression.
Antimetabolites	
Methotrexate	Hepatotoxicity, nephrotoxicity, neurotoxicity (arachnoiditis, leukomalacia), severe mucositis, rash.
Cytarabine	Fever, flulike illness, hemorrhagic conjunctivitis.
Antibiotics	
Daunorubicin, doxorubicin	Cardiotoxicity (acute and chronic).
Bleomycin	Pulmonary toxicity (chronic).
Plant products	
Vincristine	Peripheral neuropathy (foot/wrist drop, ↓ DTRs, ileus), neuritic pain → jaw pain, SIADH.
Vinblastine	Severe marrow suppression.
Etoposide	Hypotension, allergic reactions, 2° leukemia.
Others	
L-asparaginase	Coagulopathy, thrombosis, allergic reactions, pancreatitis.
Prednisone, dexamethasone	Obesity, diabetes, myopathy, avascular necrosis, behavioral changes, bone demineralization.

ONCOLOGY

493

Hemorrhagic cystitis due to cyclophosphamide and ifosfamide is prevented with MESNA.

Methotrexate toxicity is prevented with leucovorin rescue.

ONCOLOGY

> A 12-year-old girl is diagnosed with ALL. Twenty-four hours after starting chemotherapy, she has minimal urine output and describes cramping pain. Her ECG shows widened QRS complexes. What is the treatment plan for tumor lysis syndrome? Aggressive hydration with alkalinization, allopurinol, and correction of electrolyte abnormalities.

Tumor Lysis Syndrome

Metabolic abnormalities resulting from tumor cell death and release of cellular products. Presents as a triad of hyperuricemia, hyperphosphatemia, and hyperkalemia. Occurs at presentation or 12–72 hours after initiation of cytotoxic treatment (when tumor cell death occurs). Risk factors include fast-growing and/or large, disseminated tumors (most common are Burkitt's lymphoma and T-cell ALL).

SYMPTOMS/EXAM

Abdominal and back pain, vomiting, diarrhea, cramps, spasm, seizures, altered mental status, ↓ urine output.

DIAGNOSIS

- ↑ uric acid, ↑ phosphate, ↑ potassium, ↑ BUN, ↑ creatinine, ↓ calcium.
- ECG shows wide QRS and peaked T (↑ potassium) or prolonged QTc (↓ calcium).

Tumor lysis treatment—BAD Electrolytes

Block uric acid production
Alkalinization
Diuresis
Electrolyte correction

TREATMENT

- Hydration and diuresis, alkalinization, and allopurinol.
- Rasburicase degrades existing uric acid into an excretable form.
- **Correct metabolic abnormalities:**
  - ↑ **potassium:** Kayexalate, calcium gluconate, glucose with insulin.
  - ↑ **phosphate:** Aluminum hydroxide.
  - ↓ **calcium:** Calcium gluconate (but only if symptomatic; may → $CaPO_4$ precipitation).
- **Indications for dialysis:** Renal failure → anuria and volume overload; metabolic abnormalities that are not responsive to therapy.

PREVENTION

- **Hydration and diuresis:** IV fluids with bicarbonate but without potassium; maintain high urine output and low specific gravity; match input and output. Avoid furosemide (↑ stone formation).
- **Alkalinization:** Adjust bicarbonate to maintain a urine pH of 7.0–7.5 to prevent uric acid stones (occurs at pH < 7.0) and calcium phosphate stones (occurs at pH > 8).
- **Block uric acid production:** Give allopurinol (inhibits xanthine oxidase) to prevent uric acid production.

Spinal Cord Compression

Occurs in sarcoma, neuroblastoma, leukemia, lymphoma, and CNS metastasis.

SYMPTOMS/EXAM

Back pain with spinal tenderness; weakness (proximal more than distal); hyperreflexia; sensory changes; change in bowel/bladder function (loss of anal wink).

DIAGNOSIS

Spinal MRI with and without gadolinium demonstrates mass.

TREATMENT

Biopsy, dexamethasone, radiation (if known diagnosis and radiosensitive).

Superior Vena Cava Syndrome

Compression, obstruction, and thrombosis of the SVC. Occurs with mediastinal masses (leukemia, lymphoma, germ cell tumors).

SYMPTOMS/EXAM

Dyspnea, cough, dysphagia, orthopnea, hoarseness, facial swelling, plethora, cyanosis, engorged chest wall, wheezing, stridor.

DIAGNOSIS

- Mediastinal widening; anterior mediastinal mass.
- CT of the chest enables visualization of vessels and measurement of the tracheal diameter.
- Biopsy if the tumor is new.

TREATMENT

- **Tumor:** Radiation, empiric chemotherapy.
- **Clot:** Anticoagulate; consider thrombolysis.

Shortness of breath when lying down is a dangerous sign. Do not use sedation if tracheal compression is present.

BONE MARROW (HEMATOPOIETIC STEM CELL) TRANSPLANTATION

Patient and Donor Selection

- **Autologous:**
  - The patient's own stem cells are used and are collected.
  - Extremely high doses of chemotherapy are given to eradicate malignant disease, and the marrow is then rescued by stem cell infusion.
  - Used mostly for solid tumors and for leukemia if no match is found → purged marrow.
- **Allogeneic:** Stem cells are obtained from another person. Subtypes are as follows:
  - **Related HLA matched:** Identical for all six HLA alleles; associated with a one in four chance of a sibling match.
  - **Related HLA partially matched (haploidentical):** Identical for three alleles; applies to almost all parents; associated with a one in two chance of a sibling match. Donor cells/marrow must be T-cell depleted, which

will ↓ graft-versus-host disease (GVHD) risk but will delay recovery of the immune system and ↓ the chance of engraftment.

- **Unrelated HLA matched:** Associated with a one in one million chance of a match.

Indications

Indications for hematopoietic stem cell transplants are outlined in Table 16-8.

Sources of Stem Cells

- **Bone marrow:** Requires bone marrow harvest.
- **Peripheral blood:** Yields more stem cells and rapid engraftment, but takes several days of G-CSF; needs central venous access in smaller donor children, and ↑ the risk of chronic GVHD.
- **Umbilical cord blood:** An exact HLA match is unnecessary but involves a smaller number of cells, takes a longer time for engraftment and immune system recovery, and cannot be repeated.

Clinical Course of Transplantation

- **Preparative regimen (days −7 to −10):** Intensive chemotherapy/radiation therapy, fluid-electrolyte disturbances, drug toxicity.
- **Stem cell infusion (day 0):** Transfusion reaction, hypertension, bradycardia, respiratory compromise.

Peripheral blood stem collection is becoming increasingly common, as it is much less painful for the donor than a bone marrow harvest.

ONCOLOGY

TABLE 16-8. Indications for Hematopoietic Stem Cell Transplantation

GOAL OF PROCEDURE	PREPARATIVE REGIMEN	GOAL OF STEM CELL SOURCE	TYPE OF TRANSPLANT	LIMITATION	DISEASE
Eradication of refractory tumor	High intensity.	Rapid hematopoietic reconstitution.	Autologous.	Preparative-regimen acute toxicity; resistance to chemotherapy.	Neuroblastoma, Ewing's sarcoma, Wilms tumor, acute leukemia.
Management of malignant hematopoietic disease	Tumor cytoreduction; preparation for engraftment.	Hematopoietic reconstitution; graft-versus-tumor effect.	Allogeneic.	Preparative-regimen acute toxicity, GVHD, resistance to chemotherapy.	Acute leukemia, CML, high-grade lymphoma, myelodysplasia.
Replacement of a defective hematopoietically derived cell	Preparation for engraftment.	Establishment of normal function before irreversible toxicity develops.	Allogeneic.	Preparative-regimen acute toxicity, GVHD, rejection.	Aplastic anemia, Hurler disease, immunodeficiency, osteopetrosis, sickle cell anemia, thalassemia.

Reproduced, with permission, from Rudolph CD et al. *Rudolph's Pediatrics,* 21st ed. New York: McGraw-Hill, 2002:1590.)

496

- **Acute toxicity (day +1 to engraftment [days +10 to +30]):** Neutropenia (infections), thrombocytopenia (bleeding), mucositis, pulmonary edema, veno-occlusive disease, acral erythroderma.
- **Postengraftment (engraftment to day +100):** Acute GVHD (allogenic), infection from chronic immunosuppression.
- **Late transplant period (> day +100):** Chronic GVHD, recurrent infections.

Acute Complications

INFECTIONS

Table 16-9 outlines common infections encountered in stem cell transplant patients.

VENO-OCCLUSIVE DISEASE

Narrowing of terminal hepatic veins 2° to fibrin deposits and clot formation → hepatocyte damage. Due to high-dose chemotherapy and radiation. Onset is between day +20 and day +30. Risk factors include allogeneic transplant, high AST pretransplant, older age, high-dose total-body irradiation, and preparative agents (busulfan, cyclophosphamide, melphalan, etoposide).

SYMPTOMS/EXAM

Hepatomegaly, RUQ pain, jaundice, fluid retention (ascites, pulmonary edema), multisystem organ failure.

DIFFERENTIAL

Acute GVHD, sepsis.

DIAGNOSIS

Doppler ultrasound reveals hepatomegaly, ascites, and reversal of portal blood flow.

TABLE 16-9. Course of Infections in Stem Cell Transplant Patients

PHASE	UNDERLYING IMMUNODEFICIENCY	TYPE OF INFECTION
Preengraftment	Neutropenia.	Bacterial and fungal: Gram-⊖ rods, *Staphylococcus epidermidis*, streptococci, *Candida, Aspergillus.*
Postengraftment	Impaired cellular immunity.	Infections from chronic immunosuppression: EBV, CMV, adenovirus.
Late transplant period	Impaired cellular and humoral immunity.	Recurrent infections and encapsulated bacteria (pneumococcus).

TREATMENT

Supportive (balance fluid status; albumin or RBC infusion).

ACUTE GRAFT-VERSUS-HOST DISEASE

Occurs in the first 100 days; less severe in younger patients. Mediated by type 1 helper T cells → inflammation.

The classic triad of acute GVHD is hepatitis, enteritis, and rash.

SYMPTOMS/EXAM

Skin changes (pruritic maculopapular rash, desquamation, bullae), conjunctivitis, jaundice, anorexia, abdominal pain, mucoid diarrhea.

DIAGNOSIS

Biopsy, endoscopy.

TREATMENT

Steroids, antithymocyte globulin, tacrolimus, azathioprine.

PREVENTION

Prevent with methotrexate, cyclosporine, prednisone, tacrolimus, and T-cell depletion.

CHRONIC GRAFT-VERSUS-HOST DISEASE

Occurs from day 100 to two years post-transplant. Mediated by type 2 helper T cells → fibrosis.

SYMPTOMS/EXAM

Skin changes (lichen planus, atrophy, scleroderma with contractures, alopecia), conjunctivitis, photophobia, chronic lung disease, jaundice, oral dryness, malabsorption.

DIAGNOSIS

Biopsy.

TREATMENT

Steroids, antithymocyte globulin, anti-TNF, anti-IL-2 antibody, cyclosporine, mycophenolate.

COMPLICATIONS

Chronic complications include immunologic dysfunction (reconstitution takes 9–12 months; revaccinate one year post-transplant) as well as chronic lung disease, abnormal growth (hypothyroidism, growth hormone deficiency, gonadal dysfunction), 2° malignancy (↑ risk with etoposide and topotecan), and recurrence of 1° disease.

PREVENTION

Cyclosporine, methotrexate; avoid acute GVHD.

CHAPTER 17

Preventive Pediatrics, Ethics, and Epidemiology

Curtis Chan, MD, MPH
reviewed by Alan Uba, MD

Recommended Preventive Health Care Visits

Table 17-1 outlines recommendations for the scheduling of preventive health care visits in the pediatric population. Notable caveats are as follows:

- **Prenatal visit:** Recommended for the following groups:
  - Expecting parents who are experiencing high medical risks during pregnancy.
  - Those who are living under high-risk social circumstances.
  - First-time parents.
  - Any parents who request a prenatal visit.
- **Early-discharge visit:** Newborn infants who are discharged < 48 hours after delivery should be reexamined at 2–4 days of age.
- **Other recommendations:**
  - Measure head circumference at each preventive visit until 24 months of age.
  - Measure BP at every well-child visit beginning at three years of age.
  - Offer a pelvic examination to all sexually active females and as preventive health maintenance for all women 18–21 years of age.

Screening for Common Childhood Diseases

IRON DEFICIENCY ANEMIA SCREENING

Iron deficiency is the most common nutritional deficiency in the United States. Iron deficiency in children is associated with developmental delay, fatigue, and behavioral issues.

RISK FACTORS

Risk factors for iron deficiency are as follows:

- **Infancy:**
  - **Low iron stores at birth** (e.g., low-birth-weight or preterm birth; excessive blood loss during birth).
  - **Inadequate iron intake:** Low dietary intake of iron resulting from the following:
    - Use of a non-iron-fortified (low-iron) formula (rare in U.S. markets).

TABLE 17-1. Recommended Preventive Health Care Visits

AGE	RECOMMENDED VISITS
Infancy	Newborn; 2–4 days of age; 1, 2, 4, 6, 9, and 12 months of age.
Early childhood	15, 18, and 24 months of age; 3 and 4 years of age.
Middle childhood	5, 6, 8, and 10 years of age.
Adolescence	Annually from 11 to 21 years of age.

- Exclusive breast-feeding after six months of age without adding iron to the diet (e.g., iron-fortified cereal).
- Introduction of cow's milk before one year of age.
- Overconsumption of cow's milk.
  - **Blood loss** (e.g., GI blood loss).
- **Middle childhood/adolescence:** Inadequate iron intake (low dietary intake; dieting, meal skipping, eating disorders); heavy or lengthy menstrual periods; intensive physical training.

SCREENING RECOMMENDATIONS

Iron deficiency screening guidelines include two strategies: universal screening of high-risk populations and selective screening of individual children with known risk factors.

- **Whom to screen:** High-risk populations include infants and children in families with low income; those who are eligible for the Women, Infants, and Children (WIC) nutritional program; and those who are migrants or recent refugees.
- **When to screen:** At 9–12 months of age, at 15–18 months of age (six months later), and annually in children 2–5 years of age.
- **Selective screening** for iron deficiency is recommended for infants and children with **known risk factors** (see Table 17-2).
- **Additional American Academy of Pediatrics (AAP)** recommendations are as follows:
  - Screen **all** infants at 9–12 months of age, not just those at high risk or with known risk factors.
  - Screen adolescent males during their peak growth period in the course of routine physical examinations.
  - Screen adolescent females during all routine physical examinations.

TABLE 17-2. Guidelines for Iron Deficiency Screening

AGE OF SCREENING	RISK FACTOR INDICATIONS
Before six months of age	Prematurity; unfortified formula.
At 9–12 months of age (repeat at 15–18 months of age)	Above-mentioned risk factors; cow's milk before 12 months of age; insufficient dietary iron after six months of age. Consumption of > 24 ounces of milk per day after 12 months of age. Special medical conditions: - Medicines that interfere with iron absorption (calcium, phosphorus, magnesium, antacids) - Chronic infection or inflammation - Extensive blood loss
Annual screening for children 2–5 years of age	Low dietary iron, limited access to food, special medical conditions.
Adolescent females	**Every 5–10 years:** Normal health care maintenance. **Annually:** Extensive menstrual blood loss, eating disorders, meal skipping.

PREVENTION

- Breast-fed infants should receive dietary iron supplementation after six months of age.
- Iron-fortified cereal should be introduced after six months of age.
- Non-breast-fed infants should receive a formula with iron supplementation throughout the first year of life.

> A pediatrician practicing in a community with widespread exposure to lead and many older homes obtains a CBC and serum lead testing for all patients at the 12-month-old visit. One patient's lab results show a normal CBC but a blood lead level (BLL) of 24 μg/dL. What is the appropriate management for this patient, and does the patient need emergent hospitalization? A patient with a BLL of approximately 20–44 μg/dL is very likely to have chronic lead toxicity. At this level, however, the patient is not in imminent danger. The pediatrician should evaluate the patient's environment, assess nutrition, perform a physical examination, and refer to the local health department or case management. The health department will likely visit the patient's environment (e.g., school, playground) to perform an environmental evaluation and investigation. The pediatrician should order a confirmatory BLL test within one week and consult a clinician with expertise in lead toxicity. Lead chelation (EDTA, dimercaprol, penicillamine, or succimer) is typically performed for patients with BLLs > 45 μg/dL, and hospitalization is indicated for those with BLLs > 70 μg/dL.

LEAD SCREENING

The adverse effects of elevated lead levels on cognitive development have been well demonstrated. As a result, the CDC has continued to lower the threshold for diagnosing lead poisoning. The CDC currently defines an elevated lead level as > 10 μg/dL, although recent research suggests that each microgram increase in serum lead levels from 1 μg/dL to 10 μg/dL is associated with impaired cognitive development.

RISK FACTORS

Children in poor socioeconomic conditions are disproportionately affected. Additional risk factors for lead toxicity include the following:

- Living in a home with peeling or chipping paint.
- Living in a home built before 1960.
- Having household members or playmates with elevated lead levels.
- Industrial/environmental contamination.
- Parental occupational exposure.

SCREENING RECOMMENDATIONS

- Pediatricians should be aware of the risk factors for lead exposure and should understand the potential effects of lead toxicity on infant and early childhood development.
- **Whom to screen:** Local and state jurisdictions may have different recommendations for the indications and timing of serum lead level tests. However, recommendations typically follow one of two strategies:

- **Universal screening:** Screening for all children living in communities in which the risk of lead exposure is widespread.
- **Targeted screening:** Screening for children living in communities in which the risk of lead exposure is NOT widespread. Pediatricians should determine if a child is at ↑ risk of lead exposure by screening for the following risk factors:
    - Living in a specific geographic area in which > 27% of the housing was built before 1950.
    - Living in or regularly visiting a building constructed before 1950.
    - Living in or regularly visiting a building that was constructed before 1978 and has recently been renovated.
    - Living in or regularly visiting a building with peeling or chipping paint, including day care centers, preschools, or homes of babysitters.
    - Having a sibling, housemate, or playmate with ↑ serum lead levels (> 15 μg/dL).
    - Living with an adult who may be exposed to occupational lead.
    - Enrollment in public assistance programs such as WIC and Medicaid.
- **When to screen:** Appropriate times to perform serum lead level screening using the universal or targeted screening strategies include 12 months of age, 24 months of age, and 36–72 months of age if the child did not receive appropriate screening previously.

TREATMENT

Table 17-3 outlines guidelines for the treatment and disposition of lead exposure. Potential chelating agents include EDTA, penicillamine, dimercaprol, and succimer.

TABLE 17-3. Assessment and Treatment of Lead Exposure

BLL (μg/dL)	FURTHER TESTS	ACTIONS
< 5	None.	None.
5–9	None.	Environmental history; provide education.
10–19	Confirmatory BLL within one month; repeat in 2–3 months.	Environmental history; provide education.
20–44	**Confirmatory BLL within one week.**	Environmental evaluation and investigation, nutritional assessment, physical examination. Environmental history; provide education. **Referral to local health department or case management.** Consultation with a clinician with expertise in lead toxicity
45–69	Confirm BLL within two days.	Actions above; **chelation therapy.**
> 70	Confirm BLL immediately.	Actions above; chelation therapy; **hospitalization.**

Adapted, with permission, from AAP Committee on Environmental Health. Screening for elevated blood levels. *Pediatrics* 101:175, 1998.

A five-year-old Asian immigrant who had received BCG receives a PPD as part of routine screening for four- to six-year-old children entering this particular school district. Two days later, the redness has a diameter of 10 mm, and the diameter of the elevated skin is 16 mm. What is the appropriate management for this patient? An induration > 15 mm in patients > 4 years of age is considered a ⊕ TST regardless of the BCG history. A thorough history should include investigation of TB exposure, symptoms, and risk of progression to disease. A CXR should be ordered promptly. If the CXR is ⊖, the patient should take INH for nine months. The physician should report LTBIs and tuberculosis disease cases to the health department.

TUBERCULOSIS SCREENING

A latent TB infection (LTBI) is defined as a *Mycobacterium tuberculosis* infection in a person who meets all the following criteria:

- A ⊕ tuberculin skin test (TST).
- No symptoms.
- No physical evidence of disease.
- A normal CXR or evidence of healed infection (granulomas, calcification in the lung, hilar lymph nodes).

SCREENING RECOMMENDATIONS

Screening guidelines formulated by the AAP are as follows:

- **Whom to screen:** Children who are at ↑ risk of acquiring LTBI or at risk for progression to tuberculosis disease, further defined as follows:
  - **↑ risk of contracting LTBI:**
    - Contacts with people with confirmed or suspected contagious TB.
    - Children emigrating from countries with endemic TB (e.g., Asia, the Middle East, Africa, Latin America).
    - Children with a history of travel to endemic countries and/or significant contact with indigenous people from such countries.
    - Children with incidental radiographic or clinical findings suggesting possible TB.
    - Other risk groups may include children with exposure to nursing home residents or to people with HIV, the homeless, or the incarcerated.
  - **↑ risk of progression to tuberculosis disease:** Children with specific medical conditions such as type 1 DM, chronic renal failure, immunodeficiencies (including HIV), and malnutrition.
- **When to screen:**
  - **Annual TST:** Give to children infected with HIV and to incarcerated adolescents (see Table 17-4).
  - **Periodic screening for children with other risk factors** (schedule varies):
    - At 12 months of age.
    - At 4–6 years of age, before entry into kindergarten.
    - At 11–16 years of age.
  - Local health departments and school districts with a high prevalence of TB may have stricter guidelines.
- **TST caveats** include the following:

- Tuberculin reactivity appears 2–12 weeks after initial exposure. Thus, a false $\ominus$ may result if the TST is done within 12 weeks.
- The TST is approximately 90% sensitive. Thus, roughly 10% of immunocompetent children infected with TB do not initially react to a TST.
- Immunization with BCG vaccine may → a $\oplus$ TST, particularly if vaccinated recently. BCG is recommended by the World Health Organization and is used in many countries.
- In general, the interpretation of TST results in BCG recipients is the same as that for those who were not immunized.
    - All children with a $\oplus$ TST should receive a CXR regardless of BCG status.
    - Generally, BCG recipients with a $\oplus$ TST and a $\ominus$ CXR should receive nine months of INH therapy to prevent progression.
    - Some exceptions may be considered—e.g., those with recent or multiple BCG immunizations or those who have emigrated from a country with low TB prevalence.

TREATMENT

- $\oplus$ **TST:** Prompt CXR; thorough history and physical exam
    - **LTBI:** INH × 9 months is highly effective (approaching 100%) in preventing the progression of tuberculosis disease.
    - **Tuberculosis disease:** In general, a six-month regimen of 3–4 drugs is required (see the Infectious Disease chapter for details).

HEARING SCREENING AND EXAMS

Hearing loss can be congenital or acquired. Congenital causes include various genetic syndromes, TORCHeS infections, hereditary factors, severe prematurity, and anoxia. Acquired causes include infections (e.g., meningitis, otitis media), trauma, high noise levels, and ototoxic drugs.

SCREENING RECOMMENDATIONS

- Early identification and intervention, particularly within the first six months, have been shown to prevent language and learning delay.
- A newborn hearing screen is mandatory in most states. However, some cases of congenital and acquired hearing loss will not be identifiable by

TABLE 17-4. Definition of a $\oplus$ TST

INDURATION	CONSIDERED $\oplus$ TST IF THE PATIENT:
≥ 5 mm	- Is suspected of having TB. - Has close contacts with contagious cases. - Is immunosuppressed.
≥ 10 mm	- Is at ↑ risk of disseminated disease and is < 4 years of age or has a medical condition that may cause immunodeficiency. - Has ↑ exposure to TB.
≥ 15 mm	- Is ≥ 4 years of age without any risk factors.

this means. Therefore, children with suspected hearing loss should be re-screened with age-appropriate techniques.

- Hearing and language development should be assessed and documented at every well-child visit for both infants and toddlers.
- **Auditory pathway screening tests** include the following:
  - **Auditory brain-stem evoked response (ABER):** EEG response to an auditory stimulus. Motion artifact interferes with the results. Used in infants and sleeping young children. The most commonly used newborn screening test.
  - **Otoacoustic emission (OAE):** Measures the cochlea's outer hair cell response to an auditory stimulus. An effective screening measure for middle and inner ear abnormalities, but does not detect neuronal/brain abnormalities. Used for all age groups.
  - **Behavioral pure-tone audiometry:** True tests of hearing remain standard for hearing evaluation. Requires cooperation.
  - **Conditioned orientation reflex or visual reinforced audiometry:** Children 9 months to 2.5 years of age are conditioned to associate a sound with a visual stimulus (e.g., a lighted dancing doll). After the child hears the sound, he or she will look for the visual stimulus.
  - **Conditioned play audiometry:** Children approximately 2–4 years of age learn to wait and listen for a sound and then perform a simple motor task.
  - **Conventional audiometry:** Children ≥ 4 years of age should receive audiometric screening at well-child visits through adolescence.

VISION SCREENING

Table 17-5 lists important visual milestones in pediatric patients. The following are commonly administered screening tests:

- **Red reflex examination:** Should be documented in all infants during the first two months of life.
- **Periodic funduscopic exam:** May detect cataracts, glaucoma, retinal abnormalities, retinoblastoma, and systemic disease with ocular manifestations.

Amblyopia and strabismus are frequently confused by both pediatricians and parents.

- *Amblyopia is a reduction in vision in an eye that is uncorrectable by glasses.*
- *Strabismus is an ocular misalignment or deviating eye. Persistent strabismus is a cause of amblyopia.*

TABLE 17-5. Visual Milestones in the Pediatric Population

AGE GROUP	MILESTONE
Newborn	Optimal focal length 1 foot. See light and shapes; detect movement.
Three months	Focus on faces and track objects.
Four months	Eyes should be symmetrically aligned with no deviation.
Six months	Visually identify and distinguish between objects.
Two years	Vision improves rapidly between one and two years of age to ~ 20/60.
Seven to nine years	Should develop normal adult visual acuity (20/20).

- **Formal visual acuity testing:** Should begin at three years of age.
- **Unilateral cover-uncover test:** Should be performed to detect strabismus and amblyopia at all preventive visits beginning in the toddler years.

A nurse takes the BP of a three-year-old girl and finds it to be 118/78. The nurse changes from the infant blood pressure cuff to a larger one that will better fit the toddler. The nurse then notes that the follow-up BP has ↓ to 112/76. What is the appropriate management for this patient? The child's pediatricians should recheck her BP, making sure that the positioning and equipment are appropriate. If the child's BP remains 112/76, it is important for pediatricians to recognize this as hypertension. If repeated BP readings remain above the 95th percentile for height and gender, renal disease must be ruled out. Workup may include a full chemistry panel, UA, urine culture, CBC, and renal ultrasound.

BLOOD PRESSURE SCREENING

BP screening is significant for the following reasons:

- Renal disease is the most common cause of hypertension in infants and children.
- Essential hypertension is the most common cause of hypertension in adolescents.
- Both hypertension and prehypertension have become increasingly significant health issues in children because of the strong association of high BP with obesity.

SCREENING RECOMMENDATIONS

- Children > 3 years of age who are seen in a medical setting should have their BP measured.
- Significant hypertension exists if either systolic or diastolic measurements are greater than the 95th percentile for age, gender, and height (see Table 17-6).
- A BP between the 90th and 95th percentile is defined as prehypertensive and is an indication for lifestyle modification.
- BP tables based on gender, age, and height provide a precise classification of BP according to body size.
- BP ↑ with age and height.
- A BP of 120/80 in a child < 6 years of age is significant hypertension.
- A BP of 140/90 in any child is significant hypertension.

Cuff size and blood pressure:

Small → **S**ky-high BP.
Large → **L**ow BP.

TREATMENT

Evaluation is as follows:

- **Severity:**
  - **Prehypertension:** 90th–95th percentile.
  - **Stage I hypertension:** 95th–99th percentile + 5 mmHg.
  - **Stage II hypertension:** > 99th percentile + 5 mmHg.

TABLE 17-6. 95th Percentile BP for Children by Gender, Age, and Height

	MALE			FEMALE		
AGE	5% HEIGHT	50% HEIGHT	95% HEIGHT	5% HEIGHT	50% HEIGHT	95% HEIGHT
1	98/54	**101/56**	106/58	107/60	**105/60**	107/60
6	109/72	**114/74**	117/76	108/72	**111/74**	115/76
12	119/78	**123/81**	127/83	119/79	**123/81**	126/82
17	131/84	**136/87**	140/89	125/82	**129/84**	132/86

Data from 2004 National High Blood Pressure Education Program Working Group on High Blood Pressure in Children and Adolescents: The Fourth Report on the Diagnosis, Evaluation, and Treatment of High Blood Pressure in Children and Adolescents. *Pediatrics* 114 (2 Supplement):555–576, 2004.

- **Etiology:** Rule out renal disease, particularly in children.
    - Labs may include BUN, creatinine, electrolytes, UA, and urine culture.
    - CBC to rule out anemia consistent with chronic renal disease.
    - Renal ultrasound to rule out renal scarring and congenital anomalies.
- **Comorbidities:**
    - Obesity (document a BMI), sleep apnea, metabolic syndrome.
    - Consider checking fasting lipids and glucose, echocardiogram, retinal exam, and sleep study.
- **Therapies:**
    - Weight loss in obese patients, dietary changes, regular exercise.
    - Give antihypertensive medications in the presence of the following:
        - Stage 2 hypertension **or**
        - Stage 1 hypertension that (1) is refractory to lifestyle modification and weight reduction (if obese), (2) represents 2° hypertension that can be pharmacologically treated, or (3) is symptomatic.

SCREENING FOR HYPERCHOLESTEROLEMIA

Screening criteria for cholesterol measurement are as follows:

- Screen children and adolescents whose parents or grandparents have a history of coronary atherosclerosis or vascular disease at < 55 years of age.
- Screen children and adolescents if one or both parents have a history of ↑ blood cholesterol level (≥ 240 mg/dL).
- If parental history cannot be obtained, physicians may choose to measure cholesterol levels to identify patients in need of nutritional and medical advice, particularly in the presence of other risk factors.
- Screening may also be appropriate for children who are at higher risk of CAD and dyslipidemia, independent of family history—e.g., children who are overweight, are hypertensive, smoke, or consume excessive quantities of saturated fats and cholesterol.
- A blood sample should be obtained after a **12-hour overnight fast.**
- Acceptable cholesterol levels are as follows:
    - **Total cholesterol:** < 170 mg/dL.
    - **LDL cholesterol:** < 100 mg/dL.

Anticipatory Guidance

SAFETY/INJURY PREVENTION

MOTOR VEHICLES

- Motor vehicle injuries are a leading cause of death in children and young adults.
- Child safety seats and seat belts have been demonstrated to significantly ↓ the risk of serious injury and mortality in motor vehicle accidents. Child safety-seat guidelines are as follows:
  - Infants must be placed in rear-facing car seats until they are **one year of age and weigh 20 pounds.**
  - Toddlers can be placed in forward-facing car seats until they weigh 40 pounds.
  - Belt-positioning booster seats should be used for young children weighing 60–80 pounds (laws vary depending on the state).

POISON

- The AAP recommends counseling on household poisons and medications beginning at the six-month well-child visit.
- Parents should also be given the number of the local poison control center.
- Because home use of ipecac has failed to show benefit in emergency department utilization and health outcomes, ipecac is no longer recommended for home use.

DROWNING

- Drowning is the third leading cause of accidental death in the United States, with 1500 childhood fatalities per year.
- Only five minutes of hypoxia may lead to permanent neurologic sequelae.
- The epidemiology and location of pediatric drowning vary with age.
  - **Infants:** Household water tubs (e.g., bathtubs, toilets, buckets).
  - **Toddlers:** Home swimming pools, inflatable pools, Jacuzzis.
  - **Teenagers:** Pools, rivers, oceans.
- Most drownings are attributable to lack of supervision.
- Pediatricians should counsel parents with regard to water safety in a manner that is specific to the child's age, geographic area, and activities.
- The AAP recommends that children be taught to swim when they are developmentally ready, which is generally at about five years of age.

VIOLENCE

- The AAP has established statements regarding the prevention, recognition, and treatment of domestic and youth violence.
- **Domestic violence:** Pediatricians are expected to take the following measures:
  - Recognize evidence of family or intimate-partner violence in the office setting.
  - Intervene in a sensitive and skillful manner, yet in a way that maximizes the safety of women and children who may be victims.
- **Youth violence:** Homicide and suicide have become the second and third leading causes of death among teenagers. Homicide is the leading cause of death among black youth. Accordingly, pediatricians are expected to do the following:
  - Assess for high-risk situations and behaviors.

- Respond to identified problems with appropriate treatment and referrals.
- Provide violence prevention counseling and screening beginning as early as the pediatric prenatal visit and continuing into adulthood.
- Maintain familiarity with appropriate counseling and treatment services in communities.

FIREARMS

- Firearm-related deaths account for 22.5% of all injury-related deaths in children and adolescents. Injuries from firearms are the leading cause of death among black males 10–34 years of age.
- Most firearm-related injuries and deaths of children and adolescents involve a **handgun.**
- Access to guns ↑ the completion rate of suicide attempts; ↑ the number of conflict-related deaths and injuries; and ↑ the risk of serious unintentional injury and death.
- Pediatricians should counsel families on alternatives to violence, conflict resolution, and storage techniques (e.g., trigger locks, lock boxes, gun safes).
- Pediatricians should also be involved in community and policy advocacy, including educational programs for children and adolescents.
- The AAP supports firearm regulation and affirms that the most effective way to prevent firearm injuries is to ensure the absence of guns in homes and communities.

SLEEP POSITION

- Physicians should counsel all new parents about the importance of ensuring that newborn infants sleep on their backs.
- The Back to Sleep Campaign, initiated in the early 1980s, reversed the conventional sleep position from prone to supine, thereby contributing to a ↓ in SIDS rates by almost 50%, from 1.4 in 1000 to 0.8 in 1000.

> The father of an infant smokes cigarettes. Knowing that secondhand smoke, in general, is harmful to infants, the pediatrician wants to provide effective anticipatory guidance to the father. What are the known effects of second-hand smoke on children? The pediatrician should advise the father that the effects of passive smoking on children include an ↑ risk of SIDS, bronchiolitis, pneumonia, otitis media, and asthma. The pediatrician should also point out that children of smokers are themselves more likely to smoke. In addition, pediatricians should assess parents' willingness to quit and assist in smoking cessation efforts.

SMOKING AND TOBACCO USE

- Tobacco use is the most common preventable cause of disease and death in the United States.
- **Passive smoke exposure** has the following effects:
  - **Effects on the fetus:** Fetal smoke exposure ↑ the likelihood of miscarriage, fetal growth retardation, preterm delivery, and low-birth-weight babies.
  - **Effects on children:** Exposure ↑ the risk of SIDS as well as the incidence of bronchiolitis, pneumonia, otitis media, sinusitis, asthma, aller-

gic rhinitis, and hospitalization. Children with asthma have an ↑ frequency and severity of exacerbations.

- **Initiation of smoking:**
  - Almost all adult smokers began smoking before 18 years of age.
  - Children of smokers are much more likely to smoke.
  - Nicotine dependence can begin during childhood and adolescence.
- **The AAP recommends that pediatricians:**
  - Ask parents and pediatric patients about smoking.
  - Advise parents and patients about the harmful effects of passive and active smoking.
  - Determine whether the smoker is willing to quit.
  - Use motivational interviewing and repetition to encourage smokers to quit.
  - Help smokers quit by establishing a quit date and providing referral information.
  - Arrange follow-up visits to enhance motivation and prevent relapse.

SUN EXPOSURE

- Episodic high exposures to UV radiation sufficient to cause sunburn, particularly in childhood and adolescence, ↑ the risk of melanoma and other skin growths.
- Infants < 6 months of age should be kept out of direct sunlight through use of hats, clothing, and shades. The safety of sunscreen for infants < 6 months of age has not been established.
- Children and adolescents should use sun block with an SPF rating of > 15.

VITAMIN D

In an effort to prevent rickets and vitamin D deficiency in healthy infants and children, the AAP in 2003 recommended an intake of 200 IU of vitamin D per day and a supplement of 200 IU per day for the following:

- All breast-fed infants unless they are weaned to at least 500 mL per day of vitamin D–fortified formula or milk.
- All non-breast-fed infants who are ingesting < 500 mL per day of vitamin D–fortified formula or milk.
- Children and adolescents who do not get regular sunlight exposure, do not ingest at least 500 mL per day of vitamin D–fortified milk, or do not take a daily multivitamin supplement containing at least 200 IU of vitamin D.

TELEVISION

- Television viewing is associated with ↓ academic performance, ↓ reading performance, attention problems, and obesity.
- The AAP recommends that children ≤ 2 years of age not watch any television and that older children watch no more than 1–2 hours of television per day, limited to educational, nonviolent programs.
- Pediatricians should encourage parents to keep television sets out of children's bedrooms.

Breast-fed infants should take a daily vitamin D supplement. This supplementation may be provided in the form of 1 mL of a multivitamin drop.

During a well-child visit in December, a mother asks about the appropriateness of the influenza vaccine for her eight-month-old infant. The infant's past medical history is significant only for a mild skin rash that has occurred when the child has eaten eggs. Should the pediatrician recommend the influenza vaccine? What is the schedule for the vaccination? Is egg allergy a contraindication to the influenza vaccine? In addition to children with chronic conditions, the influenza vaccine is now recommended for all children 6–24 months of age. The child should receive the first dose of influenza vaccine at this visit and should then return in one month for the second dose to ↑ the likelihood of an immunologic response. The following year, the child would still be < 24 months of age and should receive a single dose. Children with severe egg allergy should not receive the vaccine. The infant in this case has a suspected egg allergy by history, but may be able to receive vaccination if allergy skin testing for egg or the influenza vaccine is ⊖.

IMMUNIZATIONS

The Immunization Action Coalition is a CDC-supported nonprofit organization that works to ↑ immunization rates and prevent disease. Its Web sites, www.immunize.org and www.vaccineinformation.org, provide excellent, accurate information for pediatricians and parents. Its quiz for pediatricians is particularly high yield for the pediatric boards. Figure 17-1 outlines the CDC's recommendations for childhood and adolescent immunizations.

HIGH-YIELD VACCINATION INFORMATION

- PCV-7 (7-valent pneumococcal vaccine):
  - The seven-serotype pneumococcal vaccine (Prevnar) is highly effective in preventing invasive pneumococcal disease, reducing cases of bacteremia by 88% and meningitis by 82% in young children.
  - The recommended PCV-7 vaccine schedule should include four doses given to all children at 2, 4, 6, and 12–15 months of age.
- Influenza:
  - The vaccine typically contains three virus strains: two type A and one type B.
  - Currently recommended for all children 6–23 months old but will likely be expanded to all children 6–59 months old.
  - Recommended for selected children with selected underlying chronic conditions.
  - Children < 9 years of age who are receiving their first influenza vaccination should receive two doses of vaccine administered one month apart to produce a satisfactory antibody response.
  - The efficacy of the vaccine in preventing culture-confirmed influenza illnesses is about 60–95%.
  - The vaccine is contraindicated in children with severe anaphylactic reaction to chickens or egg proteins.
- Pertussis Tdap:
  - Pertussis remains endemic in the U.S., despite high rates of immunization. Pertussis is highly communicable (80% transmission among nonimmune household contacts), so adolescents can transmit the disease to infants.

Vaccine ▼ / Age ▶	Birth	1 month	2 months	4 months	6 months	12 months	15 months	18 months	24 months	4–6 years	11–12 years	13–14 years	15 years	16–18 years
Hepatitis B	HepB	HepB		HepB¹		HepB					HepB Series			
Diphtheria, Tetanus, Pertussis			DTaP	DTaP	DTaP		DTaP			DTaP	Tdap	Tdap		
Haemophilus influenzae type b			Hib	Hib	Hib³	Hib								
Inactivated Poliovirus			IPV	IPV		IPV				IPV				
Measles, Mumps, Rubella						MMR				MMR	MMR			
Varicella						Varicella				Varicella				
Meningococcal											MCV4	MCV4	MCV4	
									MPSV4					
Pneumococcal			PCV	PCV	PCV	PCV				PCV	PPV			
Influenza						Influenza (Yearly)				Influenza (Yearly)				
Hepatitis A										HepA Series				

Vaccines within broken line are for selected populations

This schedule indicates the recommended ages for routine administration of currently licensed childhood vaccines, as of December 1, 2005, for children through age 18 years. Any dose not administered at the recommended age should be administered at any subsequent visit when indicated and feasible. ▨ Indicates age groups that warrant special effort to administer those vaccines not previously administered. Additional vaccines may be licensed and recommended during the year. Licensed combination vaccines may be used whenever any components of the combination are indicated and other components of the vaccine are not contraindicated and if approved by the Food and Drug Administration for that dose of the series. Providers should consult the respective ACIP statement for detailed recommendations. Clinically significant adverse events that follow immunization should be reported to the Vaccine Adverse Event Reporting System (VAERS). Guidance about how to obtain and complete a VAERS form is available at **www.vaers.hhs.gov** or by telephone, **800-822-7967**.

▨ **Range of recommended ages** ▨ **Catch-up immunization** ▨ **11–12 year old assessment**

FIGURE 17-1. Recommended childhood and adolescent immunization schedule (2006).

(Adapted from the Department of Health and Human Services, Centers for Disease Control and Prevention, www.cispimmunize.org.)

▨ Two new formulations of tetanus toxoid, reduced diphtheria toxoid and acellular pertussis vaccine (Tdap) were licensed in the U.S. in 2005, then recommended by the CDC for adolescents 11–18 years old. This replaces the old Td vaccination that did not contain the pertussis component.

▨ **Meningococcal vaccine (MCV):**
  ▨ Meningococcal conjugate vaccine (MCV4) should be given to all children at the 11- to 12-year-old visit as well as to unvaccinated adolescents at high school entry (about 15 years of age) and before college entry in those living in dormitories.
  ▨ Vaccination against invasive meningococcal disease is recommended for children and adolescents aged ≥ 2 years with terminal complement deficiencies or anatomic or functional asplenia and certain other high-risk groups. Use the polysaccharide vaccine, MPS4, for children 2–10 years old.
  ▨ Menactra (MCV4) is a conjugate vaccine, which confers longer immunity and similar efficacy compared to the older polysaccharide vaccine. The antibody levels from the MPS4 polysaccharide vaccines decreases after 2–3 years, so people at high-risk need revaccination every 3–5 years.

VACCINE CONTRAINDICATIONS

- Contraindications to vaccine use include the following (see also Table 17-7):
    - Patients with severe **egg allergy** should **not** receive influenza or yellow fever vaccination. MMR, however, can be given. (Although these vaccines are derived from chicken embryo fibroblast tissue cultures, they do not contain significant amounts of egg cross-reacting proteins.) Those with moderate egg allergies should consult their physician.
    - **Pregnant patients** should **not** receive MMR or varicella vaccine during the course of their pregnancy, but they can receive vaccine postpartum even while breast-feeding.
    - Patients with asymptomatic HIV should receive all routine vaccines, including MMR and varicella.
- The following are **not contraindications** to administering vaccine:
    - Mild to moderate local reaction (soreness, redness, or swelling).
    - Low-grade or moderate fever; mild acute illness with or without low fever.
    - Current antimicrobial therapy.
    - Convalescent phases of illness.
    - Prematurity.
    - Recent exposure to an infectious disease.
    - A history of penicillin or other nonspecific allergies.
    - Pregnancy of the mother or household contacts.
    - An unimmunized or immunodeficient household contact.
    - Breast-feeding (nursing infant or lactating mother).

VACCINE SAFETY CONCERNS

Some people in the general public have in recent years become concerned about safety issues related to vaccines. In 2000, the CDC and the NIH therefore commissioned the Institute of Medicine to convene an Immunization

TABLE 17-7. Vaccine Contraindications

VACCINE	CONTRAINDICATION
All vaccines	A previous anaphylactic reaction to specific vaccine; a specific anaphylactic reaction to a vaccine constituent.
Influenza	Anaphylactic reaction to eggs.
MMR and varicella	Pregnancy; anaphylactic reaction to neomycin or gelatin. Known altered immunodeficiency (hematologic and solid tumors, congenital immunodeficiency, long-term immunosuppressive therapy). Severe HIV infection (MMR); symptomatic HIV infection (varicella).
HBV	Anaphylactic reaction to baker's yeast.
Pneumococcal	None.
HAV	Anaphylactic reaction to 2-phenoxyethanol or alum.

Safety Review Committee for the purpose of investigating controversies surrounding immunizations. Its findings are summarized in Table 17-8.

Oral Health

Table 17-9 outlines the normal development of dentition.

The mandibular central incisors (front-bottom teeth) are the first 1° and permanent teeth to erupt, doing so at six months and six years of age, respectively (the "six rule" of tooth eruption).

PREVENTION OF DENTAL CARIES

- Dental caries is the most common chronic disease in childhood.
  - About 20% of children 2–5 years of age have at least one untreated cavity.
  - Roughly 50% of children 5–9 years of age have at least one cavity.
- **Daily maintenance to prevent caries** includes the following:
  - Community water fluoridation significantly ↓ the incidence of cavities. If there are low levels of fluoride (0.3–0.6 ppm), it is recommended that supplemental fluoride be given to children 3–16 years of age. If there is no fluoride (< 0.3 ppm), fluoride supplementation should begin at **six months of age.**
  - Babies should not be put to sleep with a bottle of milk or juice.
  - Juice should be offered in a cup, not in a bottle. The AAP recommends that no fruit juice be given to children before six months of age and that only restricted amounts be given after six months.

TABLE 17-8. Vaccine Safety Concerns and Recommendations

SAFETY CONCERN	FINDINGS	ACTIONS
MMR and autism/IBD	Evidence does not support the hypothesis that MMR vaccine causes autism or IBD.	To continue existing recommendations for MMR vaccinations.
Thimerosal preservatives in vaccines and neurodevelopmental disorders	Evidence is **inadequate** to accept or reject a causal relationship. Data on the health effects of thimerosal are inconclusive, but an association has been found to be "biologically plausible." Removal of thimerosal from vaccines was deemed to be "a prudent measure in support of the public health goal to reduce mercury exposure."	By 2002, all vaccines in the recommended childhood and adolescent immunization schedule contained no or only trace quantities of thimerosal.
Multiple immunizations and immune dysfunction	Data **reject** a causal relationship between multiple immunizations and an ↑ risk of infections and diabetes. Evidence is **inadequate** to accept or reject a causal relationship between multiple immunizations and the development of allergic disorders, particularly asthma.	No recommendations or actions taken.
HBV vaccine and demyelinating neurologic disorders	Data **reject** a causal relationship between HBV vaccine and MS and are **inadequate** to accept or reject a relationship with other demyelinating disorders.	No recommendations or actions taken.

TABLE 17-9. Development of Dentition in the Pediatric Population

VARIABLE STAGE	STAGE OF DEVELOPMENT/TIMING
Time frame in which the first teeth erupt	The mandibular central incisor erupts at six months of age. The maxillary teeth typically erupt two months after corresponding mandibular teeth.
Time frame in which all 1° teeth should have erupted	The second maxillary molar typically erupts by 24 months of age. Thus, most children will have all teeth erupted by three years of age. (The number of 1° teeth is 20 and the number of permanent teeth 32.)
Time frame in which the first permanent teeth erupt	The mandibular central incisor erupts at 6–7 years of age.
Time frame in which the wisdom teeth erupt	The third molars erupt in late adolescence (17–21 years of age). These teeth often require removal.

- Teeth should be brushed twice daily as soon as they erupt. Flossing should begin once daily as soon as teeth are in contact with one another.
- Young children should be carefully supervised to prevent the swallowing of fluoridated toothpaste (and hence the risk of fluorosis). Children < 6 years of age should not use more than a pea-sized amount of toothpaste.

PERIODIC DENTAL EXAMINATIONS

- All infants should be given oral health risk assessments by their pediatricians by six months of age.
- **Infants at higher risk of early dental caries** should be referred to a dentist as early as six months of age and no later than six months after the first tooth erupts or 12 months of age, whichever comes first.
- **Children at higher risk of early dental caries** include the following:
    - Children with special health care needs.
    - Children of mothers with a high caries rate.
    - Children with demonstrable caries, plaque, demineralization, and/or staining.
    - Children who sleep with a bottle or are breast-fed throughout the night.
    - Later-order offspring.
    - Children in families of low socioeconomic status.

ETHICS

Confidentiality

- The assurance of confidentiality facilitates a patient's disclosure of sensitive health and behavioral information, which may be essential to the provision of effective medical care.

- **Exceptions** include instances in which:
  - Disclosure would likely prevent harm to the patient or to others.
  - The patient is unable to provide informed consent because of lack of maturity or cognitive abilities.

CHILDHOOD DEVELOPMENT AND CONFIDENTIALITY

- In general, the right to confidentiality ↑ with maturity. If a child is able to provide informed consent, treatment can be given confidentially.
- **Early childhood:** The right to confidentiality for younger children is limited, as such children lack the maturity to be sufficiently informed.
- **Adolescence:** In general, adolescents should be guaranteed confidentiality. All states have statutes that allow sensitive conditions to be treated without parental involvement. Such conditions include STDs, drug- and alcohol-related issues, and family planning (states vary on the issue of abortion).

MANDATORY REPORTING

- All states mandate the reporting of child abuse.
- Some infectious diseases are reportable to state and local health departments.
- States have different guidelines for interpreting statutory rape.

Patient Autonomy

- Competent patients have the right to decide what should be done to their bodies and their health. Autonomy may be forfeited in cases in which public health is endangered or in which potential harm may be done to others.
- Competence connotes that patients can understand the potential consequences of their decisions and the available alternatives.
- Most adolescents are able to understand most decision-making processes. Thus, they are competent to be autonomous of their parents in most circumstances.

INFORMED CONSENT

- In order to be adequately informed, the patient must understand the general nature of the proposed treatment; why the treatment is necessary; the risks and benefits of treatment; and the possible alternatives.
- **Preadolescent children:** Parents generally make decisions on behalf of preadolescent children because such children are unable to become adequately informed of issues involved in the decision-making process. Thus, preadolescent children generally cannot give consent or refuse treatments. As an example:
  - A five-year-old cannot refuse his immunizations.
  - A 10-year-old cannot refuse initial treatment for leukemia or appendectomy.
- **Emergency care:** Informed consent is not required in emergency care when a patient is unable to provide consent and the delay of care would be detrimental.

- **Cultural/religious reasons for refusal of treatment:** The most common example of religion-based refusal of treatment is that of the Jehovah's Witnesses, whose followers may refuse a blood transfusion for their children.
    - In serious, life-threatening conditions requiring transfusion, the physician should first discuss the importance of the procedure with the child's parents. In many cases, parents may then allow transfusion for their child.
    - If parents do not allow the necessary transfusion, the pediatrician can ask the court to order transfusions (or other treatments) over parental objections.
    - If parents and mature adolescents both refuse treatments (e.g., blood transfusion for Jehovah's Witnesses):
        - Discuss the issue with the adolescent away from the presence of his or her parents.
        - The pediatrician may need to discuss the issue with the hospital ethics committee or consult courts.
        - In many cases, the adolescent has the right to refuse treatment and die.
        - Where feasible, alternative solutions such as erythropoietin and iron may be considered.

Beneficence

- Following the guideline of **beneficence**, physicians have the duty to act in the best interests of their patients.
- In general, patients expect physicians to provide advice, decisions, and actions that benefit their health and well-being.
- The best interests of patients supersede the interests (e.g., financial) of the physician and/or third-party payers.
- In acting in the best interests of patients, physicians should also consider any potential harms or risks.

Terminal Illnesses

RELIEF OF PAIN AND SUFFERING

- In a dying child, the child's comfort may be prioritized (ethically and legally) ahead of potential treatments and the risk of side effects. Examples are as follows:
    - A child receiving chemotherapy for an **uncomplicated**, curable leukemia should receive chemotherapy that may cause nausea and discomfort. Excessive amounts of morphine should be limited to guard against oversedation.
    - However, a child who is **dying** from advanced, incurable leukemia should **not receive chemotherapies** that are discomforting. In this instance, physicians may also provide an adequate amount of morphine (or other pain-relieving narcotics) to control pain even if the side effects lead to excessive sedation and respiratory depression.
- **Do not resuscitate (DNR) orders:**
    - Unless a DNR has been specifically ordered, the physician must attempt cardiopulmonary resuscitation regardless of the circumstances and potential consequences.

- DNR orders must be carefully discussed with the patient and family. Specific orders, consent, and the reasons for withholding resuscitation must be documented in the medical chart.
- **Futile care:** A physician is not legally or ethically obligated to provide treatments requested by the patient or parents that offer no benefit to the child.

Ethics in Research

Ethical research must ensure that:

- Subjects are adequately informed of the nature of the study.
- Subjects participate voluntarily.
- The benefits of a study outweigh the risks.
- The risks and benefits of the study are evenly distributed among the possible subject populations.

EPIDEMIOLOGY

Major Study Types

Table 17-10 outlines the major types of studies used in statistical analysis.

Test Parameters

Diagnostic test parameters measure the accuracy of a test. True disease is defined by an accepted gold standard. Test parameters include the following (see Table 17-11):

- **The sensitivity of a test:** Defined as the probability that a test will be $\oplus$ in someone with the disease. A sensitive test is "**PID,**" or Positive In Disease (think: "**PID** is a **sensitive** topic").
  - **Sensitivity** = $a/(a + c)$ = TP/TP + FN (where TP = true positives and FN = false negatives).
  - **Example:** If the sensitivity of the rapid strep test is 90%, 90 of 100 infected patients will test $\oplus$, but 10 patients will have a (false) $\ominus$ test.
  - **High sensitivity is important for screening tests.**
- **The specificity of a test:** Defined as the probability that a test will be $\ominus$ in someone who truly does not have the disease. A specific test is "**NIH,**" or Negative In Health (think: "The **NIH** requires very **specific** grant applications").
  - **Specificity** = $d/(b + d)$ = TN/FP + TN (where TN = true negatives and FP = false positives).
  - **Example:** If the specificity of the rapid strep test is 95%, 95 of 100 non-infected patients will have a $\ominus$ test, but five patients will have a (false) $\oplus$ test.
- **Positive predictive value (PPV):** The proportion of persons testing $\oplus$ who have the condition. Calculated as [TP/(TP + FP)] = $a/(a + b)$.
- **Negative predictive value (NPV):** The proportion of persons testing $\ominus$ who do not have the condition. Calculated as [TN/(TN + FN)] = $d/(c + d)$.
- **Likelihood ratio (LR):** The proportion of patients **with** a disease who have a certain test result over the proportion of patients **without** the disease in question who have the given test result (see Table 17-12).

> *Sensitivity—PID*
> "**P**ositive **I**n **D**isease"

> *Specificity—NIH*
> "**N**egative **I**n **H**ealth"

*Sensitivity and specificity are **independent** of disease prevalence in the tested population. PPV and NPV depend on disease prevalence.*

TABLE 17-10. Statistical Study Types

Study Type	Explanation	Example	Advantages	Disadvantages
Randomized controlled trial (experimental study)	Randomly assigns intervention to one group and a placebo to another (ideally **blinding** both subjects and MDs to group assignment). Outcomes are then compared between groups.	Assignment of medication or placebo to obese adolescents; assessment of the incidence of depression in each group.	Prior to the intervention, the two groups of patients should have equal susceptibility to the outcome. Minimizes **confounding.** The incidence of the outcome in each group can be compared by computing the **risk ratio.**	Expensive and time-consuming; may lack generalizability.
Cohort study (observational study)	Groups are identified by the presence of exposures or risk factors.	Following obese and nonobese children and comparing the groups' risk of depression during adolescence.	Can evaluate multiple outcomes. The incidence of the outcome in each group can be compared by computing the **risk ratio.**	Potential confounders → biased results, and it is hard to determine **causality.** May take significant time to develop outcome.
Case-control study (observational study)	Groups are identified by the presence of a case or disease outcome. The presence of exposures/risk factors is determined retrospectively.	Identification of adolescents with depression and similar adolescents without depression; determination of the presence of obesity during childhood.	Good for rare diseases. Because the outcome has already occurred, the sample size can be smaller, and the study can be quickly completed after identification of previous exposures.	Most subject to biases. Cases frequently have recall bias. The prevalence of risk factor in each group can be compared by computing the **odds ratio.**
Cross-sectional study (observational study)	Data are obtained about exposure and outcome at the same time.	A questionnaire that asks for weight and height (to calculate BMI) and symptoms of depression.	Often survey data.	Cannot detect the temporal relationship of the outcome. Causality is thus unclear.

TABLE 17-11. Sensitivity, Specificity, and Predictive Values

		DISEASE		
		+	−	
Test	+	a (TP)	b (FP)	a/(a + b) = PPV
	−	c (FN)	d (TN)	d/(c + d) = NPV
		a/(a + c) = sensitivity	d/(b + d) = specificity	

- For dichotomous test with a positive result: LR = sensitivity/(1 − specificity).
- **Example:** A rapid strep test has a sensitivity of 90% and a specificity of 95%. On the basis of the calculations in Table 17-12, the test therefore has an LR of 18. A $\oplus$ rapid strep test is 18 times more likely in patients with a streptococcal pharyngitis than in patients without streptococcal pharyngitis.

TABLE 17-12. Computation of Likelihood Ratio

	FOR A GIVEN TEST RESULT		**EXAMPLE OF RAPID STREP**
Likelihood ratio	$\dfrac{\% \textbf{ with } \text{disease}}{\% \textbf{ without } \text{disease}}$	$= \dfrac{\text{sensitivity}}{1 - \text{specificity}}$	$\dfrac{0.90}{1 - 0.95}$

CHAPTER 18

The Pulmonary System

Shannon Sullivan, MD
reviewed by Dennis Nielson, MD

A two-year-old boy presents to the clinic with five days of upper respiratory symptoms and one day of fever of 38.8°C axillary (102°F). His mother thinks that the boy's right ear hurts. On exam, the child is found to be fussy but consolable and has bulging and erythema of his right tympanic membrane (TM); the left TM is normal. You make a diagnosis of acute otitis media (AOM). What are the likely causative organisms? The most common bacterial causes are *Streptococcus pneumoniae,* nontypable *Haemophilus influenzae,* and *Moraxella catarrhalis.* What are the possible complications? Most cases of AOM will resolve with or without antibiotics. Rare complications include serous otitis media, mastoiditis, and perforation.

Otitis Media

A middle ear infection that may be bacterial or viral and is often preceded by viral illness. Some 50% of children have an episode by their first birthday. Risk factors include bottle feeding, having smokers in the home, day care, and anatomic/congenital abnormalities. Recurrent otitis media is defined as three episodes of AOM within six months or four or more episodes within one year.

SYMPTOMS

Antecedent URI; fussiness and ear pain +/– fever.

EXAM

Look for a bulging pars flaccida of the TM, exudate, erythema, loss of landmarks, and poor movement of the TM with insufflation.

DIFFERENTIAL

- Foreign body, teething, otitis externa, trauma.
- **Bullous myringitis:** A painful disorder associated with infection of the middle ear; presents with inflamed, blistering TM. Treat with a macrolide or amoxicillin.

DIAGNOSIS

- Based on the clinical history and physical exam.
- Consider a tympanogram.
- Tympanocentesis may be considered but is not routinely performed.

The most common bacterial causes of AOM are S. pneumoniae, nontypable H. influenzae, and M. catarrhalis.

TREATMENT

Recommendations vary and may range from symptomatic relief to antibiotics; because of resistance patterns, high-dose amoxicillin or amoxicillin/clavulanate (Augmentin) may be necessary.

COMPLICATIONS

- **Otitis media with effusion (OME):** The most common complication. Key points from the American Academy of Pediatrics/American Academy of Otolaryngology—Head and Neck Surgery (AAP/AAO-HNS) 2004 guidelines include the following:

- Some 40–50% of parents and children with OME report no symptoms, but symptoms may nonetheless be present and may include hearing loss, recurrent AOM, balance problems, delayed speech and development, and school problems.
- Those with craniofacial abnormalities are at special risk.
- Pediatricians should document laterality and severity and should refer to an otolaryngologist at three months if symptoms persist.
- Antihistamines and decongestants are ineffective; antibiotics and steroids do not have long-term efficacy.
- Hearing testing should occur at three months, and language testing should be conducted if hearing loss is present.
- If the patient is asymptomatic and low risk, watchful waiting with reevaluation every 3–6 months is adequate.
- If the patient is symptomatic or has hearing loss, other abnormalities (e.g., craniofacial), or effusion that is unlikely to resolve, ENT referral for tympanostomy tubes is required.
- Tonsillectomy or myringotomy alone should not be used to treat OME.
- **Mastoiditis:** Always assess for mastoid edema, erythema, and tenderness.
- **Perforation:** Exudate should be seen in the external canal. This should be painless; if not, consider foreign body or otitis externa (see below).

Otitis Externa

An infection of the external auditory canal that is often caused by *Pseudomonas* or, less commonly, by staphylococci, streptococci, or fungi. Also known as "swimmer's ear," it is less common in children < 2 years of age.

SYMPTOMS/EXAM

- Retracting pinna/pushing on the tragus → pain.
- The auditory canal is often erythematous and swollen; watery to thick discharge with debris may be present.

DIFFERENTIAL

- **Herpes zoster oticus:** Herpes infection of the geniculate ganglia (CN VII); presents as painful cutaneous herpes of the external auditory canal.
- **Cholesteatoma:** Usually painless.
- **Other:** Eczematous otitis externa, purulent otitis media with perforation of the TM, foreign body.

TREATMENT

- Avoid excess moisture and trauma.
- Symptomatic relief with analgesics.
- Acidity may be restored and inflammation reduced with 2% acetic acid solution plus hydrocortisone.
- Topical antibiotics +/– steroid drops are often used.

Cholesteatoma

A squamous epithelial cyst trapped in the mastoid, middle ear, or temporal bone that contains desquamated keratin. Although rare, it is the most com-

The hallmark of cholesteatoma is painless otorrhea +/– hearing loss.

mon growth in the middle ear. It can be congenital or acquired after AOM or trauma (even from tympanostomy tubes).

DIAGNOSIS

- TM perforation may accompany cholesteatoma in up to 90% of cases.
- Frequently, the only finding on exam will be an external auditory canal filled with granulation and drainage.
- If the TM can be seen, a **deep retraction pocket in the posterior quadrant or pars flaccida of the TM** suggests cholesteatoma.
- CT may be necessary to evaluate bony erosion.
- MRI may be needed to evaluate for dural involvement, subdural/epidural abscess, sigmoid sinus thrombosis, or cranial nerve inflammation.

TREATMENT

Treatment is surgical. Virtually all masses should be excised. Systemic antibiotics are seldom effective, and topical antibiotics may partially reduce drainage but are not curative.

COMPLICATIONS

If left untreated, cholesteatomas can destroy temporal bone and can → deafness or unilateral facial nerve paralysis. They are also associated with CNS complications such as brain abscess and meningitis.

Choanal Atresia

The absence of a connection between the external nares and nasopharynx; a complete nasal obstruction.

DIFFERENTIAL

Deviated or dislocated nasal septum, septal hematoma, teratoma/hamartoma, encephalocele.

DIAGNOSIS

- Failure to pass a suction catheter more than about 5 cm from the alar rim.
- Absence of movement of a cotton wisp placed under the nostril when the mouth is closed.
- CT scan can confirm and outline other abnormalities as well as rule out other sources of obstruction.

TREATMENT

Bilateral choanal atresia is an emergency. Insert an oral airway, an endotracheal tube, or a McGovern nipple. Ultimate correction is surgical.

Epistaxis

The most common cause is trauma/nose picking. Severe nosebleeds can be seen in **thrombocytopenia** and **Osler-Weber-Rendu syndrome (hereditary hemorrhagic telangiectasia)**.

*Choanal atresia may present as severe respiratory distress and cyanosis in the newborn and can be fatal. **Respiratory distress may be relieved when the infant cries** and takes a breath through the oropharynx.*

Diagnosis of choanal atresia— look for CHARGE anomalies

Coloboma
Heart defect
Atresia of the choanae
Retarded growth/ development
Genitourinary defects
Ear defects

Sinusitis

Infection and inflammation of the sinuses, most commonly after a viral URI. Risk factors include day care (↑ URIs), allergic rhinitis, deviated septum, midface hypoplasia, NG tube placement, CF, immotile cilia, and immunodeficiency.

SYMPTOMS/EXAM

- **Acute sinusitis:**
    - URI symptoms lasting > 10 days; nasal congestion/purulent discharge, headache, AOM (in 50% of patients), halitosis, sinus tenderness on exam, tooth pain, anosmia.
    - Fever is infrequent unless the course is severe.
    - Resolves by 30 days.
    - Causes include *S. pneumoniae*, *H. influenzae*, and *M. catarrhalis* (the same as those for AOM).
- **Recurrent acute sinusitis:** Two episodes, each lasting < 30 days, separated by 10 healthy days.
- **Subacute sinusitis:** As above, lasting 30–90 days.
- **Chronic sinusitis:**
    - Low-grade symptoms lasting > 90 days; a history of acute exacerbations with no intercurrent asymptomatic periods; **nighttime cough.**
    - Causes are usually polymicrobial, including organisms seen in acute sinusitis as well as anaerobes, *S. aureus*, and *Pseudomonas*.

TREATMENT

Treat with nasal decongestants, nasal steroids, and antibiotics (often a longer course—e.g., three weeks—than that needed for AOM).

COMPLICATIONS

Meningitis, abscess formation, orbital infection.

The ethmoid and maxillary sinuses are present at birth and → sphenoids (by five years of age), which in turn → frontal sinuses (by seven years of age; not fully formed until the teen years).

*With sinusitis unresponsive to antibiotics, think fungal—e.g., **Aspergillus**.*

FACIAL NERVE DISORDERS

Table 18-1 describes the presentation of some facial nerve disorders.

TABLE 18-1. Facial Nerve Disorders in Children

DISORDER	FEATURES
Bell's palsy	Idiopathic facial nerve paralysis. Usually unilateral; self-limited.
Bilateral facial nerve palsy	Unusual; has a limited differential that includes Lyme disease, sarcoidosis, Möbius syndrome (congenital facial nerve paralysis/cranial nerve agenesis), Guillain-Barré syndrome, basilar meningitis, and Wegener's granulomatosis.

Infection/inflammation of the parotid glands.

SYMPTOMS/EXAM

Cheeks are usually painful and swollen.

DIFFERENTIAL

- **Infection:** Mumps, strep, diphtheria, typhus.
- **Inflammation:** Sjögren syndrome → parotid swelling/xerostomia.
- **Mass:** Mucocele.
- **Other:** Sialolithiasis (stone in the salivary duct).

> *Mumps causes acute parotitis with fever and malaise and, rarely, orchitis, meningoencephalitis, Bell's palsy, and pancreatitis.*

A nine-year-old presents to the ER with sore throat of three days' duration, a fever of 38.6°F (101°F), fatigue, and poor PO intake. Throat exam reveals an erythematous oropharynx with patches of exudate over the tonsils. The remainder of the exam is significant for posterior cervical lymphadenopathy and splenomegaly. A rapid strep test is ⊖. Which other tests can be done to confirm a diagnosis of mononucleosis? A diagnosis of mononucleosis can be supported by a Monospot, EBV titers, and/or the presence of atypical lymphocytes on a peripheral smear. If mononucleosis is suspected, should penicillin be given? Why not? Penicillin can → a rash in patients with mono and should thus be avoided.

PHARYNGITIS/TONSILLITIS

Sore throat is a common complaint in pediatrics and has a variety of etiologies (see Table 18-2).

TABLE 18-2. Causes of Pharyngitis and Tonsillitis

ORGANISM	CLINICAL FEATURES	DIAGNOSIS	TREATMENT	SEQUELAE/COMPLICATIONS
Group A *S. pyogenes* (less commonly groups C and G)	Throat pain, exudative tonsillitis, palatal petechiae, sandpaper rash (scarlet fever) +/– fever and lymphadenopathy.	Rapid strep test or culture. Common.	Penicillin. Recurrent, severe strep A tonsillitis may require tonsillectomy and adenoidectomy.	Rheumatic heart disease; glomerulonephritis (incidence is **not** changed with antibiotic therapy); peritonsillar abscess (contralateral displacement of the uvula; trismus).
Neisseria gonorrhoeae	Exudative tonsillitis in sexually active patients.	Screening requires a warm Thayer-Martin plate. Less common.	Ceftriaxone, fluoroquinolones.	

TABLE 18-2. Causes of Pharyngitis and Tonsillitis *(continued)*

ORGANISM	CLINICAL FEATURES	DIAGNOSIS	TREATMENT	SEQUELAE/COMPLICATIONS
Coryne-bacterium diphtheriae	A thick gray membrane on the tonsils extending down the posterior pharynx.	Rare in the United States since the introduction of vaccine.	Antitoxin. Erythromycin may be given to ↓ bacterial load.	Airway occlusion, myocarditis.
Candida	White, cheesy patches on the tongue, buccal mucosa, and pharynx.	Commonly seen in babies or immuno-suppressed patients.	Nystatin.	Look for diaper rash as well.
Coxsackie A	"Herpangina"; papulovesicular lesions.	Clinical.	Topical and systemic analgesia; supportive care.	
Adenovirus	"Common cold" symptoms; exudative pharyngitis with conjunctivitis; also GI symptoms (watery diarrhea and emesis; abdominal pain).	Clinical; DFA if needed.	Supportive care; rehydration, fever control.	See the discussion of rhinovirus. Intussusception is a GI complication.
Rhinovirus	"Common cold" symptoms: malaise, profuse nasal discharge, fever. Generally characterized by a normal-appearing pharynx.	Generally no test is needed for the common cold; a viral culture can be performed if needed.	Supportive care, including decongestants and fever control.	Otitis media, asthma exacerbation. A possible cause of croup, bronchiolitis, and pneumonia.
EBV (mono-nucleosis)	Exudative tonsillitis and pharyngitis; associated with lymphadenopathy. Look for **posterior cervical nodes and splenomegaly,** fatigue, and low-grade fever for weeks +/–morbilliform rash.	Monospot for heterophile antibodies (low sensitivity in young children); antibody titers; atypical lymphocytes on peripheral smear.	Supportive. **Rash may develop if penicillin is given.**	Erythema nodosum, erythema multiforme, splenomegaly, splenic rupture, hepatomegaly, periorbital edema, jaundice.
HSV gingivo-stomatitis	Painful ulcerations of the tongue and inner cheeks; gingival swelling.	Clinical. Consider Tzanck smear, culture, PCR.	Supportive care. Acyclovir is controversial but may help if given within the first 48 hours.	Erythema multiforme, encephalitis, eczema herpeticum.

TABLE 18-2. Causes of Pharyngitis and Tonsillitis *(continued)*

ORGANISM	CLINICAL FEATURES	DIAGNOSIS	TREATMENT	SEQUELAE/COMPLICATIONS
Measles	The prodromal phase is characterized by red mottling on the palate and **Koplik's spots** (small, whitish spots on the buccal mucosa). Also presents with coryza, cough, conjunctivitis, and high fever.	Clinical. Antibody titers if indicated.	Supportive; antibiotics for superinfection.	Otitis, pneumonia, encephalitis.

NECK MASSES

Table 18-3 lists common neck masses and their clinical presentation.

DISORDERS OF THE LARYNX AND TRACHEA

Epiglottitis and Retropharyngeal Abscess

Table 18-4 outlines the etiology, presentation, diagnosis, and treatment of epiglottitis and retropharyngeal abscess.

TABLE 18-3. Presentation of Neck Masses

MASS	LOCATION	PRESENTATION	FEATURES
Thyroglossal duct cyst	Midline.	Usually in childhood.	Elevation upon swallowing.
Branchial cleft cyst	Lateral.	Present later, when infection occurs.	Do not elevate upon swallowing; aspirate contains cholesterol crystals.
Cystic hygroma	Variable.	Within the first 2–3 years of life.	Translucent, compressible, painless mass.
Dermoid cyst	Face, neck, and scalp; may also occur on the floor of the mouth.	Usually present at birth when on the face, neck, or scalp, but may occur later in other locations.	Soft and fluctuant; composed of epithelium.
Cervical adenitis	Not midline.	Tender and mobile; may be fluctuant or red.	Infectious (staph/strep, cat-scratch fever, atypical mycobacteria).

TABLE 18-4. Epiglottitis vs. Retropharyngeal Abscess

	EPIGLOTTITIS	RETROPHARYNGEAL ABSCESS
Definition	Inflammation of the epiglottis and nearby structures, including the aryepiglottic folds, the arytenoids, and sometimes the uvula (see Figure 18-1).	Abscess in the space posterior to the pharynx.
Etiology	Caused by *H. influenzae* type b (Hib) infection more often than strep or staph; noninfectious causes include trauma from inhalation or blind finger sweep.	**Infectious:** β-hemolytic streptococci, staphylococci, anaerobes (e.g., *Bacteroides*), gram-$\ominus$ organisms (e.g., *Haemophilus parainfluenzae*). **Noninfectious:** Trauma from intubation or foreign body.
Clinical presentation	Patients are toxic appearing and irritable with the chin hyperextended; associated with "sniffing," "tripod" positions. Drooling is also seen +/− stridor. High fever.	**< 1 year:** Fever, neck swelling, refusal to eat. **> 1 year:** Sore throat, fever, neck stiffness, pain with swallowing. Also presents with stridor, torticollis, drooling, and retropharyngeal bulge **(do not palpate!)** +/− tonsillitis/pharyngitis/AOM.
Diagnosis	Clinical; no tests are needed. If lateral neck x-ray is performed, thumbprint sign will be seen.	Clinical; lateral neck x-ray will show widening of retropharyngeal soft tissues. If x-ray is $\ominus$ with high clinical suspicion, a CT may be needed.
Treatment	Emergency airway! Apply blow-by oxygen (BBO_2), but be careful to avoid ↑ the child's anxiety. Initiate ABCs, and keep the child in view at all times. Endotracheal tube intubation should be initiated as soon as possible by the best airway person available (anesthesia if possible). IV antibiotics.	Secure the airway. Prophylactic intubation in a patient without respiratory distress is generally not indicated. Drainage of abscess in the OR; IV antibiotics.
Complications	Sudden death from airway obstruction.	Causes of mortality include airway obstruction, aspiration, mediastinitis (50% mortality), epidural abscess, jugular venous thrombosis, and erosion into the carotid artery.

An 18-month-old, fully immunized child is brought to the ER by ambulance at night after developing respiratory distress at home. The child has had a runny nose for three days and has had a fever of 39.4°C (103°F) for the past 12 hours. The parents describe a "barking" cough. Exam reveals a non-toxic-appearing patient with intermittent mild retractions and inspiratory stridor that appear to worsen with agitation. You diagnose croup. Is an x-ray indicated? A diagnosis of croup may be supported by a "steeple sign" on x-ray, but the diagnosis is usually made clinically without the need for imaging. What treatment or treatments would you provide? A child with respiratory distress from croup should be given humidified O_2 and steroids. Nebulized racemic epinephrine can also be given depending on disease severity. Avoid agitation.

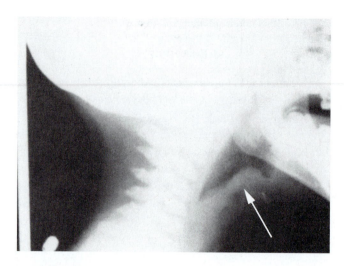

FIGURE 18-1. Epiglottitis.

(Reproduced, with permission, from Tintinalli JE et al. *Emergency Medicine: A Comprehensive Study Guide*, 6th ed. New York: McGraw-Hill, 2004:851.)

Croup

A clinical syndrome involving a hoarse, barking, seal-like cough and inspiratory stridor +/– respiratory distress. Also known as laryngotracheobronchitis. Etiologies are as follows:

- Parainfluenza virus type I is found in 60% of cases.
- Parainfluenza virus types II, III, and IV can also → croup, as can influenza, adenovirus, and RSV, among others.
- Bacterial superinfection of the trachea is sometimes seen.

SYMPTOMS/EXAM

- Presents with varying degrees of respiratory distress, including retractions and flaring.
- Inspiratory stridor is seen when patients are upset but may also occur at rest.

DIAGNOSIS

- Largely clinical.
- CBC is generally not indicated but will show a normal or ↑ WBC count and lymphocytosis.
- Hypoxemia is seen with severe disease.
- CXR and neck x-ray are unnecessary, but if taken, a PA view of the neck will show "steeple sign" in about 50% of cases (see Figure 18-2).

TREATMENT

- Cool mist; humidity.
- Aerosolized racemic epinephrine.
- Inhaled budesonide → improvement within 2–4 hours.
- Dexamethasone 0.15–0.6 mg/kg IM, IV, or PO or other corticosteroids.

Spasmodic croup is an afebrile condition consisting of sudden onset of croup symptoms that recur on a regular basis in an otherwise healthy child.

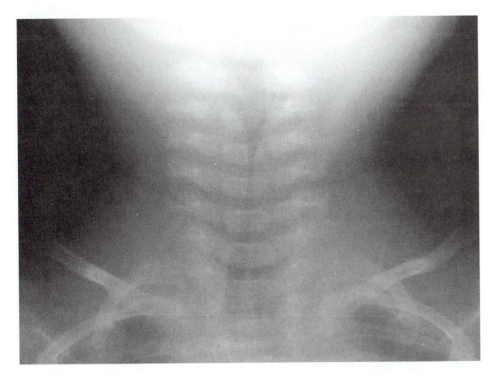

FIGURE 18-2. Croup.

The "steeple sign" of croup in a one-year-old. (Reproduced, with permission, from Stone CK, Humphries RL. *Current Emergency Diagnosis & Treatment*, 5th ed. New York: McGraw-Hill, 2004:648.)

COMPLICATIONS

Self-limiting with an excellent overall outcome, but intubation may be needed in cases of severe respiratory distress.

BRONCHIOLITIS

An acute viral infection of the lower respiratory tract (bronchioles) that is spread by **direct contact with respiratory secretions** and is most symptomatic in children < 2 years of age. It involves epithelial cell sloughing, ↑ mucus secretions, and airway edema → obstruction of the small airways. The seasonal peak differs with geographic location, ranging from the winter months to no peak at all. Bronchiolitis causes morbidity in ex-preemies and in those with chronic medical problems. Reinfection is common. Causes include the following:

- RSV (responsible for up to 85% of cases).
- Adenovirus, human metapneumovirus, parainfluenza virus, and influenza can also → bronchiolitis.

Bronchiolitis may → apnea in young infants (< 6 weeks)

Symptoms/Exam

- Fever, hypoxia, tachypnea; nasal discharge; retractions, grunting, wheezing, and crackles.
- Cyanosis is seen if hypoxia is severe (more common in young infants).

Diagnosis

- Usually clinical; no additional lab tests are necessary if the diagnosis is straightforward and the disease is mild or moderate.
- CXR shows air trapping, peribronchial cuffing, and atelectasis; patchy infiltrates may be present.
- DFA and PCR tests can be used.
- Viral cultures are less sensitive but 100% specific.

Steroids do not ↓ the likelihood of long-term wheezing or asthma following RSV infection.

Treatment

- **Hospitalization:** Required in an estimated 3% of all cases; hospitalization rate is inversely proportional to age. Indications include apnea, moderate to severe distress, dehydration/poor feeding, hypoxemia, and the need for frequent suctioning.
- **Steroids:** Systemic or inhaled; generally not useful in bronchiolitis unless the child has a history of asthma.
- **Bronchodilators:** Has no proven benefit in bronchiolitis, but may be helpful in those with a history of asthma.
- **Ribavirin:** Controversial, but may be considered in patients at high risk for severe disease, including those affected by bronchopulmonary dysplasia, prematurity, or immunodeficiency.

Complications

Bacterial coinfection (pneumonia, otitis media) may occur in bronchiolitis and is something to consider in patients who do not improve or who develop a new fever after several days of illness.

RSV-IVIG, not palivizumab, can interfere with vaccine administration.

Prevention

- AAP guidelines recommend the use of RSV immune globulin (RSV-IVIG) or palivizumab for children < 24 months of age with the following:
  - Chronic lung disease on therapy within six months of RSV season; or
  - Premature birth (32 weeks or less; or 35 weeks or less with two additional risk factors such as day care attendance, school-aged siblings, exposure to environmental air pollutants, congenital abnormalities of the airways, or severe neuromuscular disease). Those at 28 weeks' GA or less may benefit from a second season of prophylaxis.
- Palivizumab is preferred over RSV-IVIG because of its ease of administration, safety, and effectiveness. Only palivizumab is indicated for those with hemodynamically significant congenital heart disease. In addition, palivizumab does not interfere with vaccine administration.
- In general, tobacco smoke, crowds, and day care should be avoided in high-risk children.

A four-year-old boy who had a cough and runny nose two weeks ago presents with a four-day history of new fever, cough, ↓ appetite, emesis, and lethargy. His temperature is 38.6°C (101.5°F), his respiratory rate is 38, and his O_2 saturation is 96% on room air. His chest is clear to auscultation, but his CXR reveals a round opacity in the basal portion of the right lower lobe. His left lung is normal. CBC reveals a WBC count of 16,400/μL with 80% neutrophils, 15% lymphocytes, 4% monocytes, and 1% eosinophils. What is the most likely diagnosis? Pulmonary abscess, defined as a discrete, walled-off area of infection and necrosis in the lung. Pulmonary abscess can occur at any age but affects males more than females, more frequently involving the right lung than the left lung. The condition is more likely to occur in those with impaired lung defenses—e.g., those with bacterial or viral infections, anatomic abnormalities, immunodeficiency, or impaired cough. The most common pathogens are *S. aureus* and *S. pneumoniae*. Aspiration of oral bacteria can also ↑ the risk of pulmonary abscess. Anaerobic organisms can produce foul breath, and abscess spread or rupture can lead to drainage of pus into the airway, hemoptysis, and bronchopleural fistula. What would you do for this patient? Additional workup may include sputum for Gram stain and culture and a chest CT; treatment is with antibiotic therapy, typically a long course. Drainage may lead to bronchopleural fistula. Abscesses can take many months to disappear radiographically.

PNEUMONIA

Infection/inflammation of the terminal and respiratory bronchioles, alveoli, and interstitium. May occur simultaneously with laryngotracheitis or bronchiolitis. Host defenses against pneumonia include nasopharyngeal filtration, laryngeal airway protection (epiglottis, vocal cords), mucociliary clearance, cough, cellular and humoral immunity, and other immune mechanisms. Affects 4–6% of U.S. children annually; incidence and causative organisms vary by age (see also Table 18-5).

- **Neonates:** Often vertical transmission.
    - **Bacterial:**
        - **Group B strep:** Look for **pleural effusions** on CXR.
        - *E. coli.*
        - *Listeria, H. influenzae,* group D strep, *S. pneumoniae.*
        - *Ureaplasma urealyticum:* Associated with an ↑ risk of chronic lung disease. Treat with **erythromycin.**
    - **Viral:**
        - **CMV:** Does not require treatment in an otherwise healthy infant.
        - Rubella.
        - **HSV: Requires IV acyclovir.**
- **Infants:**
    - **Bacterial:**
        - *S. pneumoniae, S. aureus.*
        - *Moraxella:* Hib (less common since immunization).
        - **Pertussis:** Children < 6 months of age may not present with the classic "whoop." Diagnosis is confirmed by **PCR** (DFA and culture are only half as sensitive). **Erythromycin will ↓ transmission** but

TABLE 18-5. Special Cases of Pneumonia

MANIFESTATION	POTENTIAL DIAGNOSIS	COMMENTS
Aspiration	Often a sterile **pneumonitis,** especially in the absence of focal infiltrates. In those with **poor oral hygiene,** think **anaerobes** and *Actinomyces.*	**Up to 50%** of patients with acute aspiration pneumonia develop **2° infection** with ***S. aureus, Klebsiella,*** and ***Pseudomonas,*** among others. **Chronic aspiration** may be seen in those with poor airway protection or neuromuscular compromise.
Pleural effusion	*S. aureus.*	See the discussion of pleural effusion.
Pulmonary abscess	*S. aureus* is responsible for some 75% of 1° abscesses. Anaerobes are responsible for 2° abscesses.	
Persistent lobar density	**Foreign body;** intralobar sequestration (lower lobe).	Foreign body can present as persistent density in any lobe, as focal hyperinflation, or as recurrent cough. Decubitus and expiration films can be helpful; most often, **bronchoscopy** is needed.
Rabbit exposure	Tularemia.	Flulike; presents with skin lesions. Treat with **streptomycin.**
Rodent exposure, southwestern United States	Hantavirus.	Flulike prodrome, sudden ARDS, sometimes DIC, death.
Sheep/cattle exposure	Q fever; *Coxiella.*	From inhalation/ingestion of milk, etc. Treat with **tetracycline.**
Dog/cat exposure	Visceral larvae migrans.	Hepatomegaly. Toddlers are often affected.
Pigeon/poultry/bird exposure	Psittacosis, *Cryptococcus* (pigeon breeders).	**Psittacosis:** Headache and rash. Treat with **doxycycline.** *Cryptococcus:* Responsible for mild symptoms in the immunocompetent, but associated with significant disease in AIDS.
Exposure to the southwestern United States	Coccidioidomycosis.	May mimic TB.
Exposure to the Midwest or the Mississippi River Valley.	Histoplasmosis (history of bat or bird dung exposure), blastomycosis.	Skin lesions are common with blastomycosis, which may resolve without therapy in an immunocompetent host.
CF	*Staphylococcus, Pseudomonas, Burkholderia cepacia, Aspergillus* (allergic bronchopulmonary aspergillosis [ABPA]).	ABPA presents with a high IgE (> 1000), ⊕ IgG/RAST panels, and radiographic/PFT decline in spite of good antibiotic therapy. **Treat with steroids and antifungals.**

TABLE 18-5. Special Cases of Pneumonia (continued)

MANIFESTATION	POTENTIAL DIAGNOSIS	COMMENTS
Asthma	ABPA.	See above.
Neuromuscular compromise/tracheostomy	*Pseudomonas, Klebsiella,* gram-$\ominus$ organisms. Patients are at ↑ risk for any airway infection.	*Pseudomonas* often acquires rapid resistance; often two agents are used.
Immunodeficiency	PCP, *Nocardia, Cryptococcus,* lymphocytic interstitial pneumonitis, CMV.	*Nocardia* is often associated with **eosinophilia**; treat with **TMP-SMX**. See the discussion above for *Cryptococcus* infection.
Anemia (microcytic)	Alveolar hemorrhage.	
Foreign travel	Typhoid, TB.	
Sickle cell anemia	Acute chest.	See the Hematology chapter.

will not change the course of this toxin-mediated illness. (Think **Per**tussis is diagnosed by **PCR**; **P**revent spread with antibiotics.)
- *Chlamydia trachomatis:* Look for a peripheral **eosinophilia** and pleocytosis. Treat with **erythromycin** 50 mg/kg/day × 10 days.
- **Viral:** RSV, parainfluenza virus, influenza virus, adenovirus (requires a viral culture to diagnose; uncommonly, can → **bronchiolitis obliterans**).
- **Preschoolers:**
  - **Bacterial:** *S. pneumoniae, S. aureus, Moraxella* (Hib), *Neisseria meningitidis, Mycoplasma* (less likely in this age group than in older children).
  - **Viral: More common than bacterial in this age group:** same profile as infants
- **School-age children and teens:**
  - **Bacterial:**
    - *Mycoplasma:* Associated with headache, low-grade fever, and GI symptoms; treat with a **macrolide.**
    - *Chlamydia pneumoniae:* Associated with high fever and pharyngitis; may be difficult to distinguish from mycoplasma infection. Treat with a **macrolide.**
    - *S. pneumoniae* **and others:** Noted in the preschooler section.
    - **Viral:** Same as for preschoolers. Viruses, *Mycoplasma,* and *C. pneumoniae* make up the majority of cases of pneumonia in school-age children and beyond.

SYMPTOMS/EXAM

- Fever, tachypnea, hypoxia, retractions, grunting (neonates/infants), cough (except in neonates).
- Focal or diffuse crackles; wheezes (interstitial processes → diffuse findings).

Bacterial pneumonia in the first 24 hours of life may be confused with transient tachypnea of the newborn or RDS.

When severe and in a high-risk patient, influenza **A** may be treated with **Amantadine.**

- ■ Tactile fremitus and egophony can indicate consolidation.
- ■ Percussion may identify consolidation.
- ■ ↓ breath sounds are seen; patients may also have abdominal pain.

DIAGNOSIS

- ■ Few lab studies are helpful in the diagnosis of community-acquired pneumonia.
- ■ Outside of the neonatal period, blood cultures are rarely helpful.
- ■ CBC may be abnormal (elevated and left-shifted WBC in bacterial pneumonia, especially with strep pneumonia) but do not need to be obtained routinely. CBC is more helpful in the setting of immunodeficiency or suspected hemorrhage.
- ■ Sputum Gram stain and culture may be helpful in special populations (e.g., patients with a tracheostomy or CF).
- ■ In the febrile, nontoxic patient with a compatible exam, CXR is confirmatory and does not need to be obtained routinely.
- ■ CXR can be helpful in assessing effusion/empyema in an ill-appearing child or a child who has not improved clinically; CT may be needed to provide full detail.
- ■ Bedside cold agglutinins can confirm *Mycoplasma* pneumonia but is neither sensitive nor specific.

Cough following viral pneumonia and pertussis may last 3–4 months. Teens may be at risk for pertussis as the degree of immunity conferred by immunization wanes.

Follow-up CXRs are not necessary in an otherwise recovered child.

TUBERCULOSIS

See the Infectious Disease chapter.

OBSTRUCTIVE LUNG DISEASES

A three-year-old Caucasian girl has been followed by her 1° physician for failure to thrive. She is below the fifth percentile for weight and at the fifth percentile for height despite a seemingly normal diet. Her past medical history reveals three hospitalizations for pneumonia and frequent bouts of wheezing. Her parents and two siblings are generally healthy. What study would you order next? A sweat chloride test should be obtained to rule out CF. Are there any other questions you can ask to support this diagnosis? The parents should be asked about constipation, fat malabsorption, "floating stools," and any history of rectal prolapse.

Cystic Fibrosis (CF)

An autosomal-recessive disorder consisting of the triad of COPD, pancreatic exocrine deficiency, and abnormal sweat chloride. Delta F508 represents 70% of all CFTR mutations. CF is the most common lethal genetic disease in Caucasians; average life expectancy is 33.4 years.

SYMPTOMS/EXAM

- ■ Frequent respiratory and sinus infections.
- ■ Failure to thrive.
- ■ Constipation or loose, frequent stools.

In a child with recurrent sinopulmonary illnesses and failure to thrive, think CF.

- **Fat malabsorption:** Patients may have a history of "floating stools."
- May present early with meconium ileus.
- May also present with **rectal prolapse.**

DIAGNOSIS

- **The gold standard is the sweat chloride test.**
  - **Normal:** < 40 mmol/L.
  - **Borderline:** 40–59 mmol/L.
  - **CF:** > 59 mmol/L.
- A CF mutation panel revealing two CF mutations is also diagnostic.
- A ⊕ sweat test must be confirmed by a second sweat test or by a mutation analysis.
- Maintain a high degree of suspicion if there is a first-degree relative with CF.
- Fecal fat measurements and stool elastase are helpful but not diagnostic.
- Testing for ↑ potential differences across the nasal epithelium may be of use.

TREATMENT

Table 18-6 lists treatment guidelines for CF according to the system affected.

Think of meconium ileus if abdominal calcifications are seen on prenatal ultrasound.

The systemic immune system is not impaired in CF, and septicemia and extrasinopulmonary infections are rare.

TABLE 18-6. Manifestations and Treatment of Cystic Fibrosis

SYSTEM	SYMPTOMS/EXAM	TREATMENT	COMPLICATIONS
Sinus	Chronic sinusitis, polyps.	Nasal steroids, saline rinses, sinus surgery.	Bony erosion of sinuses.
Lungs	Obstruction of small airways with thick mucus; inflammation of small and then large airways; bronchiectasis; pulmonary infection (e.g., **Staphylococcus, Pseudomonas, B. cepacia, Stenotrophomas**); atelectasis and air trapping.	Bronchodilators; mucus clearance (chest physiotherapy/mucolytics); aggressive antibiotics for infection.	ABPA, pneumothorax, pulmonary hypertension, RVH, respiratory failure.
Hepatobiliary	Cholecystitis, cholelithiasis, cholestasis.	Treatment as needed.	Portal hypertension, cirrhosis.
Endocrine	Pancreatic insufficiency with autodigestion of pancreas; pancreatitis.	Enzyme replacement.	CF-related diabetes.
GI/metabolic	Meconium ileus or plug intussusception; rectal prolapse; distal intestinal obstruction syndrome; fat-soluble vitamin and essential fatty acid deficiencies; malnutrition and growth failure; salt deficiency, especially in hot climates.	Enzyme replacement; ADEK vitamins; high-fat diet; nutrition counseling; salt replacement.	Obstruction → microcolon (neonates) or perforation (uncommon); hyponatremic dehydration.
Reproductive	Absence of the vas deferens in males; thick cervical mucus in females. Pregnancy rates in women with CF may be somewhat lower than that of the general population.	Reproductive counseling.	

Asthma

Defined as chronic, reversible airflow obstruction characterized by airway hyperreactivity, inflammation, and excess mucus production. Etiologies are described in the discussion of cough.

SYMPTOMS

- Episodic wheezing, shortness of breath, chest tightness, hyperinflation, and cough are common.
- Often occurs in the presence of triggers, including viral infection (**most common**), environmental irritants and allergens, exercise, and cold exposure.

EXAM

All that wheezes is not asthma!

- Examination may reveal tachycardia, tachypnea, desaturation, and **pulsus paradoxus** (a drop in SBP of > 10 mmHg during inspiration).
- Wheezing, prolonged I-E ratio, ↓ aeration, difficulty speaking, and respiratory distress are also seen.
- ↑ wheezing may be heard after bronchodilator use as a result of ↑ air entry.
- **Asthma is rarely associated with clubbing!**

DIAGNOSIS

- Based largely on the history and physical exam. Disease classification is based on symptoms (see Tables 18-7 and 18-8).
- CXR may reveal hyperinflation and ↑ AP diameter.
- Spirometry; peak flow measurements.

TREATMENT

Tables 18-7 and 18-8 outline treatment guidelines for asthma delineated by the National Asthma Education and Prevention Program (NAEPP).

Classify Severity: Clinical Features Before Treatment or Adequate Control			Medications Required To Maintain Long-Term Control
	Symptoms/Day Symptoms/Night	PEF or FEV₁ PEF Variability	Daily Medications

Step 4
Severe Persistent
	Continual
	Frequent
		≤ 60%
		> 30%
			■ Preferred treatment:
			– High-dose inhaled corticosteroids
			  AND
			– Long-acting inhaled beta₂-agonists
			  AND, if needed,
			– Corticosteroid tablets or syrup long term (2 mg/kg/day, generally do not exceed 60 mg per day). (Make repeat attempts to reduce systemic corticosteroids and maintain control with high-dose inhaled corticosteroids.)

Step 3 Moderate Persistent	Daily > 1 night/week	> 60% – < 80% > 30%	■ Preferred treatment: – Low-to-medium dose inhaled corticosteroids and long-acting inhaled beta₂-agonists. ■ Alternative treatment (listed alphabetically): – Increase inhaled corticosteroids within medium-dose range OR – Low-to-medium dose inhaled corticosteroids and either leukotriene modifier or theophylline. If needed (particularly in patients with recurring severe exacerbations): ■ Preferred treatment: – Increase inhaled corticosteroids within medium-dose range and add long-acting inhaled beta₂-agonists. ■ Alternative treatment (listed alphabetically): – Increase inhaled corticosteroids within medium-dose range and add either leukotriene modifier or theophylline.
Step 2 Mild Persistent	> 2/week but < 1x/day > 2 nights/month	≥ 80% 20–30%	■ Preferred treatment: – Low-dose inhaled corticosteroids. ■ Alternative treatment (listed alphabetically): cromolyn, leukotriene modifier, nedocromil, OR sustained-release theophylline to serum concentration of 5–15 mcg/mL.
Step 1 Mild Intermittent	≤ 2 days/week ≤ 2 nights/month	≥ 80% < 20%	■ No daily medication needed. ■ Severe exacerbations may occur, separated by long periods of normal lung function and no symptoms. A course of systemic corticosteroids is recommended.
Quick Relief All Patients			■ Short-acting bronchodilator: 2–4 puffs **short-acting inhaled beta₂-agonists** as needed for symptoms. ■ Intensity of treatment will depend on severity of exacerbation; up to 3 treatments at 20-minute intervals or a single nebulizer treatment as needed. Course of systemic corticosteroids may be needed. ■ Use of short-acting beta₂-agonists >2 times a week in intermittent asthma (daily, or increasing use in persistent asthma) may indicate the need to initiate (increase) long-term-control therapy.

Step down
Review treatment every 1 to 6 months; a gradual stepwise reduction in treatment may be possible.

Step up
If control is not maintained, consider step up. First, review patient medication technique, adherence, and environmental control.

Goals of Therapy: Asthma Control

- Minimal or no chronic symptoms day or night
- Minimal or no exacerbations
- No limitations on activities; no school/work missed
- Maintain (near) normal pulmonary function
- Minimal use of short-acting inhaled beta₂-agonist
- Minimal or no adverse effects from medications

Note
- The stepwise approach is meant to assist, not replace, the clinical decisionmaking required to meet individual patient needs.
- Classify severity: assign patient to most severe step in which any feature occurs (PEF is % of personal best; FEV₁ is % predicted).
- Gain control as quickly as possible (consider a short course of systemic corticosteroids); then step down to the least medication necessary to maintain control.
- Minimize use of short-acting inhaled beta₂-agonists. Overreliance on short-acting inhaled beta₂-agonists (e.g., use of approximately one canister a month even if not using it every day) indicates inadequate control of asthma and the need to initiate or intensify long-term-control therapy.
- Provide education on self-management and controlling environmental factors that make asthma worse (e.g., allergens and irritants).
- Refer to an asthma specialist if there are difficulties controlling asthma or if step 4 care is required. Referral may be considered if step 3 care is required.

THE PULMONARY SYSTEM

TABLE 18-8. Management of Asthma in Infants and Children < 5 Years of Age.

Classify Severity: Clinical Features Before Treatment or Adequate Control	Symptoms/Day / Symptoms/Night	Medications Required To Maintain Long-Term Control — Daily Medications
Step 4 Severe Persistent	Continual / Frequent	■ Preferred treatment: – High-dose inhaled corticosteroids AND – Long-acting inhaled beta₂-agonists AND, if needed, – Corticosteroid tablets or syrup long term (2 mg/kg/day, generally do not exceed 60 mg per day). (Make repeat attempts to reduce systemic corticosteroids and maintain control with high-dose inhaled corticosteroids.)
Step 3 Moderate Persistent	Daily / > 1 night/week	■ Preferred treatments: – Low-dose inhaled corticosteroids and long-acting inhaled beta₂-agonists OR – Medium-dose inhaled corticosteroids. ■ Alternative treatment: – Low-dose inhaled corticosteroids and either leukotriene receptor antagonist or theophylline. If needed (particularly in patients with recurring severe exacerbations): ■ Preferred treatment: – Medium-dose inhaled corticosteroids and long-acting beta₂-agonists. ■ Alternative treatment: – Medium-dose inhaled corticosteroids and either leukotriene receptor antagonist or theophylline.
Step 2 Mild Persistent	> 2/week but < 1x/day / > 2 nights/month	■ Preferred treatment: – Low-dose inhaled corticosteroid (with nebulizer or MDI with holding chamber with or without face mask or DPI). ■ Alternative treatment (listed alphabetically): – Cromolyn (nebulizer is preferred or MDI with holding chamber) OR leukotriene receptor antagonist.
Step 1 Mild Intermittent	≤ 2 days/week / ≤ 2 nights/month	■ No daily medication needed.

Quick Relief — All Patients

■ Bronchodilator as needed for symptoms. Intensity of treatment will depend upon severity of exacerbation.
  – Preferred treatment: Short-acting inhaled beta₂-agonists by nebulizer or face mask and space/holding chamber
  – Alternative treatment: Oral beta₂-agonist
■ With viral respiratory infection
  – Bronchodilator q 4–6 hours up to 24 hours (longer with physician consult); in general, repeat no more than once every 6 weeks
  – Consider systemic corticosteroid if exacerbation is severe or patient has history of previous severe exacerbations
■ Use of short-acting beta₂-agonists >2 times a week in intermittent asthma (daily, or increasing use in persistent asthma) may indicate the need to initiate (increase) long-term-control therapy.

Step down
Review treatment every 1 to 6 months; a gradual stepwise reduction in treatment may be possible.

Step up
If control is not maintained, consider step up. First, review patient medication technique, adherence, and environmental control.

Goals of Therapy: Asthma Control
■ Minimal or no chronic symptoms day or night
■ Minimal or no exacerbations
■ No limitations on activities; no school/parent's work missed
■ Minimal use of short-acting inhaled beta₂-agonist
■ Minimal or no adverse effects from medications

Note
■ The stepwise approach is intended to assist, not replace, the clinical decisionmaking required to meet individual patient needs.
■ Classify severity: assign patient to most severe step in which any feature occurs.
■ There are very few studies on asthma therapy for infants.
■ Gain control as quickly as possible (a course of short systemic corticosteroids may be required), then step down to the least medication necessary to maintain control.
■ Minimize use of short-acting inhaled beta₂-agonists. Overreliance on short-acting inhaled beta₂-agonists (e.g., use of approximately one canister a month even if not using it every day) indicates inadequate control of asthma and the need to initiate or intensify long-term-control therapy.
■ Provide parent education on asthma management and controlling environmental factors that make asthma worse (e.g., allergies and irritants).
■ Consultation with an asthma specialist is recommended for patients with moderate or severe persistent asthma. Consider consultation for patients with mild persistent asthma.

Reproduced from the National Heart, Lung, and Blood Institute, National Institutes of Health, Bethesda, MD; available at www.nhlbi.nih.gov/guidelines/asthma/asthsumm.htm.

THE PULMONARY SYSTEM

Bronchopulmonary Dysplasia and Chronic Lung Disease

See the Neonatology chapter.

Other Obstructive Lung Diseases

Table 18-9 lists the etiologies, presentation, diagnosis, and treatment of other pulmonary diseases presenting with obstruction.

TABLE 18-9. Presentation and Treatment of Other Obstructive Lung Diseases

DISEASE	ETIOLOGY	PRESENTATION	DIAGNOSIS	TREATMENT/OUTCOME
Ciliary dyskinesia (Kartagener's syndrome)	Dynein arm defects → abnormal ciliary movement. Has an incidence of 1 in 16,000; males and females are affected equally. May be autosomal recessive.	Recurrent respiratory infection, otitis media, sinusitis, male infertility. Some **50% of cases are associated with situs inversus.**	Clinical suspicion. CXR may reveal hyperinflation, dextrocardia, or **bronchiectasis.** Ciliary biopsy by nasal scraping or bronchial brush.	Antibiotics, mucus clearance, sinus surgery; lobectomy in severe bronchiectasis.
ABPA	Allergic reaction to *Aspergillus* (usually *A. fumigatus*) in patients with chronic lung disease. Occurs in 1–2% of asthmatics and in 11% of those with CF. Noninvasive.	Low-grade fever, prolonged wheezing, cough. No improvement is seen with antibiotics.	Peripheral blood eosinophilia, transient infiltrates, ↑ **IgE** precipitating antibody to *Aspergillus*, bronchiectasis.	Give steroids for three months or longer. The goal is to normalize IgE.
α_1-antitrypsin (AAT) deficiency	Lack of AAT protection against proteinase damage. Incidence is 1 in 3000–5000; primarily affects Caucasians. Males and females are equally affected.	**Neonatal jaundice,** hepatomegaly, ascites. In the first two decades of life, **liver disease** is predominant. In adults, early-onset panacinar emphysema is seen.	Serum AAT levels.	Death in childhood is rare; patients usually live to the fourth or fifth decade. Death occurs much earlier in smokers.
Congenital lobar emphysema (CLE)	Usually unilobar overdistention from a variety of anatomic defects, or may be idiopathic.	Wheezing, shortness of breath, tachypnea, tachycardia, asymmetry of the chest, hyperresonance.	Prenatal ultrasound. CXR reveals hyperinflation of one lobe with mediastinal shift and compression of the remaining lung (see Figure 18-3). The left upper lobe is most commonly affected (40%). CT scan can yield more detailed information.	**Distinguish from pneumothorax!** **Large:** Lobectomy. **Small:** Watchful management; may have recurrent pain.

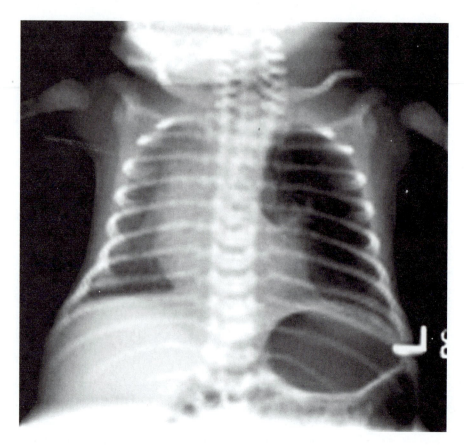

FIGURE 18-3. Congenital lobar emphysema of the left upper lobe of a two-week-old boy.

The mediastinum is shifted to the right. (Reproduced, with permission, from Brunicardi FC et al [eds]. *Schwartz's Principles of Surgery*, 8th ed. New York: McGraw-Hill, 2005:1479.)

RESTRICTIVE LUNG DISEASES

To be sure that restriction is present, TLC must also be less than normal.

Disorders in which lung volume (FVC) is reduced by a process other than obstruction (which can → 2° restriction via air trapping). See Table 18-10 for etiologies.

Bronchiolitis Obliterans Organizing Pneumonia (BOOP)

Table 18-11 outlines the presentation and treatment of BOOP.

Interstitial Diseases

In a child with a history of cardiac surgery and a diaphragmatic paralysis, think phrenic nerve injury. Stretch injury may recover; if not, diaphragmatic plication is required!

A group of **rare** disorders → **impaired gas exchange** and **fibrotic remodeling** of the distal airways and alveoli. Interstitial lung disease (ILD) is characterized as a **restrictive lung process.** Disorders are heterogenous but generally include symptoms lasting > 1 month, diffuse infiltrates on CXR, and the absence of any other known cause. Infections → ILD include the following:

- **Viral:** CMV or adenovirus.
- **Bacterial:** *Mycoplasma, Chlamydia, Legionella.*
- **Fungal:** PCP, *Aspergillus, Histoplasma.*
- **Parasitic:** Visceral larva migrans.

544

TABLE 18-10. Causes of Restrictive Lung Disease

Lung	Pleural Cavity	Chest Wall	Muscle
Resection or hypoplasia Atelectasis Fibrosis, ILD CHF: vascular congestion, ↑ interstitial fluid Tumor Pneumonia/ parenchymal lung diseases	Pleural thickening Effusion/empyema	Scoliosis Splinting due to pain Scleroderma Abdominal visceromegaly or ascites	Neuromuscular disease Diaphragmatic paralysis

SYMPTOMS

Tachypnea, retractions, exercise intolerance (75%); dry cough (75%); poor weight gain; wheezing (20–40%) +/– hemoptysis if a hemorrhagic process is involved.

EXAM

Weight loss/failure to thrive, hypoxemia, crackles, pulmonary hypertension, and RVH (loud P2).

ILD may occur in the setting of other systemic diseases, including autoimmune disorders, connective tissue disease, and vasculitides, as well as in IBD and transplant-associated disorders.

TABLE 18-11. Presentation of Bronchiolitis Obliterans Organizing Pneumonia

Etiology	Exam	Diagnosis	Treatment
Granulation in the distal airways, in particular the bronchioles. Half of all cases are idiopathic. The remaining cases are caused by **infection** (*Coxiella, Pseudomonas, Mycoplasma*), radiation, **BMT** or organ transplant, or drugs/toxins.	Hypoxia, fine crackles, shortness of breath. Unresponsive to antibiotics.	Tissue biopsy is required for precise diagnosis. CXR shows bilateral, patchy alveolar airspace consolidation that is often worse in the lower fields; air bronchograms may also be seen. Effusions are rare. PFTs show restriction and ↓ DL_{CO}. Bronchoalveolar lavage may be helpful to rule out other diagnoses; fluid shows ↑ lymphocytes.	Mortality is up to 10%. Steroids are the mainstay; if treated for < 1 year, recurrence may be seen.

<table>
<tr><td>

Causes of ILD—A SHIP'S BLIND Environment

Aspiration pneumonitis (5%); also **A**utoimmune

Storage/metabolic disorders

Hemosiderosis and **H**emorrhagic disorders (5–8%)

Infection (8–10%)

Pulmonary alveolar proteinosis

Sarcoid (2%)

BOOP

Lymphangiomatosis (4%)

Idiopathic

Neoplasia (e.g., Langerhans histiocytosis) (1%)

Drugs (anticancer drugs are often implicated, e.g., bleomycin)

Environment (13%; e.g., hypersensitivity pneumonitis, radiation)

</td></tr>
</table>

DIAGNOSIS

- Obtain a CBC.
- **UA:** If glomerulonephritis is present, think pulmonary-renal syndrome.
- **Stool guaiac:** Obtain if coincident with IBD.
- Rheumatic disease markers.
- **Angiotensin-converting enzyme (ACE) level:** Obtain if sarcoid is suspected.
- **Serum precipitants:** If hypersensitivity pneumonitis is suspected.
- Respiratory viral studies; *Mycoplasma* serologies.
- **CXR:** Useful in up to 40% of cases; look for **ground glass** and **reticular-nodular densities.**
- **CT scan:** Shows "crazy paving" and honeycombing.
- **PFTs:** DL_{CO} is ↓; **a restrictive** pattern is seen.
- ECG, echocardiography.
- Bronchoalveolar lavage.
- **Lung biopsy:** Offers the best chance of **definitive diagnosis.**

TREATMENT

- A large number of immunosuppressive agents have been tried.
- Bronchodilators and inhaled steroids if there is airway reactivity; O_2 as needed.
- In severe cases, heart-lung transplantation may be necessary.
- Survival at five years is 64%.

DEVELOPMENTAL ANOMALIES

Table 18-12 outlines common developmental anomalies with respiratory features.

You are evaluating an obese seven-year-old boy for hyperactivity. You notice on exam that he has large tonsils. His mother confirms that the boy snores loudly every night and states that it sometimes sounds as if he stops breathing. You diagnose obstructive sleep apnea. Which further studies can support your diagnosis? A sleep study should be performed. Chronic hypoventilation can be further supported by an ABG demonstrating respiratory acidosis with metabolic compensation, an ECG with RVH, and a CBC with polycythemia as a result of chronic hypoxemia.

CHRONIC HYPOVENTILATION SYNDROMES

Defined as impaired gas exchange with an ↑ in arterial P_{CO_2}. **Central hypoventilation** is rare and is usually caused by CNS dysfunction, impaired nerve conduction, or profound muscle weakness. **Obstructive hypoventilation**/sleep apnea are common in children, with tonsillar/adenoidal hypertrophy the most common cause. Less common causes include craniofacial syndromes, nasal obstruction, poor oral motor tone, and macroglossia.

SYMPTOMS/EXAM

Table 18-13 distinguishes the presentation of central hypoventilation from that of obstructive hypoventilation.

TABLE 18-12. **Developmental Anomalies**

	INCIDENCE AND EPIDEMIOLOGY	DEFINITION AND FEATURES	TREATMENT
Congenital diaphragmatic hernia	Incidence is 1 in 2000–5000. Primarily affects term males. Some 90% occur on the left.	A diaphragmatic defect occurring at 8–12 weeks' gestational age with lung compression → pulmonary hypoplasia. Also presents with respiratory distress at birth and bowel sounds in the chest (see Figure 18-4).	Avoid bag/mask ventilation and initiate immediate intubation. Surgical reduction/correction of hernia; treat pulmonary hypertension.
Pulmonary hypoplasia	Usually occurs with other abnormalities, such as oligohydramnios (Potter's syndrome: flattened face/nose; low-set ears; flexion contractures; bell-shaped chest), congenital diaphragmatic hernia, and anencephaly (↓ fetal breathing).	Varying degrees of respiratory distress; pulmonary hypertension. Lungs are small and hyperlucent on CXR.	Treat pulmonary hypertension; treat hypoxia if present. Prevent infection, especially in the first year of life, when alveolarization is still likely to occur.
Congenital cystic adenomatoid malformation (CCAM)	Associated with polyhydramnios and hydrops fetalis.	A lesion of abnormal proliferation of bronchiolar and pulmonary tissue that usually involves one lobe. Type I (large, widely spaced cysts) is most common. The mediastinum is shifted contralaterally, and the diaphragm is depressed on the CCAM side (see Figure 18-5).	Surgical resection.
Congenital lobar emphysema	Usually involves one lobe. The left upper lobe is most commonly affected (40%).	See the discussion of other obstructive lung diseases.	Lobectomy if large; if small and asymptomatic, may observe.
Pulmonary AVM	**Congenital:** May exist as a single lesion, multiple lesions, or diffuse "telangiectatic" lesions. **Acquired:** May occur in hepatopulmonary syndrome.	Arterial-to-venous connection without intervening capillary bed. Presents with desaturation and cyanosis. If located in the lower lung fields, saturation will improve with supine position.	Surgical resection if possible (delineate the lesion with angiography). If hepatopulmonary syndrome, correct the underlying liver disorder (e.g., transplant).

DIAGNOSIS

- History (loud snoring with pauses), exam (large tonsils).
- Sleep study +/− pH probe to evaluate reflux as a potentiator.
- **ABG:** Chronic arterial hypercapnia → renal wasting of H^+; ↑ serum bicarbonate brings pH closer to normal → 1° respiratory acidosis with metabolic compensation.

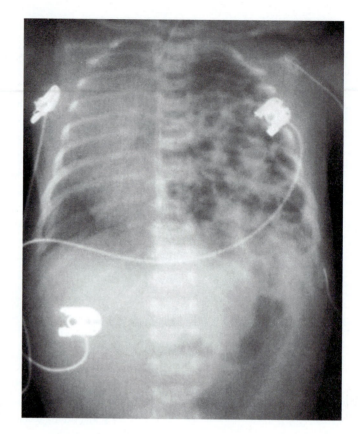

FIGURE 18-4. CXR showing a left congenital diaphragmatic hernia.

(Reproduced, with permission, from Brunicardi FC et al [eds]. *Schwartz's Principles of Surgery*, 8th ed. New York: McGraw-Hill, 2005:1478.)

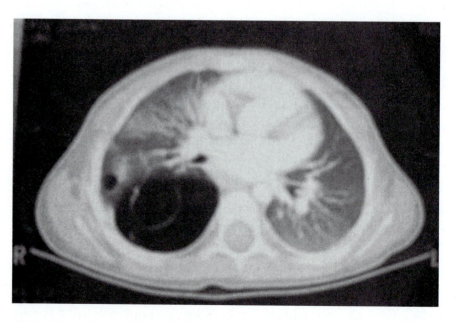

FIGURE 18-5. Congenital cystic adenomatoid malformation.

(Reproduced, with permission, from Brunicardi FC et al [eds]. *Schwartz's Principles of Surgery*, 8th ed. New York: McGraw-Hill, 2005:1479.)

TABLE 18-13. Central and Obstructive Hypoventilation

CONDITION	INCIDENCE	CENTRAL	OBSTRUCTIVE	HISTORY	TREATMENT
Nose: deviated septum, choanal stenosis, allergic rhinitis, polyp	Common	No	Yes	Trauma to the nose; patients are unable to move air through one or both nostrils.	Surgical correction; allergy treatment.
Mouth: macroglossia, poor oral pharyngeal or global tone	Seen with congenital syndromes (e.g., Down syndrome), cerebral palsy	No	Yes	Poor swallowing; large tongue; snoring.	Surgical correction; may need tracheostomy.
Tonsillar/ adenoidal hypertrophy	Most common	No	Yes	Snoring; apneic periods while sleeping; daytime sleepiness or hyperactivity. Exam reveals large tonsils +/– obesity.	Tonsillectomy and adenoidectomy. Note that there is **no direct correlation between tonsil size and severity of obstructive sleep apnea.**
Arnold-Chiari malformation	Rare	Yes	Yes, if there is vocal cord paralysis	May occur at any age and may wax and wane. Also presents with morning headache and difficulty swallowing.	Ventriculoperitoneal (VP) shunt to correct ICP; foramen magnum revision; ventilatory support; tracheotomy may be needed.
Craniofacial syndromes (e.g., Pfeiffer's, Treacher Collins syndromes)	Varies	No	Yes	Micrognathia, midface hypoplasia, macroglossia.	Surgical correction.
↑ICP (e.g., Dandy-Walker malformation)	Varies	Yes	Yes, if hypotonia is associated with the underlying condition	↑ head circumference, papilledema, seizures.	VP shunt; possibly tracheotomy and ventilation.
Congenital central hypo-ventilation syndrome (aka "Ondine's curse")	Rare	Yes	No	Presents early in life.	Ventilatory support night vs. 24 hours a day +/– phrenic nerve pacing.

THE PULMONARY SYSTEM

- **ECG/CXR:** Long-standing hypoventilation/hypercarbia may → pulmonary hypertension, RVH, and right heart failure.
- May have polycythemia due to chronic hypoxemia and resultant reticulocytosis.

TREATMENT

- **Obstructive:** Surgical correction of obstruction, noninvasive ventilation (CPAP, BiPAP), or tracheotomy.
- **Central:** Correction of foramen magnum stenosis, reduction of ICP, BiPAP, tracheotomy with ventilation.

Apnea of Prematurity

See the Neonatology chapter.

Pleural Disease

Pleural effusion is fluid in the pleural space; it may be caused by capillary leak from intraparenchymal disease, ↓ oncotic pressure, lymph disorders, or bleeding (see Table 18-14 and the mnemonic **O THINK**). Effusions may be classified as follows:

- **Uncomplicated:** Small volume of sterile fluid with PMNs.
- **Loculation/bacterial invasion:** PMNs lyse and LDH ↑. Bacteria are present. Fibrin/collagen loculations develop.
- **Empyema:** Thick, purulent fluid and cellular debris clog mechanisms for normal fluid drainage; fistulas occur. If antibiotics are started, thoracentesis fluid may be sterile.

SYMPTOMS

- Pain on inspiration +/– abdominal pain.
- Cough, shortness of breath/↑work of breathing, fever (if empyema).
- May be asymptomatic, especially if not associated with pneumonia.
- Hypoxemia/hypercapnia if large or with pneumonia.
- Mediastinal shift, ↓ venous return, ↓ cardiac output if large.

> **Causes of pleural effusions—O THINK**
>
> **O**ther (sickle cell, liver failure, etc.—3%)
> **T**rauma (7%)
> **H**eart failure (5–10%)
> **I**nfection (50–70%)
> **N**eoplasm (5–10%)
> **K**idney failure (8–10%)

TABLE 18-14. Types of Pleural Disease

TYPE	ETIOLOGY
Parapneumonic	Occurs with pneumonia, lung abscess, and/or bronchiectasis.
Empyema	Contains pus. Important to obtain fluid sample for diagnosis!
Chylothorax	Occurs from disruption of thoracic duct after surgery or trauma. High fat/triglyceride and lymphocyte content in fluid. It appears turbid or white but can be clear in neonates or fasting patients.
Hemothorax	Hematocrit of fluid is > 50% peripheral hematocrit.

Dullness to percussion, ↓ breath sounds, pleural rub in early effusion.

DIAGNOSIS

- **CXR:** Obtain PA/lateral decubitus views to look for layering.
- **Ultrasound:** To guide thoracentesis/tube; helps determine the amount of fluid.
- **CT:** Better than MRI for determining lung parenchymal or interstitial disease, pleural thickening, and mass.
- Chylothorax is more common on the right in babies.
- Tables 18-15 and 18-16 outline approaches toward the analysis of pleural fluid.

TREATMENT

- **Uncomplicated parapneumonic effusion:** Antibiotics alone.
- **Empyema/complicated pleural effusion:** Antibiotics plus drainage of infected fluid; consider video-assisted thoracoscopic surgery (VATS)/decortication. With multiple loculations, fibrinolysis with urokinase or tPA has been used but has not been fully studied and is **contraindicated in the presence of active bleeding.**
- **Chylothorax:** Formulas with medium-chain triglycerides; drain.
- **Hemothorax:** Achieve hemostasis; correct coagulopathy. Drain.
- Pleural biopsy is rarely indicated.

S. aureus is the most common cause of empyema, especially in younger children; strep is the second most common cause.

COMPLICATIONS

- Untreated parapneumonic effusions may → empyema.
- Loculations may reform even after drainage.
- Restrictive lung disease from fibrotic, damaged pleura is a long-term complication.

Stridor

Stridor indicates an **extrathoracic airway obstruction.** It is of variable pitch and is classically inspiratory, although biphasic stridor is also seen. Etiologies are as follows:

TABLE 18-15. Diagnostic Clues to Pleural Fluid Examination

APPEARANCE OF FLUID	POSSIBLE DIAGNOSIS
Light yellow	Transudate
Chalky, white	Chyle
Bloody	Infection/malignancy/trauma
Purulent	Bacterial infection
Chocolate colored	Amebiasis

TABLE 18-16. Laboratory Analysis of Pleural Fluid[a]

TYPE OF FLUID	GRAM STAIN/ CELL COUNT	pH	GLUCOSE[b]	PLEURAL-TO-SERUM (P:S) RATIOS
Exudate/empyema	PMN predominance	< 7.3	< 50% of serum level	P:S protein ≥ 0.5; P:S LDH ≥ 0.6
TB	Lymphocyte predominance		< 50% of serum level	P:S protein ≥ 0.5
Chyle	Lymphocyte predominance			P:S fat ≥ 1.0; P:S protein ≥ 0.5
Transudate	Low WBC count	≥ 7.3	> 50% of serum level	P:S protein ≥ 0.5; P: S LDH ≥ 0.6

[a] Transudate vs. exudate criteria are based on adult data and are not as reliable in children.

[b] Glucose may also be low in certain rheumatologic disorders such as RA but equal to serum levels in SLE.

- Anatomic:
  - Choanal atresia, thyroglossal cyst/lingual tonsil.
  - **Laryngomalacia (most common;** instrinsic floppiness of the supporting structures of the larynx).
  - Macroglossia (Beckwith-Weidemann syndrome, trisomy 21, congenital hypothyroidism, glycogen storage disease).
  - Micrognathia (Pierre Robin, Treacher Collins, Hallermann-Streiff syndromes).
  - Laryngeal cyst, web, laryngocele (usually present at birth or shortly thereafter).
  - Spasmodic croup.
  - **Vocal cord paresis/paralysis** (especially after **cardiac surgery** → left recurrent laryngeal nerve damage; also traumatic intubation).
  - Bulbar injury (bilateral cord paralysis in Arnold-Chiari, hydrocephalus).
  - **Subglottic stenosis** (especially with a history of **long-term intubation or a hypotensive episode while intubated**).
  - Subglottic hemangioma; cystic hygroma.
  - Laryngospasm (hypocalcemia, reflux, anesthesia).
  - Airway edema (e.g., in anaphylaxis or postextubation).
  - Extrathoracic tracheomalacia; external tracheal compression.
- **Infectious:** Laryngotracheitis (croup), tracheitis, laryngeal papilloma, epiglottitis.

DIAGNOSIS

- History is key!
- AP and lateral neck imaging may help assess the size of the tonsils and adenoids, the epiglottis, and the subglottic and tracheal anatomy.
- Airway bronchoscopy is most helpful for vocal cord paralysis and suspected laryngeal anatomic defects.

Wheezing

Wheeze means many things to many people, but for the purposes of this section, it is a high- or medium-pitched whistling noise classically heard on expiration (but may also be heard on inspiration) that indicates an **intrathoracic airway obstruction.** It may range in quality from soft and blowing to harsh and polyphonic. Etiologies are as follows:

- **Anatomic:** Tracheomalacia (lower pitch, "coarse wheeze"), tracheal stenosis, transesophageal fistula, vascular ring/sling, external compression by tumor (neuroblastoma), AAT deficiency, congenital lobar emphysema, bronchiectasis.
- **Infectious:** Bronchitis, **bronchiolitis,** visceral larva migrans.
- **Inflammatory:** Bronchopulmonary dysplasia, **CF,** ciliary dyskinesia, **asthma** (reversible), **aspiration pneumonitis.**
- **Other: Foreign body,** GERD (laryngeal chemoreceptors → bronchoconstriction), hemosiderosis, cardiac causes, hydrostatic edema, overcirculatory conditions.

DIAGNOSIS

- **Trial of bronchodilators:** Reversible airway obstruction?
- **Investigate infectious causes:** Sputum Gram stain and culture; viral studies.
- **Imaging:**
  - Modified barium swallow study for aspiration.
  - Barium swallow for vascular ring/external compression.
  - CXR for infection/mass.
  - CT scan for mass/focal parenchymal defect.
- Sweat test for CF; ciliary biopsy for ciliary function; pH probe for GERD.
- PFTs to assess for fixed airway obstruction (flow volume loop), small airway obstruction, ↑ airway resistance, and the like.
- Airway bronchoscopy +/– bronchoalveolar lavage for unusual infectious causes, dynamic airway compression/collapse, mass, or foreign body

Cough

Cough is a forceful, expiratory maneuver that helps clear mucus from the airways. It may occur acutely in the presence of infection or chronically for a variety of infectious and noninfectious reasons. Cough is under both voluntary and involuntary control. Chronic cough is defined as existing for > 3 weeks. Etiologies include the following:

- **Anatomic:** Transesophageal fistula, vascular ring.
- **Infectious:**
  - **Postnasal drip:** Viral, sinusitis.
  - **Croup:** Barking cough.
  - **Pertussis:** Whooping cough.
  - Bronchitis, bronchiolitis.
  - **Bacterial tracheitis:** Barking cough that is often associated with **inspiratory stridor. Staph** is most common. A **shaggy tracheal air column** is seen on x-ray. Infrequently, it may be an **emergency,** but up to 70% require intubation.
  - **Pneumonia:** Think *Mycoplasma* for a **dry cough.**
  - TB.

- **Inflammatory:** Postnasal drip (allergies), asthma, aspiration, postinfectious cough (up to 3–4 months), pulmonary fibrosis/autoimmune disease.
- **Other:** GERD, cardiac causes, tobacco exposure, behavioral cough, foreign body in the airway or esophagus.

SYMPTOMS/EXAM

- **History and physical** are key to determining if the patient is toxic or non-toxic.
- On examination, look for clues such as allergic shiners, nasal discharge or sinus tenderness, focal findings on chest exam, ↑ AP diameter (indicates air trapping), liver edge below costal margin, and clubbing.

DIAGNOSIS

As appropriate:

- **PFTs before and after bronchodilator or with methacholine challenge:** Asthma.
- **Lateral neck, AP neck, CXR:** Tracheitis, croup, foreign body, pneumonia, edema.
- **pH probe:** Reflux.
- **Modified barium swallow study:** Aspiration
- **Sweat chloride test:** CF.
- **Barium swallow:** Transesophageal fistula, vascular ring.
- **PPD:** TB.
- **Sinus CT:** Sinusitis (although it is reasonable to treat sinusitis on the basis of clinical suspicion).

TREATMENT

- Treat underlying illness when necessary. For cough associated with viral illness, keep in mind that if cough is due to postnasal drip, there may be a role for nasal decongestants (e.g., pseudoephedrine) Intranasal steroids appear to be safe in children down to 2–3 years and reduce rhinorrhea.
- A recent AAP policy statement states the following:
  - No well-controlled scientific studies were found that support the efficacy and safety of narcotics (including codeine) or dextromethorphan as antitussives in children.
  - Suppression of cough in many pulmonary airway diseases may be hazardous and contraindicated. Cough due to acute viral airway infections is short-lived and may be treated with fluids and humidity.
  - Dosage guidelines for cough and cold mixtures are extrapolated from adult data and clinical experience, and thus are imprecise for children. Adverse effects and overdosage associated with administration of cough and cold preparations in children are reported. Further research on the dosage, safety, and efficacy of these preparations needs to be done in children.

CHAPTER 19

The Renal System

Greg Gorman, MD, MHS
reviewed by Susan Furth, MD, PhD

Glomerular Filtration Rate (GFR)

Defined as the amount of plasma that would be entirely cleared of a substance in one minute by the amount of that substance excreted in the urine. It is usually normalized to body surface area (BSA) and expressed as mL/min/1.73 m^2. Normal GFR is > 120 mL/min/1.73 m^2. End-stage renal disease (ESRD) is < 15 mL/min/1.73 m^2.

DEVELOPMENT

- GFR is < 15 mL/min/1.73 m^2 for the first 3–5 days after birth and gradually increases to adult levels during the second year of life.
- Absolute GFR (not normed to BSA) reaches adult levels by adolescence.

MEASUREMENT

GFR is estimated in children and adolescents by the following means:

- **Schwartz formula:** $K \times$ height $\div$ serum creatinine, where $K = 0.55$ (0.7 for teenage boys; 0.45 for infants).
- Timed urine collection for creatinine clearance (which approximates GFR).
- Radionuclide study.

GFR per BSA reaches adult levels by two years of age. Absolute GFR does not reach adult levels until adolescence.

Tubular Function

Defined as the ability to modify ultrafiltrate through secretion or absorption in response to the hemodynamic and hormonal environment.

DEVELOPMENT

- Reabsorption of fluid and electrolytes (except for phosphate) is lower at birth than it is in older children and adults, developing in parallel with GFR.
- Phosphate reabsorption is higher in infants than it is in adults.
- Neonates have lower serum bicarbonate (21 mEq/L) than do adults.
- Urine concentrating ability reaches adult levels by three years of age.

MEASUREMENT

Tubular function is measured as follows:

- Fractional excretion or reabsorptive percentages (solutes).
- Osmolality (concentration).
- Urine protein electrophoresis (low-molecular-weight proteins).
- Direct measurement of substances not normally found in urine (glucose, amino acids).

Idiopathic nephrotic syndrome due to minimal change disease can be presumed without renal biopsy if the child has edema, hypoalbuminemia, normal complement, and nephrotic-range proteinuria; is 2–12 years of age; and does not have gross hematuria, hypertension, or renal insufficiency.

A 15-year-old girl has 2+ urine protein as noted by dipstick during a cheerleader physical. She has no edema and is asymptomatic. What single test will help dictate further diagnostic workup and management? Urine protein-to-creatinine ratio on a first-morning specimen. If the ratio is < 0.2, the diagnosis is likely orthostatic proteinuria and requires no further intervention unless clinical signs or symptoms develop.

Proteinuria

Defined as the excretion of > 4 mg/m^2/hr of protein in the urine, or a urine protein-to-creatinine ratio of > 0.2. Etiologies are as follows:

- **Transient:** Due to fever, illness, or exercise.
- **Orthostatic:** Proteinuria only when upright but absent when lying down.
- **Fixed:** Always pathologic.

DIAGNOSIS

Methods of testing for proteinuria are as follows (see also Table 19-1):

- **Urine dipstick:** Semiquantitative (a value of 3+ or 4+ is almost always abnormal). False ⊕s can be obtained with concentrated or high-pH urine.
- **Urine protein-to-creatinine ratio on first-morning specimen:** Quantitative.
- **Timed urine collection:** Gold standard, but difficult to collect. Ensure a properly collected specimen by making sure creatinine excretion is 15–20 mg/kg/day.
- **Microalbumin:** A highly sensitive means of obtaining urine albumin-to-creatinine ratio. Used to screen children with a high risk of developing kidney disease (e.g., diabetics).

Hematuria

Gross hematuria is visible blood; microscopic hematuria can be seen with a dipstick or microscopy. Hematuria may be urologic or glomerular in origin.

- The etiologies of gross hematuria are listed in the mnemonic **OUCH, RED URINE HURTS.**
- **Urologic:** Bleeding originating from the collecting system, bladder, or urethra.
- **Glomerular:** Etiologies include IgA nephropathy, minimal change disease (20% of cases have gross hematuria), and poststreptococcal glomerulonephritis (GN).

DIAGNOSIS

- Urine dipstick and microanalysis.
- **Urologic:** UA, urine calcium-to-creatinine ratio (normal < 0.2 for children > 1 year of age), imaging (ultrasound or CT), rarely cystoscopy.
- **Glomerular:** C3/C4, ANA, ASO, HBsAb, HCV Ab, Cr.

Causes of gross hematuria—OUCH, RED URINE HURTS

Oncologic agents (cytoxan)
Urethrorrhagia (squamous metaplasia of the urethra)
Coagulopathy
Hydronephrosis
Renal vein thrombosis
Exercise
Dead papillae (papillary necrosis)
Urolithiasis
Renal contusion
Infections (bacterial, adenovirus, schistosomiasis)
Neoplasm
External manipulation (masturbation)
Hypercalciuria
Urethral injury
Renal cysts
Trauma
Sickle cell

TABLE 19-1. Methods of Testing for Proteinuria

METHOD	COMMENT	FALSE $\oplus$	FALSE $\ominus$	NORMAL	SIGNIFICANT	NEPHROTIC RANGE
Dipstick	Albumin only; semiquantitative.	Concentrated urine or high pH.	Dilute urine or low pH.	$\ominus$ trace.	1+ to 4+.	2+ to 4 +.
Sulfosalicylic acid (SSA)	A quick test for proteinuria (including nonalbumin protein).	None.	None.	No precipitate.	Precipitate.	Precipitate.
Timed urine collection	Difficult to collect.	None.	None.	< 4 mg/m²/hr.	4–40 mg/m²/hr.	> 40 mg/m²/hr.
Protein-to-creatinine ratio	Easiest to collect.	Nonmorning specimen.	None.	< 0.2.	0.2–2.0.	> 2.0.
Microalbumin	Screening test for low levels of albuminuria. Good for screening diabetics and those at risk for renal disease.	Nonmorning specimen. Teenagers can have transient ↑ microalbumin.	None.	< 30 mg/g creatinine.	> 30 mg/g creatinine.	Not applicable.

ELECTROLYTE DISTURBANCES

Anion-Gap Metabolic Acidosis

Low serum pH with low bicarbonate and ↑ anion gap. Etiologies include excess acid in serum and organic acidemias (see also the mnemonic **MUD-PILES**).

DIAGNOSIS

- Low bicarbonate on chemistry panel; low pH on ABG.
- An anion gap (computed as $Na - [Cl + HCO_3]$) > 12.
- Search for the cause of acid load.

Non-Anion-Gap Metabolic Acidosis

Low serum pH with low bicarbonate and a normal anion gap. Etiologies include renal or GI bicarbonate wasting and failure to excrete acid in the urine (see also the mnemonic **ACCRUED**).

DIAGNOSIS

- Low bicarbonate on chemistry panel; low pH on ABG.
- An anion gap ~ 12.
- Urine anion gap (UAG, calculated as urine Na + K − Cl) distinguishes proximal RTA/GI losses (UAG < 0) from distal/type IV RTA losses (UAG > 0).

Renal Tubular Acidosis (RTA)

The subtypes and causes of RTA are outlined in Table 19-2.

Metabolic Alkalosis

High serum pH with high bicarbonate. Etiologies are as follows:

- **Volume contraction:** Chronic dehydration, diuretic use or abuse, Bartter or Gitelman syndrome.
- **Loss of acid:** Pyloric stenosis, NG tubes to suction, vomiting.
- **High mineralocorticoid states:** Hyperaldosteronism, black licorice use.

DIAGNOSIS

- High bicarbonate on chemistry panel; high pH on ABG.
- Urine chloride and BP can be used to narrow the differential.
- Urine chloride can distinguish chloride-responsive (Cl < 10) from chloride-resistant (Cl > 20) subtypes:
    - Cl < 10: GI losses, dehydration, diuretic use.
    - Cl > 20: Mineralocorticoid states, Bartter or Gitelman syndrome.
- BP distinguishes types of chloride-resistant causes:
    - **Hypertension:** Mineralocorticoid excess.
    - **Normotension:** Bartter, Gitelman.

TABLE 19-2. Types of RTA

	MECHANISM	ASSOCIATED FINDINGS	DIAGNOSTIC CLUE
Type I (distal)	Impaired acidification of urine in the distal tubule.	Nephrocalcinosis.	Alkaline urine with serum acidosis; low potassium.
Type II (proximal)	Impaired proximal tubule reabsorption of base.	Can be isolated or seen as 2° to many systemic disease (e.g., cystinosis, Wilson's disease, galactosemia, mitochondrial disorders).	Proteinuria, glucosuria, aminoaciduria.
Type IV (hypoaldosteronism)	Resistance to aldosterone.	Can be associated with obstructive uropathy.	High potassium.

Hyponatremia

Serum sodium < 135 mEq/L. The prognosis is related to the underlying etiology. Generally, the disturbance is related more to volume status than to sodium intake or sodium losses. Subtypes are as follows:

- **Hypovolemic:** Sodium and water losses (diarrhea, cerebral salt wasting, diuretic use).
- **Euvolemic:** Abnormal retention of water (SIADH, psychogenic polydipsia).
- **Hypervolemic:** Cirrhosis, nephrotic syndrome, CHF.

The diagnosis of cerebral salt wasting can be entertained only if the patient is hypovolemic.

SYMPTOMS/EXAM

- Asymptomatic if there is a slow ↓ in serum sodium.
- Presents with seizures if there is a rapid ↓ in or very low serum sodium.

TREATMENT

- Correct the underlying etiology.
    - **Hypovolemic:** Restore volume losses; replace ongoing losses; stop diuretics.
    - **Euvolemic:** Restrict water.
    - **Hypervolemic:** Improve cardiac function; administer diuretics.
- For seizures, use 3% NaCl to acutely ↑ serum sodium until seizures stop.
- Overly rapid correction of long-standing hyponatremia can → central pontine myelinolysis.

> A 12-year-old boy develops encephalitis following sinusitis. His serum sodium drops from 142 to 128 mEq/L over the next several days. He is clinically euvolemic. His serum osmolality is 278 mOsm/kg and his urine osmolality 740 mOsm/kg. What is the diagnosis—SIADH or cerebral salt wasting? SIADH, since the boy has inappropriately concentrated urine and is not hypovolemic.

Syndrome of Inappropriate Secretion of Antidiuretic Hormone (SIADH)

Defined as inappropriate release of ADH. **Appropriate ADH release** occurs with hyperosmolality and hypovolemia. **Inappropriate ADH release** is associated with cerebral conditions (encephalitis, trauma) and some tumors.

SIADH can be diagnosed only if the release of ADH is truly inappropriate (i.e., if there is no hyperosmolality and no hypovolemia, both of which are triggers for appropriate ADH release).

SYMPTOMS/EXAM

- Euvolemia.
- Can present with seizures if serum sodium is sufficiently low.

TREATMENT

Restrict fluids until serum sodium normalizes.

Hypernatremia

Serum sodium > 145 mEq/L. Etiology depends on volume status:

- **Hypovolemic:** Sodium and water losses (diarrhea, DI).
- **Hypervolemic:** Salt intoxication (e.g., adding sodium to infant formula).

SYMPTOMS/EXAM

- Clinical presentation is related to the underlying etiology.
- Venous thrombosis (cerebral or renal vein) can develop in hypovolemic states.
- An overly rapid correction of long-standing hypernatremia can → cerebral edema.

TREATMENT

- Correct the underlying etiology.
- ↓ serum sodium at a rate no faster than 10 mEq/dL per 24 hours.
- The prognosis depends on the underlying etiology and on avoidance of iatrogenic cerebral edema.

Diabetes Insipidus (DI)

Think DI when urine osmolality is low and serum osmolality is high.

Inability to concentrate the urine because of a deficiency of ADH (central DI) or resistance to the action of ADH (nephrogenic DI). Has a good prognosis if access to water is maintained. Etiologies are as follows:

- **Central:** Pituitary disorders (craniopharyngioma, pituitary tumors compressing the stalk).
- **Nephrogenic:** Lack of kidney tubule water channels (aquaporin), sickle cell nephropathy, obstructive uropathy.

SYMPTOMS/EXAM

Thirst (especially for ice-cold water); enuresis; hypernatremia and dehydration with denial of access to water (i.e., the patient is admitted to the hospital for other reasons).

Maximum urine concentrating ability (1200 mOsm/L) is not reached until three years of age.

TREATMENT

- Access to water (patients can self-regulate).
- Intranasal or oral DDAVP can be given for central DI.

Hyperkalemia

↑ serum potassium. The condition is fatal if not corrected. Etiologies are as follows:

- **Conditions with ↓ activity of the mineralocorticoid pathway:** 1° hypoaldosteronism, congenital adrenal hyperplasia, Liddle's disease (lack of aldosterone receptor), pseudohypoaldosteronism (lack of sodium channel), type IV RTA.
- **Advanced chronic kidney disease.**

SYMPTOMS/EXAM

ECG changes (peaked T waves, shortened QT, ST depression, ↑ PR, widening of the QRS); cardiac arrhythmias.

TREATMENT

- Stabilization of the myocardium with IV calcium.
- Insulin and glucose infusion (shifts potassium into cells).
- Bicarbonate infusion (shifts potassium into cells).

- Kayexalate.
- Inhaled albuterol (can drop potassium by 1 mEq/dL).
- Dialysis.

Hypokalemia

- Serum potassium < 3.0 mEq/L. Fatal in the presence of another arrhythmogenic condition.
- Etiologies are as follows:
    - **Conditions with excessive mineralocorticoid activity:** Hyperaldosteronism.
    - **Renal wasting:** Distal and proximal RTA; furosemide (Lasix) therapy; Bartter and Gitelman syndromes.
    - **GI wasting:** Diarrhea.
- **Sx/Exam:** Weakness, cardiac arrhythmia.
- **Tx:** Oral or IV supplements.

Hypocalcemia

Low ionized calcium (< 1.1 mg/dL). Etiologies include vitamin D deficiency, hypoparathyroidism, and hyperphosphatemia from tumor lysis syndrome or renal failure.

SYMPTOMS/EXAM

- Weakness, tetany.
- Widened QTc interval on ECG.
- Chvostek's sign (twitching of facial muscle with a tap on the cheekbone).
- Signs and symptoms may be masked by acidosis, since the ionized fraction of total calcium ↑ with acidosis.

TREATMENT

- Replacement of calcium (oral administration is preferred).
- Correction of the underlying etiology (vitamin D for vitamin D deficiency; ↓ phosphorus in ESRD or tumor lysis syndrome).
- Correct hypocalcemia before treating any associated acidosis.

Correcting acidosis before treating hypocalcemia will make the symptoms of hypocalcemia worse.

Hypercalcemia

- ↑ ionized calcium. Etiologies include hyperparathyroidism, sarcoidosis, vitamin D intoxication, and vitamin A intoxication.
- **Sx/Exam:** Dehydration from polyuria.
- **Tx:** Replete intravascular volume and treat the underlying etiology.

GLOMERULOPATHIES

Nephrotic Syndrome

Defined as edema, hypoalbuminemia, and heavy proteinuria (> 40 mg urine protein/m^2/hr or a urine protein-to-creatinine ratio > 2). Etiologies include the following:

- Minimal change disease (most common in children 2–12 years of age).
- Focal segmental glomerulosclerosis (more common in adolescents).
- Membranous GN (the most common cause in adults).
- Membranoproliferative GN.
- 2° causes (SLE, Henoch-Schönlein purpura, HIV).

SYMPTOMS/EXAM

- Edema (may initially be mistaken for allergies owing to eyelid swelling), frothy urine.
- **Serious complications and presentations** include thrombosis (e.g., renal vein thrombosis), pulmonary edema, and spontaneous bacterial peritonitis.

TREATMENT

- If consistent with minimal change disease, initiate a trial of steroids.
- If there is no response to steroids or the presentation is not consistent with that of minimal change disease, biopsy is indicated to make the diagnosis and guide treatment.
- The prognosis depends on the underlying etiology.

Minimal Change Disease

A glomerular condition presenting with nephrotic syndrome that has normal renal light microscopy findings. The etiology is unknown, but the condition is presumed to be immune mediated.

SYMPTOMS/EXAM

- Generally presents with nephrotic syndrome in children 2–12 years of age.
- A viral infection may precede its onset.
- Gross hematuria, hypertension, and renal insufficiency are not uncommon (~ 20%) but are considered atypical.

TREATMENT

- Response to steroid treatment is the hallmark of minimal change disease.
- Cyclosporine and cytoxan may be used for steroid-dependent or frequently relapsing cases.
- Albumin infusions are useful only if skin breakdown or pulmonary edema is present.
- Most cases relapse at least once, with relapses becoming less frequent as the child ages.
- Most patients outgrow the condition with no long-term sequelae.

Postinfectious Glomerulonephritis

Edema, hypertension, and cola-colored hematuria suggest postinfectious glomerulonephritis.

Inflammation of glomeruli following a streptococcal or other infection. Rarely, it can progress to renal failure.

SYMPTOMS/EXAM

- Presents with the triad of edema, hypertension, and gross hematuria (tea-colored urine) 1–2 weeks after infection (strep throat, impetigo, viral illness).
- Characterized by a low C3 that normalizes by eight weeks.

TREATMENT

Manage edema and hypertension with fluid restriction, a low-sodium diet, and antihypertensives (e.g., diuretics). Treat underlying infection if still present.

Focal Segmental Glomerulosclerosis

Progressive scarring or collapse of glomeruli. Although most cases are idiopathic, it may be caused by mutations in glomerular proteins (podocin) or by viral infections (HIV, CMV, parvovirus). Most commonly seen among adolescents.

SYMPTOMS/EXAM

Insidious development of edema and renal insufficiency.

TREATMENT

Steroids and cyclosporine; cytoxan can be used for refractory cases.

COMPLICATIONS

- The prognosis is poor, with most cases progressing to ESRD.
- A high rate of recurrence is found among transplant patients.

Lupus Nephropathy

Any kidney involvement with a diagnosis of SLE. The condition is autoimmune mediated, with deposition of antigen-antibody complexes in glomeruli or direct autoantigen attack.

SYMPTOMS/EXAM

- Presentation is variable, ranging from hematuria and proteinuria to nephrotic syndrome and rapid development of ARF. Proteinuria is the most common renal presentation.
- Graded histologically into five lesions:
    - **Type I:** Normal.
    - **Type II:** Mesangial.
    - **Type III:** Focal proliferative GN.
    - **Type IV:** Diffuse proliferative GN.
    - **Type V:** Membranous.

TREATMENT

- All SLE patients should have routine, regular screening for hematuria and proteinuria. Any abnormality should prompt a kidney biopsy.
- Proliferative GN (types III and IV) should be treated with steroids and cytoxan.
- Types I, II, and V require no specific treatment but warrant more frequent monitoring of renal function and proteinuria.
- The prognosis is good if the disease is adequately treated.

Membranoproliferative Glomerulonephritis

A pathologic diagnosis characterized by immune deposits in the glomerular basement membrane (GBM). May be idiopathic; HCV, SLE, and cryoglobulinemia are 2° causes.

SYMPTOMS/EXAM

- Proteinuria, hematuria.
- Hypertension is more common than in other glomerular diseases.
- A low C3 that does not recover in 6–8 weeks (as in postinfectious GN) suggests membranoproliferative GN and indicates the need for biopsy.

TREATMENT

Steroids and cytotoxic agents.

COMPLICATIONS

The prognosis is poor, with 50% of cases progressing to ESRD within five years.

Membranous Glomerulonephritis

A pathologic diagnosis characterized by a thickened GBM. Most cases in children are idiopathic; HBV is a common 2° cause.

SYMPTOMS/EXAM

- Massive proteinuria and nephrotic syndrome.
- Thrombosis and other complications of nephrotic syndrome may be more common than in other nephrotic states.

TREATMENT

- Steroids.
- Many idiopathic pediatric cases may resolve on their own.

Congenital Nephrotic Syndrome

Defined as nephrotic syndrome that is present at birth. The Finnish type is caused by a deficiency of nephrin, an integral component of the GBM (and podocyte), 2° causes include congenital syphilis and other infections, diffuse mesangial sclerosis, and Denys-Drash syndrome (associated with Wilms' tumor and ambiguous genitalia).

SYMPTOMS/EXAM

Nephrotic syndrome, placentomegaly.

TREATMENT

- Nephrectomy for congenital nephrotic syndrome of the Finnish type (to prevent massive protein losses contributing to malnutrition and the risk of infection due to immunoglobulin losses); institution of dialysis or transplantation.
- The prognosis is poor.

IgA Nephropathy

A pathologic diagnosis associated with IgA deposition in the glomeruli. The disorder is idiopathic and is responsible for the nephropathy seen in Henoch-Schönlein purpura. The most common glomerulopathy worldwide.

SYMPTOMS/EXAM

Painless gross hematuria +/– proteinuria. The classic presentation is syn-pharyngitic (gross hematuria occurring concurrently with a pharyngitis or other URI).

TREATMENT

- No treatment is necessary in the absence of significant proteinuria or renal insufficiency.
- For aggressive forms of IgA nephropathy or Henoch-Schönlein purpura nephropathy, steroids and possibly fish oil supplements can be used.
- The prognosis is varied, ranging from a benign course to the development of ESRD. Renal function at first presentation is the best predictor.

Alport Syndrome

Hearing loss and microscopic glomerular hematuria caused by a genetic absence of collagen component. The X-linked form (most common) involves type IV collagen (present in the skin, cochlea, and kidney); recessive forms involve a collagen component not found in the skin.

SYMPTOMS/EXAM

Microscopic hematuria is the earliest finding; proteinuria and renal insufficiency are later findings. High-frequency hearing loss can be detected early if tested.

TREATMENT

- ACEIs for renoprotection at the earliest sign of renal impairment (microalbuminuria, proteinuria, or an ↑ in creatinine).
- Maintain normal BP.

COMPLICATIONS

Progression to ESRD.

Lack of a family history does not entirely rule out Alport's; some families may not have any males on the maternal side or the autosomal-recessive form may be present. Do a pedigree and follow-up!

Thin Basement Membrane Disease (Benign Hereditary Nephropathy)

Hereditary microscopic hematuria. An autosomal-dominant disorder caused by a thinner-than-normal GBM.

SYMPTOMS/EXAM

- Asymptomatic microscopic hematuria.
- No family history of male relatives with ESRD or hearing loss.

DIAGNOSIS

Microscopic hematuria in a parent.

TREATMENT

None; the prognosis is excellent.

Hemolytic-Uremic Syndrome (HUS)

ARF, thrombocytopenia, and hemolytic anemia. Most cases are caused by *E. coli* O157:H7; other etiologies include pneumococcus, inherited factor H deficiency, and immunosuppressants.

SYMPTOMS/EXAM

Presents with oliguria, anemia, and petechiae several days after a hemorrhagic colitis.

TREATMENT

- Maintain euvolemia; monitor electrolytes; provide nutrition.
- Transfuse only for severe bleeding or cardiorespiratory instability.
- Dialysis (preferably peritoneal) if ARF is prolonged.

COMPLICATIONS

Persistent mild chronic kidney disease on recovery (requiring monitoring for proteinuria and renal function).

Sickle Cell Nephropathy

> **Diagnosis of sickle cell nephropathy—HIP PINCH**
>
> **H**yposthenuria
> **I**nfarction
> **P**apillary necrosis
> **P**yelonephritis
> **I**nsufficiency
> **N**ephrotic syndrome
> **C**arcinoma
> **H**ematuria

Consists of eight loosely defined conditions that share an association with sickle cell anemia: papillary necrosis, hyposthenuria (a type of nephrogenic DI), gross hematuria, nephrotic syndrome, renal medullary carcinoma, chronic renal insufficiency, renal infarction, and pyelonephritis. Caused by a sickling of RBCs that is exacerbated by the hypoxic and hypertonic environment of the kidney, especially the medulla. The associated susceptibility to cancer is not well understood.

SYMPTOMS/EXAM/TREATMENTS

Clinical presentation, diagnosis, and treatment are related to the specific manifestation.

CONGENITAL ANOMALIES AND INHERITED DISEASE

Hydronephrosis

A congenital renal abnormality (e.g., hydronephrosis and multicystic dysplastic kidney) is the most common cause of abdominal mass in a newborn.

Dilation of the renal collecting system. The most common cause of newborn abdominal mass. Etiologies are as follows:

- **Posterior urethral valves:** Thick bladder; bilateral hydronephrosis and hydroureter; residual renal insufficiency; impaired concentrating ability. A mild type IV RTA or voiding difficulties are common after surgical relief. Occurs only in boys.
- **Ureteropelvic obstruction:** Unilateral hydronephrosis.
- **Ureterovesical obstruction:** Unilateral hydronephrosis and hydroureter.
- **Acquired causes:** Stones; tumor-compressing ureter.
- **Nonobstructing hydronephrosis:** Seen with vesicoureteral reflux (VUR).

SYMPTOMS/EXAM

Pain in older children; microscopic hematuria; a thickened, palpable bladder with posterior urethral valves; weak urinary stream; renal insufficiency.

DIAGNOSIS

Diagnosed by imaging.

TREATMENT

Surgical relief. The prognosis depends on the degree of renal impairment.

Renal Dysplasia

Mesoderm that fails to develop into a normally functioning kidney. Caused by a failure in development due to dysregulated growth factors (spontaneous or related to a syndrome) or by toxins or teratogenic agents (e.g., ACEIs).

SYMPTOMS/EXAM

Unilateral dysplasia usually presents as a flank mass. Can be part of the VACTERL sequence or other syndromes or associations involving the kidneys.

TREATMENT

- Protect normal kidney tissue to the fullest extent possible (avoid dehydration and nephrotoxic drugs; prevent UTIs).
- Rule out associated VUR, especially with multicystic dysplastic kidneys.
- Monitor renal function and urine protein.
- Contact sports are a relative contraindication with a unilateral functioning kidney.

COMPLICATIONS

The prognosis depends on the amount of functional kidney tissue remaining. Patients with bilateral dysplasia often have pulmonary hypoplasia and progress to ESRD if they survive the neonatal period.

The severity of pulmonary hypoplasia associated with renal dysplasia determines the mortality risk in the newborn period.

Cystic Disease

Cysts in the kidney arising from various portions of the nephron. Etiologies include autosomal-dominant or -recessive polycystic kidney disease, medullary cystic kidney disease, multicystic dysplastic kidney, nephronophthisis, simple cysts, and acquired dialytic cysts.

SYMPTOMS/EXAM

Usually presents with symptoms and signs of associated disease. Symptoms related to the cysts themselves are pain from infection, bleeding into the cyst, or malignant carcinomatous transformation of a cyst.

DIAGNOSIS

- CT or ultrasound.
- Disease is defined and diagnosed by its location (cortical, medullary, or diffuse), time of presentation, size, laterality, and associated family or personal medical history.

TREATMENT

Treatment and prognosis are related to the underlying disease.

Autosomal-Dominant Polycystic Kidney Disease

A systemic disease with progressive cystic enlargement of kidneys accompanied by CNS, GU, and GI involvement. Caused by genetic defects in extracellular-matrix signaling and adhesion mechanisms. Cysts can develop from anywhere within the nephron.

SYMPTOMS/EXAM

- Usually present in adulthood, but can present at any time (including antenatally).
- Hypertension is prominent in children.
- Other pediatric presentations include incidental radiologic finding, abdominal pain, abdominal masses, hematuria, or UTIs. Strokes from berry aneurysms are rare in the pediatric population.

DIAGNOSIS

Diagnosed by a $\oplus$ family history plus at least one cyst seen in the kidney.

TREATMENT

- None.
- Renoprotection and BP control with ACEIs.

COMPLICATIONS

Progression of renal insufficiency. The rate is variable, and whether or when ESRD will develop cannot be predicted.

Autosomal-Recessive Polycystic Kidney Disease

Cystic disease of kidneys with hepatic fibrosis. Caused by genetic defects in extracellular-matrix signaling and adhesion mechanisms. Cysts develop from the renal collecting duct.

SYMPTOMS/EXAM

Usually presents in the neonatal period with oligohydramnios, pulmonary difficulties at birth, abdominal masses, and hypertension.

DIAGNOSIS

Clinical history and ultrasound.

TREATMENT

- None.
- Renoprotection and BP control with ACEIs; management of portal hypertension.

COMPLICATIONS

One-third of those who survive the neonatal period will have ESRD by 15 years of age.

Juvenile Nephronophthisis (JN)/Medullary Cystic Disease (MCD)

A chronic inherited sclerosing tubulointerstitial disease caused by genetic defects in various extracellular signaling mechanisms in the kidney.

SYMPTOMS/EXAM

- Insidious onset of ESRD.
- Polyuria, polydipsia, and 2° enuresis by six years of age in JN; older in MCD.
- Anemia is prominent; extrarenal associations are retinopathy (JN) and gout (MCD).

DIAGNOSIS

- Medullary cysts on ultrasound.
- Classic retinal findings in JN.

TREATMENT

- None.
- Renoprotection with ACEIs.

COMPLICATIONS

Prognosis is poor, with all cases progressing to ESRD.

Eagle-Barrett (Prune Belly) Syndrome

- A congenital anomaly marked by lack of abdominal musculature, undescended testicles, and renal dysplasia.
- **Sx/Exam:** Wrinkly abdominal skin due to lack of muscles; absent testicles in scrotum.
- **Dx:** Diagnosed by renal imaging and exam.
- **Tx:**
  - No treatment except for support of renal insufficiency if present.
  - The prognosis varies with the degree of renal insufficiency.

Posterior Urethral Valves

A congenital condition in which folds of tissue at the urethral-bladder junction obstruct urine flow. Often diagnosed prenatally.

SYMPTOMS/EXAM

- Poor urine stream; failure to thrive from renal insufficiency; oligohydramnios during gestation.
- Thickened, palpable bladder.
- Pneumothorax from pulmonary hypoplasia.

DIAGNOSIS

- Renal ultrasound.
- Voiding cystourethrogram (VCUG) (the contrast type is the only one that will show valves).
- Cystoscopy.

TREATMENT

- Urethral catheter; vesicostomy.
- Management of renal insufficiency if present.
- Management of voiding dysfunction (often present).
- The prognosis depends on the level of renal impairment and is good if creatinine is < 0.8 by one year of age.

Multicystic Dysplastic Kidneys

A form of dysplasia that presents as a unilateral nonfunctioning kidney with multiple small cysts. A common cause of a newborn abdominal mass.

SYMPTOMS/EXAM

Asymptomatic; may present with UTI given the increased risk of VUR.

DIAGNOSIS

Ultrasound.

TREATMENT

Management of comorbid VUR and UTIs. The prognosis is good if the other kidney is functional.

 A three-year-old fair-skinned boy with blond hair presents with failure to thrive, mild proteinuria, aminoaciduria and glucosuria. What is the likely diagnosis? Cystinosis.

Cystinosis

An autosomal-recessive disorder of cysteine metabolism leads to buildup of cysteine within cells. Caused by a lysosome cysteine transporter defect that usually occurs in blond, fair-skinned individuals of Northern European ancestry.

Cystinosis is the most common cause of proximal RTA.

SYMPTOMS/EXAM

Progressive renal insufficiency and ESRD, Fanconi syndrome (proximal RTA), thyroid disorders, photophobia from corneal cysteine deposits.

DIAGNOSIS

↑ WBC cysteine levels.

TREATMENT

- Cysteamine complexes cysteine and uses the lysosomal lysine channel to remove cysteine.
- Treat complications (ESRD, thyroid disease).

COMPLICATIONS

Most cases progress to ESRD.

Cystinuria

An inherited kidney stone disease resulting from loss of proximal tubule absorption of the amino acids cystine, ornithine, lysine, and arginine. Caused by a genetic defect in the dibasic amino acid transporter in the proximal tubule.

SYMPTOMS/EXAM

Recurrent kidney stones.

DIAGNOSIS

↑ urinary cystine; hexagonal urine crystals.

TREATMENT

- ↑ fluid intake; alkalinization of urine with potassium citrate.
- Cystoscopic removal of stones.

COMPLICATIONS

Associated with a lifelong risk of kidney stones.

Enuresis

Defined as inability to hold urine in the bladder until socially appropriate times. Subtypes include 1° (no history of prior continence) and 2° as well as nocturnal (nighttime only) and diurnal.

- **1° nocturnal (the most common cause):** Normal delay in development (5% of 10-year-old boys have it).
- **2° nocturnal:** Associated with polyuric states (diabetes, DI) or UTI.
- **1° diurnal:** Bladder instability or loss of bladder control; anatomic abnormalities (ectopic ureter).
- **2° diurnal:** Voluntary withholding ("busy little girl syndrome"—patients are too busy with activities to make time for the bathroom until it is too late); constipation.

Children with 1° nocturnal enuresis rarely have an organic etiology.

SYMPTOMS/EXAM

Wetting the bed; chronic wetness and odor in underpants; polydipsia or frequency in 2° nocturnal states; frequency, hesitation, bladder spasm, or sense of incomplete emptying with 1° diurnal.

DIAGNOSIS

- History (most important) and physical (e.g., stigmata of spina bifida, lower extremity reflexes).
- 1° nocturnal enuresis usually has a ⊕ family history.
- If indicated, check first-morning urine for concentrating ability, urine culture, and glucose.

TREATMENT

- Most patients outgrow 1° nocturnal enuresis as they develop.
- Behavioral techniques (e.g., double voiding, timed voiding) and alarm systems can → short-term success.
- DDAVP can be used sparingly for sleepovers and summer camps to achieve short-term dryness.

> A six-month-old boy develops fever and irritability. After a source for the fever is not found on physical exam, a UA is obtained that shows > 200 WBCs/hpf. After the UTI is treated with an appropriate antibiotic, what is the next step in management? Image the urinary tract while maintaining a high suspicion for a urinary anomaly.

URINARY TRACT INFECTIONS AND RELATED DISORDERS

Defined as > 100,000 colony-forming units (CFUs)/mL in a clean-catch urine specimen, > 10,000 CFUs/mL in a catheterized specimen, or > 0 CFU/mL in a suprapubic aspirate. Eighty percent of UTIs are due to Enterobacteriaceae (e.g., *E. coli*).

SYMPTOMS/EXAM

- In infants, fever and irritability may be the only presenting symptoms. Older children may present with abdominal pain and dysuria.
- Males with UTIs are more likely to have GU anatomic anomalies; girls have a high probability of having VUR.

DIAGNOSIS

Diagnosed by the presence of > 10 WBCs/hpf and positive urine culture.

TREATMENT

Antibiotics (IV for young children; PO for adolescents). Young children with UTIs should be evaluated for VUR.

COMPLICATIONS

Most children recover without kidney damage. Kidney damage with scarring is generally (but not always) seen with UTIs only in the presence of obstructive anomalies of the urinary tract or severe VUR.

Vesicoureteral Reflux (VUR)

Reflux of urine from the bladder into the ureter or renal pelvis. Severity is graded according to how high urine refluxes into the ureter or pelvis as well as by the presence of hydronephrosis. Associated with other urinary tract anomalies, especially multicystic dysplastic kidney and duplicated collecting systems.

SYMPTOMS/EXAM

The first UTI in a male or the second UTI in a female.

DIAGNOSIS

Diagnosis is made by contrast VCUG to provide anatomic detail. Follow-up VCUGs can be performed with radionuclides, which do not provide anatomic detail.

Reflux Nephropathy

↓ GFR, proteinuria, and hypertension from VUR. Accounts for 5% of all pediatric ESRD. Caused by renal scarring from ↑ intrarenal pressure and/or UTIs due to VUR or perhaps a developmental abnormality coexisting with VUR.

SYMPTOMS/EXAM

Proteinuria; hypertension with a history of VUR or UTIs.

TREATMENT

Preventive antibiotics for UTIs; surgical correction of VUR. Low-grade cases often resolve spontaneously over time.

Antenatal Hydronephrosis

Dilation of the fetal renal collecting system as seen on obstetric ultrasound. Caused by obstructive uropathy, VUR, or physiologic dilation due to maternal hormones.

SYMPTOMS/EXAM

Dilation > 4 mm.

TREATMENT

- Renal ultrasound after birth (at a minimum of 3–5 days of age) and VCUG if dilation is still present.
- Give prophylactic antibiotics until the urinary tract has been fully evaluated.
- The prognosis depends on the underlying condition.

Urolithiasis

Kidney stone disease associated with excess urine solute relative to urine volume (supersaturation). Etiologies are as follows:

- **Common causes:** Hypercalciuria, infection stones (struvite), hyperuricosuria.
- **Rare causes:** Medicine stones (i.e., stones made of pharmaceutical metabolites such as indinavir, triamterene), hyperoxaluria.

Distal RTA is the only form of RTA that is strongly associated with nephrocalcinosis.

SYMPTOMS/EXAM

- **Toddlers:** Presents with hematuria or dysuria, or diagnosed as an incidental finding on imaging. Pain is not a key symptom.
- **Children:** Pain, hematuria.

DIAGNOSIS

- CT is the imaging modality of choice.
- Uric acid and cystine stones do not appear on x-ray.

TREATMENT

- ↑ fluid intake; urine alkalinization.
- Lithotripsy in the presence of obstruction, large stones, or cystine/struvite stones.

↑ hydration to > 2 L/m²/day is an effective preventive therapy for stones in all causes of pediatric stone disease.

Renal Vein Thrombosis

Clot within the renal vein causing abdominal mass and pain, gross hematuria, anemia and thrombocytopenia, and occasionally hypertension and renal insufficiency. Common causes include hyperviscous or hypercoagulable states (dehydration, nephrotic syndrome [from anticoagulant urine losses], polycythemia). Infants of diabetic mothers and children with nephrotic syndrome are particularly vulnerable.

SYMPTOMS/EXAM

Abdominal mass, pain, gross hematuria, hypertension.

DIAGNOSIS

Ultrasound with Doppler flow studies.

TREATMENT

- Anticoagulation.
- Surgical declotting may be indicated.

HYPERTENSION

An antihypertensive drip can best handle a hypertensive crisis and can prevent overly rapid lowering of BP.

Hypertensive Crisis

Results from any 2° cause of hypertension. Defined as follows:

- **Emergent:** ↑ BP with evidence of neurologic or cardiac end-organ damage (encephalopathy, seizure, stroke, MI).
- **Urgent:** ↑ BP 20 mmHg or more above 90% percentile for age/sex/height without evidence of end-organ damage.

SYMPTOMS/EXAM

- BP >> 95th percentile for age, sex, and height.
- Symptoms of end-organ damage (chest pain, headache, seizure, neurologic deficits).

TREATMENT

- Do not normalize BP immediately; aim for a 10% ↓ in BP in the first 24 hours. Treatment with a drip is preferred (see Table 19-3).
- The prognosis is related to the underlying etiology.

Chronic Hypertension

BP > 95th percentile for age, sex, and height on three separate occasions using an appropriately sized cuff. The younger the child and the higher the BP, the more likely a 2° cause will be found. Such causes include the following:

- **Newborn:** Renal artery thrombosis, renal artery stenosis, renal malformation, coarctation, bronchopulmonary dysplasia.
- **Toddlers:** Renal parenchymal disease, coarctation, renal artery stenosis.
- **Children:** Renal artery stenosis, coarctation, renal scarring from UTIs, essential hypertension.

TABLE 19-3. Treatment of Emergent and Urgent Hypertensive Crisis

DRUG	MECHANISM	MAJOR SIDE EFFECTS
Nicardipine drip	Calcium channel blocker.	
Nitroprusside drip	Direct smooth muscle dilator.	Cyanide toxicity.
Labetalol	α- and β-blocker.	
Furosemide (Lasix)	Diuretic.	Hypokalemia.
Hydralazine	Direct smooth muscle dilator.	Can induce lupus-like autoantibodies.

The younger the patient with hypertension and the higher the BP, the more likely there is a 2° cause.

- **Adolescents:** Essential hypertension, obesity, GN, renal scarring from UTIs, renal parenchymal disease, obstructive sleep apnea, exogenous substances.
- Rare but needed on the differential are endocrine causes (Cushing's, hyperaldosteronism, pheochromocytoma), ↑ ICP, hyperthyroidism, and preeclampsia.

*Pheochromocytoma is **not** among the top three causes of hypertension in any age group.*

SYMPTOMS/EXAM

Often asymptomatic or may present with headaches and flushing (pertains to any type of pediatric hypertension, not just pheochromocytoma).

DIAGNOSIS

LVH on echocardiogram; narrowing and nicking of retinal vessels. Other findings depending on etiology and include renal anatomic anomalies, elevated creatinine, renal bruit, and renal mass.

Renovascular hypertension is usually severe and difficult to control medically.

TREATMENT

- Identify and correct the underlying cause (renal angiography is the preferred method of identifying and correcting renovascular hypertension).
- Salt restriction and weight loss for essential hypertension.
- Medication (see Table 19-4).

RENAL FAILURE

Acute Renal Failure (ARF)

A transient ↓ in GFR with an ↑ in creatinine. The amount of urine output does not factor into the definition. Subtypes are as follows:

- **Prerenal:** Hypovolemia, cardiogenic shock, renovascular obstruction.
- **Renal:** GN, toxins, interstitial nephritis, tumor lysis syndrome.
- **Postrenal:** Obstruction.

Doppler ultrasound and MRA are poor tools with which to detect renal artery stenosis. Angiography, despite its invasiveness, is the preferred diagnostic and therapeutic option.

SYMPTOMS/EXAM

Fluid overload; fixed urine output not related to volume status (anuria, oliguria, or polyuria).

TABLE 19-4. Classes of Antihypertensive Drugs

CLASS	EXAMPLES
β_1-blockers	Atenolol
α_2-agonists	Clonidine
α_1-blockers	Doxazosin
Combination (α_2, β_1, β_2) blockers	Carvedilol, labetalol
Direct vasodilators	Hydralazine, minoxidil
Diuretics	Furosemide, HCTZ
Calcium channel blockers	Amlodipine
ACEIs	Enalapril, lisinopril
Angiotensin receptor blockers (ARBs)	Losartan

Indications for acute dialysis—AEIOU

Acidosis
Electrolyte abnormalities (potassium, urate, phosphorus)
Ingestion or intoxication
Overload with fluid
Uremia (platelet dysfunction or mental status changes)

DIAGNOSIS

Rising creatinine; acidosis, hyperkalemia, fixed or no urine output.

Acidosis ↑ ionized calcium despite ↓ total serum calcium; correcting the acidosis before ↑ the total serum calcium can → symptomatic hypocalcemia and tetany.

TREATMENT

- Correct the underlying etiology (hydrate, improve cardiac output, treat GN).
- After correcting fluid overload or fluid depletion, balance fluids by having ins = outs (without forgetting to calculate insensible water losses from sweat and breath ~ 400 mL/m^2)
- Restrict potassium.
- Monitor for indications for dialysis.

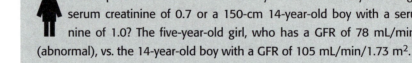

Which patient has renal insufficiency—a 100-cm five-year-old girl with a serum creatinine of 0.7 or a 150-cm 14-year-old boy with a serum creatinine of 1.0? The five-year-old girl, who has a GFR of 78 mL/min/1.73 m^2 (abnormal), vs. the 14-year-old boy with a GFR of 105 mL/min/1.73 m^2.

In an anuric patient with ESRD, volume overload is the most common cause of hypertension.

Chronic Renal Failure (End-Stage Renal Disease)

Persistent GFR < 15 mL/min/1.73 m^2 requiring dialysis or transplantation. Congenital anatomic abnormalities are the most common cause in children < 5 years of age; GN is the most common cause in children > 5 years of age.

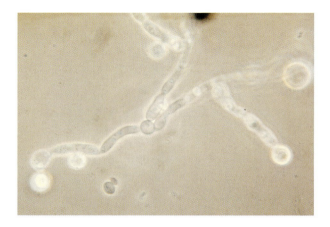

FIGURE 2-5. Pseudohyphae of candidiasis seen on vaginal secretions under KOH.

(Reproduced, with permission, from Wolff K, Johnson RA, Suurmond D. *Fitzpatrick's Color Atlas & Synopsis of Clinical Dermatology*, 5th ed. New York: McGraw-Hill, 2005:717.)

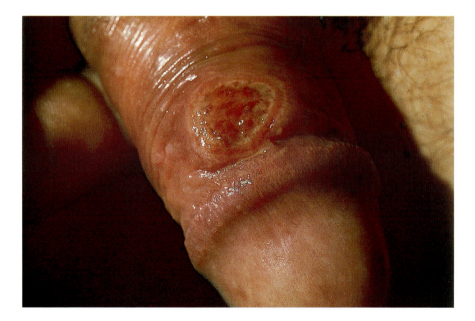

FIGURE 2-7. Chancre in primary syphilis.

(Reproduced, with permission, from Wolff K, Johnson RA, Suurmond D. *Fitzpatrick's Color Atlas & Synopsis of Clinical Dermatology*, 5th ed. New York: McGraw-Hill, 2005:915.)

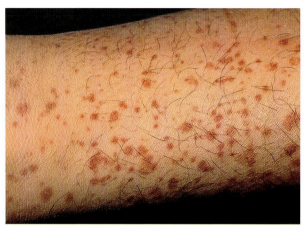
A

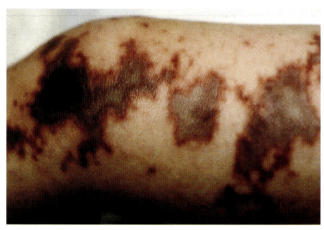
B

FIGURE 3-1. **Henoch-Schönlein purpura (A) and meningococcemia (B).**

The appearance of Henoch-Schönlein purpura, while similar to that of meningococcemia, can be distinguished because in meningococcemia purpura is more extensive, necrosis may be present, and patients appear ill. (A: Reproduced, with permission, from Rudolph CD et al. *Rudolph's Pediatrics,* 21st ed. New York: McGraw Hill, 2003: Color Plate 12; B: Reproduced, with permission, from Wolff K, Johnson RA, Suurmond D. *Fitzpatrick's Color Atlas & Synopsis of Clinical Dermatology,* 5th ed. New York: McGraw-Hill, 2005:643.)

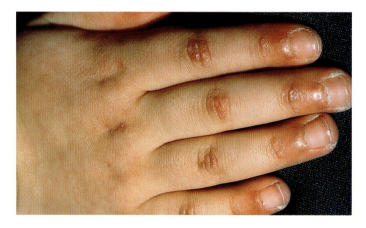

FIGURE 3-2. **Gottron's papules.**

Erythematous papules are seen overlying the knuckles. (Reproduced, with permission, from Rudolph CD et al. *Rudolph's Pediatrics,* 21st ed. New York: McGraw Hill, 2002, Color Plate 11.)

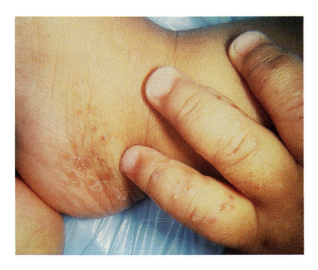

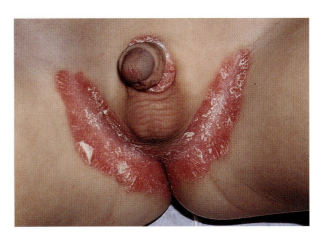

FIGURE 5-2. Psoriasis.

(Reproduced, with permission, from Weinberg S et al. *Color Atlas of Pediatric Dermatology*, 3rd ed. New York: McGraw-Hill, 1998:91.)

FIGURE 5-1. Acropustulosis of infancy.

(Reproduced, with permission, from Weinberg S et al. *Color Atlas of Pediatric Dermatology*, 3rd ed. New York: McGraw-Hill, 1998:4.)

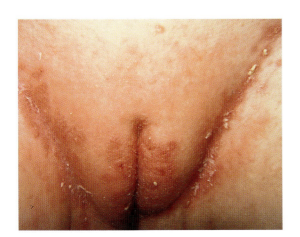

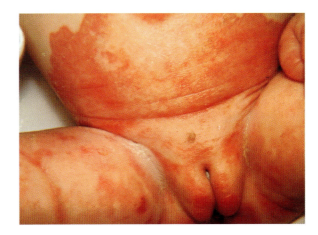

FIGURE 5-3. Langerhans cell histiocytosis.

(Reproduced, with permission, from Weinberg S et al. *Color Atlas of Pediatric Dermatology*, 3rd ed. New York: McGraw-Hill, 1998:214.)

FIGURE 5-4. Acrodermatitis enteropathica.

(Reproduced, with permission, from Weinberg S et al. *Color Atlas of Pediatric Dermatology*, 3rd ed. New York: McGraw-Hill, 1998:106.)

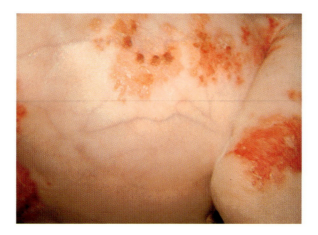

FIGURE 5-5. Herpes neonatorum.

(Reproduced, with permission, from Weinberg S et al. *Color Atlas of Pediatric Dermatology*, 3rd ed. New York: McGraw-Hill, 1998:37.)

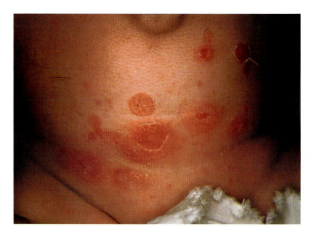

FIGURE 5-6. Bullous impetigo.

(Reproduced, with permission, from Weinberg S et al. *Color Atlas of Pediatric Dermatology*, 3rd ed. New York: McGraw-Hill, 1998:14.)

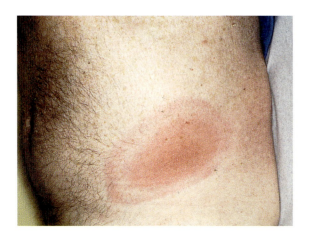

FIGURE 5-7. Erythema chronicum migrans.

(Reproduced, with permission, from Weinberg S et al. *Color Atlas of Pediatric Dermatology*, 3rd ed. New York: McGraw-Hill, 1998:25.)

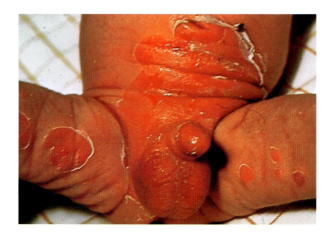

FIGURE 5-8. Staphylococcal scalded skin syndrome.

(Reproduced, with permission, from Weinberg S et al. *Color Atlas of Pediatric Dermatology*, 3rd ed. New York: McGraw-Hill, 1998:16.)

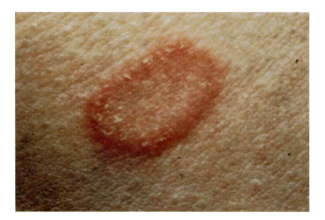

FIGURE 5-9. Tinea corporis.

(Reproduced, with permission, from Knoop K. *Emergency Atlas of Medicine*, 2nd ed. New York: McGraw-Hill, 2002, Fig. 13.26.)

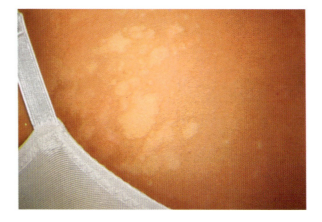

FIGURE 5-10. Tinea versicolor.

(Reproduced, with permission, from Weinberg S et al. *Color Atlas of Pediatric Dermatology*, 3rd ed. New York: McGraw-Hill, 1998:55, Fig. 178.)

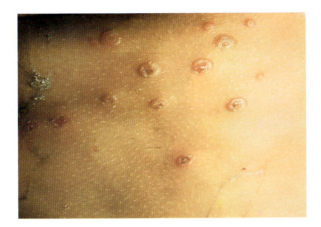

FIGURE 5-11. Molluscum contagiosum.

(Reproduced, with permission, from Weinberg S et al. *Color Atlas of Pediatric Dermatology*, 3rd ed. New York: McGraw-Hill, 1998:34.)

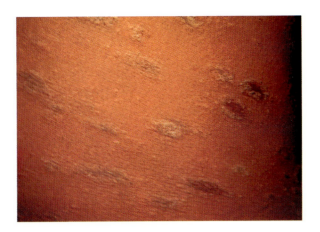

FIGURE 5-13. Pityriasis rosea.

Note the "Christmas tree" pattern of distribution. (Reproduced, with permission, from Weinberg S et al. *Color Atlas of Pediatric Dermatology*, 3rd ed. New York: McGraw-Hill, 1998:94.)

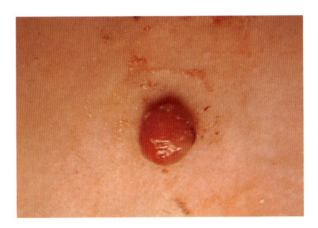

FIGURE 5-14. Pyogenic granuloma.

(Reproduced, with permission, from Weinberg S et al. *Color Atlas of Pediatric Dermatology*, 3rd ed. New York: McGraw-Hill, 1998:204.)

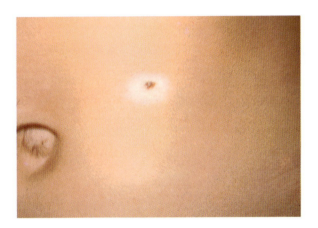

FIGURE 5-15. Halo nevus.

(Reproduced, with permission, from Weinberg S et al. *Color Atlas of Pediatric Dermatology*, 3rd ed. New York: McGraw-Hill, 1998:225.)

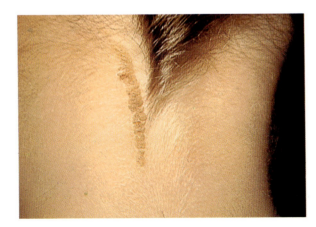

FIGURE 5-16. Epidermal nevus.

(Reproduced, with permission, from Weinberg S et al. *Color Atlas of Pediatric Dermatology*, 3rd ed. New York: McGraw-Hill, 1998:136.)

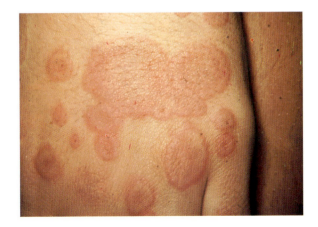

FIGURE 5-17. Erythema multiforme.

(Reproduced, with permission, from Weinberg S et al. *Color Atlas of Pediatric Dermatology*, 3rd ed. New York: McGraw-Hill, 1998:141.)

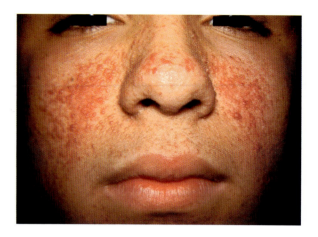

FIGURE 5-18. Sebaceous adenomas.

(Reproduced, with permission, from Weinberg S et al. *Color Atlas of Pediatric Dermatology*, 3rd ed. New York: McGraw-Hill, 1998:124.)

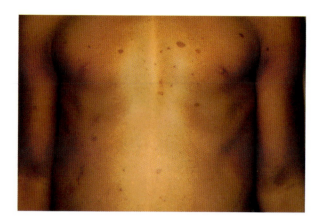

FIGURE 5-19. Café-au-lait macules.

(Reproduced, with permission, from Weinberg S et al. *Color Atlas of Pediatric Dermatology*, 3rd ed. New York: McGraw-Hill, 1998:122.)

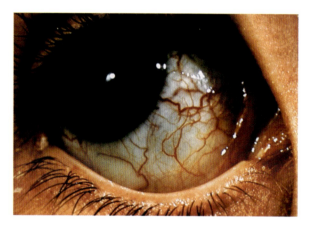

FIGURE 5-20. Telangiectasias of the bulbar conjunctiva.

(Reproduced, with permission, from Weinberg S et al. *Color Atlas of Pediatric Dermatology*, 3rd ed. New York: McGraw-Hill, 1998:117.)

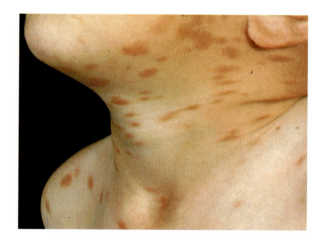

FIGURE 5-21. Urticaria pigmentosa.

(Reproduced, with permission, from Weinberg S et al. *Color Atlas of Pediatric Dermatology*, 3rd ed. New York: McGraw-Hill, 1998:186.)

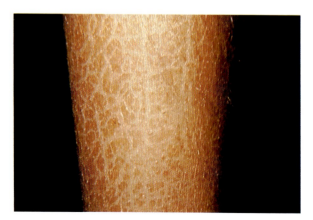

FIGURE 5-22. Ichthyosis vulgaris.

(Reproduced, with permission, from Weinberg S et al. *Color Atlas of Pediatric Dermatology*, 3rd ed. New York: McGraw-Hill, 1998:128.)

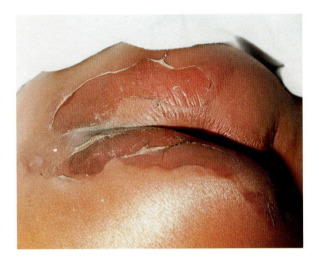

FIGURE 6-4. Burns on buttocks.

(Reproduced, with permission, from Weinberg S et al. *Color Atlas of Pediatric Dermatology*, 3rd ed. New York: McGraw-Hill, 1998:240.)

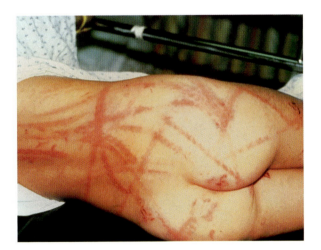

FIGURE 6-5. Loop marks from a hanger.

(Reproduced, with permission, from Weinberg S et al. *Color Atlas of Pediatric Dermatology*, 3rd ed. New York: McGraw-Hill, 1998:240.)

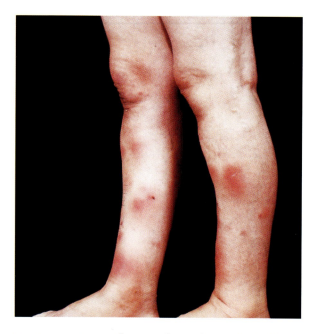

FIGURE 8-5. **Erythema nodosum in a patient with Crohn's disease.**

(Reproduced, with permission, from Freedberg IM et al. *Fitzpatrick's Dermatology in Medicine*, 6th ed. New York: McGraw-Hill, 2003:1056.)

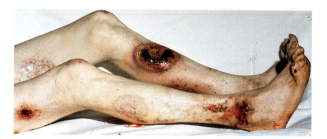

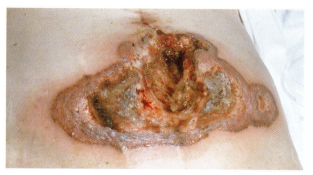

FIGURE 8-6. **Pyoderma gangrenosum in inflammatory bowel disease.**

(Reproduced, with permission, from Freedberg IM et al. *Fitzpatrick's Dermatology in Medicine*, 6th ed. New York: McGraw-Hill, 2003:971.)

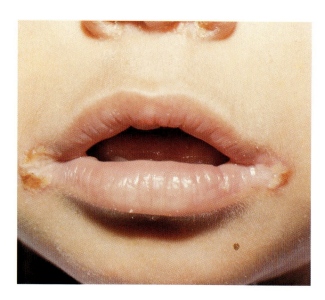

FIGURE 8-7. **Angular stomatitis associated with riboflavin deficiency.**

(Reproduced, with permission, from Freedberg IM et al. *Fitzpatrick's Dermatology in Medicine*, 6th ed. New York: McGraw-Hill, 2003:1407.)

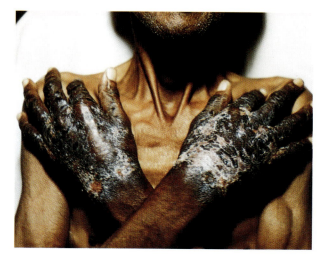

FIGURE 8-8. **Pellegra with niacin deficiency.**

(Reproduced, with permission, from Freedberg IM et al. *Fitzpatrick's Dermatology in Medicine*, 6th ed. New York: McGraw-Hill, 2003:1406.)

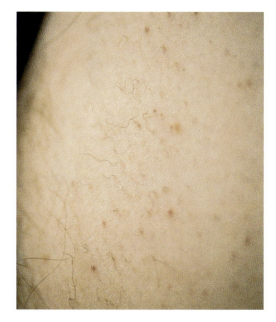

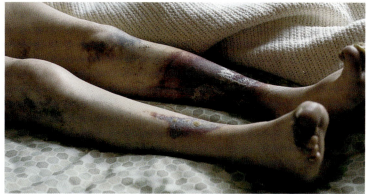

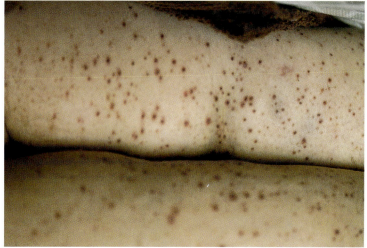

FIGURE 8-9. **Evidence of scurvy in vitamin C deficiency.**

(Reproduced, with permission, from Freedberg IM et al. *Fitzpatrick's Dermatology in Medicine,* 6th ed. New York: McGraw-Hill, 2003:1409.)

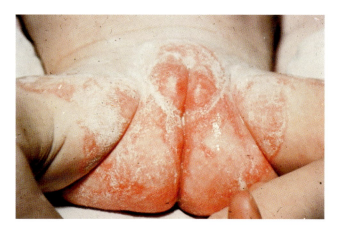

FIGURE 8-10. **Acrodermatitis enteropathica in zinc deficiency.**

(Reproduced, with permission, from Freedberg IM et al. *Fitzpatrick's Dermatology in Medicine,* 6th ed. New York: McGraw-Hill, 2003:1413.)

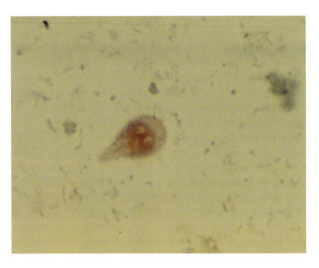

FIGURE 12-1. *Giardia* **trophozoite in stool.**

The trophozoite exhibits a classic pear shape with two nuclei imparting an owl's-eye appearance. (Reproduced, with permission, from Le T et al. *First Aid for the USMLE Step 2 CK*, 5th ed. New York: McGraw-Hill, 2006, Color Insert p. 14.)

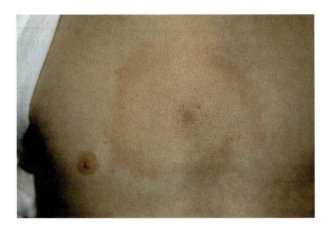

FIGURE 12-2. **"Bull's-eye" lesion of Lyme disease.**

(Reproduced, with permission, from Rudolph CD et al. *Rudolph's Pediatrics*, 21st ed. New York: McGraw-Hill, 2003, Color Plate 22.)

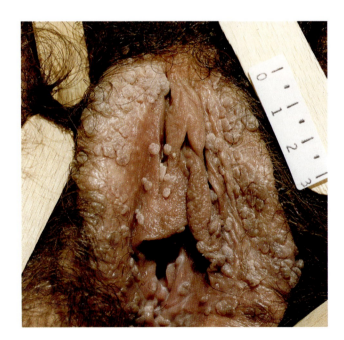

FIGURE 12-3. **Cauliflower-like lesions of HPV.**

(Reproduced, with permission, from Wolff K, Johnson RA, Suurmond D. *Fitzpatrick's Color Atlas & Synopsis of Clinical Dermatology*, 5th ed. New York: McGraw-Hill, 2005:889.)

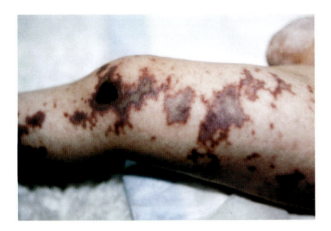

FIGURE 12-5. Characteristic rash of meningococcemia.

(Reproduced, with permission, from Freedberg IM, et al. *Fitzpatrick's Dermatology in General Medicine*, 6th ed. New York: McGraw-Hill, 2003:1898.)

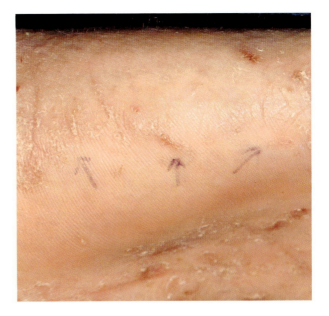

FIGURE 12-6. Characteristic lesions of scabies.

(Reproduced, with permission, from Wolff K, Johnson RA, Suurmond D. *Fitzpatrick's Color Atlas & Synopsis of Clinical Dermatology*, 5th ed. New York: McGraw-Hill, 2005:857.)

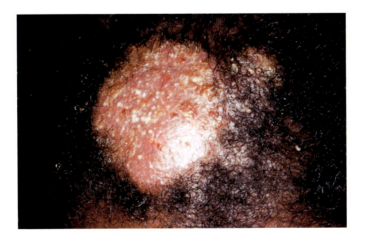

FIGURE 12-7. Characteristic lesions of tinea infection.

(Reproduced, with permission, from Freedberg IM et al. *Fitzpatrick's Dermatology in General Medicine*, 6th ed. New York: McGraw-Hill, 2003:1994.)

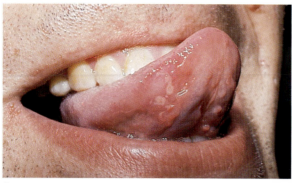

A

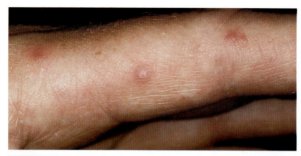

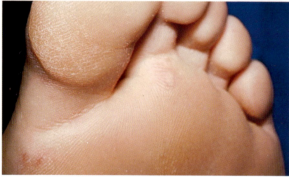

B

FIGURE 12-8. Characteristic lesions of coxsackievirus.

(A) Shallow ulcerations on the tongue. (B) Vesicular and popular lesions on the fingers and feet. (Reproduced, with permission, from Freedberg IM et al. *Fitzpatrick's Dermatology in General Medicine*, 6th ed. New York: McGraw-Hill, 2003:2050.)

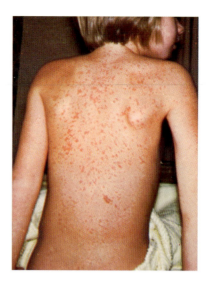

FIGURE 12-9. Generalized maculopapular rash of measles.

(Reproduced, with permission, from Freedberg IM et al. *Fitzpatrick's Dermatology in General Medicine*, 6th ed. New York: McGraw-Hill, 2003:2046.)

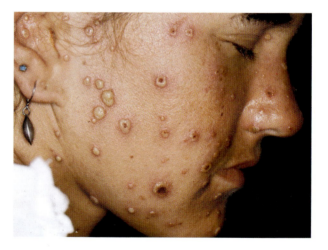

FIGURE 12-10. Characteristic rash of varicella-zoster virus.

(Reproduced, with permission, from Freedberg IM et al. *Fitzpatrick's Dermatology in General Medicine*, 6th ed. New York: McGraw-Hill, 2003:2074.)

SYMPTOMS/EXAM

- Presentation is insidious and nonspecific.
- Symptoms and signs may include anemia, growth failure, headache (from hypertension), hypocalcemia/hyperphosphatemia/hyperparathyroidism, hypertension, and acidosis.

DIAGNOSIS

- Creatinine corresponding to a GFR < 15 mL/min/1.73 m².
- Small kidneys on imaging as well as anemia and osteodystrophy support chronicity.

TREATMENT

Treatment of ESRD is as follows (see also Table 19-5):

- Transplantation (preferred) or dialysis. Survival, hospitalization rates, and quality of life are better with transplantation than with dialysis.
- Dietary management.
- Treatment of anemia, osteodystrophy, and hypertension.

COMPLICATIONS

See Table 19-6.

Transplantation is the preferred therapy for pediatric ESRD.

Focal segmental glomerulosclerosis, membranoproliferative GN type II, and nondiarrheal HUS have a high rate of recurrence after transplantation.

TABLE 19-5. Types of Renal Replacement Therapy

	MECHANISM	BENEFITS	RISKS
Transplantation	Surgical placement of deceased or living donor kidney.	Improved quality of life and survival.	Long-term immunosuppression.
Peritoneal dialysis	Ultrafiltering water and dialyzing solute using glucose solution cyclically placed in the peritoneum through an abdominal catheter.	Gentle fluid shifts; can be done at home. Minimal interference with school; dietary and fluid restrictions are less strict than in hemodialysis.	Catheter infection or peritonitis (1 per 15 months on average); hyperglycemia.
Hemodialysis	Ultrafiltering water and dialyzing solute in extracorporeal blood from a venous catheter, or surgically created subcutaneous access with a hemodialysis machine several times per week for 3–4 hours each time.	More precise control of dialysis and ultrafiltration; less reliance on patient.	Intermittent nature can → dramatic fluid shifts; requires significant time commitment away from home/school.

TABLE 19-6. Treatment of Pediatric ESRD Complications

COMPLICATION	TREATMENT
Hypertension	Fluid restriction; ACEIs and other medications.
Hyperkalemia	Dietary restriction; Kayexalate.
Growth failure	Adequate caloric intake; treatment of anemia and acidosis; growth hormone.
Uremia	Restriction of protein intake; dialysis.
Anemia	Erythropoietin; supplemental iron.
Osteodystrophy	Restrict dietary phosphorus; phosphorus binders; activated vitamin D.
Cardiovascular disease	Fluid restriction; limitation of calcium intake; treatment of hyperlipidemia, anemia, and hypertension.

Index

Marrow response, defective, 264–265
  Diamond-Blackfan anemia, 264–265
  Fanconi anemia, 265
  transient erythroblastopenia of childhood, 264
Mastocytoma, 38
  solitary, 125
Mastocytosis, 125
Mastoiditis, 525
Mayer-Rokitansky-Küster-Hauser syndrome, 12
McArdle disese, 297
McCune-Albright syndrome, 159
McMurray test, 378
Measles (rubeola), 329, 352–353, 530
Meckel's diverticulum, 194, 202, 214
Meconium aspiration syndrome, 400
Meconium ileus, 202, 408
Medial collateral ligament (MCL) tear, 378
Medial femoral torsion (femoral anteversion), 363
Medium-chain acyl-CoA dehydrogenase deficiency, 292
Medroxyprogesterone challenge, 13
Medullary cystic disease (MCD), 571
Melanoma, 117
Membranoproliferative glomerulonephritis, 565–566
Meningitis, 38, 191, 195, 313, 427, 447–449, 451
  aseptic, 448–449
  bacterial, 429, 447–448
  fungal, 448
  viral, 448
Meningococcemia, 53, 341–342
Meningococcus, 38, 43
Meningoencephalitis, chronic enteroviral, 38
Meniscal tear, 378
Menkes disease, 230
Menometrorrhagia, 14
Menorrhagia, 14
Mental health, 29–31
  anorexia nervosa, 30–31
  bulimia nervosa, 31
  depression, 29
  substance abuse, 30
  suicide, 29–30

Mental retardation, 229, 246, 285, 286, 287, 290, 451
Metabolic alkalosis, 560
Metabolic diseases, 293–300
  biotinidase deficiency, 295
  fatty oxidation disorders, 296
  galactosemia, 294
  glutaric aciduria, 296
  hepatic encephalopathy, 296
  hereditary fructose intolerance, 294
  homocystinuria, 293
  lysosomal storage diseases—lipidoses, 299–300
    Fabry disease, 300
    Gaucher disease, 299
    Krabbe disease, 300
    metachromatic leukodystrophy, 300
    Niemann-Pick disease, 299
    Tay-Sachs disease, 300
  lysosomal storage diseases—mucopolysaccharidoses (MPS), 298
    Hunter disease, 298
    Hurler disease, 298
    Maroteaux-Lamy disease, 298
    Morquio's disease, 298
    Sanfilippo's disease, 298
    Sly disease, 298
  maple syrup urine disease, 294
  nonketotic hyperglycemia, 295
  organic acidurias, 294–295
  peroxisomal diseases, 296–297
  phenylketonuria (PKU), 293
  tyrosinemia, 295–296
  urea cycle defects, 295
Metachromatic leukodystrophy, 300
Metaphyseal dysplasia, 42
Metatarsus adductus, 363
Methemoglobinemia, 137, 272
Methylene blue, 138
Methylene tetrahydrofolate reductae (MTHFR) mutation, 273
Methylmalonic acidemia (MMA), 294
Metrorrhagia, 14
Microangiopathic hemolytic anemia, 261–262
Microcephaly, 451–452
Micronutrients, functions of and clinical presentation of deficiencies, 229–230

  chromium, 229
  copper, 229
  manganese, 229
  molybdenum, 229
  selenium, 229
  zinc, 230
Micropenis, 161, 178, 185, 398
Microsporum canis, 104
Milia, 95
Miliaria, 94
Minimal change disease, 564
Mitochondrial syndromes, 281–282
Mitral regurgitation, 89
Mitral valve prolapse, 89
Molluscum contagiosum, 106, 107
  in sports participation, 373
Molybdenum, 229
Mongolian spots, 118
Mononucleosis, infectious. See Epstein-Barr virus (EBV)
Monosomy 45,X. See Turner syndrome
Moraxella, 535
Moraxella catarrhalis, 317, 347, 348, 527
Morbilliform reactions, 36
Morquio disease, 298
Movement disorders, 468–470
  Sydenham chorea, 469–470
  tics, 468–469
  Tourette syndrome, 469
Mucocutaneous disorders, 119–121
  erythema multiforme (EM), 119
  Stevens-Johnson syndrome, 120
  toxic epidermal necrolysis, 120–121
Mucopolysaccharidoses (MPS), 298
  Hunter disease, 298
  Hurler disease, 298
  Maroteaux-Lamy disease, 298
  Morquio disease, 298
  Sanfilippo disease, 298
  Sly disease, 298
Mucor, 332
Muenke syndrome, 288
Multicystic dysplastic kidneys, 572
Multiple gestation, 394–395
Mumps, 528
Muscle diseases, 461–463
  Becker muscular dystrophy, 462
  Duchenne muscular dystrophy, 461–462
  myotonic dystrophy, 462–463

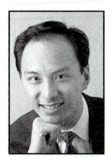
Tao Le, MD, MHS

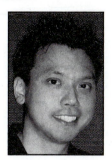
Wilbur Lam, MD

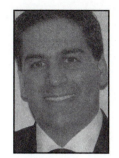
Shervin Rabizadeh, MD

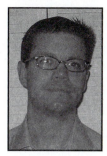
Alan Schroeder, MD

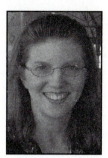
Kimberly Vera, MD

Tao Le, MD, MHS

Tao has been a well-recognized figure in medical education for the past 14 years. As senior editor, he has led the expansion of *First Aid* into a global educational series. In addition, he is the founder of the *USMLERx* online test bank series as well as a cofounder of the *Underground Clinical Vignettes* series. As a medical student, he was editor-in-chief of the University of California, San Francisco *Synapse,* a university newspaper with a weekly circulation of 9000. Tao earned his medical degree from the University of California, San Francisco, in 1996 and completed his residency training in internal medicine at Yale University and fellowship training at Johns Hopkins University. At Yale, he was a regular guest lecturer on the USMLE review courses and an adviser to the Yale University School of Medicine curriculum committee. Tao subsequently went on to cofound Medsn and served as its chief medical officer. He is currently conducting research in asthma education at the University of Louisville.

Wilbur Lam, MD

Wilbur is a clinical fellow in pediatric hematology/oncology at the University of California, San Francisco, where he also completed his residency training in pediatrics. He grew up in Texas and received his undergraduate and medical degrees through the Rice University/Baylor College of Medicine Medical Scholars program. After medical school, he moved to the Bay Area to begin his clinical training as he convalesced from severe multiorgan culture shock. Wilbur, who is board certified in pediatrics, is active in medical student and resident education at UCSF. He has twice earned UCSF's award for outstanding teaching of medical students by a resident, and subsequently the award for outstanding teaching of residents by a clinical fellow. When not in clinic, the ward, or teaching, Wilbur spends his abundant free time working toward a PhD at the UCSF/UC Berkeley Joint Graduate Group in bioengineering. His research investigates the application of state-of-the-art engineering technologies to clinical problems in pediatric cancer and blood diseases.

Shervin Rabizadeh, MD

Shervin is currently a second-year pediatric gastroenterology fellow at Johns Hopkins University. A native of Southern California, Shervin did his undergraduate work at the University of California, Los Angeles. He graduated magna cum laude with degrees in biochemistry and economics. He completed a combined MD/MBA program at the Tufts University School of Medicine in Boston. Subsequently, he finished a pediatric residency at Johns Hopkins University, where he also served as chief resident. His current research interests include the etiology and pathogenesis of inflammatory bowel disease.

Alan Schroeder, MD

Alan is currently a fellow in pediatric critical care at Lucile Packard Children's Hospital at Stanford. He was raised in the San Francisco Bay Area and received a BA in human biology from Stanford University. He attended Georgetown University for medical school, where he was elected to the Alpha Omega Alpha honor society and received the Louis Calcagni Award for Pediatrics. He then returned to Stanford to complete a residency in pediatrics. After residency, Alan worked briefly as a hospitalist and then completed a general pediatrics fellowship at UCSF. He has completed research projects on bronchiolitis and urinary tract infections in infants, and is currently the lead investigator of a randomized, controlled trial on the use of heparin to prevent catheter-related thrombosis in infants undergoing cardiac surgery. Alan was a faculty member for several "evidence-based medicine" CME courses at UCSF and is an instructor and lecturer for the Pediatric Advanced Life Support (PALS) program at Stanford.

Kimberly Vera, MD

Kimberly is currently a pediatric cardiology fellow at Vanderbilt. She was raised in Memphis, Tennessee, and attended Rhodes College, where she was a member of Phi Beta Kappa and graduated summa cum laude with a BS in biology. Kimberly attained her MD degree at the University of Tennessee and was elected to AOA. She then moved to Baltimore where she completed her pediatric residency at Johns Hopkins. She worked as a pediatric hospitalist for one year before beginning her chief residency at Johns Hopkins. During her chief year, she was involved in utilizing medical simulation as a tool for resident education.

ABOUT THE AUTHORS